# USMLE™ Step 1 Qbook
## Fourth Edition

# USMLE™ Step 1 Qbook

## Fourth Edition

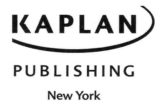

KAPLAN

PUBLISHING

New York

USMLE™ is a joint program of the Federation of State Medical Boards of the United States, Inc. and the National Board of Medical Examiners.

© 2008 by Kaplan, Inc.

Published by Kaplan Publishing, a division of Kaplan, Inc.
1 Liberty Plaza, 24th Floor
New York, NY 10006

Printed in the United States of America

September 2008
10 9 8 7 6 5 4 3 2

ISBN-13: 978-1-4195-5315-8

Kaplan Publishing books are available at special quantity discounts to use for sales promotions, employee premiums, or educational purposes. Please email our Special Sales Department to order or for more information at kaplanpublishing@kaplan.com, or write to Kaplan Publishing, 1 Liberty Plaza, 24th Floor, New York, NY 10006.

# Test-Taking and Study Strategies Guide

## Author

Steven R. Daugherty, Ph.D.
*Director of Education and Testing*
*Kaplan Medical*
*Rush Medical College*
*Chicago, IL*

## Contributor

Judy A. Schwenker, M.S.
*Director of Study Skills*
*Kaplan Medical*

# USMLE Step 1 Qbook

## Editors

Michael S. Manley, M.D.
*Director, Medical Curriculum*
*Kaplan Medical*
*Department of Neurosciences*
*University of California–San Diego*

Leslie D. Manley, Ph.D.
*Director, Medical Curriculum*
*Kaplan Medical*
*Departments of Neurosciences and Pharmacology*
*University of California–San Diego*

## Contributing Editors

Elissa Levy, M.D.
*New York, NY*

Sonia Reichert, M.D.
*New York, NY*

## Senior Vice President, Kaplan Medical

Rochelle Rothstein, M.D.

## Executive Director of Curriculum

Richard Friedland, D.P.M.

## Director of Medical Curriculum

Mark Tyler-Lloyd, M.D.

# AVAILABLE ONLINE

### Free Additional Practice

**kaptest.com/booksonline**

As owner of this guide, you are entitled to get more practice online. Log on to kaptest.com/booksonline to access additional practice questions.

Access to this selection of online USMLE™ Step 3 practice material is free of charge to purchasers of this book. When you log on, you'll be asked to input the book's ISBN number (see the bar code on the back cover). And you'll be asked for a specific password derived from the text in this book, so have your book handy when you log on.

### For any Test Changes or Late-Breaking Developments

**kaptest.com/publishing**

The material in this book is up-to-date at the time of publication. However, the USMLE™ may have instituted changes in the test after this book was published. Be sure to carefully read the materials you receive when you register for the test. If there are any important late-breaking developments—or any changes or corrections to the Kaplan test preparation materials in this book—we will post that information online at kaptest.com/publishing.

### Feedback and Comments

**kaplansurveys.com/books**

We'd love to hear your comments and suggestions about this book. We invite you to fill out our online survey form at kaplansurveys.com/books. Your feedback is extremely helpful as we continue to develop high-quality resources to meet your needs.

# Contents

Pathology and Pathophysiology

Pharmacology

Behavioral Science and Biostatistics

# Preface

Preparing for and doing well on the USMLE Step 1 are essential requirements on the road to becoming a practicing physician. The skills needed for preparation and execution on multiple-choice tests have little to do with the day-to-day practice of medicine but are necessary hurdles that you must overcome to advance in your medical career. Take heart—this task is not insurmountable; there have been many ahead of you. It only requires some knowledge of techniques, a little planning, a dash of impertinence, and above all, patience. This guidebook is intended to help you with this process.

- The first chapter, titled "Inside the USMLE Step 1 Exam," within the *Test-Taking and Study Strategies Guide* section was developed to help you gain a better understanding of the exam. It includes a thorough analysis of the question subtypes. In addition, it describes the overall purpose of the exam, as well as its structure and design, and offers crucial insights to help you do your best on test day.

- The last four chapters of the *Test-Taking and Study Strategies Guide* section offer practical suggestions to help you make the most of your preparation time and avoid common pitfalls in the exam itself. These chapters summarize the key study and test strategies that have helped thousands of students achieve their maximum score. Use these strategies and approaches as you work through the tests in this Qbook. (We also offer advice on how to use the new FRED™ software interface.) Then be sure to reread the final chapters of this guide as your exam approaches to get great advice on what to do during the weeks leading up to the exam, as well as on test day itself.

- The *Qbook Practice Tests* contain a total of 850 Step 1–style questions divided into test blocks of 50 questions each. These blocks are designed to give you a sense of how the actual exam is constructed. Each test is followed by comprehensive explanations of both the correct and incorrect answer choices. We recommend that you wait until you complete your review of a subject area before taking an exam, that you take each exam in the allotted one-hour time frame, and that you do not look at the answers until you have completed an exam in its entirety. Following each test, review why each answer is correct and why each distractor is wrong. This will provide you with the information needed to answer other similar questions on the same topic. There are two exams in Anatomy, Behavioral Science, Biochemistry, Microbiology/Immunology, Pharmacology, and Physiology. Because of the increasingly clinical nature of the exam, we have included five tests covering Pathology and Pathophysiology. A list of standard lab values can be found on pp. 447–448 for easy reference.

Best of luck on your Step 1 exam.

**Kaplan Medical**

# Test-Taking and Study Strategies Guide

# Chapter One: **Inside the USMLE Step 1 Exam**

## ABOUT THE USMLE

The United States Medical Licensing Examination (USMLE) consists of three steps designed to assess a physician's ability to apply a broad spectrum of knowledge, concepts, and principles, and to evaluate the physician's basic patient-centered skills.

The three steps are:

**Step 1 (multiple-choice exam)**—This exam is designed to test how well the examinee applies basic, integral science concepts to clinical scenarios.

**Step 2 (two separate exams)**—The Step 2 Clinical Knowledge (CK) is a multiple-choice exam designed to determine whether the examinee possesses the medical knowledge and understanding of clinical science considered essential for the provision of patient care under supervision. The Step 2 Clinical Skills (CS) is a separate "hands-on" exam that tests the examinee's clinical and communication skills through his/her ability to gather information from standardized patients, perform a physical examination, communicate the findings to the patient, and write a patient note.

**Step 3 (multiple-choice exam)**—This exam assesses the examinee's ability to apply medical knowledge and the understanding of biomedical and clinical science essential for the unsupervised practice of medicine, with emphasis on patient management in ambulatory settings.

## DESCRIPTION OF THE STEP 1 EXAM

The USMLE Step 1 is an eight-hour, computerized examination that assesses whether you understand and can apply important concepts of the sciences basic to the practice of medicine, with special emphasis on principles and mechanisms underlying health, disease, and modes of therapy. Step 1 ensures you know the science within clinical contexts to safely and competently practice medicine under supervision.

### Step 1 at a Glance

**Test Type:** Computer-based

**Examination Length:** Seven 60-minute "blocks" administered in one eight-hour testing session; each block has 50 questions; computer tutorial: 15 minutes; breaks: 45 minutes, self-scheduled

**Number of Questions:** Approximately 350

**Question Type:** Single best answer multiple-choice test items

**Average Time per Question:** Approximately 72 seconds

## How Step 1 Is Different from Other Tests

The USMLE Step 1 is different and, in many ways, broader, more difficult, and more comprehensive than any exam you have ever taken in medical school. As such, it requires a different type of preparation than most medical school exams.

More time, effort, and money go into the creation of the USMLE exams than any other exam you have taken. Items on the exam are not just questions to be answered, but problems to be solved. Good USMLE questions test the students' capacity to think about important medical knowledge and apply it in specific presented situations. *The USMLE doesn't test mere recall of facts;* it assesses students' ability to use that knowledge in clinical situations. A good knowledge base is essential, but is not sufficient. Students must know how to use the information that they know.

## HOW TO SUCCEED ON THE EXAM

You can do well on this exam, but doing your best requires forethought and preparation. This preparation must be on several levels.

**First,** you must be familiar with the types of questions you will face, as well as the overall structure of the exam itself.

**Second**, you must organize your study time efficiently to get the most out of it.

**Third**, you must know how to use the content being tested, not just recognize it. You must be able to apply it in hypothetical situations.

**Fourth**, you must physically and mentally prepare yourself for the task at hand.

In short, you must know the exam, master the material tested, and be prepared to handle yourself during this stressful time. In this chapter and the chapters ahead, we'll help you tackle these tasks.

## WHAT IS TESTED ON STEP 1

Step 1 consists of multiple-choice questions designed to measure basic science knowledge, including questions in anatomy, behavioral sciences, biochemistry, microbiology, pathology, pharmacology, physiology, and interdisciplinary topics, such as nutrition, genetics, and aging.

Some questions test what you know per se, but the majority of questions require you to analyze and interpret written, graphic, and tabular material. You'll be called upon to identify gross and microscopic pathologic and normal specimens and to solve problems through application of basic science principles.

Step 1 organizes the basic science content tested according to general principles and individual organ systems. Test questions are classified in one of these major areas, depending on whether they focus on concepts and principles that are important across organ systems or within individual organ systems.

## Step 1 Content

**Step 1 includes test items in the following content areas:**
- Anatomy
- Behavioral sciences
- Biochemistry
- Microbiology
- Pathology
- Pharmacology

**Note**

Familiarize yourself with the test tutorial on the USMLE website at usmle.org at home and save 15 minutes for breaktime on test day.

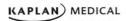

- Physiology
- Interdisciplinary topics, such as nutrition, genetics, and aging

**Step 1 Tasks**

Step 1 is a broadly based, integrated examination.
Test items commonly require you to perform one or more of the following tasks:
- Interpret graphic and tabular material
- Identify gross and microscopic pathologic and normal specimens
- Apply basic science knowledge to clinical problems

**The Step 1 System**

Step 1 classifies test items along two dimensions, system and process:
- 40–50% General principles
- 50–60% Individual organ systems

# ONE BEST ANSWER QUESTIONS

Step 1 includes only single multiple-choice questions with one best answer. This is the traditional, most frequently used multiple-choice format, except that USMLE questions can have up to eleven answer choices. USMLE test items consist of a statement or question followed by three to eleven response options arranged in alphabetical or logical order. Some of the questions require interpretation of graphic or pictorial materials. The response options for all questions are lettered (A, B, C, D, E, etc.). Your job is to select the best answer to the question. Other options may be partially correct, but there is only *one best* answer.

The most important thing to remember is that these questions require you to select not only a good answer, but the *best* answer from the choices given. One answer is always better than the others. Therefore, it is critical that you read through all of the options before making your choice. Remember, you don't get any points for selecting the second best answer. If an answer choice seems partially correct, then it is entirely wrong.

**Strategy Tip**

You are not looking for a good answer; you are looking for the single best answer.

# USMLE STEP 1 QUESTION TYPES

This book contains examples of each of the question types discussed below. As you practice and review, pay attention to the way the questions are constructed, as well as to the content issues tested.

Be aware that the test maker has moved away from questions that require simple basic science recall such as:

> Which of the following areas of the heart is supplied by the right coronary artery?

and toward questions that require an application of knowledge such as:

> A 77-year-old woman is admitted with angina pectoris. An angiogram is performed and reveals a 90 percent blockage of the right coronary artery. Blood supply is most likely to be diminished to which of the following areas?

You'll notice the same objective lies within both questions. The first question is a direct request for a fact. The second question, the kind that is now more common, asks for the same fact in the context of a clinical presentation.

## Question Subtypes

There are a number of different subtypes of one best answer questions. Most students find it useful to classify these subtypes as follows:

1. Positively worded questions ("most likely")
2. Clinical case questions (long clinical cases)
3. "Two-step" (double-jump) questions
4. "Bait and switch" questions
5. Conjunction questions
6. "True/False"questions
7. Visual questions

## Positively Worded Questions

Positively worded questions ask you to select the answer that is "most likely" to be true. Note that all of the options given may be somewhat likely. Your job is to select the one that is most likely. An example of this type of question is as follows:

> An 85-year-old man has had urinary frequency, difficulty initiating stream, and dysuria for the last two months. A rectal exam reveals an enlarged prostate. Prostate-specific antigen (PSA) is not elevated. Which part of the prostate is most likely affected in this patient's condition?
>
> (A) Peripheral zone
> (B) Prostatic capsule
> (C) Prostatic urethra
> (D) Posterior lobe of the prostate
> (E) Transitional/central zone

*(Answer: A)*

## Clinical Case Questions

Clinical case questions are distinguished by a fairly lengthy presentation of a patient's history, physical exam findings, and maybe even lab results. Your task is to read through this detailed information and arrive at the best answer to the question being asked.

The most important part of the clinical case question is the last sentence. This is the sentence that actually poses the question. Until this point, you cannot be sure exactly what you will be asked. Many students are tempted to simply skip to this last line, and then skim the case looking for necessary information to formulate an answer. Generally, this is not the best strategy.

Clinical case questions are often constructed by first writing a classic case, and then including one or two extra details. These details, by themselves, may suggest one or the other of the given answer options. To answer these questions correctly, you must read the whole case and treat all the information given as a whole. The total gestalt of the case is what is crucial, not any one individual fact.

Question writers know that because of the length of the questions, candidates do not want to read the whole question if they can help it. They know that some test takers are scanning for that one critical piece of information. Because of this, single pieces of information may lead you away from the right answer to one of the incorrect distractors. Avoid this trap. You need to focus on the meaning of the case as a whole, not any one piece of it.

**Strategy Tip**

Negatively worded questions, those that ask for the option that is "least likely," are no longer used on the Step 1 exam. Don't waste your time mastering the techniques for handling them.

**Strategy Tip**

You need to understand the case as a whole to avoid fixating on single pieces of information that lead to a wrong answer choice.

**Strategy Tip**

Paraphrase to help you understand the question and note important information and key symptoms.

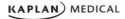

When reading through the case, choose what is important. Paraphrase the question and note key factors and symptoms as they are presented. This will help you remember them when formulating your answer. Then select the answer that best matches not some but all of the facts presented. An example of this clinical case type of question follows:

A 24-year-old woman presents with a fever and myalgias. She experienced brief, self-limited diarrhea 24 hours after attending a barbecue two weeks earlier. She remained asymptomatic until the day prior to presentation when she developed a fever of 39.4 C (103 F), conjunctivitis, and severe muscle pain. On physical examination she appears acutely ill and has a fever of 39.4 C. There is a diffuse maculopapular rash and generalized muscular tenderness. Several hemorrhages are noted beneath the fingernails. Admission hemogram reveals a white blood cell count of 15,000/mm$^3$ with 25 percent eosinophils. The infectious form of the most likely causative agent is a(n)

(A) cyst
(B) cysticerci
(C) encysted larvae
(D) ovum
(E) rhabditiform larvae

(*Answer: C*)

A pair of brothers (35 and 38 years old) present with fairly dramatic pneumonias. On lung exam, rales are easily heard. Chest x-rays of both men reveal bilateral and diffuse infiltrates. The brothers spent a day together two weeks ago hiking in a mountainous area of Virginia where they entered a dusty cave. The most likely causative agent is

(A) *Blastomyces dermatidis*
(B) *Chlamydia trachomatis*
(C) *Coccidioides immitis*
(D) Coxsackie A virus
(E) *Haemophilus ducrey*
(F) *Haemophilus influenzae*
(G) *Histoplasma capsulatum*
(H) Influenza B virus
(I) *Neisseria gonorrhoea*
(J) *Neisseria meningitidis*
(K) *Streptococcus pyogenes*

(*Answer: G*)

Some test takers find these questions with a large number of options to be anxiety producing. They need not be. Some examinees feel that questions with many options are easier and actually take less time to do. The real danger with these types of questions is that students will waste too much time reading back and forth through the list of options. The correct method of approaching these questions is to think of an answer, look for that answer, and then pick it. If none of the options look appealing, then take a guess and move to the next question. This is the same strategy we recommend for all questions, but it is most critical when there are a large number of options.

## Two-Step (Double-Jump) Questions

Two-Step (also called double-jump) questions require several cognitive step to arrive at a correct answer. Consider this question when finding the correct answer requires you to formulate a proper diagnosis and then select the most appropriate pharmacologic treatment. Note that you get no credit for the intermediate step of diagnosis. The correct answer is found only by reasoning all the way through to the treatment.

> A 46-year-old, bright, energetic, and overweight man loves to talk and to give his opinion on the world around him. He is always quick with a joke and seems to love a good laugh. Yet, whenever he has to talk in front of more than three or four people, he reports sweating, heart palpitations, and trembling hands. "My mind just goes blank," he says, "and I feel that I'm going to say something so stupid that I would rather die." The most appropriate treatment for this man would be
>
> (A) Alprazolam
> (B) Atenolol
> (C) Clonadine
> (D) Diazepam
> (E) Phenelzine

*(Answer: B)*

In this next question, you must reason your way to the additional characteristics of the organism in mind by first correctly identifying what the organism is based on the laboratory data. Again, you get no credit for identifying the correct organism but only for "two-stepping" to the additional characteristic.

> A 71-year-old man was admitted from his extended care facility because of recent aggravation of an exfoliative skin condition that has plagued him for several years. He had been receiving a variety of antibiotic regimens, including many topical preparations over the last year or two. He now has a temperature of 38.9 C (102 F). The skin of upper chest, extremities, and neck shows erythema with diffuse epidermal peeling and many pustular lesions. Cultures obtained from these lesions are reported back from the laboratory as yielding a gram-positive organism that is highly salt (NaCl) tolerant. This organism is also most likely
>
> (A) bacitracin sensitive
> (B) bile soluble
> (C) coagulase positive
> (D) optochin sensitive
> (E) novobiacin sensitive

*(Answer: C)*

Note that you need to make two correct decisions to arrive at the correct answer, hence the name "two-step." The goal is to guide you away from simple memorization in your learning. Instead, the exam wants you to be able to use the information you have memorized to reason through to a correct answer.

The correct process for answering these questions is not "read, answer," but "read, think, answer." You'll definitely see your share of these two-step (and even three-step) questions on the Step 1 exam.

## Bait and Switch Questions

Sometimes what you first think the question is about is not what the question is really asking. Have you ever begun reading a question thinking that the core focus is physiology and discover at the end of the question that the real issue is pharmacology? Have you ever read a clinical case collecting evidence for a diagnosis and discover that at the end of the question they give you the diagnosis, but want to know something about treatment options? If you have had these experiences, then you have run into bait and switch questions.

Bait and switch questions begin by presenting material that may lead you to think about content in one direction, but then shift you to another line of thought at the end; a sort of mental sleight of hand. The key question is always given in the last line of the question stem. Everything else before the last line is simply a setup. You cannot tell for certain what information is useful and what information in unnecessary until you get to the end of the stem and encounter the actual question.

Because of this, some students make a habit of reading the last line of the question stem, and then scan the rest of the presented information looking for pertinent material. This strategy may have worked on other tests, but has some pitfalls on the USMLE Step 1. If you have the discipline to read the question line and then return to read the rest of the stem in detail, this is not a bad strategy for this type of question. However, experience suggests that this is not the best strategy for most students.

There are two problems with reading the last line of the stem first:

- You do not know that you are faced with a bait and switch question until you read through the whole question. In other words, you often can't tell that this strategy will work until you have already read the question.

- Many people do not have the discipline to read the last line and then return to read through the rest of the question stem. Once they read the question line, many students move directly to the options without adequately evaluating the information presented in the question stem. Alternatively, students scan the question stem looking for one single piece of information to help them answer the question. Looking only for one key fact often means you will miss another key detail and, therefore, end up with a wrong answer.

The best advice is to read the last line of the question first only if you then read through the rest of the question. Read the last line before reading the rest of the question, not in place of reading the rest of the question. Reading the last line first to avoid reading the entire question is a low-yield strategy and results in an increased error rate.

> A generally healthy, 65-year-old man was in a car accident and broke several ribs on his left side. His medical record shows a history of mild diabetes and treatment in the past year for gonorrhea. Approximately 12 days after the car accident, the patient developed a painful, well-circumscribed vesicular rash over his left rib cage. The rash persisted for several weeks. What is the rash due to?
>
> (A)  Primary infection with herpes B virus
>
> (B)  Primary infection with herpes simplex virus type 1

(C) Primary infection with herpes simplex virus type 2

(D) Reactivation of latent Epstein-Barr virus

(E) Reactivation of latent varicella-zoster virus

*(Answer: E)*

A 59-year-old man with a history of hypertension and cigarette smoking survived a myocardial infarction two years ago. He has been reluctant to follow the diet prescribed by his physician, but as part of his recovery program, he has taken up running. Following an early morning run, he consumes a breakfast consisting of cereal, eggs, bacon, sausage, pancakes with maple syrup, doughnuts, and coffee with cream and sugar. Which of the following proteins will most likely be activated in his liver after breakfast?

(A) Glycogen phosphorylase

(B) PEP carboxykinase

(C) Hydroxymethylglutaryl-CoA reductase

(D) Glycogen synthase

(E) Carnitine acyltransferase

*(Answer: D)*

## Conjunction Questions

In the same manner as two-step questions, conjunction questions require two correct choices to arrive at the best answer. Options are presented as sets of terms or facts linked by a conjunction (usually the word "and"). The best answer is the one in which both parts of the option are correct.

By using this type of question, the examiners are able to move beyond asking for a single piece of information, asking instead which two pieces of information satisfy the question criterion. Most commonly, students are asked to detect two overlapping disease states, or which are the two best interventions to be performed next.

A 66-year-old man has been brought to his physician's office by his wife who expresses concern that "something is just not right." During neurologic examination, both recent and long-term memory appear unimpaired. However, the patient seems to have difficulty concentrating. He asks repeatedly where he is and what he is doing there. He has difficulty with simple arithmetic and in writing simple sentences. He has no difficulty outlining or reproducing presented figures, but on a discrimination task, he confuses his right and left hands. This patient is most likely suffering from lesions affecting which of the following?

(A) Dominant parietal and frontal lobes

(B) Dominant parietal and dominant temporal lobes

(C) Dominant temporal and frontal lobes

(D) Nondominant parietal and dominant temporal lobes

(E) Nondominant parietal and nondominant temporal lobes

*(Answer: A)*

The best method for handling a conjunction question is to treat it as two separate questions. Answer the question twice, once for each part of the response option. Cognitively, it is difficult to hold the two parts of the option in mind at the same time. By splitting the task into two simpler choices, you are less likely to become confused or make mental mistakes. For example, in the above question, first notice that some of the symptoms are suggestive of a frontal lobe lesion; then as a second step, focus on those that suggest a dominant parietal lobe dysfunction.

## True/False Questions

True/false questions ask you to read a set of options and select the one that is most likely to be a statement of fact. These questions are becoming increasingly rare on the USMLE exams. They are useful for testing recall of basic facts, but are less helpful in testing your capacity for reasoning and applying learned knowledge.

The basic form of the question is: "Which of the following is true?" You must select the statement that is likely to be the correct answer in most situations. Special care must be taken if the question describes a specific situation. In this case, you must select the option that is most likely true in the specific situation presented.

For true/false questions, you must pay careful attention to the exact wording of the options. The question writer usually constructs true/false questions by writing out a series of true statements and then changing a word or two to make all but one of the statements false. Unlike other USMLE questions, your attention here should be directed to the options (which is one reason why these questions are so rarely used).

The mechanism of action of heparin includes

(A) binding to antithrombin III and inducing a conformational change in it to potentiate its action

(B) binding to heparin and the complex activating antithrombin III

(C) enhancing the activity of antithrombin III with coagulation factors by acting as a template

(D) inhibition of regeneration of vitamin K quinone

(E) the formation IgG antibodies leading to thrombocytopenia

*(Answer: A)*

Two different manufacturers prepare ibuprofen 200-mg tablets. The two batches of tablets are said to be bioequivalent if

(A) they have the same shape and color

(B) the area under the curve is the same after a single dose

(C) the relative bioavailability = 1

(D) they have the same volume of distribution

(E) they have the same and volume of distribution

(F) they have the same $C_{max}$ after a single dose

(G) they have the same rate of absorption and elimination

(H) the tablets break apart at the same time

(I) they have the same half-life of elimination

(J) their plasma concentrations are above the minimum effective level

*(Answer: B)*

## Visual Questions

As a computer-based test, the USMLE makes use of visual materials, including pictures, histology slides, and MRI and CT scan results as a part of questions. Many candidates are uneasy about these types of questions but need not be. The images presented for the Step 1 exam will be of fairly common phenomena; things you have probably seen before. Your first task when faced with a visual question is to stay calm. Deal with these questions just as you would any other question. When you come to a visual question, look at the presented image and also read any accompanying text. A substantial portion of the visual questions can be answered from hints included in the text.

To prepare for visual questions, review images and then tell yourself what you are looking at. Many students study incorrectly by starting with a concept and then looking at the matching image. The exam always requires you to select the concept that matches the image, not to find the image that matches the concept. The key here is to know what you are looking at when it is presented.

**Experimental Questions**

A number of questions on each exam are experimental and don't count toward your score, but you won't know which ones. Don't assume that a question doesn't count.

## Primacy and Recency Effects

Information that appears early in a question stem and information that appears at the end of the question stem exerts a strong influence on the examinee. Early and late information forms your cognitive set, which makes finding the correct answer either easier or harder. Information at the start of the question stem has a primacy effect, which controls your thinking by determining what you start thinking about. Information at the end of the question stem has a recency effect, which controls your thinking by providing the jumping off point for selecting the correct answer.

If the key information for the question appears in the primacy or recency spots, you will be led to the correct answer. The difficulty comes when the key information lies somewhere in between. Primacy and recency information can blind you to other essential content. Examinees sometimes fixate on early or late information and miss other important information given in the question stem.

For example, if a question begins by describing a patient as having a generalized anxiety disorder, all of the information that follows will tend to be seen in that context, even though the anxiety disorder diagnosis may not be directly pertinent to the correct answer for that question.

Primacy or recency effects seem most pronounced when the beginning or ending information in a question stem is something with which you are unfamiliar. We all have a special tendency to fixate on unknown content.

If you suspect that primacy or recency information is distorting your reading of a given question, try changing the order in which you read the question. Skip the initial content, read the rest of the question first, and see if this changes your perspective. Remember, no one single piece of information is the key; you must deal with each question as a whole. Avoid fixating on one word or concept you do not know, and focus on the parts of the question you do know.

## Multimedia Questions

New changes to the USMLE exams include the addition of multimedia to selected multiple choice questions. Approximately 5 items with associated media clips will appear in a single examination. Multimedia is in the form of a video or an audio file and typically relates to a physical finding that relates to the case described in the question. Physical findings include heart and lung sounds, reflexes, characteristic tremors, or other distinctive physical examination findings.

# Understanding Distractors

To deal most effectively with exam questions, you need to have some understanding of how the questions are constructed. Getting a question correct means selecting the best answer. Incorrect options are called "distractors." Their purpose is to distract; that is, to get you to pick them rather than the best answer. Each distractor will be selected by some examinees, or it would not be included as an option. Every option fools somebody. Your job is to not be misled.

In general, distractors will seem plausible and few will stand out as obviously incorrect. Distractors may be partially right answers but not the best answer. Common misconceptions, incomplete knowledge, and faulty reasoning will cause you to select a distractor.

The test maker tells his or  question writers that their distractors must follow these five rules:

1. They must be homogeneous. For example, they will be all laboratory tests or all therapies, not a mix of the two.

2. They must be incorrect or definitely inferior to the correct answer. There will be enough of a difference between the right answer and the distractors to allow a distinction. For example, if estimating the percentage of a population with a disease, the options will differ by more than 5 percent.

3. They must not contain any hints as to the right answer. Distractors are meant to induce you to an incorrect choice, not give you clues as to the correct one.

4. They must seem plausible and attractive to the uninformed. If you are not sufficiently familiar with a topic, you may well find that all of the options look good.

5. They must be similar to the correct answer in construction and length. Thus, trying to "psych out" the question by looking for flaws in its construction is not a useful strategy.

Answer choices that do not adhere to these rules are not used on the exam. All options are meant to distract you, but often one of the distractors will seem better than the others, the so-called "preferred distractor." While still incorrect, this is the wrong answer chosen most often. Preferred distractors are why you can often get yourself down to two choices: the correct answer versus the preferred distractor.

Selecting the correct answer is not a matter of splitting hairs. The correct answer will be clearly correct. If you think two answers are so close that you cannot reasonably choose between them, then the odds are that neither one is correct; you need to look carefully at a different option.

Many students have learned test-wise strategies and used them effectively on their medical school exams. These strategies will not help you on the USMLE. Worse, focusing on these test-wise strategies actually hurts you because it distracts you from doing the mental work you need to do to recall the proper content and think through the question.

This means that you should break yourself of the habit of looking for:

1. *Grammatical cues*: where one or more distractors does not follow grammatically from the stem. For example, a stem ends in "an" and only some options begin with a vowel.

2. *Logical cues*: where a subset of options is logically exhaustive, indicating that the answer is one of the subset. For example, including the three options: "greater than," "same as," and "less than" in a five-option question. You will also not find logically exhaustive options when one of the options is nonsensical.

3. *Absolute terms*: terms such as "always" and "never," which wise test-takers avoid, will not be used in this exam.

4. *Long correct answers*: options will be the same in construction and level of detail. Efforts are made to ensure that the correct answer is not longer, more specific, or more complex than the other options.

5. *Word repeats*: where the same word or phrase is included in both the stem and the correct answer.

6. *Word association links*: where the correct answer can be arrived at by simple word association without a deeper understanding of the topic. For example, Vietnam veteran and post-traumatic stress can be associated. However, in a diagnostic stem about a Vietnam veteran, the correct answer may well be some other condition.

7. *Convergence strategy*: where the correct answer includes most of the elements in common with the other options. For example, consider the following question:

> The 16th president of the United States was
>
> A. Julius Lincoln
> B. Abraham Smith
> C. Abraham Lincoln
> D. Vladimir Lenin
> E. Andrew Jackson

By the convergence strategy, the correct answer is "C" (two Lincolns and two Abrahams).

The USMLE will no longer feature the types of flaws mentioned above. If you're thinking of using these strategies, don't. Tricks don't work on the USMLE. They distract you from the high-power cognitive strategies that are much more likely to lead to a correct answer.

## THE COMPUTER-BASED TEST

**Note**

For more information about the new FRED software, which replaced the previous testing interface for the Step 1 exam in 2005, refer to pages 31–32 in Chapter 3, "Tackling the Exam."

Although you'll receive a tutorial on using the computer on test day, be sure you're comfortable with this format by running the tutorial and sample materials on the USMLE website prior to your test date. You'll see that the Step 1 examination consists of questions presented in standard multiple-choice format divided into "blocks". A normal laboratory values table, including Standard International conversions, will be available as an online reference when you take the examination. Other computer interface features include clickable icons for marking questions to be reviewed, automated review of marked and incomplete questions, a clock indicating the time remaining, and a help application.

During the alloted time to complete the items in each block, you may answer the items in any order, review your responses, and change answers. After you exit the block, or when time expires, you can no longer review test items or change answers.

## SCORE REPORTING

The USMLE program recommends a minimum passing score for each Step exam. Currently, the passing score as set by the USMLE program is 182 for Step 1. This corresponds to answering 60–70 percent of the items correctly. The mean score for first-time examinees from accredited medical schools in the United States is in the range of 200 to 220, and the standard deviation is approximately 20. Your score report includes the mean and standard deviation for recent administrations of the exam.

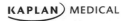

There will also be a two-digit score on your score report. This two-digit score is derived from the three-digit score and is used in score reporting to meet requirements of some medical licensing authorities that the passing score be reported as 75.

The graphical profiles which appear on the back of your individual score report are provided as an assessment tool for your benefit and will not be reported to any third party. The profiles summarize relative areas of strength and weakness to aid in self-assessment.

There's no "curve" on the USMLE exams, so percentiles are not provided. You are competing against the test, not other students.

# ELIGIBILITY

To be eligible to take the Step 1, you must be in one of the following categories at the time of application and on test day:

- A medical student officially enrolled in, or a graduate of, a U.S. or Canadian medical school program leading to the M.D. degree that is accredited by the Liaison Committee on Medical Education (LCME)
- A medical student officially enrolled in, or a graduate of, a U.S. medical school program leading to the D.O. degree that is accredited by the American Osteopathic Association (AOA)
- A medical student officially enrolled in, or a graduate of, a medical school outside the United States and Canada and eligible for examination by the ECFMG for its certificate

# USMLE EXAM SEQUENCING

- Students and graduates medical schools may take Step 1, Step 2 CK, and Step 2 CS in any sequence.

# REGISTRATION AND SCHEDULING FOR THE STEP 1 EXAM

Students and graduates of medical schools in the United States and Canada accredited by the Liaison Committee on Medical Education or the American Osteopathic Association may register for the Step 1 through:

**NBME**
Examinee Support Services
3750 Market Street
Philadelphia, PA 19104-3190
Website: http://www.nbme.org
Telephone: (215) 590-9700
Fax: (215) 590-9457
Email: webmail@nbme.org

You may use one application to apply for Step 1 and both components of Step 2 at the same time.

Students and graduates of medical schools outside the United States and Canada may register for the Step 2 CS through:

> **ECFMG**
> 3624 Market St.
> Philadelphia, PA 19104-2685
> Application materials:
> Website: http://www.ecfmg.org
> Telephone: (215) 386-5900
> Fax: (215) 386-9196
> Email: info@ecfmg.org

International students may also complete a paper application (Form 106S). You can download the Form 106S from the ECFMG website or request a photocopy from ECFMG.

## ELIGIBILITY PERIODS

When applying for Step 1, you must select a three-month period during which you would like to take the test. A Scheduling Permit with instructions for making an appointment at a Prometric Test Center will be sent to you after your registration is processed. The Scheduling Permit specifies the three-month eligibility period during which you must complete the examination.

### The Steps to Take Step 1

Obtain application materials from the appropriate registration entity.

Complete your application materials and submit them to the registration entity.

Receive a Scheduling Permit verifying your eligibility and authorizing you to schedule the examination.

Follow the instructions on your Scheduling Permit to schedule your test date at a Prometric test center. Center locations are available at www.prometric.com.

Bring your Scheduling Permit and identification as described on your Scheduling Permit to the Prometric test center on the scheduled date and time to take the examination.

## TESTING REGIONS

Step 1 is administered in the United States and Canada and in more than 50 other countries by Prometric. You can contact Prometric's central scheduling office known as the "Regional Registration Center" to schedule test dates at **www.prometric.com**. Use the Prometric Test Center Locator for up-to-date information on the locations of Prometric Test Centers.

## ON EXAMINATION DAY

- Arrive at the Prometric Test Center 30 minutes before your scheduled testing time on your testing day. If you arrive more than 30 minutes after your scheduled testing time, you will not be admitted.

- When you arrive at the test center, you must present your Scheduling Permit and the required identification described on your Scheduling Permit. Your identification must contain both your signature and photograph. Acceptable forms of identification include the following forms of unexpired identification:
    - Passport
    - Driver's license with photograph,
    - National identity card
    - Other form of unexpired, government-issued identification,
    - ECFMG-issued identification card

- Your name as it appears on your Scheduling Permit must match the name on your form(s) of identification exactly.

- Upon arrival at the test center, you must present the required identification, sign a test center log, be photographed, and store your personal belongings in your assigned locker.

- You will receive a marker and laminated writing surfaces for use during the test. If you fill the laminated writing surface provided, please inform test center staff. Replacement laminated writing surfaces will be provided. You will not be provided with material to erase the laminated writing surfaces; do not wipe them clean yourself.

- Center personnel will escort you to your assigned testing station and provide brief instructions on use of the computer equipment. You may then take a brief tutorial prior to starting the first test block.

- Fifteen minutes is allotted to complete the tutorial and 45 minutes for break time. The 45 minutes for breaks can be divided in any manner, according to your preference. For example, you can take a short break at your seat after you complete a block, or you can take a longer break for a meal outside the test center after you complete a few blocks.

- Once you begin a block of the test, no breaks are provided during the block. Each block lasts approximately 60 minutes. During blocks, the clock continues to run even if you leave the testing room for a personal emergency. Each block ends when its time expires or when you exit from it.

- As you progress through the blocks of the test, you should monitor how many blocks are remaining and how much break time is remaining. If you take too much break time and exceed the allocated or accumulated break time, your time to complete the last block(s) in the testing session will be reduced.

- The test session ends when you have started and exited all sections or the total time for the test expires.

## EXAMINEES WITH DISABILITIES

Reasonable accommodations will be made for USMLE examinees with disabilities who are covered under the Americans with Disabilities Act (ADA). If you wish to apply for test accommodations, you must send your official request and documentation at the same time that you apply for the exam. See the USMLE website for more information.

## FOR MORE INFORMATION

- See the USMLE *Bulletin of Information* and the USMLE website at usmle.org. Changes can occur after the *Bulletin* is released, so monitor the USMLE website for the most current information about the test.

- Refer to the website of your registration entity (Educational Commission for Foreign Medical Graduates [ECFMG®] for students and graduates of international medical schools; the National Board of Medical Examiners® [NBME®] for students and graduates of U.S. and Canadian medical schools).

- Run the sample Step 1 test materials and tutorials provided at the USMLE website.

# Chapter Two: **Study Techniques**

## ACTIVE LEARNING

Active use of material increases retention and facilitates recall. Repetition makes memories. Each instance of recall produces a new memory trace, linking it to another moment of life and increasing the chance for recall in the future. Memory is dynamic. Recall actually changes neuronal structures. To be truly useful, a piece of information needs to be triangulated, connected to a number of other concepts or, better yet, experiences. For the USMLE Step 1 exam, meaning, not mere information, is your goal.

Rereading textbooks from cover to cover and underlining—yet again, in a different color— every line on every page is not an efficient way to learn. You need to focus on the material most likely to be on the examination. Studying that material through active application is the best way to enhance your understanding and retention of the information.

The following study techniques will help you develop better ways to prepare for the exam, but remember, learning for retention and use requires active involvement.

**Remember**

Active use of the study material is the key to successful studying.

## CHOOSING WHAT TO STUDY (AND WHAT TO IGNORE)

How can you possibly know what is likely to be on your examination? There are a number of approaches.

1.  Talk to medical school faculty. They often have seen past exams or have reviewed an item analysis and can tell you the topics most likely to appear on the examination. They should be able to direct you to what is essential knowledge in their field and what is less important.

2.  Talk to students and colleagues who took the examination in past years. Do they remember some topics being particularly "hard hit"? Was there a "flavor" to the exam? For example, did there seem to be a lot of Pathology?

    Students who took the exam in the past cannot tell you what will be on the exam that you will take, but they can direct you to the high-yield content areas that you must make sure to master. It's highly recommended to talk with people who have taken the exam. However, be cautious. Candidates typically overestimate how much of their weakest area was on the exam. They are most likely to recall tested content that they got wrong.

3.  Download test materials from NBME website *(www.nbms.org)* and take advantage of the CD-ROM practice disk sent with your Step 1 application confirmation. These questions can also be downloaded from the USMLE's website *(www.usmle.org)*. In the long term, these practice questions will indicate the content structure of the exam, but each exam may have sections not covered. Every year new topics are added to the content outline, and some older ones are eliminated. These changes are likely to indicate new questions that you will not hear about from any other source, so be sure to check out these sources.

4.  Certain topics are standard. Others appear as trends. Recently, there have been many questions on AIDS, infectious disease, genetic disorders, toxicology, pregnancy and prenatal care, ethics, nutrition, aging, and increasingly, molecular biology. Pay special attention to these topics when you plan your studying. In general, topics begin to appear on the exam two to three years after they reach prominence in the scientific/lay community. Any interesting medical topic that appeared in the literature at least two years ago is a candidate for inclusion on the exam.

5.  Beware of the trap of "studying for the last exam"—exam content differs from year to year. This year's exams will be different from last year's. And within any given year, your exam will be different from that of others. This is especially true since the exam is computerized.

## CHOOSING HOW TO STUDY

Mastering the material you must learn for this exam is a three stage process. These stages parallel the functional organization of memory.

### Basic Terms and Definitions

You must learn basic terms and definitions. This provides the core vocabulary to understand the content being tested. This stage is a matter of simple recognition and memorization. Terms and definitions are learned by the use of associational memory. This is the level where mnemonics can be useful.

### Central Concepts

You must learn central concepts for each of the seven subject areas. This stage is a matter of being able to explain the meaning of concepts, how they are used, and how they connect with other concepts. Understanding the cross-linkages within subjects and across subjects will serve you well over the course of the exam.

Your basic mental task here is that of reconstructive memory, learning to recall concepts in terms of how things fit together. At this stage, the practice of recalling one concept facilitates the recall of other related ideas. Patterns begin to emerge. This is the level at which diagrams, tables, and pictures can be most helpful.

### Application

You must be able to apply the concepts in presented clinical settings and recognize what concepts are most important in mini-case presentations. This is the hardest stage of preparation, and the one that most students neglect. Achieving your best possible score depends on knowing not only what concepts mean, but also how they are applied in a given medical situation.

The task at this level is that of reasoning, understanding the implications of presented information and being able to choose the appropriate action from the available options. At this level, study/discussion groups and doing practice questions can be most helpful.

Your method of study and your study schedule should be arranged to allow you to master each of these stages in turn. As you make your decisions about how you will study, the following suggestions may be helpful:

**Remember**

Use a number of different sources of information when deciding what to study.

**Remember**

You must be able to recognize concepts, understand their importance, and apply them in presented situations.

- Be organized. Set up an organized study schedule and adhere to it. The biggest danger when preparing for the exam is spending too much time on one area or ignoring one subject altogether. Decide how much time you will study each day and put your time in like it is a job. Schedule regular breaks and keep them.

- Decide what your weak areas are by taking pretests, a diagnostic exam, using information from your coursework, or using the questions in each book. Begin your study plan with your weak areas and plan to cover those at least twice before the exam.

- Do not entirely neglect your strong areas, but allocate less time to them. This can be difficult. Research suggests that, left on their own, most students study what they know best and give less time to subjects that make them uncomfortable. Reverse this process and spend the most time on the subjects that make you the most uncomfortable.

- Emphasize integration by reviewing subjects together and/or by organ system. This will greatly aid your preparation for USMLE, which emphasizes the integration of basic sciences. This type of review is best conducted in a group with other people. Other people may look at the same material differently than you and help you expand your perspective and your understanding.

- Review materials in related clusters. For example, take the anemias and review how each might present, the basic epidemiology, what lab tests would differentiate, the underlying mechanisms, and initial therapies for each. Using this strategy allow you to "preview" questions and anticipate both the correct answer and the most likely distractors.

- Keep your sessions short; no more than an hour to an hour and a half with at least a 15-minute break. Your concentration declines significantly after an hour or so. Sitting longer will provide only minimal extra return. In addition, the break time allows the short-term memory to be consolidated into long-term memory.

- Do not reread textbooks. Use review books that consolidate the information for you.

- Limit the number of information sources from which you study. Select one main review book for each subject. If you have several books, use one as your primary study material and the others as back-up to clarify points as needed. Too many study sources creates overload, and overload stifles comprehension.

## HIGHLY EFFECTIVE STUDY METHODS

Each person has his or her own preferred way of studying. You will have to decide what will work the best for you. High yield study methods all have one feature in common: The more active you are with the material, the more content you will ultimately retain. Remember, your goal in studying is not just to put in the most time, but to be efficient. Many of the best students make use of the following techniques:

### Ask Yourself Questions

One of the best study techniques is to pose questions to yourself as you review material. Perhaps you'll want to jot them down on index cards to share with others and to practice later. By asking yourself questions, you are framing the material, challenging yourself to focus on key areas, and preparing for questions you may well see on the examination. Your goal is not to learn knowledge for general use, but to be able to answer multiple-choice exam questions.

This strategy will move you from thinking like a student answering questions to thinking like a faculty member who is writing questions. By this process, you "get into" the head of the question writers and begin to understand what makes a good question and the basic science issues likely to be at the core of presented questions.

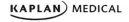

## Use Graphs and Charts

Many common graphs and charts appear repeatedly on the exam. Practice reading graphs, charts, and tables. Try abstracting the salient facts quickly from a graph or chart. This may be expedited by using a plain sheet of paper to cover unneeded information and to focus your attention on selected information.

Drawing the graph yourself seems to help you remember it more than just looking at it multiple times. Drawing a graph from memory will give you the confidence that you've truly mastered the material. The more active you are with the material, the more likely you are to both remember it and understand important nuances.

## Paraphrase

Practice paraphrasing material to highlight important information. Paraphrasing means processing the material you have read; telling yourself what is important and unimportant as you read through it, and summarizing the key content in your own words.

Pretend that you are the teacher who is in charge of presenting the content. What would you choose to emphasize? What would you leave out if you were short on time? How would you explain the concept to someone new to the field? Remember, if you can say it in your own words, then you really know it.

The art of paraphrasing will allow you to answer questions with extensive information in the stem, such as case histories, much more efficiently. Many students say the most difficult part of the USMLE is getting through the large volume of reading required for each question. When you are paraphrasing, you do not treat every piece of information with the same emphasis, but decide what is important and what is not. Developing this skill will also be helpful as you progress through your medical career.

## Summary Notes

Creating summary notes is a great study technique and will reinforce your paraphrasing skills. Summary notes are your personal representation of key points in the material written in a way that makes sense to you. Summary notes should run parallel to your primary study material and should serve to annotate, illustrate, and amplify the key points of that material. The physical action of simply writing the notes tends to reinforce learning and aid long-term retention. Once completed, summary notes provide a ready guide for those times when you review the material.

## Study Groups

Study with friends or colleagues in groups of four or five. The best groups comprise people with a range of expertise. Try to form a group where each person's weakness is complemented by someone else's strengths.

The goal of these study groups is not to show your colleagues how much you know. Rather, it's to find the holes in your knowledge while you still have time to correct those gaps. Don't be afraid to tackle the tough topics. With the aid of your study group, things will make sense much sooner than they will on your own. Challenge each other. Pose hypothetical situations and seek agreement as to the best answers.

**Study Tip**

You'll see lots of tables, graphs, and charts on the exam, so practice using these tools.

**Study Tip**

Putting content in your own words will make you a better test-taker.

## Plan Your Study Time

For most efficient studying, avoid cramming and plan to re-review key material on a regular basis. Repeated exposure to material over time leads to more thorough retention than one massive concentrated exposure.

In your final reviews, remember that active learning is best. This means avoiding simply reading the same page of notes over and over. Instead, use key words as mental triggers and tell yourself as much as you can about the topic you are studying. For example, don't simply re-read the Krebs cycle. Rather, tell yourself about it as if you were explaining it to someone else, and then check your explanation against your notes.

Re-review is also the time to begin to make links among different sections of your material. What does your understanding of the physiology of the cardiovascular system tell you about common pathology or pharmacologic intervention? The threads of common diseases weave through each of the basic science subjects; tie them together and provide a framework that aids in retention.

## Practice with Testlike Practice Questions

Doing practice questions is essential in your preparation for taking a multiple-choice exam. Your goal here is to test yourself and also to learn good question-answering habits. As you do questions, examine whether you got them right, but more importantly, look at why you got the question right or wrong. Did you not know the content? Then that's your cue that more study is needed. Did you misread the question? Then evaluate how you misread it and learn how the question writer wants you to read it.

### Sources of Multiple-Choice Errors

| Problem Type | Source of Errors |
|---|---|
| Format problems | Particular question subtypes |
| Anxiety problems | Questions containing numbers, or done early in the review session |
| Fatigue problems | Questions done late in review session |
| Reading errors | More common in long questions |
| Directionality errors | Questions that ask prediction of consequences |
| Group delineation errors | Questions that present material in a unique context |

When you do your practice questions, do them under a time limit similar to the actual exam. In general, your rule should be one minute per question. This is roughly the amount of time (72 seconds) you will have during the real exam. Get used to the time constraint. It is one of the unchangeable realities of the USMLE.

When doing practice questions, avoid these common mistakes:

1. **Do not do questions without preparatory studying.** Review material first until you feel you know it, and then use questions to test yourself. If you study by doing questions before you are ready, you will erode your self-confidence and fail to develop key linkages within the material.

2. **Do not get into the habit of lingering over a question**. You do not have this luxury on the real exam. Remember that you have just over one minute per question. You should spend about 75 percent of that time reading and analyzing the question stem, and the other 25 percent selecting an answer. Be honest when you do not know an answer; move on, and look it up when you are finished.

3.  **So-called "retired questions" and many published questions in review books are not representative of questions featured on the current USMLE Step 1**. They are a reasonable way to review content, but often do not reflect the length or form of the questions on the current exam.

4.  **Do not do questions individually**. Do them in clusters under time pressure, with 5 to 10 as a minimum. This will get you used to moving from question to question. Do not look up answers after each question. Instead, check yourself after you have done the full set of questions.

5.  **When you start working on questions, do not panic if you do not get the correct answers**. Learn from your mistakes. Questions are a part of the study process; they help you see what else you need to learn. You will get better at questions as your studying continues.

## TRY THIS QUESTION-MASTERING EXERCISE

Cover up the options to the question and read the question stem. Pause at each period and paraphrase what you have read. When you finish reading the question, cover the question and reveal the options. Select from the options without looking back at the question stem.

With practice, you will get faster, and this strategy will become a habit. This strategy forces you to get the information out of the question as you read it and does not allow you to waste time by going back and re-reading. Remember, you only have time to read each question once. Learn to make your reading time as efficient as possible.

# Chapter Three: **Tackling the Exam**

## STEP 1 TEST STRATEGIES

Some students have their own personal strategies for dealing with multiple-choice exams. If you have a method that you are comfortable with, stick with it. However, many people find the following set of recommendations helpful. Our experience shows that your best strategy is to follow this advice:

- **Start with the beginning of the question block and work your way to the back of it.** This means start with the first question and do each question, in order, until you come to the last question. The idea here is to get into a rhythm that will carry you through the exam. This rhythm will help create what one psychologist calls a "flow" experience. The flow experience is a state of optimal concentration and maximal performance.

- **Do not skip any questions.** If you don't know the answer when you come to it, you are not likely to know it later. Skipping around wastes time and can end up confusing you as to where you are in the exam. Deal with each question as you come to it. Answer it as best you can, and move on to the next question.

- **Limit your use of the question-marking feature to no more than two questions in each block of 50.** The marking feature lets you return to review and reconsider questions where you would like more time. However, marking more than a couple of questions makes it hard to keep track of how many you want to revisit. You simply may not have time to go back and look at questions you have marked, especially if you mark a lot of them. Keep track of the questions you do mark by writing down the question number and any option you have been considering on your whiteboard. Use the marking feature to keep yourself from getting bogged down, not to hold yourself back.

- **Remember that you can only return to questions within the current question block.** Once the time has expired on any given question block, you can no longer access any of the questions within it.

- **Be cautious about changing answers.** In general, your odds of changing a correct answer to a wrong one are so much higher than the reverse that it is simply not worth the risk. If you change an answer, you are most likely making it wrong! Your first impulse is usually the correct one. Stay with it unless some clear insight occurs to you. If you are not sure, leave your first answer.

- **If you finish a question block with time left over, go back and "check" only those answers that you have previously marked.** Checking almost always leads to changing and tends to reduce your score. If you have a spare moment, make sure that you have entered an answer for every question in the block and then relax. Sit, take a break, and mentally prepare yourself for the next block of questions. Focus on the questions to come, not the ones that are past.

### Test-Taking Tip

Used correctly, marking will let you double-check questions where you have a high probability of getting the answer correct. Misused, marking can cause you to not give a question your full attention the first time around.

### Remember

Effective time management is key to getting your best score.

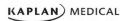

- **Segment your time so that you know how much you have left, and so that you do not find yourself rushed at the end.** You have just over one minute per question (72 seconds). Some questions will take more time and some less. Work on your pacing from the beginning of the question block. Check your watch every 10 questions to make sure you are on the correct pace to finish. If you pace yourself throughout the block, you should not be squeezed for time at the end.

- **Do not spend a lot of time on individual questions.** Research has shown that students spend the most time on questions that they get wrong. If you find yourself spending a lot of time on a question, this is your indication that you do not know the answer. How will you know if you are spending too long on any one question? If you find yourself thinking, "Maybe I'm taking too long on this question," you are. As soon as you think this, stop, mark your best guess, and move on to the next question.

- **During the breaks between question blocks, try to relax and not think back over the exam.** The desire to recall questions is strong but not helpful. Those questions are in the past; you will never see them again. Focus on relaxing and making the most of your break. Remember, you will always tend to remember those questions you got wrong. Thinking back over these questions will hurt your self-confidence and make the remainder of the exam more difficult. Be glad one set of questions is behind you. Forget about them, and think about something more pleasant.

**Remember**

Keep moving forward through the exam. There is always another question coming.

## A PROVEN ROUTINE FOR HANDLING EACH QUESTION

The Step 1 exam is not just about regurgitating facts, but about applying those facts in a clinical context. To handle these types of questions, your response pattern must not simply be "read, answer," but instead "read, think, answer."

**Strategy Tip**

Read, *think,* answer.

## Take a Moment to Think

You must train yourself to take this crucial moment of thought on each question. Give yourself time to reflect and call to mind the key facts that will help you answer the question. Many questions require you to make multiple determinations to arrive at a correct answer. You must take a reflective moment on each question to allow yourself the time for this cognitive processing. Read the question, call to mind what you know, and then proceed to select an answer. Approach each question with the assumption that you know the answer, and then muster your knowledge to attack it.

## Make Your Choice in the Time Allotted

The mental task of selecting an answer on a multiple-choice exam is different than the task you face when you make decisions in clinical medicine. In the day-to-day practice of medicine, when selecting a laboratory test, arriving at a diagnosis, or finding the best treatment option, you want to carefully consider all of the options and be sure about your choice. A patient's health, and perhaps life, is in your hands. Before making a choice, most people report that they want to feel as close to one hundred percent certainty as they can.

For the USMLE exams, you do not have the time to wait for this level of certainty. You must train yourself to make your choice within the time allotted. This often means choosing an answer, even when you are not completely sure. If you wait for that absolute feeling of inner certainty, you will take too long. Make your choice as soon as you have identified a clear best guess. Then move on to the next question. Remember, there is always another question coming next.

# THE KAPLAN METHOD: THREE TRIES FOR AN ANSWER

You have three chances to get each question right. If you cannot get a clear answer using these three attempts, you do not know the answer. Mark your favorite letter and move on to the next question. The key to this strategy is that you always know what you are going to do next. This helps you feel in control and reduces anxiety.

**Step 1: Read the Question.** This may seem trivial, but studies have shown that most students look at the answers first. Questions cause anxiety and answers provide the solution, so many people go right for the solution. However, you cannot pick the correct answer until you know what you are being asked.

Superior students generally spend about 45 seconds reading the question and about 15 to 20 seconds choosing from the given options. Poorer students tend to reverse this time allocation, spending less time on the question and more on the options. Time reading the question is time well spent. More time on the question means more time spent thinking.

- Read the question and pick out key words. Key words are diagnostic information, abnormal values, indications of gender or race, and any qualifying terms.
- Read carefully enough so that you only have to read the question once. Going back over the question takes time. Read for comprehension the first time.

**Paraphrasing is the key to effective reading.** Because the exam is administered on computer, you can no longer underline key facts, circle abnormal findings, or make notes in the margins. To compensate, superior test takers continuously summarize the key information in a brief fashion while reading the question. This allows you to look to the options with a sharp focus on the key elements and lessens the need to go back to reread it while examining the choices. Look at the following question to see how this is done.

A 75-year-old smoker and alcohol abuser is hospitalized for evaluation of a squamous cell carcinoma of the larynx. On his second hospital day, he complains of sweating, tremors, and vague gastrointestinal distress. On physical examination, he is anxious with a temperature of 101 F, heart rate of 104, BP of 150/100, and a respiratory rate of 22 breaths per minute. Later that day, he has three generalized tonic-clonic seizures. Which of the following is the most likely cause of his seizures?

(A) Alcohol withdrawal

(B) Brain metastasis

(C) Febrile seizure

(D) Hypocalcemia

(E) Subdural hematoma

Answer: A

The mental paraphrasing for this question might be as follows:

An old man with laryngeal cancer who smokes and drinks too much has sweats, tremor, anxiety, and some GI problems—he has three seizures a few days after admission. What's causing the seizures?

**Paraphrasing is the mental equivalent of underlining**. It helps you select what's important and keep those key facts in mind while you are evaluating possible answers. Like most test-taking skills, it also takes practice. If you practice paraphrasing material when you study, you will find that you have developed the basics to answer questions. Paraphrase each time you work with questions to gain skill and confidence.

**Step 2: The Prediction Pass.** After reading the question, stop. Before looking at the options, try to come up with an answer. We call this the prediction pass because you are trying to think like the question writer and predict the correct answer. By the USMLE's own rules, questions are written so that any expert in the field can come up with the correct answer without having any options present.

With the correct answer in mind, you are less likely to be led astray by distractors. Remember, they are supposed to distract you and convince you to pick the wrong answer. If you see the answer you thought of, scan the other answers to be sure that it is the best. Then pick it and move on to the next question.

**Step 3: The Selection Pass.** After reading the question, look down through all of the distractors, in order (A, B, C, D, E, F, G, etc.). If you see a correct answer, pick it. This is the selection pass. If the answer seems obvious and direct, good. Do not trick yourself into thinking the question must be tricky or more difficult.

Most answers will be clearly correct. If you find yourself making up a long story why one option is better than another, stop yourself. You are probably wrong. **The correct answer should be clearly correct.** If two answers seem to be almost the same, then neither one is correct. Once you have identified what looks like the best answer, choose it and move on to the next question.

**Step 4: The Final Pass**. If, after reading through the options, you are still not sure of the answer, you have one final try: the final pass. At this stage, rather than trying for a correct answer, you are eliminating those you know to be incorrect. Using this strategy, you can usually eliminate all but two of the options.

When you have narrowed your choices down to only two options, you have now arrived at the most crucial moment of the exam. The correct action at this point is to pick one of the two answers and move on to the next question. If you are really unsure of the correct answer, which one you pick does not matter. With two options to choose from you have a 50 percent chance of getting the question correct rather than the 20 percent chance you started with.

**Make a choice.** Many people waste time at this point by not choosing. Some people, when they have eliminated all but two answers, go back and reread the question in hopes of finding some information that will help them choose between the two options. Time spent talking with students and watching their thought processes during the exam suggests that this is the wrong strategy. When students reread a question at this point, they tend to add to it or pick out single features that help them feel better about choosing one of the answers. However, it does not help them pick the right answer. By adding assumptions to the question, students may feel more confident, but they are really mentally rewriting the question to be one that they feel more comfortable answering. The answer they pick is then the right answer to the question that they envision, but not for the actual question presented.

If after these three passes *1)* Prediction Pass, *2)* Selection Pass and *3)* Final Pass you still are not sure of the answer, your best option is to guess. At this point, mark any letter and move on to the next question. No answer counts the same as a wrong answer.

Questions with a large number of options should be handled the same way as all one-best-answer questions. The only difference is that you should not do a Final Pass as it would eat up too much time. That means these questions usually take less time to handle if done correctly.

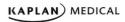

Remember, the key to doing well on this exam is to train yourself to make choices. If you do not know an answer, admit it, make your best guess, and move on to the next question. Don't be afraid to use common sense, but watch out for "myths." Myths are options that most people might think are true, but are not.

## TIPS FOR THE WEEK BEFORE THE EXAM

During the last few days before the exam you should be tapering off your studying and getting into mental and physical shape.

1. This is not the time for cramming in new material, but time to organize and integrate what you already know. Work on making what you know more accessible.

2. Review keywords, phrases, and concepts. Look over your summary notes one more time. This is the time to drill yourself on essential information. The key is to practice recall, not simply read over the material again. What you need to know is probably already in your head. Your task now is to train yourself to access the information when you need it. Doing practice questions is a good way to reinforce your recall skills. Remember, practice questions are often harder than the questions on the real exam, so do not panic if you do not get them right. Use them to clarify your understanding of key details.

3. Have an honest conversation with yourself and decide what you do not know. No one can know everything that is asked on this exam. Be honest with yourself about what you do and do not know. Knowing that you do not know something gives you more of a sense of control on the exam and makes you less likely to panic when you encounter the material and/or waste time on questions you are not likely to get correct. When you come to a question that you know that you do not know, simply mark your favorite letter and move on!

4. Get yourself onto the right time schedule. Wake up every day at the same time you will need to on the day of the exam. This will get your circadian rhythm coordinated with the exam schedule. Do not nap between 8:00 a.m. and 5:00 p.m. Otherwise, you will accustom your body to shutting down during critical exam hours.

5. You should be getting a sufficient amount of sleep. For most people that means at least 6 to 7 hours a night. Sleep is an essential time for your brain to consolidate what you have learned. You need sleep; it makes you a more efficient learner when you are awake.

6. Take some time each day to relax. Have a good meal. Take a walk in the fresh air. Find time for exercise. The change of pace will refresh you and the physical activity will help you relax and sleep at night.

7. Consider the impact of your personal relationships on your preparation. Family responsibilities and obligations can be very distracting. The week before the exam you should avoid family confrontations and any stressful relationships. Your focus should be on the exam and nothing else. The other parts of your life can wait.

8. If you haven't done so already, visit the Prometric Center where you will be taking the exam. It will be indicated on your exam entry ticket. This will ensure you know how to get there and how much time you should allow for the commute. You can see where you should park, and see what the computer set-up is like.

9. If you have not yet done so, review the tutorial on the official USMLE CD-ROM. Become familiar with the interface, the location of key information on the screen, and how to navigate between screens. If you walk into the exam familiar with the exam, you will not have to use any of your valuable break time to do this on Test Day.

### Remember

Use the time before the exam for review, not for trying to learn new material.

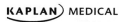

## THE DAY BEFORE THE EXAM

1.  Take the day off from all studying. This is your day to relax and gather your strength before the main event. Get out of bed at the same time you will have to get up the next day, and then treat this day as a vacation day to reward yourself for all your hard work. If you must study, limit yourself to reviewing your own notes and flashcards.

2.  Have some fun. Go for a walk. Listen to your favorite music. Go see a good comedy or an action movie that will allow cathartic release. Go shopping. Spend time with a significant other. Do whatever you like. You have worked hard and deserve it.

3.  Make sure that you have checked out the basics for the exam:
    *   Have you worked through the USMLE CD-ROM tutorial?
    *   Do you know where the exam is being given, and how to get there?
    *   Do you have alternative transportation if, for example, your car does not start?
    *   Do you trust your alarm clock to wake you up in time? If not, make arrangements with friends as a back up. You want to be sure to wake up rested, refreshed, and on time.

4.  Lay out what you'll need for your exam before you go to sleep. This includes your photo identification, scheduling permit, and confirmation number, as well as any personal items like eyeglasses. While you're at it, don't forget to pack a lunch!

5.  Call your friends and classmates and make some plans to celebrate after the exam is over. You'll need to blow off some steam anyhow, and talking with colleagues will remind you that you are not in this by yourself.

6.  Be sure to do some physical activity. Just taking a walk for an hour will help relax you.

7.  Get a good night's sleep. To help you sleep, consider a hot bath or warm milk. Avoid taking sleeping medication as it may leave you groggy in the morning.

## THE DAY OF THE EXAM

This is not the most important day of your career, but just another hurdle on your way to becoming a licensed physician. Keep it in perspective. Treat the exam like what it is, a routine mechanical exercise. You are not a doctor for this day, but an assembly line worker. Rather than making cars or toasters, you are answering questions. Deal with each question as you come to it, make your choice, and then move on.

No matter how well prepared you are for the USMLE Step 1 exam, you will get many questions wrong. This is not an exam where you should expect to know every answer. Remember, 70 percent correct puts you well over the mean! Knowing this, your test-taking strategy should be somewhat different than it may be when you take other exams.

Doing well on this exam means spending your time on those questions you are most likely to get correct, and not wasting time on questions you are likely to get wrong. Two minutes spent on a question that you get wrong is two minutes wasted. Approach every question assuming that you will be able to answer it correctly. If you discover that you can not arrive at a clear answer, admit it, make a choice, and move on to the next question. The core idea is a simple one. You know you will get some questions wrong. Therefore, admit which ones they are and spend your time on those questions for which your probability of a correct answer is higher.

## TEST-TAKING TIPS

Try to arrive 30 minutes early to the Prometric Center so you are not rushed and have time to get organized. You will be given a locker to store your personal items and then assigned a computer station. Remember that you have a total of 8 hours to complete 350 questions in 50-question blocks. You will have one hour for each block of questions, and a total of one hour to be used throughout the day for breaks and lunch. You will be required to sign out when taking breaks.

To cope with fatigue, you will need to schedule breaks. Our recommended schedule for the exam is:

| Question Block | Break Time at End of Block |
| --- | --- |
| Block 1 | No break |
| Block 2 | 5-minute break |
| Block 3 | 5-minute break |
| Block 4 | 30-minute lunch break |
| Block 5 | No break |
| Block 6 | 10-minute break |
| Block 7 | Done! |

This allows you 10 minutes extra to use as needed. You should also be aware that if you leave the exam room during a block, it will be marked as an irregularity in your testing session. So consider after each block whether you want to take a bathroom break during your break time.

## UNDERSTANDING FRED™: HOW TO USE THE USMLE™ SOFTWARE

### Show Answers Window

A window down the left-hand side of the screen lists the question number and any answer given to each question in the block. This enables students to track where they are in the block and provides an easy way to make sure they have answered every question in the block.

### Highlighting feature

When HIGHLIGHT is turned on, you can use your mouse to highlight in yellow a section of text. This yellow highlighting will remain even after you move your mouse onto something else.

Used appropriately, highlighting can also keep you engaged and make sure you are actually taking content out of the question rather than just reading without retention. Highlighting can help to draw you into the details and avoid the mental mistake of skimming over the question without focusing on the presented details.

### Strikeout feature

When STRIKEOUT is turned on, text in options that you click on with your mouse will be faded from black to a grayish color. This moves them to the background (while not completely removing it from view) and provides a clear visual indication that you have ruled out that option as a choice. If you can read the options and select the best answer directly, you will not need to use the strikeout feature. If one answer looks best, pick it and move on.

**Note**

Highlighting can be very useful when creating a symptom list in a long clinical case item or for making sure that some significant feature of the presented information is remembered at the end of the question.

**Note**

Don't use the strikeout feature on every question, but only on the questions where you are trying to improve your odds by eliminating options.

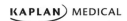

**Note**

The annotation window is probably more trouble than it's worth. It takes time to write a note. Your best approach is always to deal with each question as you come to it and then move on. Look forward, not backward.

**Note**

If you do not know your normal lab values, spend five minutes a day on these until they are part of your reflexive knowledge base. You need to know these for the exam, but also for medical practice. Committing these lab values to memory will facilitate your performance in both arenas.

## Annotation Window

FRED software provides a window in which you can write question-specific comments. You can use this annotation feature to create a symptom list or to remind yourself of something if you desire to revisit the question.

## Categorized Lab Values

The test interface gives you the ability to look up the reference ranges for standard laboratory values, which may be presented as a part of your question stem. FRED groups the lab values into categories such as blood, cerebrospinal, hematologic, and sweat and urine. When you click on each category, you will be shown the lab values and reference ranges only for that category. This reduces the size of the list you have to scan and makes a particular value easier to find.

Every time you click on the LAB VALUES button, you are pulling yourself away from your focus on the question. Our advice, therefore, is *learn your normal lab values so you do not have to look them up*. You should know these already before you walk into the exam. If you forget a reference range, the LAB VALUES button is there to help you. But consider this button a safety net. It is there to bail you out if you need it, but do not plan to use it.

# Chapter Four: **Physical and Mental Preparation**

The USMLE Step 1 is a big event. Like an athlete preparing for a big race, you want to approach it fully prepared—both physically and mentally. The following information consists of training tips to help you prepare for your test-taking marathon.

## PHYSICAL PREPARATION

All-day examinations are physically stressful. What can you do to help decrease this stress?

**Get in training.** At least one month before the exam, begin the plan described below.

1. **Get enough rest.** Although you may be tempted to study late into the night and right up to the moment before the examination, this strategy can backfire and hurt you. The brain needs rest. By shutting off factual input, you foster the assimilation of information into long-term memory and allow time for making connections that help the integration, retention, and recall of information. In the week before the exam, you should be getting at least 6 1/2 hours of sleep a night.

2. **Eat right.** While preparing for the exam, have good solid meals. Protein, carbohydrates, and some fats are all important. However, do not overeat or eat very late, since this will impair your sleep. Breakfast on the big day should be light; complex carbohydrates like fruit and cereal work well. Avoid anything greasy or unusual. Likewise, keep sugar or simple carbohydrate equivalents, such as candy, to a minimum at this time. Hard candy, not chocolate, can be useful as a pick-me-up during the examination. If you normally drink coffee in the morning, drink coffee the morning of the exam. You don't want to trigger a caffeine withdrawal headache. Eat light lunches, salads, simple sandwiches, and nonalcoholic drinks to avoid after-lunch sleepiness.

   a. Some students report that vitamin B complex, especially B6, can help with stress reduction.

   b. Schedule and eat meals as a part of your study time. These meals serve as breaks which give you a chance to recharge and be more efficient in your studies.

3. **Get some exercise.** The exam requires you to be in good physical condition, since you will be sitting for long periods of time and want to avoid muscle fatigue resulting in neck, back, or leg aches. As part of your preparation, start an exercise program and stick with it, no matter how difficult. Your regimen should include stretching and aerobic exercise, such as brisk walking or bike riding. The night before the exam, exercise, on a more moderate scale, should continue. Besides the physical benefit, exercise can also help to decrease your anxiety.

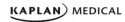

# MENTAL/EMOTIONAL PREPARATION

People differ tremendously in their reaction to test situations. Some appear to sail through—confident and calm—while others experience mental and physiologic symptoms of test anxiety such as insomnia, nausea, muscle twitching, or increasing inability to concentrate. If you have serious concerns about test anxiety, don't wait until the day before to seek help. Deal with the problem so anxiety doesn't increase as exam day approaches and your options for dealing with it decrease to zero. This is a situational problem and effective treatment is available.

Here are some suggestions for how to deal with test anxiety and some exercises that may help you to cope.

1. **Avoid negative thoughts and feelings.** Negative self talk such as, "There is no way I can pass this exam" can be distracting and produce more anxiety about the test. Focusing on avoiding failure is a recipe for failure. Focus instead on achieving success.

2. **Make anxiety your friend.** A degree of anxiety on the day of the examination is not only natural, but also beneficial. How often have you heard of people responding well beyond their daily abilities when pushed to the limits psychologically? However, there is no need for you to push yourself to the limits, you simply need be a little tense and anticipatory on exam day. Incapacitating anxiety will destroy your ability to pass. We have heard many individuals say, "I knew everything, I even taught my peers, but I didn't pass. I don't understand it." Anxiety may do this to you!

3. **Seek help if necessary.** If you find that your studying is being overwhelmed by your anxiety, the most useful thing you can do may be to seek counseling. Talking to someone about your anxiety is not a waste of time if your study time is unproductive due to that anxiety. Get help to be more productive.

4. **Be aware of obsessive thoughts.** If you find yourself focusing on your inability to answer questions, the volume of material, or doubts about your ability to pass the exam, try giving yourself something else to think about. Keeping your mind focused on a small task at hand, such as the information you are currently studying, will help you avoid letting obsessive thoughts distract you.

5. **Make a study schedule.** Purchase a calendar and write out which subjects you will study and a time frame for each. Leave room for breaks and "free time." This helps you gain control over your life and your studying. Following a schedule gives you structure, which makes you more efficient and reduces stress.

6. **Improve your attention control.** Awareness is like a searchlight. Whatever you direct your attention to is pretty clear, but other things and events tend to fade into the periphery. Try directing your attention separately to sights, sounds, the feelings in your hands, feet, etc. Your awareness can shift very quickly from one focus to another; however, you can only be fully aware of whatever is in your realm of focus at one particular moment. Use this fact to redirect your wandering thoughts and feelings by focusing your attention. In time this will allow you to quickly de-emphasize extraneous thoughts by redirecting them to simple bodily functions. Keep in mind how attention works:

   a. You can attend to only one thing at a time.

   b. Attention is voluntary and immediate, focusing on NOW. The future has no role to play.

   c. You can monitor your own attention.

   d. Attention can be redirected.

   e. Focusing on other things that are more relevant can redirect irrelevant attention.

   f. You cannot pay attention continuously to one thing without breaks.

7. **Use visualization.** Spend a few moments thinking back to a crisis situation that you handled beautifully. Perhaps it was a medical emergency or a family quarrel where you intervened and helped solve the issue. It can be any type of crisis in which you took charge successfully. Recall how strong and in control you felt, how effectively you controlled a bad scene, even what the setting was like. Reflect on the event to recall it in as much detail as you can. Each day while you are studying, spend 5–10 minutes re-visiting this past event until you are able to bring it back in your mind with great clarity and detail. Now, when you feel an anxious feeling welling up, take a mental time out and re-visit this scene. When you do, all the emotions of that day will also return and replace those anxious feelings.

8. **Use an Affirmation Card.** Take 30 minutes or so to write a series of statements on an index card. The statements should describe what you believe are your greatest personal strengths, character traits, and talents. You might state that you are a deeply empathetic person, or that you are very good at solving problems. It doesn't matter what you write down, as long as you believe each statement is true and that you are proud of that skill, personality aspect, or talent. Once you have created the card, keep it with you as you study and practice with test questions. When anxious feelings begin to intrude, take out the card and read through it slowly, realizing the truth of what you have written. With practice, this process will help focus you and lessen negative thoughts.

9. **Take a mental "time out."** If anxious or angry thoughts interfere while you are practicing with questions, try this exercise. Close your eyes, take some slow, deep breaths, and flex, then relax first the muscles in your neck, then your shoulders, then your lower limbs. Use a 1-2-3 count for each inhaled and exhaled breath to keep your breathing deep and even. The whole process will only take a few minutes and will help you reduce the physical symptoms of anxiety and allow you to return to the test with a calm, focused state of mind.

10. **Learn and practice deep breathing techniques.** It can be difficult to focus your attention when you are anxious, but deep breathing can help. With enough practice during stressful events, this technique will become second nature during the exam.

11. **Use "time out" during the exam.** If necessary, to break the anxiety loop during the exam, back away from the mouse and keyboard and take a few deep breaths. Thirty seconds of rest will seem like 30 minutes in the middle of the exam. Try timing yourself and see how long it feels. By taking very little time away, you get a lot of mental rest. When the exam becomes too much, the best strategy is not to push yourself to concentrate harder, but to back off and rest for a few moments. You will find that when you return to the exam, your anxiety will be reduced, and the questions will make more sense.

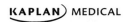

# Chapter Five: **Summary Pointers**

The USMLE Step 1 is an all-day exam. The day can seem long and tiring. You need to have a clear goal in mind and a clear plan for reaching that goal. You need to be in good mental and physical shape for the exam.

## REMEMBER

1.  Not every question counts. (Although you can't tell which ones do and which ones do not.)

2.  You need to be prepared in all of the seven core subjects: Anatomy, Behavioral Sciences, Biochemistry, Microbiology/Immunology, Pathology, Pharmacology, and Physiology. A question in one subject counts just as much as one in another.

3.  Become familiar with the basic single best answer question types: positively worded, two-step, bait and switch, true/false, clinical case, and conjunction questions.

4.  You must be able to answer questions regarding material presented as either basic knowledge or as applied to clinical tasks. Increasingly, for this exam, application of knowledge is the key.

5.  Spend some time becoming familiar with what is likely to be tested, but be careful of the mistake of "studying for last year's exam."

6.  Be organized and plan your study time. Kaplan has a variety of resources ranging from home study materials to live lecture review courses that you may find useful in this regard. Make a study plan and stick to it!

7.  Strongly consider forming a study group and helping each other review information. Presenting to each other is one of the best ways to learn to use the material you have studied.

8.  Practice questions only after mastering the underlying material. Always do questions in clusters and within a time limit.

9.  Taper off your preparation before the exam to give yourself a chance to rest up mentally and physically.

10. During the exam, read each question and answer them in order. Never change an answer. Segment your time to be sure you are not squeezed at the end of the exam.

11. Do not linger over questions you do not know. Move on and use the time to answer questions you do know.

12. You have three chances to get every question right: recall, selection, and final passes. If you can't get a good answer after these three tries, guess and move on.

13. Consider using any of the time-tested behavioral strategies, especially taking a "time out" for coping with anxiety and distracting negative thoughts during the exam.

14. Take care of yourself. Suffering doesn't help anyone.

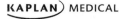

# THE USMLE STEP 1 EXAMINATION: DOS AND DON'TS

## DOs

**DO** remember the content of the computer-based exam (CBT) will be similar to previous exams as will the amount of time per question (just over one minute).

**DO** take advantage of the CD-ROM computer-based testing practice disk that will be sent with your Step 1 application confirmation.

**DO** be organized. Set up an organized study schedule and adhere to it. Plan your work and work the plan.

**DO** be sure to make up questions while you study (use index cards) and form a study group to review important content.

**DO** use graphs and charts in texts to speed up your comprehension of the material. A picture is worth a thousand words, and the exam will test you using similar images.

**DO** practice questions under a time limit similar to the actual exam. In general, your rule should be one minute per question.

**DO** understand that there is material tested that you will either be unfamiliar with or never really fully understood. Don't panic! Guess and move on.

**DO** know that you are not required to pass each subsection (physio, biochem, etc.) of the exam separately, but only to answer enough questions correctly to attain an overall passing score.

**DO** understand that you will only need to get about 70 percent of the questions right to receive a passing score.

**DO** realize you'll probably see more pictures than in past exams. They are only intended to test you on core basic science content.

**DO** know that not all of the questions on the exam will count! Anywhere from 30 to 35 questions on the exam are included so they can be pretested and evaluated for use in later exams. In addition, as many as 10 to 15 other questions may be eliminated from the scored pool after the exam results are reviewed.

**DO** make sure your selected answer matches *all* the information presented in the question. All answers are somewhat likely; you want to pick the one *most* likely.

**DO** be prepared for two-step questions, where you will need to make two correct decisions to arrive at the correct answer (e.g., come up with a diagnosis, then decide what the treatment should be).

**DO** remember when you have the question down to two choices, you need to pick one and move on. Lingering over the question tends to result in making the wrong choice.

# DON'Ts

**DON'T** just practice questions without preparatory studying. Review material first until you feel you know it, and then use questions to test yourself.

**DON'T** do practice questions individually. **DO** them in clusters with five to ten as a minimum to get yourself used to moving from question to question, and **DON'T** look up answers after each question.

**DON'T** get into the habit of lingering over a question or thinking about it for an extended period of time. You **DON'T** have this luxury on the real exam.

**DON'T** just memorize material! Learn and understand how to apply the content in presented scenarios. Very little of the exam will test rote memory for basic facts, and that's not enough to pass this exam.

**DON'T** reread your textbooks from cover to cover. You need to focus on the material most likely to be on the examination. Talk to others who have taken the exam to see how they prepared. Talk to faculty. Use the NBME booklet as a study guide.

**DON'T** assume commercial review books and practice exams are current. A good rule of thumb is that whatever appears in most of the review books is probably important, and whatever appears in just one book is most likely peripheral.

**DON'T** be afraid to face your weak or least-liked areas. Take pretests and/or diagnostic exams to help you narrow down strengths and weaknesses. Begin your study plan with your weak areas and plan to cover those at least twice before the exam. **DON'T** entirely neglect your strong areas, but leave them to a time closer to the examination.

**DON'T** expect traditional exam "tricks," short cuts, or buzz words to point you to the correct answer. The USMLE has put great effort into eliminating these cues from the exam.

**DON'T** get caught by distractors. They may be partially right answers, but not the best answer. Common misconceptions, incomplete knowledge, and faulty reasoning will cause you to select a distractor.

**DON'T** substitute reading the last line of the question for reading the whole question. This can cause you to miss important information or point you to distractors intended to confuse the issue.

**DON'T** skip any questions. If you don't know it when you come to it, you are not likely to know it later. Deal with each question as you come to it, answer it as best you can, and move on to the next question.

**DON'T** change an answer. Your odds of changing a correct answer to a wrong one are so much higher than the reverse that it is simply not worth the risk.

## A FINAL COMMENT

This is not a test of your intelligence or even of how good a doctor you will be. This is a test of your capacity to identify and apply core principles within the constraints of the multiple-choice format. Planning, preparation, practice, perseverance, and patience will lead you to your best score. Good luck, and remember, we're here to help!

# Qbook Practice Tests

# Anatomy: **Test One**

1. A 75-year-old man with a 40-pack-year history of smoking and hypercholesterolemia is diagnosed with severe atherosclerosis. Atherosclerotic occlusion of which of the following arteries would result in insufficient perfusion of the urinary bladder?

   (A) External iliac

   (B) Inferior epigastric

   (C) Internal iliac

   (D) Internal pudendal

   (E) Lateral sacral

2. A 36-year-old woman is hospitalized for treatment of a stomach ulcer that has been getting progressively worse over several months. Radiographic studies reveal the site of involvement to be along the greater curvature, approximately 4 cm away from the pyloric sphincter. That night, the ulcer perforates, and there is considerable intra-abdominal bleeding. Surgery reveals that the ulcer has eroded through the stomach wall and has damaged the artery supplying the involved region of the stomach. Which artery was likely involved?

   (A) Left gastric

   (B) Left gastroepiploic

   (C) Right gastric

   (D) Right gastroepiploic

   (E) Short gastric

3. A woman who recently gave birth has elevated prolactin levels. The gland responsible for secretion of this hormone is derived from which of the following structures?

   (A) Cerebral vesicle

   (B) Infundibulum

   (C) Neurohypophysis

   (D) Proctodeum

   (E) Rathke's pouch

4. A previously normal 56-year-old woman comes to the emergency department because of a "flu-like" illness. She complains of nausea and vomiting, unilateral tingling in the leg, and a headache involving the eye and forehead. She is alert and fully oriented. Motor, sensory, gait, and coordination examinations are normal. Cranial nerve examination is normal, aside from the visual field disorder indicated in the plot below.

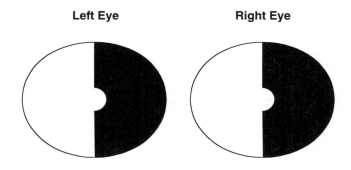

**Left Eye**          **Right Eye**

The neurologic examination suggests an occlusion of which of the following vessels?

   (A) Left middle cerebral artery

   (B) Left posterior cerebral artery

   (C) Right middle cerebral artery

   (D) Right posterior cerebral artery

   (E) Posterior communicating artery

5. A 49-year-old Vietnamese man is diagnosed with tuberculosis. On physical examination, large flocculent masses are noted over the lateral lumbar back, and a similar mass is located in the ipsilateral groin. This pattern of involvement strongly suggests an abscess tracking along which of the following muscles?

   (A) Adductor longus
   (B) Gluteus maximus
   (C) Gluteus minimus
   (D) Piriformis
   (E) Psoas major

6. A 24-year-old man is stabbed in the neck. Neurologic examination reveals left-sided hemiparesis. There is complete loss of discriminatory joint position and vibration sensation below C8 on the left side. On the right side, there is loss of pain and temperature sensation below C8. It can be expected that an MRI of the cervical spinal cord will show which of the following findings?

   (A) A complete transection of the spinal cord
   (B) A hemisection of the left side of the cord
   (C) A lesion of the dorsal columns of the cord on the left side
   (D) A lesion of the lateral funiculus on the left side
   (E) Damage to cervical dorsal roots on left side

7. A 2-year-old boy is brought to the pediatrician by his mother because he has had several episodes of rectal bleeding. Evaluation with a technetium-99m perfusion scan reveals a 3-cm ileal outpouching located 60 cm from the ileocecal valve. This structure most likely contains which of the following types of ectopic tissue?

   (A) Duodenal
   (B) Esophageal
   (C) Gastric
   (D) Hepatic
   (E) Jejunal

8. A 34-year-old man is examined in the prison infirmary after sustaining a superficial stab wound to the superolateral aspect of the thoracic wall at the level of the third rib. There is little bleeding and no difficulty breathing; however, the medial border of the scapula on the injured side pulls away from the body wall when the arm is raised. In addition, the arm cannot be abducted above the horizontal. Which of the following muscles is paralyzed?

   (A) Levator scapulae
   (B) Pectoralis minor
   (C) Rhomboid major
   (D) Serratus anterior
   (E) Supraspinatus

9. A histologist is examining cells arrested at various stages of oogenesis. He discovers a follicle within the stroma of the ovary that has developed an antrum. This follicle would be classified as

   (A) Graafian
   (B) primary
   (C) primordial
   (D) secondary

10. A 54-year-old man has cirrhosis, with obstruction of the portal circulation within the liver. Portal blood could still be conveyed to the caval system via which of the following?

    (A) Azygos and hemiazygos veins
    (B) Gonadal veins
    (C) External iliac veins
    (D) Splenic vein
    (E) Vesical venous plexus

11. A 47-year-old man presents to his neurologist with an unsteady, broad-based gait and slow, slurred speech. Neurologic examination reveals dysdiadochokinesia, intention tremor, hypotonia, and nystagmus. The patient's lesion is in a brain structure that derives from which of the following embryonic structures?

    (A) Diencephalon
    (B) Mesencephalon
    (C) Metencephalon
    (D) Myelencephalon
    (E) Telencephalon

12. A 47-year-old woman with a history of rheumatic fever is examined by her physician. Physical examination is significant for a low-pitched, rumbling, diastolic murmur preceded by an opening snap. The affected valve can be best evaluated by auscultation at which of the following locations?

    (A) Left second intercostal space
    (B) Left fifth intercostal space
    (C) Left lower sternal body border
    (D) Right second intercostal space
    (E) Right fifth intercostal space

13. A newborn girl is noted to have abnormal accommodation of the lens. Further evaluation reveals an abnormal production of aqueous humor. A malformation of the structure responsible for these functions that is continuous posteriorly with the choroid might be due to abnormal development of

    (A) axons of retinal ganglion cells
    (B) choroid fissure of the optic stalk
    (C) mesoderm surrounding the optic cup
    (D) mesoderm surrounding the optic stalk
    (E) neuroectoderm of the optic cup

14. A neuroscientist decides to perform a study that requires him to increase the concentration of norepinephrine in the cortex of an animal subject. He does this by electrically stimulating a nucleus in the brain. Which of the following nuclei is the most important source of noradrenergic innervation to the cerebral cortex?

    (A) Basal nucleus of Meynert
    (B) Caudate nucleus
    (C) Locus caeruleus
    (D) Raphe nucleus
    (E) Substantia nigra
    (F) Ventral tegmental area

15. A surgeon tells a medical student to tap the side of the face of a patient who just had thyroid surgery. The surgeon is most worried about damage to which of the following vessels?

    (A) Common carotid artery
    (B) External carotid artery
    (C) Facial vein
    (D) Internal jugular vein
    (E) Superior and inferior thyroid arteries

16. A 45-year-old man comes into the emergency department with abdominal pain that has progressively worsened since the previous night. He also notes nausea and vomiting, but is afebrile. Upper gastrointestinal radiographic studies reveal that a loop of small intestine has passed through the epiploic foramen into the omental bursa and is constricted by the margins of the foramen as the intestine fills. The constriction should not be surgically relieved by opening the epiploic foramen because this procedure would risk cutting the

    (A) abdominal aorta
    (B) hepatic artery
    (C) hepatic vein
    (D) hypogastric plexus
    (E) pancreatic duct

17. A 26-year-old man is stabbed in the left chest during a bar brawl. Several days after he is treated, he returns to the physician complaining of decreased function in his left arm. Physical examination reveals a winged left scapula and an inability to raise his left arm above the horizontal. Which of the following nerves is most likely affected?

    (A) Axillary
    (B) Long thoracic
    (C) Lower subscapular
    (D) Suprascapular
    (E) Thoracodorsal

18. A patient is transported to the emergency department with a knife wound to the right fifth intercostal space at the midaxillary line. Which of the following structures is likely to have been damaged?

    (A) Liver
    (B) Right atrium
    (C) Right pulmonary artery
    (D) Superior vena cava
    (E) Upper lobe of right lung

19. A couple comes to the physician for advice about contraception and family planning. The physician provides advice about various methods of birth control. While discussing the option of using an intrauterine device, a discussion of the process of implantation comes up. At what stage of embryonic development does an embryo normally begin to implant in the endometrium?

    (A) Blastocyst
    (B) Four-cell stage
    (C) Morula
    (D) Trilaminar embryo
    (E) Zygote

20. A newborn male is found to have urethral openings along the ventral surface of the penis. The physician explains to the parents that the bilateral structures that should have fused in the midline failed to fuse completely, and this resulted in the defect. The parents are very concerned, but the physician reassures them that this can easily be surgically corrected. Which of the following structures in a female normally develop from the same structures that failed to fuse in this boy?

    (A) Round ligaments of the uterus
    (B) Crura of the clitoris
    (C) Labia majora
    (D) Labia minora
    (E) Ovarian ligaments

21. A 19-year-old woman comes to the emergency department after falling while on roller-blades. There is a 3-cm laceration over the lateral aspect of the knee penetrating so deep that the head of the fibula is apparent. A radiograph of the leg is negative for any fractures. A noticeable foot-drop occurs while the patient walks. Further examination reveals inability to dorsiflex or evert the foot. Which of the following best explains her injury?

    (A) The common peroneal nerve was severed
    (B) The peroneal muscles were detached from the head of the fibula
    (C) The superficial peroneal nerve was severed
    (D) The tibial nerve was severed

22. A resident physician is performing a pelvic examination on a young woman. The fingers of one of her hands are in the patient's vagina, palpating the cervix. The other hand is pressing on the abdomen. With the palm of this hand, the physician feels a bony structure in the lower midline. This structure is most likely the

    (A) coccyx
    (B) ilium
    (C) ischium
    (D) pubis
    (E) sacrum

23. A 45-year-old man with a history of stable angina presents to the emergency department with an episode of chest pain that is not relieved by rest or nitroglycerin. After stabilization in the telemetry unit for 2 days, he undergoes a thallium stress test. The results show reduced perfusion of the lateral wall of the left ventricle. Which artery is most likely occluded?

    (A) Left anterior descending
    (B) Left circumflex
    (C) Left main coronary
    (D) Right coronary

24. A 41-year-old man is injured in a motorcycle accident. He is taken to the hospital by a rescue helicopter and treated for abdominal, spinal, and head injuries. Three weeks later he is examined by a neurologist, who notes that the patient has left-sided facial swelling and discoloration, slight drooping of the left eyelid, and a constricted pupil on the left side. There are no other motor or sensory abnormalities. Which of the following is the most likely cause of this patient's ocular disorder?

    (A) A lesion of cranial nerve VI
    (B) A lesion of the midbrain
    (C) A lesion of the oculomotor nerve
    (D) A lesion of the thoracic spinal cord
    (E) Myasthenia gravis

25. A 4-day-old boy is brought to the pediatric clinic because of breathing difficulties and poor feeding. He coughs, chokes, and spits up milk very soon after beginning to suckle. Physical examination and radiographs reveal the presence of the most common type of tracheoesophageal fistula. The infant's defect likely resulted from

    (A) failure of the buccopharyngeal membrane to rupture
    (B) failure of the tracheoesophageal ridges to fuse
    (C) incomplete formation of the septum secundum
    (D) incomplete recanalization of the larynx
    (E) patent thyroglossal duct

26. A 40-year-old man complains of loss of sensation over the right scrotum and on the medial right thigh. Damage to which of the following nerves would result in such symptoms?

    (A) Genitofemoral
    (B) Iliohypogastric
    (C) Ilioinguinal
    (D) Lateral cutaneous
    (E) Pudendal

27. A neonate has a prominent defect at the base of his spine through which his meninges and spinal cord protrude. A failure of which of the following processes is the most common cause of this type of defect?

    (A) Development of the body
    (B) Development of the pedicle
    (C) Development of primary vertebral ossification centers
    (D) Development of the superior articular process
    (E) Fusion of the vertebral arches

28. A surgeon is first on the scene after a serious automobile accident. He finds a passenger bleeding profusely from the neck and correctly surmises that the bleeding is from the carotid artery. To control the bleeding, the surgeon can compress the carotid artery against the anterior tubercle of which of the following vertebrae?

    (A) Second cervical
    (B) Third cervical
    (C) Fourth cervical
    (D) Fifth cervical
    (E) Sixth cervical

29. An intravenous pyelogram is performed on a patient to evaluate the function and structure of her kidneys. Examination of the resulting radiographs reveals that the left kidney is normal but that there is a duplication of the ureter and renal pelvis on the right side. Further testing reveals that kidney function is normal. This variation is a result of abnormal development of which of the following structures?

    (A) Allantoic duct
    (B) Metanephric blastema
    (C) Mesonephric duct
    (D) Mesonephric tubules
    (E) Ureteric bud

30. MRI reveals that a 62-year-old man has a brain tumor growing in his interhemispheric fissure at the level of the central sulcus. The tumor produces neurologic dysfunction of the cerebral cortex on either side of the tumor. A neurologic examination of this patient would most likely reveal

    (A) ataxia
    (B) hemiplegia
    (C) paraplegia
    (D) quadriplegia
    (E) rigidity

31. Brunner's glands secrete an alkaline product that helps achieve optimal pH for the activity of pancreatic enzymes. Where are these glands located?

    (A) At the base of villi throughout the small intestine
    (B) In the epithelium of the ampulla of Vater
    (C) In the mucosa and submucosa of the jejunum
    (D) In the submucosa of the duodenum
    (E) In the submucosa of the ileum

32. A 24-year-old man presents with pain in his right wrist that resulted when he fell hard on his outstretched hand. Radiographic studies indicate an anterior dislocation of a proximal row carpal bone that articulates with the most lateral proximal row carpal bone. Which of the following bones was dislocated?

    (A) Capitate
    (B) Lunate
    (C) Scaphoid
    (D) Trapezoid
    (E) Triquetrum

33. The femoral triangle is bounded superiorly by the inguinal ligament. Which of the following structures form the lateral and medial borders of the femoral triangle?

    (A) Adductor longus and gracilis

    (B) Adductor longus and sartorius

    (C) Gracilis and pectineus

    (D) Gracilis and sartorius

    (E) Pectineus and sartorius

34. A 43-year-old woman is diagnosed with a condition that causes excruciating pain near her nose and mouth. The involved nerve innervates which of the following branchial arches?

    (A) First

    (B) Second

    (C) Third

    (D) Fourth

35. An infant is born with an abnormally developed falciform ligament. The hepatogastric and hepatoduodenal ligaments are also malformed. These developmental anomalies are most likely due to abnormal development of the

    (A) dorsal mesoduodenum

    (B) dorsal mesogastrium

    (C) pericardioperitoneal canal

    (D) pleuropericardial membranes

    (E) ventral mesentery

36. An autopsy is performed on a man who died of an unknown cause. The pathologist discovers that the man has a small atrial septal defect. The defect is seen in the portion of the atrial septum near the upper border of the fossa ovalis. Which of the following was the likely functional manifestation of this defect during life?

    (A) No cyanosis occurred prenatally or postnatally

    (B) Postnatal cyanosis due to a shunt of blood from the left atrium to the right atrium

    (C) Postnatal cyanosis due to a shunt of blood from the right atrium to the left atrium

    (D) Prenatal cyanosis due to a shunt of blood from the right atrium to the left atrium

    (E) Prenatal cyanosis due to a shunt of blood from the left atrium to the right atrium

37. A 6-year-old boy is brought to the office for evaluation of a neck mass. His mother reports that he first developed the mass 3 days ago, and it has not resolved. Further questioning reveals that he has recently recovered from a viral upper respiratory infection. He is otherwise healthy and is up to date on all recommended vaccinations. Physical examination shows a 2-cm neck mass in the midline immediately above the thyroid cartilage notch. The mass elevates when he sticks his tongue out of his mouth. Which of the following is the most likely diagnosis?

    (A) Reactive lymph node

    (B) Branchial cleft cyst

    (C) Thyroglossal duct cyst

    (D) Head and neck neoplasm

    (E) Thyroid nodule

38. When removing an impacted mandibular third molar, the oral surgeon must warn the patient of possible lasting numbness of the tip of the tongue. This loss of general sensation is due to damage to the

    (A) auriculotemporal nerve

    (B) chorda tympani

    (C) lingual nerve

    (D) mental nerve

    (E) mylohyoid nerve

39. A resident physician is demonstrating the correct technique for inserting a subclavian central venous line. He has a medical student palpate the clavicle, then the chest wall below it. The first bony structure that can be palpated below the inferior margin of the medial portion of the clavicle is the

    (A) acromion

    (B) atlas

    (C) first rib

    (D) manubrium

    (E) second rib

40. A 34-year-old woman bursts through the doors of the emergency department. She is straining to take a breath but can only mouth the phrase: "I can't br—" before collapsing. She is placed on a stretcher. Her tongue is swollen and protruding from her mouth. The patient has only minimal air movement with bag-mask ventilation. Oxygen saturation is approximately 80%. Attempts at oral intubation are unsuccessful due to massive soft tissue edema of her pharynx. A decision is made to perform a cricothyrotomy. The necessary instrument tray is collected, and the patient's neck is quickly prepped. After palpating the neck to identify the appropriate landmarks, an incision should be made at which of the following locations?

    (A) The cricothyroid membrane, which is located at the junction of the clavicle and the sternum

    (B) The cricothyroid membrane, which is located between the thyroid cartilage and the cricoid cartilage below

    (C) The thyrohyoid membrane, which is located between the thyroid cartilage (Adam's apple) and the hyoid bone above

    (D) The sternal notch, which is located at the junction of the clavicle and the sternum

    (E) The trachea, which is located below the cricoid cartilage

41. An infant born to an alcoholic mother had microcephaly and cardiac abnormalities and died despite resuscitative efforts. During which of the following periods of pregnancy is alcohol most teratogenic?

    (A) First 2 weeks

    (B) Third through ninth weeks

    (C) Ninth through twelfth weeks

    (D) Twelfth through sixteenth weeks

    (E) Sixteenth through twentieth weeks

42. A 15-year-old girl with a history of chronic rhinitis, allergy, asthma, and nasal polyposis presents with fever and dental pain. She is diagnosed with maxillary sinusitis. Mucopurulent exudate would be most likely to drain through an ostium in the

    (A) bulla ethmoidalis

    (B) hiatus semilunaris

    (C) inferior nasal meatus

    (D) sphenoethmoidal recess

    (E) superior nasal meatus

43. A patient presents to the physician complaining of "something wrong with her foot" that causes her to trip and fall. Physical examination reveals an inability to dorsiflex (extend) the foot and a loss of sensation between the first and second toes. There is no other motor or sensory loss. Which of the following nerves was most likely injured?

    (A) Deep peroneal

    (B) Femoral

    (C) Superficial peroneal

    (D) Sural

    (E) Tibial

44. During a routine physical examination, a 71-year-old man is found to have a 7-cm pulsatile mass deep in the abdomen, between the xiphoid and the umbilicus. He has a history of untreated hypertension. The endothelial lining of the affected structure is composed of which of the following tissue types?

    (A) Pseudostratified epithelium

    (B) Simple columnar epithelium

    (C) Simple cuboidal epithelium

    (D) Simple squamous epithelium

    (E) Stratified columnar epithelium

    (F) Stratified cuboidal epithelium

    (G) Stratified squamous epithelium

45. One week following a sexual encounter at a ski resort in Colorado, a young woman develops a painful, swollen knee joint. The emergency department physician suspects gonococcal arthritis and wants to confirm this by sending joint fluid for bacterial culture. He uses the standard suprapatellar approach and passes a needle from the lateral aspect of the thigh into the region immediately proximal to the patella. Through which of the following muscles does the needle pass?

    (A) Adductor magnus

    (B) Gracilis

    (C) Iliacus

    (D) Sartorius

    (E) Vastus lateralis

46. A 67-year-old man has an abnormal neurologic exam. An electroencephalogram is subsequently performed and reveals delta waves over his left frontal lobe. Which of the following was the most likely abnormal finding on his neurologic exam?

    (A) Left hemiparesis
    (B) Left hemisensory loss
    (C) Left homonymous hemianopia
    (D) Right hemiparesis
    (E) Right hemisensory loss
    (F) Right homonymous hemianopia

47. A 23-year-old woman wearing high-heeled shoes inverts and sprains her ankle while running down a flight of stairs. Which of the following ligaments did she most likely injure?

    (A) Anterior talotibial
    (B) Calcaneofibular
    (C) Calcaneotibial
    (D) Deltoid
    (E) Medial collateral

48. A surgeon performing an appendectomy makes an incision through the ventrolateral abdominal wall. The layers of the abdominal wall are shown below.

    1. Internal oblique
    2. External oblique
    3. Peritoneum
    4. Transversus abdominis

    Which of the following corresponds to the order of penetration of the layers of the abdominal wall?

    (A) 1-3-4-2
    (B) 2-1-3-4
    (C) 2-1-4-3
    (D) 4-1-2-3
    (E) 4-2-1-3

49. A 49-year-old woman comes to the emergency department because of right upper quadrant pain, nausea, vomiting, and fever. She also complains of pain in her right shoulder. A right upper quadrant ultrasound reveals multiple gallstones and pericholecystic fluid. Which of the following dermatomes is most likely involved in her shoulder pain?

    (A) C1-C2
    (B) C3-C5
    (C) C6-C8
    (D) T1-T3
    (E) T4-T6

50. A 57-year-old man has hematuria and left-sided flank pain. Diagnostic studies show a left-sided renal mass with extension into the renal vein. A radical nephrectomy is performed, and the specimen is sent for pathologic evaluation. Which of the following structures present in this patient's specimen is lined with epithelium derived from mesoderm of the ureteric bud?

    (A) Bowman capsule
    (B) Distal convoluted tubule
    (C) Loop of Henle
    (D) Proximal convoluted tubule
    (E) Ureter

# Anatomy Test One: **Answers and Explanations**

## ANSWER KEY

| | | | |
|---|---|---|---|
| 1. | C | 26. | C |
| 2. | D | 27. | E |
| 3. | E | 28. | E |
| 4. | B | 29. | E |
| 5. | E | 30. | C |
| 6. | B | 31. | D |
| 7. | C | 32. | B |
| 8. | D | 33. | B |
| 9. | D | 34. | A |
| 10. | A | 35. | E |
| 11. | C | 36. | A |
| 12. | B | 37. | C |
| 13. | E | 38. | C |
| 14. | C | 39. | E |
| 15. | E | 40. | B |
| 16. | B | 41. | B |
| 17. | B | 42. | B |
| 18. | A | 43. | A |
| 19. | A | 44. | D |
| 20. | D | 45. | E |
| 21. | A | 46. | D |
| 22. | D | 47. | B |
| 23. | B | 48. | C |
| 24. | D | 49. | B |
| 25. | B | 50. | E |

1.  **The correct answer is C.** The bladder is supplied by the vesicular branches of the internal iliac arteries. The internal iliacs arise from the common iliac artery. Note that this is a simple fact question (Which artery supplies the urinary bladder?) embedded in a clinical scenario.

    The external iliac (**choice A**) also arises from the common iliac artery. It makes no contribution to the blood supply of the bladder.

    The inferior epigastric (**choice B**) is a branch of the external iliac artery. It serves as a landmark in the inguinal region. Indirect inguinal hernias lie lateral to the inferior epigastric arteries, whereas direct inguinal hernias lie medial to these vessels. A good mnemonic is MDs don't LIe. (Medial-Direct, Lateral-Indirect).

    The internal pudendal (**choice D**) is a branch of the anterior division of the internal iliac artery. It gives rise to the inferior rectal artery, perineal artery, artery of the bulb in men, urethral artery, deep artery of the penis or clitoris, and dorsal artery of the penis or clitoris.

    The lateral sacral (**choice E**) is a branch of the posterior division of the internal iliac artery. It supplies sacral structures.

2.  **The correct answer is D.** The right gastroepiploic artery, off the gastroduodenal artery, supplies the right half of the greater curvature of the stomach and could be directly affected by ulceration of the greater curvature of the stomach at a site this close (4 cm) to the pyloric sphincter.

    The left gastric artery (**choice A**), off the celiac trunk, supplies the left half of the lesser curvature of the stomach.

    The left gastroepiploic artery (**choice B**), off the splenic artery, supplies the left half of the greater curvature of the stomach. Although it anastomoses with the right gastroepiploic artery, it is unlikely that this artery would be directly damaged by ulceration of the stomach near the pyloric sphincter.

    The right gastric artery (**choice C**), off the proper hepatic artery, supplies the right half of the lesser curvature of the stomach.

    The short gastric artery (**choice E**), actually one of several (4-5) short gastric arteries, off the splenic artery (occasionally the left gastroepiploic), supplies the fundus of the stomach, which is most distant from the pylorus.

3.  **The correct answer is E.** The anterior pituitary produces prolactin. The structure originates from Rathke's pouch, which is itself a diverticulum of the roof of the stomodeum.

    The cerebral vesicle (**choice A**) lies close to Rathke's pouch.

    The infundibulum (**choice B**) comes in contact with Rathke's pouch at the fifth week of development.

    The neurohypophysis (**choice C**) gives rise to the posterior pituitary.

    The proctodeum (**choice D**) is also known as the anal pit.

4.  **The correct answer is B.** The visual field defect can be described as a right homonymous hemianopsia with macular sparing. Macular sparing is characteristic of lesions of the calcarine cortex. Because of the reorganization of optic nerve fibers that takes place in the optic chiasm, the visual pathways and visual cortex on one side of the brain carry information from the contralateral visual field. Because the patient had a defect of the right half of the visual field, the lesion must be in the *left* hemisphere. The posterior cerebral artery (PCA) is the vessel that supplies blood to the occipital lobe. Consequently, the ischemic lesion in this patient must involve the left PCA, not the right (**choice D**).

    The middle cerebral artery (**choices A and C**) is the largest cerebral artery and supplies blood to most of the lateral surface of the hemisphere. However, it does not extend to the visual cortex.

    The posterior communicating artery (**choice E**) is part of the circle of Willis and does not supply the cerebral cortex.

5.  **The correct answer is E.** This is the classic presentation of a psoas abscess. This clinical entity was formerly a fairly common complication of vertebral tuberculosis, but is now rare in clinical practice in this country. The psoas muscle is covered by a fibrous sheath known as the psoas fascia. This sheath is open superiorly, permitting an infection involving the soft tissues around the spine to enter the sheath, then track down to the groin.

    The adductor longus (**choice A**) is a muscle of the medial thigh and is not related to the lumbar portion of the back.

    The gluteus maximus (**choice B**), gluteus minimus (**choice C**), and piriformis (**choice D**) are muscles of the buttock with no relationship to the groin.

6.  **The correct answer is B.** A hemisection of the cord produces Brown-Sequard syndrome. Below the level of the lesion there is ipsilateral hemiparesis, ipsilateral loss of discriminatory touch sensation, and contralateral loss of pain and temperature sensation. A hemisection of the left half of the spinal cord will transect the fibers of the corticospinal tract on the left side, resulting in left-sided motor paralysis. (These motor fibers originate in the contralateral cortex, decussate in the medulla, and descend in the lateral funiculus of the spinal cord.) The hemisection will also transect the ascending fibers of the dorsal column pathway that carry sensory information concerning discriminatory touch, vibration, and joint position from the same side. (This tract will subsequently cross in the medulla and end in the contralateral cerebral cortex.) In contrast, the fibers carrying information about pain and temperature decussate segmentally in the spinal cord and form the spinothalamic tract, which ascends in the lateral funiculus. Damaging the spinothalamic tract on the left side impairs sensation arising from the right side of the body.

    A complete transection of the spinal cord (**choice A**) will cause loss of sensation and motor function bilaterally below the transection.

    Transection of the dorsal columns on the left side (**choice C**) will interfere only with fine touch, vibration, and joint position sense. A lesion of the lateral funiculus (**choice D**) will produce deficits in motor function and in pain and temperature sensation but not in discriminatory touch.

    Lesions of the cervical dorsal roots on the left side (**choice E**) will produce anesthesia to discriminatory touch, as well as pain and temperature on the left side. Only the dermatomal areas supplied by those roots will be affected. Such lesions will not produce hemiparesis because motor fibers exit the spinal cord in the ventral roots.

7.  **The correct answer is C.** This child has a Meckel diverticulum, an ileal outpocketing typically located within 50 to 75 cm of the ileocecal valve. It is a congenital anomaly resulting from the persistence of the vitelline (omphalomesenteric) duct. Approximately half cause ulceration, inflammation, and gastrointestinal bleeding because of the presence of ectopic acid-secreting gastric epithelium. Pancreatic tissue may sometimes occur in these diverticula as well. Note that this is the most common type of congenital gastrointestinal anomaly.

    Something else to keep in mind: A favorite question attendings ask on the wards is the rule of 2s associated with Meckel diverticulum: it occurs in about 2% of children, occurs within approximately 2 feet of the ileocecal valve, contains 2 types of ectopic mucosa (gastric and pancreatic), and its symptoms usually occur by age 2.

    None of the other answer choices has a relationship to Meckel diverticulum.

8.  **The correct answer is D.** The serratus anterior plays a major role in holding the scapula against the body wall. If paralyzed, the primary clinical sign is "winging" of the scapula, especially when raising the arm or pushing the body away from a wall. In addition, it aids in rotation of the scapula, raising the glenoid cavity when the arm is abducted beyond the horizontal. The serratus anterior is innervated by the long thoracic nerve, which runs very superficially on the superolateral thoracic wall, where it is especially prone to injury.

    The levator scapulae (**choice A**) elevates the scapula. It is not involved in holding the scapula against the body wall. Its innervation, derived from the cervical plexus (C3, C4), is not damaged by injury to the superolateral thoracic wall.

    Although the pectoralis minor (**choice B**) has a scapular attachment (to the coracoid process), it is not involved in holding the scapula against the body wall. Its innervation, the medial pectoral nerve, is not likely to be damaged by injury to the superolateral thoracic wall.

    The rhomboid major (**choice C**) primarily retracts the scapula. It does not have an important role in holding the scapula against the body wall. Its innervation, the dorsal scapular nerve, is not easily damaged by injury to the superolateral thoracic wall.

    Although the supraspinatus (**choice E**) plays a role in arm abduction, it is essential to the initiation of this movement (the first 20-30 degrees) before there is significant rotation of the scapula. It is not involved in holding the scapula against the body wall (although it is important in holding the head of the humerus against the glenoid fossa). Its innervation, the suprascapular nerve, would not be damaged by injury to the superolateral thoracic wall.

9.  **The correct answer is D.** During the growth of the primary follicle, there is a proliferation of follicular cells, an increase in the size of the oocyte, and formation of a connective tissue capsule around the follicle by the follicular cells. Soon thereafter, small spaces begin to appear in the follicular mass. These spaces fuse to form the follicular cavity, or antrum. Once the antrum develops, the follicle is termed a secondary follicle.

    The Graafian follicle (**choice A**) is the mature follicle that extends through the entire cortex and bulges out at the ovarian surface.

    The primary follicles (**choice B**) are relatively small and spherical, with a central oocyte and one or more layers of cuboidal-like follicular cells.

The primary oocytes, which are arrested in prophase of their first meiotic division, are contained within the primordial follicles (**choice C**) as inactive reserve follicles.

Recall the sequence of oogenesis:

Primordial follicle (contain primary oocytes) → Primary follicle → Secondary follicle → Graafian follicle

10. **The correct answer is A.** The esophageal venous plexus, which drains into the azygos and hemiazygos veins within the thorax, has anastomoses with branches of the left gastric vein. Thus, following blockage of the portal vein, portal blood may enter the superior vena cava via the azygos system. Other important portacaval connections include the superior rectal vein with the middle and inferior rectal veins; paraumbilical veins with epigastric veins (engorgement of these vessels results in *caput medusae*); and the colic and splenic veins with renal veins and veins of the posterior body wall.

The gonadal veins (**choice B**) exclusively drain the gonads (although in the female, the ovarian vein communicates with the uterovaginal plexus). These vessels have no anastomoses with portal vessels.

The external iliac veins (**choice C**), which drain much of the inferior extremities, have no demonstrated portal anastomoses.

The splenic vein (**choice D**) is incorrect because it is itself a component of the portal venous system.

The vesical venous plexus (**choice E**), which is situated well within the pelvis and drains the bladder and the prostate (or uterus and vagina), has no association with portal vessels.

11. **The correct answer is C.** The patient has a cerebellar lesion. Cerebellar dysfunction can lead to a variety of motor dysfunctions, including truncal ataxia (appearing similar to the gait of an intoxicated individual), intention tremor (uncontrolled shaking of affected extremity present only with purposeful movement), dysdiadochokinesia (the inability to perform rapid and regular alternating movements), dysmetria (inability to stop movements at the desired point), dysarthria (ataxic speech), hypotonia, and nystagmus.

During the fourth week of embryonic development, the anterior end of the neural tube develops three vesicles: the prosencephalon (forebrain), the mesencephalon (midbrain), and the rhombencephalon (hindbrain). By the sixth week, 5 vesicles (listed in the answer options) have developed. The rhombencephalon has now developed into the metencephalon and myelencephalon. The cerebellum and pons derive from the metencephalon.

The diencephalon (**choice A**), which is derived from the prosencephalon, develops into the thalamus, hypothalamus, epithalamus, subthalamus (everything with the word "thalamus"), posterior lobe of the pituitary, and neural retina.

The mesencephalon (**choice B**), or midbrain, is the only brain vesicle that does not produce a secondary vesicle; it remains the mesencephalon.

The myelencephalon (**choice D**), which is derived from the rhombencephalon, develops into the medulla oblongata.

The telencephalon (**choice E**), which is derived from the prosencephalon, develops into the cerebral hemispheres (cerebral cortex, basal ganglia, and deep white matter).

12. **The correct answer is B.** Solid knowledge of cardiac anatomy and its clinical correlations are crucial for performing physical examinations (and answering USMLE questions). This question tests two facts. First it requires that you recognize the patient has mitral stenosis. Classic clues to this diagnosis are "low-pitched, rumbling, diastolic murmur," "opening snap," and "rheumatic fever." The mitral valve is the most commonly affected valve in rheumatic fever, followed by the aortic and tricuspid valves. The question then asks you where sounds generated by a faulty mitral valve will be best heard on physical exam. The mitral valve is most audible over the left fifth intercostal space at the midclavicular line.

The pulmonary valve is most audible over the left second intercostal space (**choice A**). Pulmonic stenosis is associated with tetralogy of Fallot, a common cyanotic congenital heart disease.

The tricuspid valve is most audible over the left lower sternal border (**choice C**). This valve is primarily affected in IV drug abusers with endocarditis.

The aortic valve is most audible over the right second intercostal space (**choice D**). Aortic stenosis is associated with angina, syncope, and congestive heart failure. A systolic murmur that radiates to the carotids is heard on exam, along with a systolic ejection click.

No particular structure is best heard over the right fifth intercostal space (**choice E**).

13. **The correct answer is E.** The optic cups derive from the optic vesicles, which are evaginations of the diencephalon. The anterior two layers of the optic cup (neurectoderm), in association with choroidal mesoderm, give rise to the ciliary body and the iris. The optic cup also gives rise to the neural and pigment layers of the retina.

Retinal ganglion cell axons (**choice A**), which run in the optic stalk, become the nerve fibers of the optic nerve.

Closure of the choroid fissure in the optic stalk (**choice B**) occurs during the seventh week of development. The former optic stalk is then called the optic nerve.

Mesoderm surrounding the optic cup (**choice C**) becomes the sclera and choroid of the eye.

Mesoderm surrounding the optic stalk (**choice D**) gives rise to the meninges surrounding the optic nerve.

14. **The correct answer is C.** The locus caeruleus is a dense collection of neuromelanin-containing cells in the rostral pons, near the lateral edge of the floor of the fourth ventricle. The fact that it appears blue-black in unstained brain tissue gave rise to its name, which means "blue spot" in Latin. These cells, which contain norepinephrine, provide the majority of noradrenergic innervation to the forebrain, including the cerebral cortex.

The basal nucleus of Meynert (**choice A**), a part of the substantia innominata, is a major collection of forebrain cholinergic neurons. These neurons (together with neurons in septal nuclei) innervate the neocortex, hippocampal formation, and the amygdala. The basal nucleus is one of the structures that degenerates in Alzheimer disease.

The caudate nucleus (**choice B**) is part of the basal ganglia, located immediately lateral to the lateral ventricles. There are at least two important cell types in the caudate. GABAergic projection neurons (the majority) innervate the globus pallidus and substantia nigra pars reticulata. The GABAergic neurons degenerate in Huntington disease, leading to enlarged lateral ventricles that are clearly visible on MRI. The caudate also contains cholinergic interneurons, which provide most of the acetylcholine to the striatum (caudate and putamen). The balance of striatal acetylcholine and dopamine is important for the treatment of patients with extrapyramidal symptoms, such as Parkinson disease or parkinsonism accompanying therapy with antipsychotic medications.

The raphe nuclei (**choice D**) are located in the midline at most levels of the brainstem. They contain serotonergic cell bodies that innervate virtually every part of the CNS.

The substantia nigra (**choice E**) is located in the midbrain and consists of the substantia nigra pars compacta and the substantia nigra pars reticulata. The substantia nigra pars compacta contains the nigrostriatal neurons that are the source of striatal dopamine. This cell group degenerates in Parkinson disease or in response to neurotoxic agents such as MPTP. The substantia nigra pars reticulata consists predominately of GABAergic neurons that innervate the thalamus.

The ventral tegmental area (**choice F**) is located in the midbrain and is an important source of dopamine for the limbic and cortical areas. These cells are called mesolimbic and mesocortical neurons. Overactivity of this cell group is a popular theory of the etiology of schizophrenia and is the basis for the administration of antipsychotic agents (dopamine receptor antagonists).

15. **The correct answer is E.** The surgeon has asked the medical student to test for tetany, which can occur if the blood supply to the parathyroid glands (through the superior and inferior thyroid arteries) is disrupted during thyroid surgery. Specifically, the medical student is being asked to tap with his fingers the muscles of mastication, notably the masseter, which because of its strength is a sensitive indicator of tetany. Tetany will be seen as an abnormally strong jerk or contraction related to the hypocalcemia that can develop if secretion of parathyroid hormone is inadequate.

16. **The correct answer is B.** The hepatic artery is one component of the portal triad: the hepatic artery, common bile duct, and portal vein. These structures constitute the porta hepatis and lie in the free edge of the lesser omentum as it forms the epiploic foramen. Opening the epiploic foramen would therefore involve cutting the porta hepatis and, possibly, the hepatic artery and/or other components of the portal triad.

The abdominal aorta (**choice A**) is retroperitoneal, posterior to the omental bursa. It is not associated with the epiploic foramen and would not likely be damaged by surgery to open the foramen.

The hepatic vein (**choice C**) returns blood from the liver to the inferior vena cava and is not associated with the epiploic foramen. In contrast, the portal vein, part of the portal triad, brings venous blood to the liver.

The hypogastric plexus (**choice D**) is a plexus of autonomic nerves found in the superior pelvis and the posterior abdominal wall in the inferior abdomen. This plexus is not close to the epiploic foramen, so it is unlikely to be injured by surgery in that region.

The pancreatic duct (**choice E**) is not a boundary of the epiploic foramen.

17. **The correct answer is B.** The serratus anterior, innervated by the long thoracic nerve, is responsible for stabilization of the scapula during abduction of the arm from 90 to 180 degrees. When the long thoracic nerve is damaged, it is difficult to elevate the arm above the horizontal. This nerve arises from C5, C6, and C7. Remember: a "winged scapula" is a classic clue for long thoracic nerve injury.

Note that the supraspinatus muscle, innervated by the suprascapular nerve (**choice D**), is responsible for abducting the arm from 0 degrees to about 30 degrees. The rest of the motion to 180 degrees is performed by the deltoid muscle, which is innervated by the axillary nerve (**choice A**). However, the motion from 90 to 180 degrees also requires a stable scapula and therefore depends on the long thoracic nerve.

The axillary nerve (**choice A**) is a branch of the posterior cord of the brachial plexus (C5, C6). It is particularly susceptible to injury in shoulder dislocations that displace the humeral head or in fracture of the surgical neck of the humerus. A poorly placed crutch may also damage this nerve, causing paralysis of the teres minor and deltoid muscles. Arm abduction is impaired, and there is associated loss of sensation over the lower half of the deltoid.

The lower subscapular nerve (**choice C**) innervates the teres major, which is responsible for adducting and medially rotating the arm. It is a branch of the posterior cord (C5, C6) of the brachial plexus.

The suprascapular nerve (**choice D**) innervates the supraspinatus and infraspinatus muscles, which are responsible for abduction and lateral rotation of the arm. The nerve is derived from the C5 and C6 nerve roots.

The thoracodorsal nerve (**choice E**) innervates the latissimus dorsi muscle, which is responsible for adduction and extension of the arm. The nerve arises from the posterior cord (C5, C6, C7) of the brachial plexus.

18. **The correct answer is A.** Any perforating wound occurring below the level of the fourth intercostal space on the right side may damage the liver, which is protected by the rib cage, although it is an abdominal organ lying inferior to the diaphragm.

At its most lateral aspect, the right atrium (**choice B**) forms the right border of the heart, which extends from the third costal cartilage to the sixth costal cartilage just to the right of the sternum.

The right pulmonary artery (**choice C**) enters the hilus of the lung at the level of the T5 vertebra. Since the ribs are angled downward as they pass forward, this entry occurs above the level of the fifth intercostal space at the midaxillary line.

The superior vena cava (**choice D**) enters the right atrium at the level of the third costal cartilage.

At the midaxillary line, the oblique fissure of the right lung (**choice E**) passes between the inferior and middle lobes.

19. **The correct answer is A.** After fertilization, the fertilized ovum begins to divide as it migrates through the uterine tube. It reaches the blastocyst stage (approximately 110 cells) at about day 5, and it enters the uterus at about day 6. Implantation normally begins on day 6 with the syncytiotrophoblast of the embryonic pole of the blastocyst eroding into the endometrium.

After fertilization, cleavage divisions of the zygote begin. These are mitotic divisions that result in an increase in the number of cells but not an increase in the total cytoplasmic mass. The zygote divides into the two-cell embryo, and these cells then divide to form the four-cell embryo (**choice B**). The embryo is still in the upper end of the uterine tube at this stage of development, and it is surrounded by the zona pellucida, which prevents it from implanting.

Cleavage divisions continue to eventually result in a solid ball of cells called the morula (**choice C**) at about day 4. The morula is still in the uterine tube but is close to entering the uterus. It is still surrounded by the zona pellucida.

The trilaminar embryo (**choice D**) is formed during the third week. This results from gastrulation, the process of cells from the epiblast migrating though the primitive streak to form the mesoderm and notochord. This occurs well after implantation has occurred.

The zygote (**choice E**) is the single-cell embryo that is created at fertilization after the union of the male and female pronucleus. This is considered day 1 of development and typically occurs in the ampulla of the uterine tube.

20. **The correct answer is D.** The urethral folds in the female do not fuse, and they develop into the labia minora. The space between the folds becomes the vestibule of the vagina. In the male, the urethral folds normally fuse to become the ventral surface of the penis. A failure of these folds to fuse normally in the male results in hypospadia, the presence of openings of the urethra along the ventral surface of the penis.

The round ligaments of the uterus (**choice A**) are the adult remnants in the female of the caudal portions of the caudal genital ligaments. In the male, these structures become the caudal portions of the gubernaculum testis. The gubernaculum testis attaches the testis to the wall of the scrotum. The round ligaments of the uterus in the female attach the uterus to the fascia of the labia majora. The round ligaments pass through the inguinal canals in the female.

The crura of the clitoris (**choice B**) are erectile bodies that fuse together to form the clitoris. In the male, the same structures are the crura of the penis, which are erectile bodies that are continuous with the corpora cavernosa of the penis. The penis and the clitoris develop from the genital tubercle.

The labia majora (**choice C**) in the female develop from the genital swellings (or labioscrotal folds) of the embryo. In the male, the same structures fuse in the midline to develop into the scrotum.

The ovarian ligaments (**choice E**) in the female develop from the rostral portion of the caudal genital ligament. The ovarian ligament connects the ovary to the uterus. In the male, the same structure forms the rostral portion of the gubernaculum testis. Thus, in the male the caudal genital ligament becomes one structure, the gubernaculum testis. In the female, this ligament becomes two structures: the ovarian ligament and the round ligament of the uterus.

21. **The correct answer is A.** The common peroneal nerve wraps around the lateral aspect of the head of the fibula and is highly susceptible to damage during lacerations or blunt injuries to the lateral knee. Foot-drop with loss of dorsiflexion or eversion is characteristic.

Only the peroneus longus completely attaches to the fibular head (**choice B**). Other muscles that attach in other places along the tibia and fibula provide dorsiflexion and eversion for the foot (e.g., extensor digitorum longus, peroneus brevis, extensor hallucis longus, and tibialis anterior).

The common peroneal nerve then branches into the superficial (**choice C**) and deep peroneal nerves, which supply the muscles of the anterior compartment of the leg and cutaneous areas of the distal anterior leg, dorsum of the foot, and most of the digits.

The tibial nerve (**choice D**) supplies all the muscles in the posterior compartment of the leg (e.g., tibialis posterior, flexor digitorum longus, gastrocnemius, and soleus).

22. **The correct answer is D.** The resident is feeling the two pubic bones, which are joined at the midline by the symphysis pubis. Experienced obstetrician/gynecologists can often perceive the softening of the symphysis pubis that occurs during late pregnancy as a "springiness" of the pubic bones during palpation.

The coccyx (**choice A**) is the caudal terminus of the vertebral column, generally formed by the fusion of four rudimentary vertebral bodies. It is also called the tailbone.

The ilium (**choice B**) is one of the two "wings" that form the lateral sides of the pelvic cavity and support the abdominal contents.

The ischium (**choice C**) is the portion of the pelvis on which a person sits.

The sacrum (**choice E**) is the triangular bone situated just beneath the lumbar vertebrae.

23. **The correct answer is B.** In some patients with coronary artery disease, thallium stress tests may be performed instead of cardiac catheterization to determine the vessels involved and the extent of occlusion. The left circumflex (LCx) branch supplies the lateral wall of the left ventricle; in 10% of the population, it also supplies the posterior wall and AV node.

The left anterior descending (LAD) branch of the left coronary artery (**choice A**) supplies the anterior wall of the left ventricle and the anterior portion of the interventricular septum.

The left main coronary artery (**choice C**) gives rise to both the LCx and the LAD.

The right coronary artery (RCA; **choice D**) supplies the right ventricle; in 90% of the population, it supplies the AV node and posterior and inferior walls of the left ventricle.

24. **The correct answer is D.** The pupillary dilator muscle is innervated by the sympathetic nervous system. Preganglionic fibers originating at spinal cord levels T1 through T5 ascend to the superior cervical ganglion, from which postganglionic fibers travel to the eye. Mueller's muscle in the upper eyelid is also innervated by sympathetic fibers originating in the upper thoracic spinal cord. Disruption of the sympathetic supply to the eye, as has apparently occurred in this patient, causes ptosis and miosis due to unopposed action of the pupillary constrictor muscle. Interruption of sympathetic supply to the eye is known as Horner syndrome.

The abducens nerve (CN VI; **choice A**) does not innervate the muscles of the pupil or eyelid. It innervates the lateral rectus muscle, and a lesion would result in medial deviation of the eye.

The oculomotor nerve (**choice C**) contains parasympathetic fibers that innervate the pupillary constrictor fibers. Lesion of this nerve, or of its origin in oculomotor complex of the midbrain (**choice B**), results in mydriasis because action of the pupillary dilator muscle is unopposed.

Myasthenia gravis (**choice E**) is an autoimmune disease in which antibodies attack acetylcholine receptors at the neuromuscular junction, producing skeletal muscle fatigability. The ptosis that is observed in this disease is bilateral and accompanied by weakness of other parts of the locomotor system.

25. **The correct answer is B.** The tracheoesophageal ridges are two longitudinal ridges that separate the respiratory diverticulum from the foregut. Eventually, they fuse to form a septum separating the esophagus (dorsal) from the trachea (ventral) and lung buds, maintaining

a communication only rostrally at the pharynx. Incomplete formation of the tracheoesophageal septum (by fusion of ridges) results in the most common type of tracheoesophageal fistula, whereby the proximal part of the esophagus ends as a blind sac (esophageal atresia), while the distal part is connected to the trachea by a narrow canal just above the bifurcation. This defect occurs in approximately 1 in 2500 births.

The buccopharyngeal membrane is a bilaminar membrane (ectoderm externally, endoderm internally) separating the stomodeum (mouth) from the pharynx. The membrane ruptures at about 4 weeks. The buccopharyngeal membrane is not involved in formation of the esophagus and trachea; therefore, failure to rupture (**choice A**) would not lead to tracheoesophageal fistula.

The septum secundum is a membrane that forms on the right side of the developing interatrial wall of the heart. It is not associated with formation of the esophagus and trachea; therefore, failure to close would not lead to tracheoesophageal fistula. Failure of formation of the septum secundum (**choice C**) leads to a patent foramen ovale, a relatively common atrial septal defect.

Incomplete recanalization of the larynx (**choice D**) is relatively rare and results in a membrane (laryngeal web) that may partially obstruct the airway. Though there may be difficulty breathing, there should be little problem with swallowing and keeping milk down.

The thyroid gland forms from a primordium associated with development of the tongue that eventually descends into the neck. For a short time, it remains connected to the tongue by a narrow canal called the thyroglossal duct. Although the duct normally closes, it occasionally remains patent (**choice E**) or develops cysts, which are usually asymptomatic unless they become infected. They do not interfere with breathing or feeding and do not involve the trachea or esophagus.

26. **The correct answer is C.** This question allows us to review the sensory innervation of the perineum and vicinity. The ilioinguinal nerve supplies the skin of the scrotum and the medial thigh with sensory fibers.

    The genitofemoral nerve (**choice A**) supplies motor fibers to the cremaster muscle and a small area of skin on the thigh, giving rise to the cremasteric reflex.

    The iliohypogastric nerve (**choice B**) supplies the skin of the anterior lower abdominal wall.

    The lateral cutaneous nerve (**choice D**) of the thigh supplies the skin over the lateral surface of the thigh.

    The pudendal nerve (**choice E**) gives off branches that supply the external anal sphincter, the lower half of the anal canal, perianal skin, and skin on the posterior surface of the scrotum.

27. **The correct answer is E.** The condition described is spina bifida with myelomeningocele. A failure of the posteriorly located vertebral arches to fuse posteriorly causes spina bifida, which can vary in severity from a completely asymptomatic minor abnormality to protrusion of the spinal cord and roots through an open skin defect, with a very real risk of minor trauma or infection causing paralysis.

    The bodies of the vertebrae (**choice A**) are the stacking ovoid structures on the anterior aspect of the spinal canal.

    The pedicles (**choice B**) attach the bony ring that surrounds the spinal canal to the body of the vertebrae.

    Failure of development of one of the paired primary ossification centers (**choice C**) of the body can produce very severe scoliosis.

    The superior articular process (**choice D**) articulates with the inferior articular facet of the vertebra above it.

28. **The correct answer is E.** The sixth cervical vertebra is a critical boundary of the root of the neck. To enter the neck from the chest, the vascular structures pass through a ringlike opening bounded by the scalene muscles laterally, the sternum and first ribs anteriorly, and the vertebrae (notably C6).

29. **The correct answer is E.** The ureteric bud forms the ureter, renal pelvis, major and minor calyces, and collecting tubules of the kidney. The ureteric bud is an outgrowth of the mesonephric duct that grows toward the metanephric blastema and induces the metanephric blastema to develop into the nephrons of the kidney. The caudal end of the mesonephric duct becomes incorporated into the trigone of the urinary bladder. Thus, the ureteric bud drains urine from the filtration portion of the kidney into the bladder.

    The allantoic duct (**choice A**) is an endodermally lined vestigial structure that extends from the caudal portion of the gut tube into the umbilical cord. In lower vertebrates, the allantois carries excretions from the embryo; in humans, it does not function. It normally becomes the urachus, a fibrous cord that extends from the bladder into the umbilical cord. If it remains patent, it results in a urachal fistula that allows urine to drain from the bladder through the umbilicus.

    The metanephric blastema (**choice B**) is the caudal portion of the urogenital ridge that becomes the metanephros after the more rostral mesonephros ceases functioning as a kidney. The metanephric blastema is induced to become the metanephros by the ingrowth of the ureteric bud. The metanephric blastema forms the filtration portion of the kidney, i.e., the glomeruli and the nephrons.

The mesonephric duct (**choice C**) initially serves as the drainage duct for the mesonephros, the embryonic kidney. The mesonephros functions as a kidney during the second month of development. While the mesonephros functions as a kidney, the mesonephric duct drains urine into the cloaca, the caudal portion of the gut tube. Subsequently, the mesonephric duct becomes adapted to form the ductus deferens in the male, and it degenerates in the female.

The mesonephric tubules (**choice D**) carry urine from the mesonephros into the mesonephric duct while the mesonephros functions as a kidney. Subsequently, the mesonephric tubules become the efferent ductules of the testis in the male and carry spermatozoa from the seminiferous tubules of the testis to the epididymis. In the female, most of the mesonephric tubules degenerate. Those few that remain contribute to the vestigial epoophoron that may be found in the broad ligament.

30. **The correct answer is C.** Knowledge of the motor homunculus of the precentral gyrus (primary motor cortex) is necessary to answer this question. The parts of the cortex that control the legs are buried within the interhemispheric fissure. Paraplegia indicates weakness of both legs.

Ataxia (**choice A**) is clumsiness or incoordination that is not caused by weakness or sensory loss. It is most commonly caused by a lesion of the cerebellum or of the dentatorubrothalamic tract.

Hemiplegia (**choice B**) is weakness of an arm and leg. This could be caused by a very large lesion on one-half of the motor strip. It would include the cortex inside the interhemispheric fissure (controlling the legs) and the area of cortex present on the medial and superior aspect of the motor strip (controlling the arms).

Quadriplegia (**choice D**) is weakness of all four extremities. If the lesion were present in the motor strip, it would have to extend from the interhemispheric portion of both motor strips to the medial and superior aspects of both motor strips.

Rigidity (**choice E**) is hypertonia that is uniform throughout passive movement. This type of dysfunction is caused by lesions of the basal ganglia, most commonly the nigrostriatal dopaminergic pathway.

31. **The correct answer is D.** Brunner's glands are located in the submucosa of the duodenum. These glands are connected to the intestinal lumen by ducts that open into certain crypts. They secrete an alkaline product that protects the duodenal mucosa from the acidic chyme and helps achieve optimal pH for pancreatic enzymes.

Note that if you did not recall the location of Brunner's glands, the question's description of their function allowed you to deduce it, on the basis of your knowledge of the anatomy of the small intestine. You should have immediately ruled out **choices C and E** because they are too far from the pancreas. **Choices B and D** would therefore remain as the best possible answers because of their proximity to the pancreas. If you remembered the structure and function of the ampulla of Vater, you were left with the correct answer.

Let's review some other key features of intestinal histology by way of the wrong answer choices.

The small intestinal villi (**choice A**) are outgrowths of the mucosa into the lumen. Their epithelium contains columnar absorptive cells and goblet cells (which produce acid glycoproteins that protect and lubricate the lining of the intestine). Near the base of each villus are tubular glands called crypts, whose lining is continuous with the simple columnar epithelium of the villus. The crypts include Paneth cells, which produce acidophilic cytoplasmic granules containing bactericidal enzymes. The lamina propria of the small intestine penetrates the core of the villi and is composed of blood vessels, lymphatics, fibroblasts, and smooth muscle cells.

The ampulla of Vater (**choice B**) receives bile from the common bile duct and the main pancreatic duct, delivering it to the duodenum through the major duodenal papilla.

The mucosa and submucosa of the jejunum (**choice C**) are both included in the permanent folds called the plica circulares.

The submucosa of the ileum (**choice E**) is the home of Peyer's patches, which are large aggregates of lymphoid nodules.

32. **The correct answer is B.** The lunate is in the proximal row and articulates with the scaphoid laterally (this being the most lateral of the proximal row). The lunate is the most commonly dislocated carpal bone. It is usually displaced anteriorly by rotation on its proximal, convex surface (where it articulates with the radius). The displaced bone may compress the median nerve in the carpal tunnel, leading to pain, sensory loss, and/or paralysis.

The capitate (**choice A**) is a carpal bone in the distal row. It articulates with the hamate (the most medial of this row).

The scaphoid (**choice C**), the most commonly fractured carpal bone, is the most lateral bone of the proximal row. Patients with scaphoid fractures have an increased risk for avascular necrosis.

The trapezoid (**choice D**) is a carpal bone of the distal row and articulates with the most lateral of this row (trapezium).

The triquetrum (**choice E**), although in the proximal row of carpal bones, is the most medial carpal bone of the proximal row.

33. **The correct answer is B.** You should know the boundaries of the femoral triangle: the inguinal ligament above, the medial border of the sartorius laterally, and the medial border of the adductor longus on the inner aspect of the thigh.

    The gracilis muscle (**choices A, C, and D**) runs roughly parallel to the adductor longus but is not usually considered part of the triangle.

    The pectineus muscle (**choices C and E**) is found on the floor of the femoral triangle.

34. **The correct answer is A.** The clinical history suggests trigeminal neuralgia, which is characterized by extreme pain along the distributions of the maxillary and mandibular subdivisions of the fifth cranial nerve. The trigeminal nerve innervates the first branchial arch.

    The second branchial arch (**choice B**) gives rise to the muscles of facial expression and is innervated by the facial nerve, cranial nerve VII.

    The third branchial arch (**choice C**) is innervated by the ninth cranial nerve, the glossopharyngeal, which innervates the stylopharyngeus muscle.

    The fourth branchial arch (**choice D**) gives rise to most pharyngeal constrictor muscles and is innervated by the tenth cranial nerve, the vagus nerve.

35. **The correct answer is E.** The ventral mesentery forms the falciform ligament and lesser omentum, which can be divided into the hepatogastric and hepatoduodenal ligament.

    The dorsal mesoduodenum (**choice A**) is the mesentery of the developing duodenum, which later disappears so that the duodenum and pancreas lie retroperitoneally.

    The greater omentum is derived from the dorsal mesogastrium (**choice B**), which is the mesentery of the stomach region.

    The pericardioperitoneal canal (**choice C**) embryologically connects the thoracic and peritoneal cavities.

    The pleuropericardial membranes (**choice D**) become the pericardium and contribute to the diaphragm.

36. **The correct answer is A.** Atrial septal defect is a noncyanotic defect. This defect will result in postnatal shunting of blood from the left to the right atrium. Because the left atrium contains oxygenated blood, this shunt results in oxygenated blood being sent back to the pulmonary circuit. Cyanosis is the result of deoxygenated blood being sent to the systemic circuit. Heart defects that result in postnatal shunts from right to left are cyanotic defects because deoxygenated blood on the right side of the heart is shunted to the left side of the heart, which sends blood into the systemic circulation.

    A postnatal shunt from the left atrium to the right atrium (**choice B**) is noncyanotic because oxygenated blood is shunting to the pulmonary circuit.

    An atrial septal defect does not typically result in postnatal shunting of blood from the right atrium to the left atrium (**choice C**) because the pressure is higher on the left than on the right and the shunt of blood follows the pressure gradient. Thus, a postnatal atrial septal defect usually results in a left-to-right shunt.

    Prenatally, there is normally a shunt from the right atrium to the left atrium (**choice D**) that occurs through the foramen ovale. Prenatally, the right atrium receives oxygenated blood through the inferior vena cava, which receives venous return from the placenta through the umbilical vein. The placenta is the source of oxygenated blood in the fetus. Thus, the normal right-to-left shunt that occurs prenatally is shunting oxygenated blood into the systemic circulation.

    Prenatally, the shunts through an atrial septal defect—whether the normal shunt through the foramen oval or an abnormal shunt through an atrial septal defect—will be a right-to-left shunt, not a left-to-right shunt (**choice E**) because the pressure is higher on the right than on the left due to the large volume of blood entering the right atrium from the entire embryo plus the placenta and the small volume of blood entering the left atrium from the lungs. Most of the pulmonary circuit is bypassed through the ductus arteriosus because of the high vascular resistance in the prenatal lungs.

37. **The correct answer is C.** Thyroglossal duct cysts are derived from the remnant of the thyroglossal duct. The thyroglossal duct extends from the foramen cecum of the tongue base to the thyroid gland during the embryologic development of the thyroid gland, and it typically degenerates completely. If a portion of the duct remains, it can develop into a cyst and enlarge, presenting as a midline neck mass. The pathognomonic finding of a thyroglossal duct is elevation during protrusion of the tongue, which is true in this case.

    **Choice A** (reactive lymph node), **choice B** (branchial cleft cyst), **and choice D** (head and neck neoplasm) would all typically present as lateral neck masses. **Choice E** (thyroid nodule) would most likely be in the usual location of the thyroid gland, which would be far below the thyroid cartilage and just above the sternal notch. Therefore, choices A, B, D, and E are not correct.

38. **The correct answer is C.** The lingual nerve is a branch of the mandibular division of the trigeminal nerve that conveys general sensation from the anterior two-thirds of the tongue. It enters the oral cavity by passing just under the mandibular third molar between the medial pterygoid muscle and the mandibular ramus.

    The auriculotemporal nerve (**choice A**) is a branch of V3 that passes from the infratemporal fossa to the parotid region. It contains sensory fibers from the region in front of the ear and the temporomandibular joint, and also conveys postganglionic parasympathetic fibers to the parotid salivary gland.

    The chorda tympani (**choice B**) is a branch of CN VII that travels with the lingual nerve in the floor of the mouth. It carries taste fibers from the anterior two-thirds of the tongue and preganglionic parasympathetic fibers that synapse in the submandibular ganglion.

    The mental nerve (**choice D**) is a sensory branch of the inferior alveolar nerve that supplies the skin of the chin and lower lip.

    The mylohyoid nerve (**choice E**) is a motor branch of the inferior alveolar nerve that supplies the mylohyoid and anterior belly of the digastric muscles.

39. **The correct answer is E.** The palpable space immediately inferior to the clavicle is the first intercostal space, and the bone below it is the second rib.

    The acromion (**choice A**) is the lateral extension of the scapular spine.

    The atlas (**choice B**) is the first cervical vertebra, articulating with the occipital bone above and the axis below.

    The first rib (**choice C**) is hidden under the clavicle.

    The manubrium (**choice D**) is the most superior portion of the sternum.

40. **The correct answer is B.** A cricothyrotomy is performed at the cricothyroid membrane, which is correctly located between the thyroid cartilage (Adam's apple) and the cricoid cartilage below.

    **Choice A** is incorrect because the junction of the clavicle and the sternum is the sternal notch, not the cricothyroid membrane.

    **Choices C, D, and E** have matching descriptions and names of specific neck landmarks. However, these choices are incorrect because none of them is the proper site for this procedure.

41. **The correct answer is B.** Embryonic tissue is most susceptible to teratogens during the third through ninth weeks of pregnancy. This is when organogenesis, as well

as most major congenital anomalies, occur. Because brain development occurs throughout pregnancy, however, it is wisest for a pregnant woman to avoid alcohol for all 9 months of gestation.

The first 2 weeks (**choice A**) of pregnancy are not generally associated with teratogenicity, unless so many of the cells of the conceptus are irreversibly damaged that death results. Otherwise, the abundance of undifferentiated cells present can compensate for the damage.

The ninth through twelfth weeks (**choice C**) are associated with minor congenital anomalies, including those of the eyes, palate, teeth, and ears.

The twelfth through sixteenth weeks (**choice D**) and sixteenth through twentieth weeks (**choice E**) are associated with minor congenital anomalies, including those of the eyes, teeth, ears, and external genitalia. Minor CNS anomalies may occur during the twentieth week.

42. **The correct answer is B.** This patient has two risk factors for sinusitis: chronic rhinitis and allergy. She probably also has aspirin allergy, which is associated with the triad of nasal polyps, asthma, and sinusitis. In maxillary sinusitis, exudate may drain into the middle meatus through an ostium in the hiatus semilunaris, which contains openings to the frontal and maxillary sinuses and anterior ethmoidal cells.

    The bulla ethmoidalis (**choice A**), also part of the middle meatus, contains an opening to the middle ethmoidal air cells.

    The inferior nasal meatus (**choice C**) receives fluid from the nasolacrimal duct, which drains tears from the medial aspect of the orbit to the nasal cavity.

    The sphenoethmoidal recess (**choice D**) is located above the superior concha and contains an opening for the sphenoid sinus.

    The superior nasal meatus (**choice E**) is located above the superior concha and contains an opening for the posterior ethmoidal air cells.

43. **The correct answer is A.** The deep peroneal nerve arises from the common peroneal nerve (L4-S2). It innervates the muscles of the anterior compartment of the leg, which dorsiflex (extend) the foot. Damage to the nerve therefore produces "foot-drop"—a classic clue to deep peroneal nerve pathology. The nerve gives rise to many branches, one of which innervates the skin between the first and second toes.

    The femoral nerve (**choice B**) contains fibers from L2-L4. It supplies flexor muscles of the thigh, extensors at the knee joint, and cutaneous areas of the thigh. The saphenous nerve branches off it and supplies the knee joint and the skin on the medial aspect of the foot.

**KAPLAN**) MEDICAL

The superficial peroneal nerve (**choice C**) supplies the muscles of the lateral compartment of the leg and is responsible for foot eversion. It also conveys sensory information from most of the dorsal surface of the foot.

The sural nerve (**choice D**) arises from the common peroneal and tibial nerves and innervates the skin of the calf.

The tibial nerve (**choice E**) innervates the hamstrings, as well as muscles of the calf and sole of the foot.

44. **The correct answer is D.** Endothelium lines the cardiovascular and lymphatic vessels and is composed of simple squamous epithelium. The mesothelium that lines the pleural, pericardial, and peritoneal cavities is also composed of a single layer of simple squamous epithelium.

    Pseudostratified epithelium (**choice A**) is found in the epithelial lining of the respiratory tract, as well as in the transitional epithelium of the urinary system.

    In simple columnar epithelium (**choice B**), the cells are taller than they are wide. This epithelium can be found in the intestinal absorptive surface.

    Simple cuboidal epithelium (**choice C**) can be found in the ducts of many glands.

    Stratified columnar epithelium (**choice E**) can be found in portions of the male urethra.

    Stratified cuboidal epithelium (**choice F**) is found in the ducts of the salivary glands.

    The epidermis of the skin is composed of keratinizing stratified squamous epithelium (**choice G**). Nonkeratinizing stratified squamous epithelium can be found in the oral cavity, esophagus, and vagina.

45. **The correct answer is E.** This route passes through the vastus lateralis to penetrate the knee joint via the suprapatellar bursa, allowing aspiration of joint fluid for culture. The vastus lateralis, together with the vastus medialis, vastus intermedius, and rectus femoris, forms the quadriceps muscle.

    The adductor magnus (**choice A**) is on the inner and anterior aspect of the upper thigh.

    The gracilis (**choice B**) is on the inner aspect of the thigh.

    The iliacus (**choice C**) is mostly in the false pelvis.

    The sartorius (**choice D**) passes diagonally from the lateral hip to the medial knee.

46. **The correct answer is D.** A normal waking adult characteristically shows alpha activity over the posterior regions of the head, some beta activity in the fronto-central regions, and few (if any) theta waves over the temporal areas. Delta waves are not present in normal adults during wakefulness. The delta waves over his left

frontal lobe indicate a lesion in this area. The left primary motor cortex resides in this region and would produce a right hemiparesis if damaged.

A left hemiparesis (**choice A**) could be caused by a lesion of the right primary motor cortex, located in the frontal lobe.

A left hemisensory loss (**choice B**) could be produced by a lesion of the right primary somatosensory cortex, located in the parietal lobe.

A left homonymous hemianopia (**choice C**) could be caused by a lesion in the visual pathway after the optic chiasm (right optic tract, right optic radiations, right visual cortex).

A right hemisensory loss (**choice E**) could be produced by a lesion of the left primary somatosensory cortex, located in the parietal lobe.

A right homonymous hemianopia (**choice F**) could be caused by a lesion in the visual pathway after the optic chiasm (left optic tract, left optic radiations, left visual cortex).

47. **The correct answer is B.** The most common type of ankle sprain is lateral, which occurs as a result of excessive inversion of the foot and plantar flexion of the ankle. The calcaneofibular (not calcaneotibial [**choice C**]) and anterior talofibular (not talotibial [**choice A**]) ligaments may tear, producing marked swelling and pain. These two ligaments combined with the posterior talofibular ligament constitute the lateral ligament of the ankle.

    The deltoid ligament (**choice D**), also known as the medial ligament of the ankle, is a very strong, thick structure located at the medial malleolus. Excessive eversion would be the most likely mechanism of injury.

    The medial collateral ligament (**choice E**) is damaged in lateral blows to the knee.

48. **The correct answer is C.** Questions like these are particularly amenable to the use of test-taking strategies because even if you don't know 100% of the answer, you will be able to eliminate some answer choices on the basis of knowledge you do have. For example, you probably are aware that the peritoneum does not lie superficial to the transversus abdominis muscle, enabling you to eliminate choice A and increase your chances of answering correctly by 20%. Note that this is a question surgeons love to ask students, so keep this information in mind in the operating room!

49. **The correct answer is B.** Pain in the liver and gallbladder can be referred to C3-C5 dermatomes of the right shoulder. Many people are familiar with the projection of cardiac pain to the left shoulder, which is a similar

phenomenon. Pancreatic disease can also produce left shoulder pain. On physical examination, referred pain can usually be distinguished from pain truly originating in the perceived area by palpation and manipulation of the area. Local physical manipulation does not usually alter the character or intensity of referred pain, but it does alter those features of skin, joint, or muscle pain truly localized to the region.

50. **The correct answer is E.** The transitional epithelium that lines the ureter, the renal pelvis, and the major and minor calyces is derived from mesoderm of the ureteric bud. Similarly, the cuboidal epithelium of the collecting tubules derives from ureteric bud mesoderm.

The simple squamous epithelium lining Bowman capsule (**choice A**) is derived from mesoderm of the metanephros.

The simple cuboidal epithelium lining the distal convoluted tubule (**choice B**) is derived from mesoderm of the metanephros.

The simple squamous epithelium lining the loop of Henle (**choice C**) is derived from mesoderm of the metanephros.

The proximal convoluted tubule (**choice D**) is lined with simple columnar epithelium derived from mesoderm of the metanephros.

# Anatomy: **Test Two**

1. A woman comes to the physician for a prenatal visit. Examination reveals that her uterus is considerably larger than her gestational age would predict. An ultrasound examination is ordered and reveals that she has polyhydramnios. Which of the following congenital defects of the fetus would be most likely to be associated with this abnormality?

   (A) Atrial septal defect

   (B) Esophageal atresia

   (C) Lung hypoplasia

   (D) Meckel diverticulum

   (E) Renal agenesis

2. A gastric biopsy is performed on a 42-year-old man. As the pathologist inspects the specimen, he observes numerous, normal cuboidal-to-columnar cells with apical membrane-bound secretion granules in the gastric glands. From which area of the stomach was the biopsy specimen most likely taken?

   (A) Cardiac region

   (B) Columns of Morgagni

   (C) Fundic region

   (D) Greater omentum

   (E) Pyloric region

3. During a football game, a player sustains a powerful blow to the lateral side of his weight-bearing leg. He experiences excruciating knee pain and is unable to walk. The three structures most likely to be injured are the

   (A) anterior cruciate and lateral collateral ligaments and the lateral meniscus

   (B) anterior cruciate and medial collateral ligaments and the medial meniscus

   (C) posterior cruciate and lateral collateral ligaments and the lateral meniscus

   (D) posterior cruciate and medial collateral ligaments and the lateral meniscus

   (E) posterior cruciate and medial collateral ligaments and medial meniscus

4. A mother brings her 5-year-old daughter to the physician complaining that the child still seems to regularly wet herself despite having been toilet-trained. The physician orders an IV pyelogram, which demonstrates a complete duplication of the ureter on the right side. Although one ureter opens normally into the bladder, the other opens ectopically into the vagina. This congenital anomaly is caused by

   (A) duplication of the proximal mesonephric (Wolffian) duct

   (B) early division of the ureteric bud

   (C) ectopic growth of the pronephros

   (D) improper union of excretory tubules and collecting tubules

   (E) persistence of embryonic ureters as the kidney ascends from the pelvis to the superior abdomen

5. A newborn baby is observed to be cyanotic immediately after birth. Diagnostic studies, including an ultrasound, reveal that the baby has persistent truncus arteriosus. Which of the following additional defects is this baby most likely to have?

   (A) Dextrocardia

   (B) Membranous ventricular septal defect

   (C) Secundum-type atrial septal defect

   (D) Tetralogy of Fallot

   (E) Transposition of the great arteries

6. A 61-year-old woman undergoes surgery to remove a solitary painless mass just anterior to the tragus of her left ear. Pathologic examination shows a well-circumscribed, yellowish-white tumor with a proliferation of epithelial and myoepithelial cells in duct formations within a background of loose myxoid tissue. During the surgery, particular attention is paid to the nerve that exits the skull via the stylomastoid foramen, passes lateral to the styloid process, and then enters this affected structure. Injury to the lower division of this nerve during surgery will most likely result in

   (A) inability to furrow the brow (to frown) on the same side

   (B) numbness over the angle and mental region of the jaw on the same side

   (C) ptosis of the eye on the same side

   (D) weakness in closing the eye on the same side

   (E) weakness of the lower lip on the same side

7. An arteriogram is performed on a patient with atherosclerosis. Luminal narrowing of which of the following vessels would compromise blood flow through the renal arteries?

   (A) Abdominal aorta

   (B) Celiac trunk

   (C) Common iliac artery

   (D) Inferior mesenteric artery

   (E) Superior mesenteric artery

8. Nissl bodies correspond to which of the following cytoplasmic organelles?

   (A) Golgi apparatus

   (B) Mitochondria

   (C) Nucleoli

   (D) Rough endoplasmic reticulum

   (E) Smooth endoplasmic reticulum

9. A 42-year-old man undergoes surgery for medullary carcinoma of the thyroid. After the surgery, he complains of a "noisy quality" to his voice. This condition was most likely caused by damage to the

   (A) internal laryngeal nerve

   (B) recurrent laryngeal nerve

   (C) thyroarytenoid muscle

   (D) vestibular folds

   (E) vocal folds

10. After an amniocentesis, a 29-year-old woman who is carrying twins learns that one fetus has XY chromosomes and the other has XX chromosomes. At 37 weeks' gestation, the woman delivers two healthy babies. Which of the following structures is likely to be present in the baby with the XY chromosomes but not in the one with XX chromosomes?

    (A) Bulbospongiosus muscle

    (B) Bulbourethral gland

    (C) Corpus cavernosum

    (D) Membranous urethra

    (E) Perineal body

11. During an automobile accident, a person sustains a "broken neck" and dies after a small bony fragment is driven into his spinal cord. From which of the following bones was this fragment most likely derived?

    (A) Atlas

    (B) Axis

    (C) Seventh cervical vertebrae

    (D) Sixth cervical vertebrae

    (E) Fifth cervical vertebrae

12. A patient is complaining of difficulty swallowing. A barium contrast x-ray shows a constriction of the esophagus at the level of the third thoracic vertebra. An aortogram shows that the patient has a double aortic arch. Which of the following developmental abnormalities explains this finding?

    (A) Abnormal persistence of the right dorsal aorta

    (B) Abnormal persistence of the right fourth aortic arch

    (C) Abnormal persistence of the right seventh intersegmental artery

    (D) Abnormal persistence of the right sixth aortic arch

    (E) Abnormal persistence of the right third aortic arch

13. Because she is too weak to go to the cafeteria, a 93-year-old nursing-home resident on a liquid diet is fed in bed. She refuses to sit up, so the aide has to feed her while she is lying on her back. Halfway through the feeding, the patient aspirates the liquid and subsequently develops pneumonia. Which of the following is the most likely site of this pneumonia?

    (A) Anterior segment of the right upper lobe

    (B) Apical segment of the right lower lobe

    (C) Inferior lingular segment of the left upper lobe

    (D) Lateral segment of the right middle lobe

    (E) Superior lingular segment of the left upper lobe

14. A patient has a tiny (0.2 cm) but exquisitely painful tumor under the nail of her index finger. Local anesthetic block to a branch of which of the following nerves would be most likely to provide adequate anesthesia for the surgical removal of the mass?

    (A) Axillary

    (B) Median

    (C) Musculocutaneous

    (D) Radial

    (E) Ulnar

15. A 3-year-old boy has repeated episodes of sore throat and fever. He undergoes surgery to remove collections of lymphoid tissue that lie on each side of the oropharynx between the palatoglossal and palatopharyngeal arches. The removed structures developed from which of the following pharyngeal pouches?

    (A) First

    (B) Second

    (C) Third

    (D) Fourth

    (E) Fifth

16. A 35-year-old woman with severe dysmenorrhea and prolonged menstrual periods due to large uterine fibroids undergoes a hysterectomy. Which of the following structures is the gynecologist most likely to inadvertently ligate during surgery?

    (A) Internal iliac artery

    (B) Internal iliac vein

    (C) Ovarian artery

    (D) Ureter

    (E) Uterine vein

17. A pregnant woman comes to her physician with questions about the effect that ingested substances may have on her unborn child. The physician explains that large molecules do not pass between the mother and fetus because of the placental barrier. The physician adds that fetal blood is in the fetal blood vessels of the villi of the placenta and the mother's blood is in the maternal blood vessels, and that these blood vessels do not connect. The placental villi are formed from which of the following cells?

    (A) Cytotrophoblast

    (B) Embryoblast

    (C) Endometrium

    (D) Epiblast

    (E) Syncytiotrophoblast

18. A 32-year-old man complains of progressive, severe, generalized headaches that began 3 months ago, are worse in the mornings, and lately have been accompanied by projectile vomiting. He has also lost his upper gaze, and on physical examination the upper part of the sclera is visible above the downward looking irises. Which of the following is the most likely diagnosis?

    (A) Brain tumor affecting the frontal lobe

    (B) Nelson syndrome

    (C) Pituitary apoplexy

    (D) Posterior fossa tumor

    (E) Tumor in the area of the pineal gland

19. A prostate-specific antigen (PSA) level is drawn from a 54-year-old man as part of a routine health evaluation. Which of the following embryonic structures gives rise to the organ being screened for carcinoma?

    (A) Genital tubercle

    (B) Processus vaginalis

    (C) Testis cords

    (D) Tunica albuginea

    (E) Urogenital sinus

20. A football player is examined by the team physician following a shoulder injury during a game. Preliminary x-ray films show an inferior dislocation of the humerus. On further examination, there is weakness in lateral rotation and abduction of the arm. The nerve most likely affected is the

    (A) axillary
    (B) dorsal scapular
    (C) radial
    (D) suprascapular
    (E) thoracodorsal

21. During anatomy laboratory, a first-year medical student is dissecting the atrial chambers of the heart. At the upper border of the fossa ovalis, she discovers a small opening through which the tip of her probe can be passed from the right into the left atrium. The laboratory instructor identifies this as a probe patency of the atrial septum. This probe patency resulted from which of the following developmental events?

    (A) Excessive resorption of the septum primum
    (B) Failure of the endocardial cushions to form
    (C) Failure of postnatal fusion of septum primum and septum secundum
    (D) Failure of the right and left conotruncal ridges to fuse
    (E) Failure of the septum primum to fuse with the endocardial cushions

22. A 20-year-old man is stabbed immediately to the left of the body of the sternum at the fifth intercostal space. The knife most likely penetrated the

    (A) left atrium
    (B) left ventricle
    (C) right atrium
    (D) right ventricle
    (E) stomach

23. A 5-month old girl has fatigue on exertion. She was born at full-term with a birth weight of 9 lb and had an uncomplicated perinatal period. She has been bottle-fed, and there have been no feeding problems. She is alert and appears well. Physical examination reveals a loud holosystolic murmur in the left parasternal region with an associated systolic thrill. The first and second heart sounds are normal. There is no gallop or diastolic murmur. Her blood pressure is normal in all four extremities, and she has palpable peripheral pulses. There is no peripheral edema or cyanosis. Which of the following is the most likely diagnosis?

    (A) Atrial septal defect
    (B) Patent ductus arteriosus
    (C) Patent foramen ovale
    (D) Pulmonic stenosis
    (E) Ventricular septal defect

24. An elderly woman with osteoporosis is taken to the emergency department following a fall. One of her legs appears shortened and is externally rotated. A fracture of which part of the femur is suggested by these findings?

    (A) Greater trochanter
    (B) Lateral epicondyle
    (C) Medial epicondyle
    (D) Neck
    (E) Shaft

25. An otherwise healthy first-year medical student visits the student health office for a physical examination. He is taking no medications. He is concerned because he has noticed several painless uniform "large bumps" at the back of his tongue. These are most likely

    (A) aphthous ulcers
    (B) candidal colonies
    (C) circumvallate papillae
    (D) filiform papillae
    (E) fungiform papillae

26. An oblique x-ray view of a patient with right middle lobar pneumonia demonstrates an area of consolidation bounded by sharp, intersecting, relatively straight lines above and below. These lines correspond to which of the following?

    (A) Diaphragm above and oblique fissure below

    (B) Oblique fissure above and breast shadow below

    (C) Oblique fissure above and transverse fissure below

    (D) Transverse fissure above and diaphragm below

    (E) Transverse fissure above and oblique fissure below

27. During an interview, a 34-year-old psychiatric patient suddenly becomes aggressive. The patient is quickly taken to a quiet, private room and given an intramuscular injection of haloperidol in the upper outer quadrant of the buttock. The injection is given at this specific location to prevent damage to which of the following nerves?

    (A) Common peroneal

    (B) Lateral femoral cutaneous

    (C) Obturator

    (D) Sciatic

    (E) Superior gluteal

28. A 21-year-old man is brought to the hospital by emergency medical technicians after he was involved in a car accident. Examination reveals a clear fluid draining from his left ear. Laboratory studies confirm that the fluid is cerebrospinal fluid. Which of the following is the most likely site of trauma that has resulted in the leakage of this fluid?

    (A) Fracture in the region of the internal auditory meatus, along with rupture of the tympanic membrane

    (B) Fracture in the region of the jugular foramen, along with rupture of the tympanic membrane

    (C) Fracture of the external ear canal, along with rupture of the tympanic membrane

    (D) Fracture of the floor of the anterior cranial fossa, along with rupture of the tympanic membrane

    (E) Fracture of the floor of the middle cranial fossa, along with rupture of the tympanic membrane

29. During a bar fight, a 20-year-old man is stabbed with an ice pick. The weapon passes through the superior orbital fissure. Which of the following is most likely to be severed as the ice pick passes through this fissure?

    (A) Abducens nerve

    (B) Facial nerve

    (C) Mandibular nerve

    (D) Maxillary nerve

    (E) Middle meningeal artery

    (F) Ophthalmic artery

    (G) Optic nerve

30. A patient presents to the emergency department after sustaining a laceration of the first web space of his hand in a rock-climbing accident. Which of the following structures is also likely to be injured?

    (A) Deep branch of radial nerve

    (B) Opponens pollicis

    (C) Radial artery

    (D) Recurrent branch of median nerve

    (E) Superficial palmar arch

31. After a motor vehicle accident, a patient is brought to the emergency room. X-rays reveal that she has fractures of her left ninth and tenth ribs. She has a rapid heart rate and low blood pressure. Peritoneal lavage reveals free blood in the peritoneal cavity. A surgeon is able to stop the bleeding by placing a clamp across which of the following structures?

    (A) Broad ligament

    (B) Falciform ligament

    (C) Gastrosplenic ligament

    (D) Hepatoduodenal ligament

    (E) Splenorenal ligament

32. A football player experiences an anterior dislocation of the shoulder. Cutaneous sensation over the lower half of the deltoid muscle is impaired. These findings suggest damage to which of the following nerves?

    (A) Axillary

    (B) Median

    (C) Musculocutaneous

    (D) Radial

    (E) Ulnar

33. A 45-year-old garbage collector has severe neck pain and weakness in his left upper extremity. He has gotten no relief from over-the-counter medications. He denies any history of trauma. On examination the patient is thin and walks with his neck tilted to the left side. The patient has limited neck flexion and extension secondary to pain. The patient has a normal motor and sensory examination of all extremities, with the exception of the left upper extremity. His left radial forearm and thumb are numb to the touch (decreased sensation to light touch). The patient has a decreased brachioradialis reflex and slight weakness of his wrist extensors. Plain radiographs appear normal. Which of the following is the most likely diagnosis?

    (A) Compression of his left C6 nerve root
    (B) Compression of his left thoracic first nerve root (T1)
    (C) Compression of his right T1 nerve root
    (D) A tumor in his lumbar spine
    (E) A tumor in his sacral spine

34. A patient with a left adrenal mass is scheduled for surgery. The surgeon is planning to approach the suprarenal area by removing the twelfth rib. With this approach, the surgeon should take particular care to avoid damaging which of the following structures?

    (A) Aorta
    (B) Diaphragm
    (C) Pancreas
    (D) Stomach
    (E) Vena cava

35. A 45-year-old man has an obvious mass on the right side of his face. It is determined that he has a benign tumor of the parotid gland, and the tumor is excised. After surgical excision of the tumor, it is noted that the patient's mouth droops on the right side and, when asked to smile, his smile is asymmetrical. The patient is able to open and close both eyes normally and can wrinkle his forehead symmetrically and raise both eyebrows. Sensation is normal on both sides of his face. Which of the following is the most likely cause of the findings?

    (A) Damage to branches of the mental nerve
    (B) Damage to branches of the infraorbital nerve
    (C) Damage to branches of the facial nerve
    (D) Damage to branches of the glossopharyngeal nerve
    (E) Damage to branches of the hypoglossal nerve

36. During anatomy lab, a medical student notes a fibrous band that runs on the visceral surface of the liver. It is attached on one end to the inferior vena cava and on the other end to the left branch of the portal vein. In the embryo, this structure corresponds to the

    (A) ductus venosus
    (B) ligamentum teres
    (C) ligamentum venosum
    (D) umbilical arteries
    (E) umbilical vein

37. While examining a newborn baby in the nursery, a physician notes that urine is draining from the umbilicus. Contrast dye is introduced into the bladder through the urethra, and it is confirmed radiologically that dye is passing to the umbilicus. Which of the following embryonic structures has abnormally persisted in this patient?

    (A) Allantoic duct
    (B) Mesonephric duct
    (C) Mesonephric tubules
    (D) Ureteric bud
    (E) Urorectal septum

38. A 4-year-old boy with recurrent urinary tract infections is evaluated for renal/urinary tract abnormalities with a voiding cystourethrogram (VCUG). Reflux is discovered, so an intravenous pyelogram (IVP) is performed. The renal anatomy appears normal. On the IVP, which of the following structures would have been seen emptying into the renal pelvis?

    (A) Major calyx
    (B) Minor calyx
    (C) Renal pyramid
    (D) Ureter

39. A neonate is observed to have a small notch in the transitional zone and a vermillion border of the lip. Which of the following is the most likely etiology of this malformation?

    (A) Abnormal development of the third and fourth pharyngeal pouches
    (B) Bony defects of the malar bone and mandible
    (C) Failure of the maxillary processes and medial nasal swellings to fuse
    (D) Incomplete joining of the palatine shelves
    (E) Insufficient migration of neural crest cells

40. A patient's left hypoglossal nerve (CN XII) is injured during a carotid endarterectomy. Which of the following would most likely result from this injury?

    (A) Decreased gag reflex on the left

    (B) Decreased salivation from the left submandibular and sublingual salivary glands

    (C) Deviation of the tongue to the left on protrusion

    (D) Inability to elevate the pharynx on the left during swallowing

    (E) Inability to perceive sweet and salt taste sensation on the anterior part of the left side of the tongue

41. During a physical examination a physician elicits a pupillary light reflex by shining a light into a patient's eye. The iris contracts, thereby constricting the pupil. Where are the cell bodies of the preganglionic neurons found that are responsible for this response?

    (A) Oculomotor nucleus

    (B) Edinger-Westphal nucleus

    (C) Ciliary ganglion

    (D) Precentral gyrus

    (E) Geniculate ganglion

42. A 69-year-old woman fractures her humerus during a motor vehicle accident. Which of these types of bone will most likely be seen in a biopsy taken from the healing area?

    (A) Cancellous

    (B) Compact

    (C) Spongy

    (D) Trabecular

    (E) Woven

43. A 58-year-old man with lymphoma has shortness of breath and chest pain. A chest x-ray shows bilateral blunting of the costophrenic angle. A thoracocentesis is performed. During this procedure, it is important to pass the needle immediately above the rib to prevent damage to which of the following structures in the subcostal groove?

    (A) Intercostal artery and vein

    (B) Intercostal nerve

    (C) Intercostal nerve and artery

    (D) Intercostal nerve and vein

    (E) Intercostal nerve, artery, and vein

44. A newborn boy does not pass meconium until 48 hours after his birth. Several weeks later his mother complains that he has not been passing stool regularly. Anorectal manometry reveals increased internal anal sphincter pressure on rectal distention with a balloon. The patient's disorder may be attributed to

    (A) defective recanalization of the colon

    (B) failure of neural crest cells to migrate into the colonic wall

    (C) herniation of abdominal contents into the umbilical cord

    (D) persistence of the proximal end of the yolk stalk

    (E) presence of a rectourinary fistula

45. A 38-year-old woman slips on an icy sidewalk and falls, hitting the ground with her right elbow. She reports that she is experiencing severe pain in her upper limb. Examination reveals that she cannot extend her hand at the wrist. She has diminished sensation on the lateral portion of the dorsum of her hand. Which of the following is the most likely site of her fracture?

    (A) Scaphoid

    (B) Distal end of the radius

    (C) Medial epicondyle of the humerus

    (D) Midportion of the shaft of the humerus

    (E) Surgical neck of the humerus

46. An infant is brought to the emergency department with a temperature of 40° C (104° F). The physician notes that the infant has a "bulging anterior fontanelle." The third-year medical student reads the physician's note and wants to evaluate this physical finding, but she forgot where the anterior fontanelle is. In evaluating this finding, the medical student should look for which of the following anatomic landmarks?

    (A) Bregma

    (B) Coronal suture

    (C) Lambda

    (D) Pterion

    (E) Sagittal suture

47. A 63-year-old man has blood-streaked stools and constipation. Barium enema shows a right-sided obstructing
lesion. Surgery is performed, and pathologic evaluation
reveals a well-differentiated, colonic adenocarcinoma.
Observation of a hematoxylin and eosin-stained microscopic slide from the specimen reveals that the nuclei of
the cells are blue. What is the basis for this observation?

   (A) Eosin binds to carbohydrates
   (B) Eosin binds to lipids
   (C) Eosin binds to nucleic acids
   (D) Hematoxylin binds to lipids
   (E) Hematoxylin binds to nucleic acids

48. On physical examination, the upper body of a 7-year-
old boy appears much more developed than his lower
body. Blood pressure in the upper extremities exceeds
that of the lower extremities. On cardiac examination,
there is a midsystolic murmur over the anterior chest
and back. The child's lower extremities are cold, and
femoral pulses are absent. The part of the vascular system
that is affected in this disorder is derived from which of
the following embryologic structures?

   (A) Bulbus cordis
   (B) Ductus arteriosus
   (C) Left horn of sinus venosus
   (D) Right common cardinal vein
   (E) Right horn of sinus venosus
   (F) Third, fourth, and sixth aortic arches

49. A urologist performs a cystoscopy to examine the bladder and the openings of the ureters into the bladder.
After distention of the bladder with air, the physician
slowly passes the cystoscope up the urethra into the
bladder. In which direction should she turn the head of
the cystoscope to see the ureteric orifices and examine
for blockage?

   (A) Anterior and inferior
   (B) Anterior and superior
   (C) Posterior and inferior
   (D) Posterior and superior

50. After receiving a punch to the left eye, a 16-year-old boy
complains of double vision. During clinical testing, he has
difficulty when asked to look medially, inferolaterally,
superolaterally, and superomedially. The affected muscles
are derived from which of the following structures?

   (A) Branchial arches
   (B) Optic cup ectoderm
   (C) Somites
   (D) Somitomeres
   (E) Splanchnic mesoderm

# Anatomy Test Two: **Answers and Explanations**

## ANSWER KEY

| | | | | |
|---|---|---|---|---|
| 1. | B | | 26. | E |
| 2. | C | | 27. | D |
| 3. | B | | 28. | E |
| 4. | B | | 29. | A |
| 5. | B | | 30. | C |
| 6. | E | | 31. | E |
| 7. | A | | 32. | A |
| 8. | D | | 33. | A |
| 9. | B | | 34. | B |
| 10. | B | | 35. | C |
| 11. | B | | 36. | A |
| 12. | A | | 37. | A |
| 13. | B | | 38. | A |
| 14. | B | | 39. | C |
| 15. | B | | 40. | C |
| 16. | D | | 41. | B |
| 17. | E | | 42. | E |
| 18. | E | | 43. | E |
| 19. | E | | 44. | B |
| 20. | A | | 45. | D |
| 21. | C | | 46. | A |
| 22. | D | | 47. | E |
| 23. | E | | 48. | F |
| 24. | D | | 49. | C |
| 25. | C | | 50. | D |

1. **The correct answer is B.** Polyhydramnios is the presence of excess amniotic fluid. Because amniotic fluid is normally swallowed by the fetus, esophageal atresia, an obstruction of the esophagus that prevents the fetus from swallowing the amniotic fluid, causes an excess of fluid to be retained in the amniotic cavity.

   An atrial septal defect (**choice A**) is a common acyanotic heart defect. This defect has no relationship to abnormalities in amniotic fluid volume.

   Renal agenesis (**choice E**) is a failure of the kidneys to develop. Because the amniotic fluid is augmented by fetal urine production, the absence of the kidneys results in reduced amniotic fluid (oligohydramnios).

   Lung hypoplasia (**choice C**) is an underdevelopment of the lungs. This condition is associated with oligohydramnios. The fetus normally produces respiratory movements and "inhales" amniotic fluid into the lungs. This fluid in the lungs assists the lungs to develop normally. Reduced amniotic fluid is therefore associated with underdevelopment of the lungs. Other developmental abnormalities associated with oligohydramnios include skeletal defects such as clubfoot, presumably because the fetus has inadequate space for normal skeletal development.

   Meckel diverticulum (**choice D**) is an abnormal persistence of the proximal portion of the vitelline duct. The vitelline duct connects the embryonic gut tube to the yolk sac. Normally, the yolk sac and vitelline duct disappear. When the small portion of the duct remains connected to the gut tube, this results in Meckel diverticulum. This is found in about 2% of the population and is often asymptomatic. It is connected to the ileum of the small intestine.

2. **The correct answer is C.** The pathologist saw normal chief cells, which are abundant in the body and fundus of the stomach. Chief cells secrete pepsinogen, which is stored in apical membrane-bound granules. The body and fundus of the stomach contain high concentrations of four other types of cells in the epithelium. The parietal (oxyntic) cells are large, pyramidal, and acidophilic with central nuclei (like a "fried egg"). They make and secrete HCl. The mucous neck cells secrete mucus and appear clear. The enteroendocrine cells have affinity for silver stains and exhibit a positive chromaffin reaction; these cells synthesize amines, polypeptides, or proteins.

   The cardiac region (**choice A**) is a narrow, circular band at the transition between the esophagus and stomach, consisting of shallow gastric pits and mucous glands. It does not normally contain an abundance of chief cells.

   The columns of Morgagni (**choice B**) are found in the rectum, not in the stomach. These are mucous membrane infoldings in the submucosa of the proximal anal canal. They would not contain chief cells.

   The greater omentum (**choice D**) is a four-layered fold of peritoneum that hangs from the greater curvature of the stomach and attaches to the transverse colon. It would not contain chief cells.

   The pyloric region (**choice E**) has deep gastric pits into which tubular glands open. The predominant secretion is mucus. It does not normally contain an abundance of chief cells.

   Note that in this question you could have automatically eliminated choices B and D, since they are not gastric structures. If nothing else, you would have improved your guessing odds to 33%.

3. **The correct answer is B.** The anterior cruciate and medial collateral ligaments and the medial meniscus are sometimes called the "unhappy triad," because they are commonly injured in lateral blows to the knee that forcefully abduct the tibia. A good mnemonic is "MAMM" (for Medial collateral, Anterior cruciate, and Medial Meniscus). Damage to the anterior cruciate ligament is characterized by the ability to push the tibia too far forward on the femur.

   Damage to the lateral collateral ligaments and lateral menisci are very uncommon (**choices A and C**) and would be expected if the tibia were forcefully adducted.

   Damage to the posterior cruciate ligaments (**choices C, D, E**) is extremely rare and is characterized by the ability to push the tibia too far backward on the femur.

4. **The correct answer is B.** The collecting system of the kidney, including the ureters, develops from an outgrowth of the distal mesonephric duct called the ureteric bud. The ureteric bud grows into the metanephros and induces the formation of the excretory system (nephrons). Early splitting of the ureteric bud may result in partial or complete duplication of the ureter. One of the buds typically opens into the bladder. The lower, abnormal bud usually opens more inferiorly and may communicate with the vagina or urethra in females.

   The mesonephric duct (**choice A**) is the drainage system of the mesonephros (the second "incarnation" of the kidney). The mesonephros, like the pronephros, eventually degenerates and almost completely disappears (to be replaced by metanephros) by the second month of gestation. With the mesonephros gone, the duct no longer functions in urine drainage. In females it also degenerates, whereas in males it persists to become the epididymis and ductus deferens.

   The pronephros (**choice C**) is the first "incarnation" of the kidney. It rapidly regresses so that by 4 weeks postfertilization, all indications of it have completely disappeared.

During normal kidney formation there is union of the excretory tubules derived from the metanephros and the collecting tubules derived from the mesonephric duct. However, when the union does not occur properly (**choice D**), the outcome is not incontinence but rather the formation of renal cysts.

Renal arterial branches of the abdominal aorta form and then degenerate as the kidney ascends from the pelvis to the superior abdomen; one or more supernumerary renal arteries may persist. The ureters do not undergo a similar process during development (**choice E**); once formed, the embryonic ureters persist and continue to develop into the adult ureters.

5.  **The correct answer is B.** Persistent truncus arteriosus results from failure of the aorticopulmonary septum to form. Normally, the aorticopulmonary septum divides the truncus arteriosus into the ascending aorta and the pulmonary trunk. The aorticopulmonary septum also contributes to the formation of the membranous portion of the interventricular septum. When the aorticopulmonary septum does not form, the truncus arteriosus persists rather than being divided, and the membranous interventricular septum is incomplete. Because neural crest cells contribute to the formation of the aorticopulmonary septum, it is believed that this defect may result from a defect in migration of neural crest cells.

    Dextrocardia (**choice A**) is having the heart on the right side of the chest midline instead of the left side. This results from the heart tube forming a loop to the right instead of the left. Blood flow though the heart is normal, and there is no functional defect of the heart. This defect is not related to the aorticopulmonary septum.

    A secundum-type atrial septal defect (**choice C**) results from the foramen secundum in the septum primum being too big, probably due to excessive resorption of the septum primum, such that the septum secundum is not able to cover the foramen secundum. This prevents normal closure of the foramen ovale when the baby is born, and the pressure in the left atrium rises above the pressure in the right atrium. The aorticopulmonary septum is not involved in this defect.

    Tetralogy of Fallot (**choice D**) results from the aorticopulmonary septum forming in the wrong location. Instead of dividing the truncus arteriosus into an aorta and pulmonary trunk of equal sizes, the displacement of the septum results in the aorta being too large and the pulmonary trunk being too small. Thus, the elements of tetralogy of Fallot include pulmonary stenosis and overriding aorta. The other elements are ventricular septal

defect and right ventricular hypertrophy. Because there is an aorticopulmonary septum, it is not possible to have both tetralogy of Fallot and persistent truncus arteriosus.

Transposition of the great arteries (**choice E**) is when the ascending aorta emerges from the right ventricle and the pulmonary trunk emerges from the left ventricle. This is a cyanotic heart defect that results from the aorticopulmonary septum forming without having its normal 180-degree spiral. Thus, the truncus arteriosus is divided, but the vessel that should be on the left is on the right and vice versa. Because there is an aorticopulmonary septum, it will contribute to the formation of the membranous ventricular septum.

6.  **The correct answer is E.** The motor component (special visceral efferent) of the facial nerve (CN VII) exits the skull via the stylomastoid foramen, passes lateral to the styloid process, and then enters the parotid gland. Within the gland, two divisions can usually be identified (upper and lower), which in turn give off five named branches that innervate the muscles of the face. The upper division gives rise to the temporal and zygomatic branches, which collectively innervate the frontalis, corrugator, and orbicularis oculi muscles. The lower division gives off the buccal, mandibular, and cervical branches. The largest, the buccal, innervates the muscles attaching to the upper lip, including the orbicularis oris and the levators, as well as the buccinator and the muscles of the nose. The mandibular branches innervate the muscles of the lower lip and of the chin, whereas the cervical branch innervates the platysma muscle. There are usually communicating branches between the named terminal nerves so that overlapping innervation of the muscles occurs. If the lower division is injured, there will be weakness (not frank paralysis because of the innervation overlap) of the muscles that attach to the lower lip.

    An inability to furrow the brow (**choice A**) would be caused be denervation of the corrugator supercilii and frontalis muscles, which are innervated by the upper division of the facial nerve.

    **Choice B** is wrong because once the facial nerve emerges from the stylomastoid foramen, it is a pure motor nerve (special visceral efferent, or branchiomotor nerve). It carries no sensory nerve fibers.

    Ptosis (a drooping of the upper eyelid; **choice C**) is the result of a paralysis of the levator palpebrae muscle, which is innervated by the oculomotor (CN III) nerve.

    **Choice D** is not correct because the orbicularis oculi muscle is innervated by branches from the upper division of the facial nerve.

7. **The correct answer is A.** The renal arteries emerge from the abdominal aorta at about the level of the L1/L2 intervertebral disk and travel at nearly right angles to it (on the right, passing posterior to the inferior vena cava) to enter the hilum of the kidney.

The celiac trunk (**choice B**) gives off the common hepatic, splenic, and left gastric arteries.

The common iliac artery (**choice C**) gives off the internal and external iliac arteries. Occasionally, a persistent, supernumerary renal artery may be seen arising from the junction of the abdominal aorta and the common iliac artery. In addition, an unascended pelvic kidney may be supplied by the common iliac artery.

The inferior mesenteric artery (**choice D**) gives off the superior rectal, sigmoid, and left colic arteries.

The superior mesenteric artery (**choice E**) gives off the inferior pancreaticoduodenal, intestinal (ileal and jejunal), right colic, middle colic, and ileocolic arteries.

8. **The correct answer is D.** This is a straightforward question relating to the definition of Nissl bodies. Rough endoplasmic reticulum present in neurons is called Nissl substance, or Nissl bodies. Nissl bodies stain intensely with basic dyes and are found in the cell body and proximal dendrites, but not in the axon hillock or axon.

9. **The correct answer is B.** The recurrent laryngeal nerves are branches of the vagus (CN X), and supply all intrinsic muscles of the larynx except the cricothyroid. The right recurrent laryngeal nerve recurs around the right subclavian artery. The left recurrent laryngeal nerve recurs in the thorax around the arch of the aorta and ligamentum arteriosum. Both nerves ascend to the larynx by passing between the trachea and esophagus, close to the thyroid gland.

The internal laryngeal (**choice A**) nerve is a purely sensory branch of the superior laryngeal nerve.

The thyroarytenoid (**choice C**) is an intrinsic muscle of the larynx; its inner fibers are specialized as the vocalis muscle, which is related to the vocal ligament. It is not usually at risk during thyroid surgery.

The vestibular folds (**choice D**), or false vocal folds, are located superior to the true vocal folds inside the larynx. They are not concerned with phonation.

The vocal folds (**choice E**) form the boundaries of the rima glottidis inside the larynx and are not vulnerable during thyroidectomy.

10. **The correct answer is B.** The bulbourethral glands are paired structures located within the deep perineal pouch, embedded within the sphincter urethrae. Their ducts pass to the spongy urethra. The homologous female structures are the greater vestibular (Bartholin's) glands, which are located in the superficial perineal pouch.

The bulbospongiosus muscles (**choice A**) lie superficial to the bulb of the penis in males and to the bulbs of the vestibule in females.

The corpora cavernosa (**choice C**) are paired structures, consisting of cavernous erectile tissue, that form a large portion of the penile shaft in males and of the body of the clitoris in females.

The membranous urethra (**choice D**) is the portion of the urethra that passes through the urogenital diaphragm in both males and females.

The perineal body (**choice E**) is the centrally located tendinous structure that provides attachment for perineal musculature in both males and females. It separates the urogenital area from the anal area and is an important obstetric landmark.

11. **The correct answer is B.** The odontoid process is the part of the axis (second cervical vertebrae) that fits into and articulates with the atlas (first cervical vertebrae). It is susceptible to traumatic fracture, and bony fragments can injure the spinal cord. The scenario presented is unfortunately realistic, and a similar mechanism is thought to cause deaths by execution-style hanging.

The atlas (**choice A**) is the first cervical vertebra; it receives the odontoid process of the axis.

Fracture of the lower cervical vertebrae (**choices C, D, and E**) does not usually cause sudden death, but may cause paralysis of any or all limbs depending on the amount of damage done.

12. **The correct answer is A.** Each pharyngeal arch has an aortic arch that passes through it. The aortic arches connect the aortic sac with the right and left dorsal aortas. Normally, the left fourth aortic arch is retained as the definitive aortic arch. The right fourth aortic arch normally forms the proximal part of the right subclavian artery. The distal part of this artery is formed by the right seventh intersegmental artery. Normally, most of the right dorsal aorta between these two vessels disappears. The presence of a right aortic arch in addition to the normal left aortic arch indicates that the portion of the right dorsal aorta that should have disappeared did not.

The right fourth aortic arch (**choice B**) normally persists. It forms the proximal part of the right subclavian artery.

The right seventh intersegmental artery (**choice C**) normally persists. It forms the distal part of the right subclavian artery.

The proximal part of the right sixth aortic arch (**choice D**) normally persists. It forms the right pulmonary artery. The distal part of this arch on the right disappears. On the left, the proximal part of the sixth aortic arch becomes the left pulmonary artery, and the distal part persists to become the ductus arteriosus in the fetus and the ligamentum arteriosum postnatally.

The third aortic arches (**choice E**) normally persist. They form the common carotid arteries and the proximal parts of the internal carotid arteries. The distal parts of the internal carotid arteries are formed by the cranial parts of the dorsal aortas. The external carotid arteries arise as branches of the third aortic arches.

13. **The correct answer is B.** Aspiration pneumonia is a common complication observed in nursing home patients. The most probable site of the pneumonia can be anticipated by knowing the anatomy of the bronchial tree, since the aspirated fluid usually flows downhill. In a supine or nearly supine patient, the fluid flows into the trachea and then into either of the (typically the right) main bronchi. The first posteriorly located branch is the one leading to the apical aspect of (either) lower lobe. The lateral and posterior segments of the lower lobes are also supplied by posteriorly branching segmental bronchi. In contrast, the posterior aspects of the upper lobes are somewhat protected by an initial anteriorly directed bifurcation before their segmental bronchi arise. All other segments of the bronchial tree and their corresponding portions of lung are more anterior.

14. **The correct answer is B.** The tumor in question is probably a benign glomus tumor, which is notorious for producing pain far out of proportion to its small size. The question is a little tricky (but important clinically for obvious reasons) because the most distal aspect of the dorsal skin of the fingers, including the nail beds, is innervated by the palmar digital nerves rather than the dorsal digital nerves. Specifically, the median nerve, through its palmar digital nerves, supplies the nail beds of the thumb, index finger, middle finger, and half ring finger.

The axillary nerve (**choice A**), musculocutaneous nerve (**choice C**), and radial nerve (**choice D**) do not supply the nail beds. The radial nerve does supply the more proximal skin of the back of the index finger.

The ulnar nerve (**choice E**) supplies the nail beds of the small finger and half the ring finger.

15. **The correct answer is B.** The epithelial lining of the second pharyngeal pouch buds into the mesenchyme to form the palatine tonsil. Part of the pouch remains in the adult as the tonsillar fossa.

It is important to review the other choices, since pharyngeal pouch derivatives are typically tested on the USMLE Step 1:

The first pharyngeal pouch (**choice A**) develops into the middle ear cavity and eustachian tube.

The third pharyngeal pouch (**choice C**) develops into the thymus and the inferior parathyroid glands.

The fourth pharyngeal pouch (**choice D**) gives rise to the superior parathyroid glands. Recall that abnormal development of the third and fourth pouches leads to DiGeorge syndrome and results in hypocalcemia, as well as abnormal cellular immunity and consequent susceptibility to viral and fungal illnesses.

There is no fifth pharyngeal pouch (**choice E**).

16. **The correct answer is D.** The ureter passes directly inferior to the uterine artery, lateral to the body of the uterus near its junction with the cervix ("water flows under the bridge"). During a hysterectomy, therefore, the ureter (instead of the uterine artery) may be inadvertently ligated.

The internal iliac artery (**choice A**) gives rise to the uterine artery, the primary blood supply of the uterus.

The internal iliac vein (**choice B**) receives blood from the uterine vein (**choice E**), the primary venous drainage of the uterus.

The ovarian artery (**choice C**) arises from the abdominal aorta and is the primary blood supply of the ovaries.

17. **The correct answer is E.** The syncytiotrophoblasts are cells that form a syncytium and invade the endometrium. These cells form the placental villi. The syncytiotrophoblast arises from cells of the cytotrophoblast. The trophoblasts are the outer cells of the blastocyst. Fetal blood and fetal blood vessels develop within the placental villi. These blood vessels later communicate with intraembryonic blood vessels and thereby provide communication between the embryo and the placenta. Maternal blood is found in the intervillous spaces of the placenta. The cells and extracellular matrix of the placental villi form the placental barrier.

The cytotrophoblast (**choice A**) is composed of the mitotically active cells of the outer cell layer of the blastocyst. The cytotrophoblast cells give rise to more cytotrophoblast cells and to syncytiotrophoblast cells. The syncytiotrophoblast cells lose their cell boundaries and thereby form a syncytium. The cytotrophoblast remains mitotically active, whereas the syncytiotrophoblast is mitotically inactive.

The embryoblast (**choice B**) is the name given to the inner cell mass of the blastocyst. These cells form the future embryo, whereas the trophoblast cells of the blastocyst form the fetal portion of the placenta. The embryoblast cells will organize themselves into two layers, called the epiblast and hypoblast.

The endometrium (**choice C**) is the inner lining of the uterus. This is composed entirely of maternal tissue. Implantation occurs when the syncytiotrophoblast cells invade the endometrium.

The epiblast (**choice D**) is the upper layer of embryonic cells in the two-layer embryo. The two-layer embryo forms during the second week of development. The epiblast and hypoblast form from the inner cell mass. All cells of the future embryo are found in the epiblast.

18. **The correct answer is E.** The first two lines of the question clearly suggest a brain tumor. The additional ocular findings (loss of upper gaze and "sunset eyes"—the upper part of the sclera is visible above the downward-looking irises) locate it to the pineal gland area.

The frontal lobe (**choice A**), when pressed on by tumors, produces changes in social behavior and olfactory and visual deficits.

Nelson syndrome (**choice B**) occurs in people who have had bilateral adrenalectomies performed for Cushing disease secondary to a nonresected pituitary microadenoma. The symptom is that of pressure on the chiasma (hemianopsia).

Pituitary apoplexy (**choice C**) occurs when bleeding into an adenoma destroys the pituitary gland. Besides sudden headache, the most notable finding would be shock from adrenal insufficiency.

Posterior fossa tumors (**choice D**) affect equilibrium and gait, in addition to producing visual symptoms.

19. **The correct answer is E.** It is recommended that PSA (prostate-specific antigen) levels be measured annually in men older than 50 to screen for prostatic carcinoma (and to record a baseline level). The prostate is immediately derived from the prostatic urethra, which is derived from the urogenital sinus.

The genital tubercle (**choice A**) gives rise to the glans penis.

The processus vaginalis (**choice B**) is a coelomic extension into the scrotal swelling that carries with it extensions of the body wall to form the inguinal canal during the descent of the testes.

The testis cords (**choice C**) are composed of primitive germ cells, which give rise to spermatogonia, and sex cord cells, which differentiate into Sertoli cells.

The tunica albuginea (**choice D**) is derived from mesenchyme and condenses to form the fibrous connective tissue capsule of the testis.

20. **The correct answer is A.** Because of the proximity of the axillary nerve to the glenohumeral joint, a fracture of the surgical neck of the humerus or an inferior dislocation of the humerus could damage the nerve. The axillary nerve innervates the deltoid muscle. The deltoid abducts, adducts, flexes, extends, and rotates the arm medially. The axillary nerve also innervates the teres minor, which rotates the arm laterally.

The dorsal scapular nerve (**choice B**) innervates both the major and minor rhomboid muscles. These muscles raise the medial border of the scapula upward and retract the scapula.

The radial nerve (**choice C**) innervates muscles involved in extension of the forearm and hand.

The suprascapular nerve (**choice D**) innervates the supraspinatus and infraspinatus. The supraspinatus abducts the arm, whereas the infraspinatus rotates the arm laterally. This nerve travels along the posterior aspect of the scapula and would not easily be subjected to injury in a dislocation of the shoulder joint.

The thoracodorsal nerve (**choice E**) innervates the latissimus dorsi, which adducts, extends, and rotates the arm medially.

21. **The correct answer is C.** The normal atrial septum is formed from the septum primum and septum secundum. The septum secundum covers the foramen secundum within the septum primum. Normally, the prenatal pressure gradient in the atria is from right to left, resulting in a patent foramen ovale. Normally, at birth the pressure gradient reverses and becomes a left-to-right gradient. This causes the septum primum to be pressed against the septum secundum, thus closing the foramen ovale. Fusion of the two septa does not immediately occur. In most people, the two septa eventually fuse; however, the foramen ovale is functionally closed regardless of whether there is fusion or not. When fusion does not occur completely (approximately 10 to 15% of the population), a probe patency of the atrial septum can be found. There is normally no functional significance to this finding inasmuch as there is no shunting of blood across the septum.

Excessive resorption of the septum primum (**choice A**) results in a secundum-type atrial septal defect, a noncyanotic heart defect that results in a postnatal shunting of blood from the left atrium to the right atrium. This shunting may lead to pulmonary hypertension. Normally, a portion of the septum primum is resorbed to form the foramen secundum. This foramen is covered by the septum secundum. If the foramen secundum is too large due to excessive resorption, the septum secundum does not completely cover it, resulting in a secundum-type atrial septal defect.

The endocardial cushions (**choice B**) are ingrowths into the heart tube found at the atrioventricular canal. They cause a narrowing of the wall at this point, resulting in the canals between the atria and the ventricles. The endocardial cushions contribute to the formation of the valves of the heart. They also contribute to the atrial and ventricular septa. Neural crest cells contribute to the endocardial cushions.

The right and left conotruncal ridges (**choice D**) grow in from the wall of the heart tube in the region of the bulbus cordis, and the truncus arteriosus and fuse with one another to form the aorticopulmonary septum. This septum divides the single outflow of the heart, the truncus arteriosus, into two outflow vessels: the ascending aorta and the pulmonary trunk. A failure of the ridges to form and fuse results in a persistent truncus arteriosus, a cyanotic heart defect.

The endocardial cushions fuse with the septum primum of the atrial septum (**choice E**), which thereby closes the foramen primum. Failure of this fusion to occur results in a primum-type atrial septal defect. Because the endocardial cushions also contribute to the valves, there is a high correlation between a primum-type atrial septal defect and a valvular defect.

22. **The correct answer is D.** The right ventricle comprises most of the anterior surface of the heart.

The left atrium (**choice A**) and the left ventricle (**choice B**) are located more posteriorly.

The right atrium (**choice C**) is located more to the right of the sternum.

The stomach (**choice E**) is located more inferiorly and to the left.

23. **The correct response is E.** A ventricular septal defect is the most common congenital cardiac defect and is associated with a loud, holosystolic murmur and is often associated with a thrill.

Patients with atrial septal defects (**choice A**) typically have a systolic flow murmur and a widely split and fixed second heart sound.

Although it can occur in full-term infants, a patent ductus arteriosus (**choice B**) is more commonly seen in premature babies and in cases if maternal rubella infection. Physical findings typically include a continuous murmur and hyperdynamic peripheral pulses.

Typically, children with isolated patent foramen ovale (**choice C**) are asymptomatic and have no physical findings.

Pulmonic stenosis (**choice D**) causes a loud ejection systolic murmur at the upper left sternal border. The pulmonary vascularity is not increased with pulmonic stenosis.

24. **The correct answer is D.** This is the classic presentation of a fracture of the neck of the femur. This type of fracture typically occurs in postmenopausal women with significant bone resorption due to osteoporosis. Dislocation of the head of the femur can produce a similar effect. The change in the position of the leg is due to the action of the gluteal muscles, particularly the gluteus maximus.

Fracture of the femur at the greater trochanter (**choice A**) produces a less dramatic effect, because only the gluteus medius and gluteus minimus attach to it, and the overall structure of the femur remains intact.

Fractures occurring lower in the femur, involving the epicondyles (**choices B and C**) or shaft (**choice E**), would not produce outward rotation of the entire limb.

25. **The correct answer is C.** This medical student has apparently not yet studied the anatomy of the tongue. Otherwise, he would have recognized the large bumps at the back of his tongue as circumvallate papillae. These are large circular structures surrounded by moatlike depressions. The lateral surfaces of these papillae contain taste buds.

Aphthous ulcers (**choice A**) are small, white or red mouth lesions.

Candidal colonies (**choice B**) appear in thrush, which occurs more commonly in the immunocompromised host or in those taking antibacterial drugs. You are told that the patient is healthy and not taking medications, making this condition unlikely.

Filiform papillae (**choice D**) are the most numerous papillae of the tongue. They are elongated cones that create the tongue's rough texture. They do not contain taste buds.

Fungiform papillae (**choice E**) are mushroom-shaped structures scattered among the filiform papillae. They frequently contain taste buds.

26. **The correct answer is E.** The transverse fissure above (between the right upper and right middle lobes) and the oblique fissure below (between the right middle and right lower lobes) are often strikingly visible on the oblique view in patients with right middle lobar pneumonia. The diaphragm and the breast may also be seen but do not overlap the middle lobe on the oblique view.

27. **The correct answer is D.** Injections are given in the upper, outer quadrant of the buttocks to prevent damage to the sciatic nerve, which is present in the lower quadrant. The other nerves listed are not particularly vulnerable to injections into the buttocks.

The common peroneal nerve (**choice A**) is a branch of the sciatic nerve that diverges from it in the popliteal fossa. It then divides into the superficial and deep peroneal nerves.

The lateral femoral cutaneous nerve (**choice B**) derives from the lumbar plexus, emerges slightly below the anterior superior iliac spine, and supplies the skin of the anterior thigh down to the knee.

The obturator nerve (**choice C**) derives from the lumbar plexus, diverges from the femoral nerve in the psoas muscle, and passes medially along the lateral pelvic wall to run in the obturator canal, where it divides into anterior and posterior divisions. The anterior division generally supplies the gracilis, adductor brevis, and adductor longus; the posterior division generally supplies the obturator externus and the adductor part of the adductor magnus.

The superior gluteal nerve (**choice E**) is a branch of the sacral plexus. It supplies the gluteus minimus and medius and the tensor fascia lata. Only small branches of this nerve are likely to be encountered in the upper outer quadrant of the buttock, making injection here relatively safe.

28. **The correct answer is E.** The leakage of cerebrospinal fluid is called otorrhea. This patient's fluid leaked from the subarachnoid space of the middle cranial fossa into the middle ear cavity. From the middle ear cavity, it passed through the ruptured tympanic membrane into the external ear canal. The roof of the middle ear cavity (tegmen tympani) is the floor of the middle cranial fossa along the anterior surface of the petrous portion of the temporal bone. Along with the bony fracture, the dura and underlying arachnoid are torn, providing a direct communication between the subarachnoid space, where the cerebrospinal fluid is found, and the middle ear cavity. The rupture of the tympanic membrane provided access to outside the body. Because of this open communication, there is risk of infection in the cranial cavity.

The internal auditory meatus (**choice A**) is in the posterior cranial fossa, on the posterior surface of the petrous portion of the temporal bone. The internal auditory meatus passes from the posterior cranial fossa to the inner ear. It does not communicate with the middle ear. The seventh and eighth cranial nerves and the labyrinthine artery pass through the internal auditory meatus.

The jugular foramen (**choice B**) is in the floor of the posterior cranial fossa. It is not related to the roof of the middle-ear cavity. The ninth, tenth, and eleventh cranial nerves and the sigmoid sinus and inferior petrosal sinus all pass through the jugular foramen. The jugular foramen communicates between the posterior cranial fossa and the neck.

The external ear canal (**choice C**) does not communicate with the cranial cavity, and a fracture of its wall will not create a communication with the subarachnoid space. The external ear canal is partly cartilaginous and partly bony. It terminates at its medial end, at the tympanic membrane. The canal is the adult derivative of the first pharyngeal cleft.

A fracture of the floor of the anterior cranial fossa (**choice D**) may result in rhinorrhea, a leakage of cerebrospinal fluid into the nasal cavity, if the fracture is near the midline in the region of the cribriform plate. The cribriform plate is the roof of the nasal cavity and part of the floor of the anterior cranial fossa.

29. **The correct answer is A.** A good way to remember what goes through the superior orbital fissure is that everything that innervates orbital structures, other than the optic nerve, passes through this fissure. This includes the oculomotor nerve (CN III), the trochlear nerve (CN IV), the ophthalmic nerve (V1), and the abducens nerve (CN VI).

The facial nerve (CN VII; **choice B**) passes through the internal auditory meatus.

The mandibular nerve (V3; **choice C**) passes through the foramen ovale.

The maxillary nerve (V2; **choice D**) passes through the foramen rotundum.

The middle meningeal artery (**choice E**) passes through the foramen spinosum.

The ophthalmic artery (**choice F**) passes through the optic canal.

The optic nerve (**choice G**) passes through the optic canal.

30. **The correct answer is C.** After crossing the floor of the anatomic snuff box, the radial artery passes deep to the tendon of extensor pollicis longus to enter the palm deeply in the space between the first and second metacarpals (first web space). Within this space, it contributes to the formation of the deep palmar arterial arch.

The deep branch of the radial nerve (**choice A**), or posterior interosseous nerve, supplies the deep muscles of the extensor forearm. It does not enter the palm. The superficial branch of the radial nerve conveys sensory information from the dorsum of the hand, particularly from the skin of the first web space.

The opponens pollicis (**choice B**) arises from the trapezium and the flexor retinaculum. It inserts on the lateral aspect of the first metacarpal and lies deep to abductor pollicis brevis and flexor pollicis brevis in the thenar eminence.

The recurrent branch of the median nerve (**choice D**) supplies the muscles of the thenar eminence. It leaves the median nerve following that nerve's passage through the carpal tunnel, and passes between abductor pollicis brevis and flexor pollicis brevis. It supplies both of these muscles and the opponens pollicis, which lies deep to them. The median nerve also supplies the first two lumbrical muscles.

The superficial palmar arch (**choice E**) is formed mainly by the ulnar artery, with a contribution from the radial artery. It lies more distally in the palm than the deep palmar arch.

31. **The correct answer is E.** This patient has a ruptured spleen. The splenic artery and vein reach the spleen by passing through the splenorenal ligament. A clamp across this ligament will stop the flow of blood to the spleen. The spleen lies under cover of the left ninth, tenth, and eleventh ribs. Fractures of these ribs may cause laceration of the spleen and bleeding into the peritoneal cavity.

The broad ligament (**choice A**) is in the pelvis of the female. It encloses the uterus and contains the uterine tubes and the ovaries. The uterine arteries cross the base of the broad ligament to pass from the internal iliac artery to the cervix of the uterus.

The falciform ligament (**choice B**) is the remnant of the ventral mesentery between the liver and the anterior body wall. During prenatal life, the umbilical vein passes within the falciform ligament. After birth, the umbilical vein becomes fibrous and is called the ligamentum teres.

The gastrosplenic ligament (**choice C**) is the portion of the dorsal mesogastrium between the greater curvature of the stomach and the spleen. There are no major blood vessels passing through the gastrosplenic ligament. This allows the ligament to be used as a surgical access portal into the omental bursa.

The hepatoduodenal ligament (**choice D**) is the portion of the lesser omentum that is along its right free edge. It is attached to the liver and the duodenum. Within the hepatoduodenal ligament are the hepatic artery, portal vein, and common bile duct. Clamping of this ligament will stop blood flow to the liver. This may be done when a patient has a lacerated liver.

32. **The correct answer is A.** The axillary nerve can be damaged during anterior dislocation of the shoulder, causing loss of sensation in the skin overlying the lower half of the deltoid muscle.

The median nerve (**choice B**) supplies sensation to the anterior arm, palm, and distal aspects of the lateral three-and-a-half fingers.

The musculocutaneous nerve (**choice C**) supplies sensation to the lateral surface of the arm and forearm.

The radial nerve (**choice D**) supplies sensation to the back of the arm, forearm, and hand.

The ulnar nerve (**choice E**) supplies sensation to the medial side of the arm, forearm, and hand.

33. **The correct answer is A.** This anatomy question demonstrates the importance of knowing a basic neurologic examination and appropriate sensory dermatomes. This patient has decreased sensation in his C6 dermatome and an asymmetric brachioradialis reflex (C6). Although the C6 root contributes to many different motor functions, wrist extension and elbow flexion are included among them. Motor findings are unilateral for this patient, so only the left C6 root is being compressed. There are other causes of radicular findings, but compression by a cervical disc is by far the most common.

The T1 nerve root supplies sensation to the medial (ulnar) aspect of the arm. It has no reflex to test but does supply the hand intrinsic musculature (interossei). This patient has no findings to suggest T1 (left or right) nerve root compression (**choices B and C**).

The patient has no evidence to suggest a lumbar or sacral tumor, as findings are all in a cervical root distribution (**choices D and E**).

34. **The correct answer is B.** The diaphragm is at particular risk because it is closely related to both the twelfth rib and the suprarenal area. Surgeons sometimes call this the "perilous pleura" because of the care they must exercise with this approach. The close physical relationship also accounts for the pleural effusions seen in some patients with kidney infections. The other structures listed in the answers are not particularly vulnerable during the suggested surgical approach.

35. **The correct answer is C.** The facial nerve passes through the parotid gland and may be injured during a parotidectomy. The facial nerve divides into branches as it passes through the gland. The branches innervate the muscles of facial expression. The branches injured in this patient are likely the buccal and mandibular branches because of the abnormalities seen in the region of the mouth. The zygomatic and temporal branches are probably intact because the patient has normal function in the muscles around the eye and in the forehead.

The mental nerve (**choice A**) is a branch of the mandibular division of the trigeminal nerve and a terminal branch of the inferior alveolar nerve. The mental nerve emerges through the mental foramen in the mandible and provides sensory innervation to the skin of the lower jaw. This patient has normal sensory function, so this nerve was not injured. This nerve is not endangered during a parotidectomy.

The infraorbital nerve (**choice B**) is the terminal branch of the maxillary division of the trigeminal nerve. The maxillary division carries only sensory nerve fibers. The infraorbital nerve emerges through the infraorbital foramen in the maxilla below the orbit and provides sensory innervation to the skin below the eye, above the mouth, and to the lateral side of the nose. This nerve does not pass through the parotid gland.

The glossopharyngeal nerve (**choice D**) provides sensory innervation to the mucosa of the pharynx, the mucosa of the middle ear and the Eustachian tube, and the mucosa of the posterior one third of the tongue. It also provides taste sensation to the posterior one third of the tongue. The glossopharyngeal nerve innervates one skeletal muscle, the stylopharyngeus, which is an elevator of the pharynx. The glossopharyngeal nerve contains preganglionic parasympathetic fibers responsible for the autonomic innervation of the parotid gland. These fibers synapse in the otic ganglion in the infratemporal fossa. The postganglionic parasympathetic nerve fibers from the ganglion reach the parotid gland by traveling with the auriculotemporal nerve, a branch of the mandibular division of the trigeminal nerve.

The hypoglossal nerve (**choice E**) provides motor innervation to the skeletal muscles of the tongue. Injury to this nerve causes the patient to have difficulty in moving the tongue, such as protrusion of the tongue. The nerve does not pass through the parotid gland.

36. **The correct answer is A.** This question could have tricked you if you didn't catch the key words, "in the embryo." If you read the question too quickly and thought you were going to be asked to identify the structure described, you probably chose **choice C** (ligamentum venosum), since that is indeed the structure in question. In the embryo, however, this fibrous band is actually the ductus venosus. The ductus venosus is an embryonic vessel that allows blood to bypass the fetal liver; this prevents the depletion of oxygen and nutrient-rich blood in the hepatic sinusoids.

The embryonic umbilical arteries (**choice D**) become the medial umbilical ligaments.

The embryonic umbilical vein (**choice E**) actually becomes the fibrous ligamentum teres (**choice B**). The ligamentum teres is located in the free margin of the falciform ligament.

37. **The correct answer is A.** The allantoic duct (or allantois) is an evagination of the caudal end of the gut tube. This part of the gut tube becomes the cloaca. The allantoic duct extends into the umbilical cord and, in lower species, serves as a pathway for waste. In humans, it does not serve this function and is vestigial. The anterior portion of the cloaca forms the urinary bladder, and the allantoic duct passes from the bladder into the umbilical cord. Normally, this duct becomes a fibrous cord called the urachus and persists in the adult as the median umbilical ligament. If it remains patent as a duct, urine may pass from the urinary bladder through the duct to the umbilicus. This is called a urachal fistula.

The mesonephric duct (**choice B**) initially serves to carry urine from the embryonic mesonephros to the cloaca. After the formation of the definitive kidney from the metanephric blastema and the ureteric bud, the mesonephric duct no longer serves a function in the urinary system. In the male, it becomes the ductus deferens. In the female, it regresses and has no adult functional remnant.

The mesonephric tubules (**choice C**) are the functional units of the mesonephros when it serves as the embryonic kidney. Later in development, they form the efferent ductules of the male testis and carry spermatozoa from the testis to the epididymis. In the female, they regress and have no functional remnants.

The ureteric bud (**choice D**) is an outgrowth from the caudal end of the mesonephric duct that grows toward the metanephric blastema. The ureteric bud becomes the ureter, renal pelvis, major and minor calyces, and collecting tubules of the kidney. The portion of the mesonephric duct from which the ureteric bud evaginates becomes incorporated into the urinary bladder. Thus, the derivatives of the ureteric bud carry urine from the kidney to the bladder.

The urorectal septum (**choice E**) is a mesodermal septum that grows down into the wall of the caudal gut tube to divide the cloaca into the rectum posteriorly and the urogenital sinus anteriorly.

38. **The correct answer is A.** Children with recurrent urinary tract infections should be further evaluated for renal/urinary tract abnormalities with a voiding cystourethrogram (VCUG). If the VCUG shows no urinary reflux, an ultrasound should be performed to evaluate the upper urinary tract and kidney. If reflux is present, an intravenous pyelogram (IVP) or radionuclide scan may be performed to detect renal scarring. (Note that the number one cause of urinary reflux in children is posterior urethral valves.) A normal IVP would be expected to display normal renal anatomy, in which two cup-shaped major calyces unite to form the renal pelvis.

The minor calyces (**choice B**), of which there are usually 7 to 14, first unite into 2 (sometimes 3) major calyces before emptying into the renal pelvis.

The renal pyramids (**choice C**) represent the region where the collecting tubules of the kidney are located (separated from each other by renal columns in which glomeruli and convoluted tubules are located). At their apices (renal papilla), the collecting tubules constituting the renal pyramids discharge urine into the minor calyces. These collecting tubules are too small to be filled by contrast material in pyelograms; hence, the renal papilla are seen on the IVP as dark, unfilled indentations of the minor calyces.

The ureter (**choice D**) receives urine from the renal pelvis, not the other way around.

39. **The correct answer is C.** Cleft lip is caused by the failure of the maxillary processes to fuse with the medial nasal swellings.

Abnormal development of the third and fourth pharyngeal pouches (**choice A**) can give rise to DiGeorge syndrome, which is characterized by underdevelopment or absence of several structures, including the thymus and parathyroids.

Bony defects of the malar bone and mandible (**choice B**) are associated with mandibulofacial dysostosis, which is mainly due to abnormal development of derivatives of the first arch. This condition is characterized by downward sloping palpebral fissures; hypoplasia of the malar and mandibular bones; macrostomia; high or cleft palate; abnormally shaped, low-set ears; and unusual hair growth patterns. If pits or clefts appear between the mouth and ear, the condition is called Franceschetti syndrome. If the condition is limited to the orbit and malar region, it is termed Treacher-Collins syndrome. Insufficient migration of neural crest cells (**choice E**) is an important factor as well.

When the palatine shelves fail to join together (**choice D**), cleft palate results. Cleft lip and cleft palate commonly co-occur.

40. **The correct answer is C.** The hypoglossal nerve is a pure motor nerve (general somatic efferent) to the intrinsic muscles of the tongue. If the nerve is damaged, denervation atrophy of the affected side will permit the intact musculature of the opposite side to operate unopposed, thereby protruding the tongue to the side of the injury.

The gag reflex (**choice A**) is mediated by the glossopharyngeal nerve (CN IX; afferent limb) and the vagus nerve (CN X; efferent limb).

**Choice B** is incorrect because the preganglionic parasympathetic fibers that regulate these two salivary glands are carried by the chorda tympani (which joins with the lingual nerve) to the submandibular ganglion. Postganglionic fibers are then distributed to these glands.

The muscles responsible for elevation of the pharynx (**choice D**) are innervated primarily by the vagus nerve (CN X).

**Choice E** is incorrect because taste fibers for the anterior two-thirds of the tongue are carried via the chorda tympani to the facial nerve (CN VII) and hence to the brainstem.

41. **The correct answer is B.** The Edinger-Westphal nucleus is found in the midbrain and contains preganglionic parasympathetic cell bodies. The axons of these neurons leave the brain stem with the oculomotor nerve and travel with this nerve through the cavernous sinus to the superior orbital fissure. At the fissure, the oculomotor nerve divides into a superior and inferior division. The preganglionic parasympathetic axons continue with the inferior division. They enter the ciliary ganglion through the motor root of the ganglion and synapse on postganglionic parasympathetic neurons. These postganglionic parasympathetic neurons innervate the smooth muscle of the sphincter pupillae found in the iris.

The oculomotor nucleus (**choice A**) is in the midbrain and contains cell bodies of somatic motor neurons that innervate skeletal muscle cells of several extraocular muscles. The superior division of the oculomotor nerve innervates the superior rectus muscle and the levator palpebrae superioris muscle. The inferior division of the oculomotor nerve innervates the inferior rectus muscle, the medial rectus muscle, and the inferior oblique muscle.

The ciliary ganglion (**choice C**) is found in the orbit lateral to the optic nerve. The ganglion contains postganglionic parasympathetic cell bodies. These neurons are synapsed upon by preganglionic neurons from the Edinger-Westphal nucleus. The postganglionic neurons have axons that leave the ciliary ganglion through the short ciliary nerves and go to the eyeball. Within the eye these neurons innervate the smooth muscle of the sphincter pupillae muscle of the iris, which are responsible for pupillary constriction, and the smooth muscle of the ciliary muscles in the ciliary bodies, which are responsible for accommodation of the lens.

The precentral gyrus (**choice D**) is in the cerebral cortex. The neurons of the precentral gyrus are the upper motor neurons responsible for volitional control of skeletal muscle. The axons from these neurons descend through the corticospinal and corticobulbar tracts to the lower motor neurons in the spinal cord and brain stem, respectively.

The geniculate ganglion (**choice E**) is the sensory ganglion of the facial nerve. The ganglion is found in the temporal bone. The geniculate ganglion contains pseudounipolar cell bodies of the sensory neurons found in the facial nerve. These sensory neurons provide general sensory innervation to the skin on the posterior side of the external ear; special sensory taste innervation to the anterior two thirds of the tongue; and visceral afferent innervation from the submandibular, sublingual, and lacrimal glands and the mucosal glands of the oral, nasal, and pharyngeal mucosa.

42. **The correct answer is E.** Bone is formed by type I collagen fibers, ground substance, and hydroxyapatite crystals. The collagen is oriented in a layered or lamellar fashion. It can be parallel (trabecular bone and periosteum) or concentric (Haversian system). When bone is formed quickly, as in a healing fracture site, metabolic bone disease, or tumor, the collagen is randomly oriented and is called woven bone.

    Compact bone (**choice B**) is the dense calcified external part of the bone. It is lamellar bone.

    Cancellous (**choice A**), spongy (**choice C**), and trabecular (**choice D**) bone are all synonymous terms for the thinner network of bone within the cortex. These are also lamellar bone.

43. **The correct answer is E.** All three structures lie in the subcostal groove below a rib. Third- and fourth-year students are sometimes offered the chance to help tap a patient's pleural effusion, and can look a little foolish if the resident has to stop them because they have forgotten this basic anatomic point and have entered the intercostal space in the middle or upper region.

44. **The correct answer is B.** The infant has Hirschsprung disease (more common in males), a diagnosis that should spring to mind in an infant who fails to pass meconium soon after birth and presents with chronic constipation. Diagnosis is made most easily and most reliably by anal manometry and/or rectal biopsy. On manometry, internal anal sphincter pressure increases on rectal balloon distention in patients with Hirschsprung disease (normally, pressure decreases with distention). Rectal biopsy reveals an absence of ganglion cells (which are derived from neural crest cells) in a portion of the colonic wall. Barium enema would show a transition zone between the aganglionic area of bowel (narrow) and the region of normal bowel proximal to it (dilated).

    Defective recanalization of the colon (**choice A**) results in rectal atresia. In this condition, there is no communication between the rectum and anal canal. Therefore, neither meconium nor stool can be passed.

    Herniation of abdominal contents into the umbilical cord (**choice C**) describes a congenital omphalocele. This occurs because of the failure of all or part of the intestines to return into the abdominal cavity during the tenth week of gestation.

Persistence of the proximal end of the yolk stalk (**choice D**) results in Meckel diverticulum, an ileal outpouching that is more prevalent in males. It usually contains ectopic gastric mucosa, which can cause ulceration and bleeding. Inflammation of the diverticulum may produce symptoms and signs similar to appendicitis.

The presence of a rectourinary fistula (**choice E**) would result in the passage of meconium, stool, and gas into the urine.

45. **The correct answer is D.** The clinical findings indicate that the radial nerve has been injured. The radial nerve innervates all of the posterior muscles of the forearm. The paralysis of these muscles prevents the patient from extending the hand at the wrist. The radial nerve also provides sensory innervation to the skin of the dorsum of the hand in the region of the lateral three and one-half digits. The radial nerve injury results in the diminished sensation in this region. The radial nerve passes through the arm in close proximity to the midshaft of the radius. The musculospiral groove of the radius has the radial nerve and the deep brachial artery lying in it. Fracture of the midshaft of the humerus endangers the radial nerve.

    The scaphoid (**choice A**) is a carpal bone. It is the most lateral of the proximal row of carpal bones. The scaphoid articulates with the distal end of the radius and is the most commonly fractured carpal bone. The injury typically occurs when the patient falls on the outstretched hand and force is transferred from the hand across the scaphoid to the radius. Nerve injuries do not typically accompany this fracture. Avascular necrosis of the proximal head of the scaphoid is a clinical concern with this type of fracture.

    Fracture of the distal end of the radius (**choice B**) is often called a Colles fracture. This fracture usually occurs by falling on the outstretched hand. Nerve injuries do not typically accompany this fracture, but if a nerve is injured, it is likely to be the median nerve.

    The nerve in close proximity to the medial epicondyle of the humerus (**choice C**) is the ulnar nerve. The ulnar nerve can be injured by direct blunt trauma to the medial side of the elbow. If the ulnar nerve is injured at this site, the patient would be able to extend at the wrist but would have weakness in flexing the wrist, and the hand would deviate radially upon flexion at the wrist. The patient would have normal sensation on the lateral portion of the dorsum of the hand but diminished sensation on the medial portion of the dorsal and palmar aspect of the hand.

    Fracture of the surgical neck of the humerus (**choice E**) would endanger the axillary nerve, which lies against the surgical neck as it passes through the posterior wall of the axilla. The axillary nerve innervates the deltoid muscle. Injury to this nerve would result in weakness in abduction at the shoulder and a region of diminished sensation on the skin overlying the deltoid muscle.

46. **The correct answer is A.** Bregma represents the point where the coronal and sagittal sutures intersect; it is the site of the anterior fontanelle.

    The coronal suture (**choice B**) lies between the frontal and parietal bones.

    Lambda (**choice C**) represents the point where the sagittal and lambdoid sutures intersect; it is the site of the posterior fontanelle in infants.

    The pterion (**choice D**) is the point on the lateral aspect of the skull where the greater wing of the sphenoid, parietal, frontal, and temporal bones converge. Recall that the pterion is the landmark for the middle meningeal artery and that a blow to the temple (e.g., as could occur in boxing) can lead to a middle meningeal arterial bleed and an epidural hemorrhage.

    The sagittal suture (**choice E**) is located between the two parietal bones.

47. **The correct answer is E.** Blue hematoxylin binds to polyanions such as RNA and DNA. Nuclei contain large amounts of DNA and RNA, and they are consequently almost always blue. The nuclei of dysplastic and cancerous cells are often enlarged and hyperchromatic (e.g., darker blue) compared with normal cells of similar cell lines, because these altered cells often have extra DNA (are aneuploid) and/or RNA (are metabolically active).

    Pink eosin binds relatively nonselectively to cellular components, particularly proteins. Cytoplasm of different cell lines can be pink, purple, or blue, depending principally on the number of ribosomes in the cytoplasm. Consequently, blue-tinged cytoplasm tends to suggest high synthetic activity (i.e., abundant ribosomes).

48. **The correct answer is F.** This patient has coarctation of the aorta (constriction of the ascending aorta), which is suggested by a midsystolic murmur over the anterior part of the chest and back, hypertension in the upper extremities, and absent or delayed pulsations in the femoral arteries. The upper extremities and thorax may be more developed than the lower extremities. Patients with coarctation of the aorta may experience symptoms such as cold extremities as a result of tissue ischemia. The truncus arteriosus gives rise to the proximal portions of the ascending aorta and the pulmonary trunk. The third, fourth, and sixth aortic arches and the right and left dorsal aortae contribute to the remainder of the aorta.

The bulbus cordis (**choice A**) gives rise to the right ventricle and the aortic outflow tract.

In 98% of cases, coarctation of the aorta takes place immediately distal to the offshoot of the left subclavian artery, close to the junction of the ductus arteriosus (**choice B**) with the aorta.

The left horn of the sinus venosus (**choice C**) gives rise to the coronary sinus.

The right common cardinal vein (**choice D**) gives rise to the superior vena cava.

The right horn of the sinus venosus (**choice E**) gives rise to the smooth part of the right atrium.

49. **The correct answer is C.** The submucosa and mucosa lining the inside of the bladder are highly folded when the bladder is empty, but are loosely adherent to the underlying muscle and move against each other, smoothing the folds of the bladder wall as it fills. The only site where the attachment of mucosa to muscle is tight is the triangularly shaped trigone of the bladder, located on the posterior bladder floor (i.e., posterior and inferior). The internal wall here is smooth even when the bladder is empty. All ducts that open into the bladder (including the internal ureteric orifices) do so at the angles of the trigone; hence, they are not stretched or pulled by the movement of the bladder wall as the bladder fills. In the distended bladder, the internal ureteric openings are approximately 5 cm apart.

50. **The correct answer is D.** The somitomeres are specialized masses of mesoderm found in the head region that give rise to the muscles of the head. The extraocular muscles are derived from somitomeres 1, 2, 3, and 5.

    The branchial arches (**choice A**) give rise to muscles of mastication (arch 1), muscles of facial expression (arch 2), and muscles of the pharynx and larynx (arches 3-6), as well as additional small muscles.

    The optic cup ectoderm (**choice B**) gives rise to the muscles of the iris (sphincter and dilator pupillae). These are the only muscles not formed from mesoderm.

    Somites (**choice C**) give rise to the inferior muscles of the neck.

    Splanchnic mesoderm (**choice E**) gives rise to smooth muscle of the viscera and the heart muscle.

# Physiology: **Test One**

1. A 42-year-old woman complains of a burning pain in the upper middle region of her abdomen. The pain usually occurs about 2 hours after a meal and frequently awakens her at night. Antacids can usually relieve the pain within a few minutes. An x-ray film reveals a typical duodenal ulcer identified as a discrete crater in the proximal portion of the duodenal bulb. Because the woman does not have a history of chronic use of aspirin or other nonsteroidal antiinflammatory drugs (NSAIDs), the bacterium *Helicobacter pylori* is assumed to be the major factor in the etiology of the ulcer. Which of the following is likely to be normal in this woman?

   (A) Basal acid output

   (B) Fasting serum gastrin

   (C) Gastrin response to a meal

   (D) Maximal acid output

   (E) Parietal cell mass

   (F) Pepsin secretion

2. A series of photographs taken of a middle-aged man over a period of 2 decades demonstrates gradual coarsening of facial features and progressive protrusion of the brows. Upon questioning, the patient reports having to wear larger shoes than he did as a young man. Which of the following pair of hormones normally regulates the hormone responsible for these changes?

   (A) Dopamine and norepinephrine

   (B) LH and hCG

   (C) Prolactin and FSH

   (D) Somatostatin and GHRH

   (E) TSH and ACTH

3. Given these data below, what is the net filtration pressure at the glomerulus?

   Glomerular hydrostatic pressure = 44 mm Hg
   Bowman's capsule hydrostatic pressure = 9 mm Hg
   Osmotic pressure of plasma = 28 mm Hg
   Osmotic pressure of tubular fluid = 0

   (A) −5 mm Hg

   (B) 7 mm Hg

   (C) 25 mm Hg

   (D) 63 mm Hg

   (E) 81 mm Hg

4. A 50-year-old woman undergoes surgery to remove a large abdominal tumor. Histologic findings show that the mass contains a large number of blood vessels. Several metastases were found 2 months after surgery. A decrease in which of the following is the most likely cause for the development of metastases after the removal of the large tumor?

   (A) Basic fibroblast growth factor (bFGF)

   (B) Endostatin

   (C) Growth hormone

   (D) Platelet-derived growth factor (PDGF)

   (E) Transforming growth factor (TGF-β)

   (F) Vascular endothelial growth factor (VEGF)

5. A 48-year-old man presents to the emergency department with chest pain that radiates to his jaw and left shoulder. Angina pectoris is suspected, and he is sent for an angiogram. The test reveals an atherosclerotic coronary artery that is 50% occluded. The maximal blood flow through this artery is reduced by

   (A) 1/2

   (B) 1/4

   (C) 1/8

   (D) 1/16

   (E) 1/32

6. A 24-year-old man becomes paraplegic after he severs his spinal cord at T1 in an automobile accident. Chronic constipation is a problem, but he wants to be as independent as possible in its treatment. His physician advises him to distend the rectum digitally on a regular schedule to initiate the defecation reflex. Rectal distention causes which of the following in this patient?

   (A) A deep breath

   (B) Closure of the glottis

   (C) Contraction of the internal anal sphincter

   (D) Increased abdominal pressure

   (E) Increased peristaltic waves

   (F) Relaxation of the external anal sphincter

7. A 14-year-old boy has a craniotomy performed under general endotracheal anesthesia for removal of a craniopharyngioma. The anesthetic agent used is halothane, and when he is fully awake in the recovery room, he is extubated and sent to the floor. Five percent dextrose in one-third normal saline was dripping in his intravenous line at a rate of 125 mL/h. Four hours later, the nurses report that he cannot be roused from a deep sleep. They also point out that his urinary output in each of those 4 hours was 1050, 1100, 980, and 1250 mL, respectively. Laboratory studies show:

   | | |
   |---|---|
   | Sodium | 156 mEq/L |
   | Osmolarity | 312 mOsm/L |
   | pH | 7.55 |
   | $p_{CO_2}$ | 28 mm Hg |
   | Bicarbonate | 24 mEq/L |

   Which of the following best explains these findings?

   (A) Brain edema

   (B) Nephrogenic diabetes insipidus

   (C) Respiratory depression induced by unmetabolized anesthetic

   (D) Surgical trauma to the posterior pituitary

   (E) Water retention

8. A 26-year-old woman is stranded for more than a week when her hiking trip is interrupted by an avalanche. Because she expected to be gone for only a few hours, she did not bring along any food. Which of the following substances can be converted to glucose to supply the needs of the brain during this period?

   (A) Acetoacetate

   (B) Acetone

   (C) Amino acids

   (D) Beta-hydroxybutyrate

   (E) Fatty acids

9. A 54-year-old man is seen in clinic with complaints of palpitations and light-headedness. Physical examination is remarkable for a heart rate of greater than 200/min and a blood pressure of 75/40 mm Hg. Which of the following adjustments have probably occurred in the cardiac cycle?

   (A) Diastolic time has decreased and systolic time has increased

   (B) Diastolic time has decreased but systolic time has decreased more

   (C) Systolic time has decreased and diastolic time has increased

   (D) Systolic time has decreased but diastolic time has decreased more

   (E) Systolic time has decreased but diastolic time has not changed

10. A 25-year-old man visits a friend living in a mountain cabin at an altitude of 5000 meters. After 5 days, he has an increase in ventilation rate and a decrease in arterial $P_{CO_2}$. Which of the following physiologic changes is also expected?

   (A) Decreased production of erythropoietin

   (B) Decreased 2,3-diphosphoglycerate (2,3-DPG)

   (C) Increased renal excretion of $H^+$ ions

   (D) Increased renal excretion of $HCO_3^-$

   (E) Pulmonary vasodilation

11. As part of an experimental study, a volunteer agrees to have 10 g mannitol injected intravenously. After sufficient time for equilibration, blood is drawn, and the concentration of mannitol in the plasma is found to be 65 mg/100 mL. Urinalysis reveals that 10% of the mannitol had been excreted into the urine during this time period. What is the approximate extracellular fluid volume of this volunteer?

    (A) 10 L

    (B) 14 L

    (C) 22 L

    (D) 30 L

    (E) 42 L

12. A neurophysiologist is studying the functional properties of various receptor subtypes, using whole-cell voltage clamp recordings made from coronal brain slices. At a holding potential of –70 mV, bath application of receptor agonists for four different receptor types consistently elicited either excitatory postsynaptic currents or inhibitory postsynaptic currents. During the study of one receptor, however, agonist application failed to elicit a postsynaptic response at –70 mV but did elicit a reliable response at a holding potential of 0 mV. This receptor is most likely which of the following?

    (A) Gamma-amino-butyric acid $(GABA)_A$

    (B) Kainate

    (C) Nicotinic acetylcholine

    (D) *N*-methyl-D-aspartate (NMDA)

    (E) Serotonin 3 $(5-HT_3)$

13. A researcher is carrying out an experiment on an anesthetized animal to study the cardiovascular and neural responses to various types of stimuli. His experimental setup allows him to measure blood pressure and monitor the electrocardiogram. He carefully isolates the afferent nerves from the carotid sinus and aortic arch and implants microelectrodes to record nerve activity. After taking baseline measurements, he massages the right carotid artery for 60 seconds. Which of the following data sets corresponds best to his experimental findings during the carotid massage?

    (HR = heart rate, BP = blood pressure, FR IX = firing rate of glossopharyngeal afferents, FR X = firing rate of vagal afferents)

**(A)**
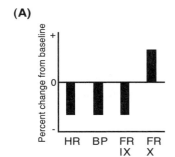

**(B)**
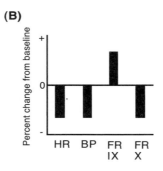

**(C)**
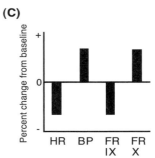

**(D)**
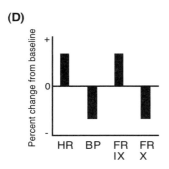

**(E)**
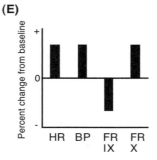

**(F)**
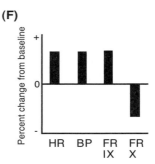

14. In clinical trials, an experimental drug is found to cause impotence in a large percentage of male patients. Inhibition of which of the following could be responsible for this side effect?

    (A) Conversion of DHT to testosterone

    (B) Forward motility factor

    (C) Nitric oxide synthase (NOS)

    (D) Oxytocin

    (E) Prostaglandins

15. A healthy 22-year-old female medical student has an exercise stress test at a local health club. Which of the following is most likely to decrease in her skeletal muscles during exercise?

    (A) Arteriolar resistance

    (B) Carbon dioxide concentration

    (C) Lactic acid concentration

    (D) Sympathetic nervous activity

    (E) Vascular conductance

16. A young man goes to the gym on his way home from work. He runs on the treadmill for 30 minutes, lifts weights for 20 minutes, and does push-ups and sit-ups for 10 minutes. Which of the following is quantitatively the most important method for transporting the $CO_2$ in the blood that is produced by his muscles?

    (A) As carbaminohemoglobin

    (B) As $CO_2$ in gas bubbles

    (C) As $CO_2$ in physical solution

    (D) As bicarbonate in red cells

    (E) As bicarbonate in serum

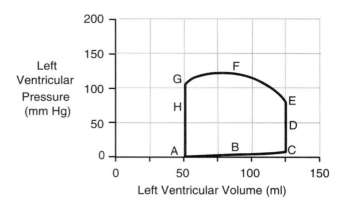

17. A volume-pressure diagram of the left ventricle during one cardiac cycle of a normal heart is shown above. Which point on the diagram marks the beginning of ventricular systole?

    (A) A

    (B) B

    (C) C

    (D) D

    (E) E

    (F) F

    (G) G

    (H) H

18. A 43-year-old man with a recurrent history of ulcer disease associated with diarrhea and a strong family history of duodenal ulcer disease is suspected of having Zollinger-Ellison syndrome (gastrinoma). Secretin (1 U/kg) is given as a rapid intravenous injection to test for gastrinoma. Which of the following results would support the existence of gastrinoma following secretin administration?

    (A) Gastrin release from antrum

    (B) Increased serum gastrin

    (C) Inhibition of gastric emptying

    (D) Inhibition of gastric secretion

    (E) Stimulation of pancreatic $HCO_3^-$ secretion

19. Medical students are studying the clearance of inulin by the kidneys on a computer-simulated patient. The professor programs the computer so that the patient's ratio of urinary concentration to plasma concentration of inulin ([U/P] inulin) decreases. Which of the following is true if the glomerular filtration rate remains constant?

    (A) Aldosterone levels have increased

    (B) Inulin clearance has decreased

    (C) Positive free water clearance has decreased

    (D) Reabsorption of inulin has increased

    (E) Urine flow rate has increased

20. Blood is drawn from a 14-year-old boy with bacterial meningitis for a complete blood count. The leukocyte count is elevated. Which of the following is released by the predominant type of white blood cell present?

    (A) Histamine

    (B) Leukotrienes

    (C) Lysozyme

    (D) Peroxidase

    (E) Vasoactive amines

21. A 21-year-old man is competing in a weight-lifting competition. He lifts 325 lb over his head and holds it there for 5 seconds. Suddenly, his arms give way and he drops the weight to the floor. Which of the following receptors is responsible for this sudden muscle relaxation?

    (A) Free nerve ending

    (B) Golgi tendon organ

    (C) Merkel disk

    (D) Muscle spindle

    (E) Pacinian corpuscle

22. A 16-year-old type 1 diabetic is noncompliant with his required insulin therapy and develops hyperglycemia after eating several pieces of hard candy. The release of which of the following intestinal hormones would most likely be stimulated?

    (A) Gastric inhibitory peptide (GIP)

    (B) Gastrin

    (C) Motilin

    (D) Secretin

    (E) Somatostatin

    (F) Substance P

    (G) Vasoactive intestinal polypeptide (VIP)

23. A 69-year-old alcoholic has had severe, progressively increasing epigastric pain for the past 24 hours. He has been nauseous, and he vomited three times. Laboratory studies show hypocalcemia and metabolic hypochloremic alkalosis. The primary metabolic effect of the principal hormone secreted by the alpha cells of this organ is

    (A) augmentation of calcium deposition in bone

    (B) increase of amino acid storage in the liver

    (C) promotion of lipogenesis in liver and adipose tissue

    (D) inhibition of gluconeogenesis

    (E) stimulation of glycogenolysis

24. A researcher is studying the substance para-aminohippuric acid (PAH) and its interaction with the kidneys. She injects a volunteer with the substance. She finds that which of the following can be determined by calculating the clearance of PAH?

    (A) Extracellular fluid (ECF) volume

    (B) Effective renal plasma flow (ERPF)

    (C) Glomerular filtration rate (GFR)

    (D) Plasma volume

    (E) Total body water (TBW)

25. A 57-year-old woman with a 30-year history of alcoholism and liver disease visits her physician complaining of abdominal swelling and shortness of breath. The physician determines that she has severe ascites. Which of the following factors contributes to the accumulation of fluid in the abdominal cavity?

    (A) Decreased plasma epinephrine and norepinephrine

    (B) Decreased plasma volume

    (C) Increased hepatic lymph flow

    (D) Increased hydrostatic pressure in splanchnic capillary beds

    (E) Increased natriuresis

    (F) Increased plasma albumin concentration

    (G) Increased plasma oncotic pressure

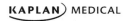

26. A 33-year-old man complains that his chest hurts when he eats, especially when he eats meat. An x-ray film shows a dilated esophagus, and achalasia is suspected. Esophageal manometry is used to confirm the diagnosis. Swallowing induced relaxation is reduced at which anatomic location in this man?

    (A) Lower esophageal sphincter
    (B) Lower esophagus
    (C) Middle esophagus
    (D) Pharynx
    (E) Upper esophageal sphincter
    (F) Upper esophagus

27. A substance that is filtered, but not secreted or reabsorbed (substance X), is infused into a volunteer until a steady state plasma level of 0.1 mg/mL is achieved. The subject then empties his bladder and waits 1 hour, at which time he urinates again. The volume of urine in the second specimen is 60 mL, and the concentration of substance X is 10 mg/mL. What is the glomerular filtration rate (GFR) in this individual?

    (A) 30 mL/min
    (B) 60 mL/min
    (C) 100 mL/min
    (D) 300 mL/min
    (E) 600 mL/min

28. A 40-year-old man with sleep apnea participates in a sleep study. During his evaluation, normal sawtooth waves are observed on his EEG tracing. This pattern is associated with which period of sleep?

    (A) REM
    (B) Stage 1
    (C) Stage 2
    (D) Stage 3
    (E) Stage 4

29. A 48-year-old white female secretary presents with progressive difficulty typing over the past month. She also notes that her hands begin to feel numb and weak after typing for long periods of time. On testing, which of the following deficits would be predicted?

    (A) Difficulty in abducting the fifth finger
    (B) Difficulty in adducting the thumb
    (C) Difficulty in flexing digits two and three at the metacarpophalangeal joints
    (D) Loss of sensation over the lateral half of the dorsum of the hand
    (E) Loss of sensation over the lateral half of the palm
    (F) Loss of sensation over the medial half of the dorsum of the hand
    (G) Loss of sensation over the medial half of the palm

30. A 70-year-old woman undergoes a gastrectomy for Zollinger-Ellison syndrome. Her physician informs her that she will need to take intramuscular vitamin $B_{12}$ shots for the rest of her life. Absence of which of the following cell types is responsible for this vitamin replacement requirement?

    (A) Chief cells
    (B) G cells
    (C) Goblet cells
    (D) Mucous neck cells
    (E) Parietal cells

31. A 32-year-old man visits the physician for a periodic health maintenance examination. He has no complaints at this time. He is 170 cm (5 ft 7 in) tall and weighs 75 kg (165 lb). Physical examination is unremarkable. In this patient, the volumes of total body water, intracellular fluid, and extracellular fluid are, respectively,

    (A) 40 L, 30 L, 10 L
    (B) 45 L, 30 L, 15 L
    (C) 45 L, 35 L, 10 L
    (D) 50 L, 25 L, 25 L
    (E) 50 L, 35 L, 15 L

32. A 35-year-old, sexually active woman visits her gynecologist complaining of mild, right-sided, lower abdominal pain but no other symptoms. There are no peritoneal signs. Her surgical history is significant for an appendectomy at age 10. Her last period occurred 14 days ago. Which of the following endometrial changes corresponds to this stage of the patient's menstrual cycle?

(A) Apical movement of secretions in the glandular cells

(B) Degeneration of the glandular structures

(C) Glandular glycogen accumulation in the functionalis

(D) Growth of the spiral arteries

(E) Tissue expansion by cellular hypertrophy

33. A 71-year-old woman undergoes an elective sigmoid resection for recurrent diverticulitis. On the second postoperative day, it is noted that her urinary output is averaging only 35 to 45 mL/h. She is receiving 5% dextrose in half normal saline at a rate of 100 mL/h. The intravenous rate of infusion is increased to 125 mL/h. Two days later, her urinary output becomes 15 to 25 mL/h. A sample of urine shows a urinary sodium concentration of 85 mEq/L. Laboratory studies show the systemic arterial values as follows:

| | |
|---|---|
| pH | 7.25 |
| $pCO_2$ | 30 mm Hg |
| Bicarbonate | 15 mEq/L |
| Potassium | 5.8 mEq/L |
| BUN | 85 mg/dL |
| Creatinine | 5.1 mg/dL |

Which of the following is the most likely diagnosis?

(A) Acute renal failure

(B) Excessive sodium intake

(C) Fluid volume deficit

(D) Surgical ligation of both ureters

(E) Ureteroenteric fistula

34. A 47-year-old recent immigrant from Africa has significant edema of the left lower extremity. A polymerase chain reaction assay for DNA of *Wucheria bancrofti* is positive. Which sequence of the numbered statements below correctly describes the pathway of the flow from the affected system on the affected side of the body?

1) Junction of left internal jugular and left subclavian

2) Lymph capillaries

3) Thin lymph vessels

4) Thoracic duct

(A) 2-1-3-4

(B) 2-3-1-4

(C) 2-3-4-1

(D) 2-4-1-3

(E) 2-4-3-1

35. The following data were collected from a normal patient before and after an intervention. Assume that plasma osmolarity and glomerular filtration rate remain constant.

| | **Before** | **After** |
|---|---|---|
| Urine osmolarity (mOsm/L) | 900 | 250 |
| Urine flow rate (mL/min) | 0.65 | 2.3 |
| Fractional clearance of sodium | 1% | 1% |
| Osmolar clearance (mL/min) | 2.0 | 2.0 |

The intervention that would best account for the observed changes is

(A) administration of furosemide

(B) administration of hydrochlorothiazide

(C) administration of lithium

(D) a high dietary intake of potassium

(E) a transfusion of 2 L isotonic saline

36. An unlabeled container of blood product is left in a laboratory. The technician must determine whether the sample is serum or plasma. An elevated level of which of the following substances would identify the specimen as plasma?

    (A) Albumin

    (B) Erythrocytes

    (C) Fibrinogen

    (D) Granulocytes

    (E) Serotonin

37. A Swan-Ganz catheter inserted into a patient with acute respiratory distress syndrome (ARDS) records a pulmonary artery wedge pressure of 6 mm Hg. The same pressure would be expected in which of the following structures?

    (A) Aorta

    (B) Left atrium

    (C) Left ventricle

    (D) Right atrium

    (E) Systemic veins

38. A hysterical patient is hyperventilating and doubles his alveolar ventilation. If his initial alveolar $P_{A}CO_2$ was 40 mm Hg, and his $CO_2$ production remains unchanged, what will his alveolar $P_{CO_2}$ be on hyperventilation?

    (A) 80 mm Hg

    (B) 60 mm Hg

    (C) 20 mm Hg

    (D) 10 mm Hg

    (E) 4 mm Hg

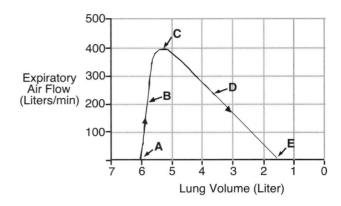

39. The maximum expiratory flow-volume curve shown above was obtained from a normal, healthy volunteer. Which point on the curve represents residual volume?

    (A) A

    (B) B

    (C) C

    (D) D

    (E) E

40. A 42-year-old obese woman experiences episodic abdominal pain. She notes that the pain increases after the ingestion of a fatty meal. The action of which of the following hormones is responsible for the postprandial intensification of her symptoms?

    (A) Cholecystokinin (CCK)

    (B) Gastrin

    (C) Pepsin

    (D) Secretin

    (E) Somatostatin

41. In a normal patient, if renal vascular resistance is decreased to 50% of its initial value, with no change in renal artery or renal vein pressure, which of the following combinations of changes will occur?

|  | Renal Blood Flow | Renal Artery [$O_2$] | Renal $O_2$ Use |
|---|---|---|---|
| (A) | double | increase | no change |
| (B) | double | no change | increase |
| (C) | increase 50% | decrease | increase |
| (D) | increase 50% | increase | no change |
| (E) | decrease 50% | no change | decrease |

42. A 61-year-old woman develops purple striae on her abdomen and a rounded facial appearance. She has smoked two packs of cigarettes a day for the past 40 years. Chest x-ray shows a 4-cm, centrally located lung mass. This mass is most likely producing a hormone that promotes the production of cortisol by stimulating which of the following reactions?

    (A) 11-Deoxycortisol to cortisol

    (B) 17-Hydroxyprogesterone to 11-deoxycortisol

    (C) Cholesterol to pregnenolone

    (D) Pregnenolone to progesterone

    (E) Progesterone to 17-hydroxyprogesterone

43. A 69-year-old man presents with unilateral hearing loss. A lesion in which of the following structures could be responsible for this loss?

    (A) Inferior colliculus

    (B) Lateral lemniscus

    (C) Medial geniculate body

    (D) Medial lemniscus

    (E) Organ of Corti

    (F) Superior olivary nucleus

44. A young boy presents with failure to thrive. Biochemical analysis of a duodenal aspirate after a meal reveals a deficiency of enteropeptidase (enterokinase). The levels of which the following digestive enzymes would be affected?

    (A) Amylase

    (B) Colipase

    (C) Lactase

    (D) Pepsin

    (E) Trypsin

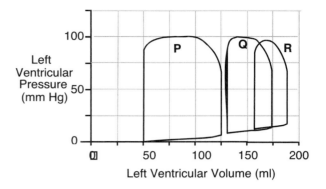

45. Above are volume-pressure diagrams (work diagrams) depicting changes in left ventricular volume and pressure during one cardiac cycle for a normal heart, a failing heart, and a failing heart after treatment with digitalis. Which of the following best describes the relationship of the volume-pressure diagrams with the stated conditions?

|  | Normal | Before Digitalis | After Digitalis |
|---|---|---|---|
| (A) | P | Q | R |
| (B) | P | R | Q |
| (C) | Q | R | P |
| (D) | R | P | Q |
| (E) | R | Q | P |

46. A 45-year-old man has a blood pressure reading of 160/100 mm Hg on three separate visits. He refuses to take antihypertensive medication but is willing to modify his lifestyle in an effort to lower his blood pressure. He quits smoking, joins a health club, and greatly reduces salt from his diet. Which of the following areas of the adrenal gland would be expected to increase in activity because of his diet?

    (A) Adrenal medulla

    (B) Zona fasciculata of the adrenal cortex

    (C) Zona glomerulosa of the adrenal cortex

    (D) Zona reticularis of the adrenal cortex

47. A medical student is studying the fluid exchange in skeletal muscle capillaries in a laboratory animal. He determines that fluid is being forced out of a capillary with a net filtration pressure of 8 mm Hg, and he obtains the following laboratory values:

| | |
|---|---|
| Capillary hydrostatic pressure | 24 mm Hg |
| Capillary colloid osmotic pressure | 17 mm Hg |
| Interstitial hydrostatic pressure | 7 mm Hg |

Which of the following is the interstitial osmotic pressure?

(A) −9 mm Hg

(B) −6 mm Hg

(C) 6 mm Hg

(D) 8 mm Hg

(E) 9 mm Hg

48. A 37-year-old woman has been trying to get pregnant for the past 16 months. Just as she is about to schedule an appointment with a fertility specialist, she gets a premonition that she is pregnant, despite a negative home pregnancy test 7 days earlier. By the time of implantation in the uterine endometrium, the typical fertilized ovum has divided into how many cells?

(A) 2

(B) 4

(C) 8

(D) 16

(E) >50

49. A 24-year-old woman suffers from epistaxis, gingival bleeding, and menorrhagia. Her mother and grandmother have similar symptoms, and her brother has incisional bleeding after surgery and dental extractions. They all have similar laboratory findings, including a prolonged bleeding time, reduced levels of factor VIII antigen, normal platelet aggregation, and reduced ristocetin cofactor activity. This family has disorder characterized by a deficient or defective protein. In normal patients, which of the following binds to the affected protein at the platelet membrane?

(A) Adenosine diphosphate (ADP)

(B) Calcium

(C) Glycoprotein GPIb

(D) Platelet factor 3 (PF3)

(E) Prostacyclin

(F) Serotonin

(G) Thromboplastin

(H) Thromboxane $A_2$

50. A 25-year-old woman involved in an automobile accident is admitted as an emergency patient. A major artery severed in her leg caused an estimated 600 mL blood to be lost. Her blood pressure is 90/60 mm Hg. Which of the following would be expected to increase in response to hemorrhage?

(A) Arteriolar diameter in skeletal muscle

(B) Sodium excretion

(C) Sympathetic nerve activity

(D) Vagal nerve activity

(E) Water excretion

# Physiology Test One: **Answers and Explanations**

## ANSWER KEY

| | | | |
|---|---|---|---|
| 1. | B | 26. | A |
| 2. | D | 27. | C |
| 3. | B | 28. | A |
| 4. | B | 29. | C |
| 5. | D | 30. | E |
| 6. | E | 31. | B |
| 7. | D | 32. | D |
| 8. | C | 33. | A |
| 9. | D | 34. | C |
| 10. | D | 35. | C |
| 11. | B | 36. | C |
| 12. | D | 37. | B |
| 13. | B | 38. | C |
| 14. | C | 39. | E |
| 15. | A | 40. | A |
| 16. | E | 41. | B |
| 17. | C | 42. | C |
| 18. | B | 43. | E |
| 19. | E | 44. | E |
| 20. | C | 45. | B |
| 21. | B | 46. | C |
| 22. | A | 47. | D |
| 23. | E | 48. | E |
| 24. | B | 49. | C |
| 25. | D | 50. | C |

1.  **The correct answer is B.** The fasting serum gastrin is normal in patients with duodenal ulcer (DU); however, the gastrin response to a meal (**choice C**) is increased. The increase in serum gastrin following a meal occurs, in part, because acid suppresses gastrin release less effectively in DU patients compared with controls.

    DU patients have an increase in parietal cell mass (**choice E**), which may be caused by the trophic (growth promoting) effects of gastrin.

    Patients with DU have an increased basal acid output (**choice A**) that totally disappears following eradication of the *H. pylori* infection.

    However, the increase in maximal acid output (**choice D**), which occurs in response to IV gastrin, can remain following eradication of the *H. pylori* infection and is likely to result from the increased parietal cell mass.

    The secretion of pepsin (**choice F**) is usually doubled in DU patients.

2.  **The correct answer is D.** The disease is acromegaly, which is typically produced by a growth hormone-secreting pituitary adenoma. Growth hormone synthesis is predominately regulated by hypothalamic GHRH (growth hormone releasing hormone), and its pulsatile secretion is predominately regulated by hypothalamic somatostatin.

    **Choice A:** Dopamine and norepinephrine are catecholamines that regulate smooth muscle tone and cardiac function.

    **Choice B:** Luteinizing hormone (LH) regulates sex steroid hormone production by both testes and ovaries. Human chorionic gonadotropin (hCG) is produced by the placenta and has actions similar to LH.

    **Choice C:** Prolactin regulates menstruation and lactation. Follicle stimulating hormone (FSH) regulates ovarian and testicular function.

    **Choice E:** Thyroid stimulating hormone (TSH) regulates secretion of thyroid hormones. Adrenocorticotropin (ACTH) regulates glucocorticoid and adrenal androgen secretion.

3.  **The correct answer is B.** There is more than one way to think about this question. One way is to determine which of each of the descriptions corresponds to $P_c$, $P_i$, $\pi_c$, and $\pi_i$ and then to use the Starling equation for net filtration pressure: $(P_c - P_i) - (\pi_c - \pi_i)$. Perhaps faster and more intuitive is to just envision that the filtration pressure will be the difference between the forces pushing fluid out and the forces pulling fluid back into the glomerulus. The pushing forces are the hydrostatic pressure of the glomerulus (44 mm Hg) and the osmotic pressure of the tubular fluid (0). So the total pressure

forcing fluid from the glomerulus into the tubular fluid is 44 mm Hg. The forces pulling the fluid back are the hydrostatic pressure of the Bowman's capsule (9 mm Hg) and the osmotic pressure of the plasma (28 mm Hg). The total pressure pushing the fluid back into the glomerulus is $9 + 28 = 37$ mm Hg. The difference between the forces favoring filtration and those opposing it is therefore $44 - 37 = 7$ mm Hg.

4.  **The correct answer is B.** Tumors produce both angiogenic and anti-angiogenic factors (also called angiostatic factors). Angiogenic factors stimulate the growth of blood vessels (angiogenesis), whereas angiostatic factors inhibit blood vessel growth (anti-angiogenesis). Angiogenic factors such as VEGF and bFGF have relatively long half-lives in the blood compared with angiostatic factors such as endostatin or angiostatin. Large tumors often produce sufficient amounts of angiostatic factors to suppress the growth of blood vessels in small, undetectable tumors present elsewhere in the body. This suppression of angiogenesis in the smaller tumors also suppresses the overall growth of the tumors, because the small tumors cannot grow without an adequate blood supply, i.e., tumor growth is angiogenesis-dependent. When the large tumor is removed, the blood levels of angiostatic factor (endostatin) decrease, allowing angiogenesis to occur in the smaller tumors. The smaller tumors grow rapidly as a consequence of this angiogenesis and can be detected within a few weeks. Endostatin is a fragment of collagen XVIII, which inhibits angiogenesis and shrinks tumors. It shows promising behavior as an anticancer agent in early, preclinical trials.

    The astute student may wonder how angiogenesis can occur in large tumors in the presence of angiostatic factors. The answer is that angiogenesis occurs when the levels (or activities) of angiogenic factors become greater compared with the levels of angiostatic factors, i.e., both angiogenic and angiostatic factors may be present in a tumor, but angiogenesis occurs when the influence of angiogenic factors predominates. The student may also ask how a large tumor can suppress angiogenesis in small tumors when both angiostatic and angiogenic factors are released from the large tumor. The answer is that angiostatic factors have long half-lives in the blood compared with that of angiogenic factors, as discussed above. Thus, the smaller tumors "see" higher levels of angiostatic factors compared with angiogenic factors.

    Basic fibroblast growth factor (bFGF; **choice A**) is a powerful angiogenic agent, both in vitro and in vivo, and is produced by many different types of cells. bFGF is also a potent mitogen for cells of mesenchymal, neural, and epithelial origin. Overexpression of bFGF can result in tumor production.

Growth hormone (**choice C**) has a general effect to cause growth of all, or almost all, tissues of the body, but does not appear to stimulate angiogenesis to a significant extent in solid tumors.

Platelet-derived growth factor (PDGF; **choice D**) is actually three molecules, each of which is a dimeric combination of two distinct but structurally related peptide chains. PDGF isoforms are potent mitogens for connective tissue cells, smooth muscle cells, and some epithelial and endothelial cells. PDGF is thought to have a role in neoplastic transformation and tumor pathogenesis.

Transforming growth factor (TGF-β; **choice E**) is a polypeptide growth factor. It is generally stimulatory for cells of mesenchymal origin and inhibitory for cells of epithelial or neuroectodermal origin. It is an important mediator of the formation of extracellular matrix.

Vascular endothelial growth factor (VEGF; **choice F**) is a heparin-binding glycoprotein that increases endothelial cell proliferation in vitro as well as capillary growth (i.e., angiogenesis) in vivo. Unlike most other growth factors, VEGF has unique target cell specificity for vascular endothelial cells. VEGF is overexpressed in some solid tumors, as well as in ischemic areas of the heart and retina of the eye. VEGF levels are also reversibly increased in a variety of normal and transformed cells exposed to a hypoxic environment. These characteristics of VEGF make it an ideal candidate as a regulator of angiogenesis in physiologic and pathophysiologic situations where vessel growth is preceded by deficient perfusion of the tissues.

5. **The correct answer is D.** According to the equation, $R = 8\eta l/\pi r^4$, where R is resistance, $\eta$ is viscosity of blood, l is the length of the blood vessel, and $r^4$ is the radius of the blood vessel wall to the fourth power, the resistance is inversely proportional to the fourth power of the radius. In other words, if the radius is reduced by one-half, the resistance is multiplied by 16. In addition, blood flow can be expressed as the following: $Q = \Delta P/R$, where Q is blood flow, DP is the pressure gradient at both ends of the vessel, and R is the resistance. Blood flow is inversely proportional to resistance. So when the resistance is increased by 16-fold, blood flow must decrease by 16-fold.

6. **The correct answer is E.** Defecation is initiated by defecation reflexes. An intrinsic reflex mediated entirely by the local enteric nervous system is stimulated when feces enters the rectum. Distention of the rectum initiates afferent signals that spread through the myenteric plexus to initiate peristaltic contractions in the descending colon, sigmoid, and rectum and force the feces toward the anus.

The internal anal sphincter is relaxed (compare with **choice C**), and, if the external anal sphincter (**choice F**) is *voluntarily* relaxed at the same time, defecation will occur. This intrinsic defecation reflex works together with a more powerful reflex that involves the sacral elements of the spinal cord. The cord reflex is also initiated by distention of the rectum, which transmits afferent signals to the sacral cord and then back to the descending colon, sigmoid, rectum, and anus by way of parasympathetic fibers in the pelvic nerves. These parasympathetic signals greatly intensify the peristaltic contractions, adding considerable power to the defecation process. The lower neurons of the second, third, and fourth sacral roots, which provide the sensory and motor fibers for the defecation reflex, are intact when the spinal cord is injured at a higher level.

However, the afferent signals entering the spinal cord initiate other effects that require an intact spinal cord. These include taking a deep breath (**choice A**), closing the glottis (**choice B**), and increasing abdominal pressure (**choice D**), all of which together move the fecal contents downward. Voluntary relaxation of the external anal sphincter then allows the feces to be expelled from the body. Loss of voluntary aid to the defecation process following spinal transection or injury can make defecation a difficult process; however, excitation of the cord defecation reflex (either digitally or with an enema) can usually produce adequate defecation.

7. **The correct answer is D.** The clinical and laboratory picture is that of diabetes insipidus. His surgical procedure took place in the vicinity of the pituitary gland (where craniopharyngiomas are typically located); thus, the most likely scenario is that of inadvertent damage to the posterior pituitary or the stalk.

Brain edema (**choice A**) would be expected as a consequence of rapid water retention, in which case the serum sodium concentration and the osmolarity would be significantly less than normal.

Nephrogenic diabetes insipidus (**choice B**) is a good alternative choice that could have occurred if the anesthetic agent had been Penthrane. Because that was not the drug used and the surgery was near the pituitary, damage to the latter is a more likely scenario.

Respiratory depression (**choice C**) is completely wrong. He is in fact hyperventilating, as evidenced by his low $p_{CO_2}$.

Water retention (**choice E**) is equally wrong, given his high serum sodium concentration and osmolarity.

8. **The correct answer is C.** During starvation, the diet is inadequate to provide sufficient glucose to maintain the brain, yet the brain requires glucose as an energy

source. Glucose used in the brain during starvation is synthesized from amino acids, primarily derived from muscle protein. This use of amino acids in starvation leads to profound muscle wasting.

The ketone bodies (acetoacetate, **choice A**; acetone, **choice B**; and beta-hydroxybutyrate, **choice D**) produced during starvation and diabetic ketoacidosis are derived from adipose triacylglycerols. Although these compounds can be used in biochemical pathways in the brain, they cannot completely replace glucose in that organ. Furthermore, glucose cannot be synthesized from these precursors.

Fatty acid (**choice E**) degradation cannot be used to produce glucose. It can be used, however, to produce ketone bodies that can be used by the brain as a source of intermediates for some synthetic pathways.

9. **The correct answer is D.** Under normal conditions, one-third of the cardiac cycle is spent in systole and two-thirds spent in diastole. As heart rate increases dramatically, the time spent in diastole falls precipitously but the time spent in systole falls to a lesser extent.

A large increase in heart rate must produce a decrease in both diastole and systole (compare with **choice A**).

The major change with increased heart rate is in diastole, not systole (compare with **choice B**).

Heart rate cannot increase if diastolic time increases (**choice C**).

An increase in heart rate must be accompanied by a decrease in diastolic time (compare with **choice E**).

10. **The correct answer is D.** Compensation for high altitude includes an increase in the renal excretion of bicarbonate. The diminished barometric pressure found at high altitude causes arterial hypoxia, which is sensed by peripheral chemoreceptors. The ventilation rate increases, thereby causing a respiratory alkalosis. The kidney then compensates by increasing the excretion of $HCO_3^-$.

Erythropoietin is increased, not decreased, in chronic hypoxia and at high altitude (**choice A**). Increased erythropoietin leads to an increased hematocrit.

Another adaptation to high altitude is increased 2,3-DPG (compare with **choice B**), which shifts the oxygen dissociation curve to the right.

High altitude leads to respiratory alkalosis. The renal compensation is a metabolic acidosis characterized by decreased $H^+$ excretion and increased $HCO_3^-$ excretion. Respiratory acidosis is renally compensated with a metabolic alkalosis that would include increases in $H^+$ excretion (**choice C**).

Pulmonary vasoconstriction, not vasodilation (**choice E**), occurs in response to alveolar hypoxia, such as would occur at high altitudes.

11. **The correct answer is B.** Volume = amount/concentration.

The amount of mannitol in the volunteer is equal to the amount injected minus the amount excreted: 10 g – 1 g = 9 g = 9000 mg. Therefore,

$$\text{Volume} = \frac{9000}{65 \text{ mg}/100 \text{ mL}} = 13.8 \text{ L}$$

12. **The correct answer is D.** The NMDA receptor, a type of glutamate receptor, is unique in that it is both voltage- and ligand-gated. In other words, it requires both an agonist and neuronal depolarization to be activated. The NMDA receptor is an ion channel that allows the passage of $Na^+$ and $Ca^{2+}$ when open. At resting membrane potential, the channel is plugged by a $Mg^{2+}$ ion. Depolarization (and agonist activation) causes the $Mg^{2+}$ ion to dislodge, allowing the receptor to be functional.

The $GABA_A$ receptor (**choice A**) is a ligand-gated chloride channel.

The kainate receptor (**choice B**), a type of glutamate receptor, the nicotinic acetylcholine receptor (**choice C**), and the 5-$HT_3$ receptor (**choice E**) are ligand-gated $Na^+$ channels.

13. **The correct answer is B.** This is actually a straightforward question. The fastest way to approach it is to predict the physiologic responses that would occur as a result of a carotid massage and identify the appropriate graph, rather than spending the time to read all of the graphs.

During a carotid massage, the carotid sinus baroreceptors sense the distortion of the vessel wall. This leads to an increase in afferent traffic (firing rate) in the glossopharyngeal nerve. A signal indicating high blood pressure travels to the nucleus of the solitary tract (NTS) in the medulla, and a baroreceptor reflex occurs. The animal is "tricked" into thinking it has high blood pressure, so it decreases sympathetic outflow and increases parasympathetic outflow, leading to decreases in blood pressure and heart rate. Meanwhile, the aortic arch baroreceptors, which are innervated by the vagus nerve, correctly sense that the blood pressure has decreased. This decreases afferent traffic along the vagus nerve to the brainstem.

If you simply knew that a carotid massage leads to a decrease in blood pressure and heart rate, you could immediately narrow your choices to A and B. Knowledge of baroreceptor physiology allows you to distinguish between A and B.

14. **The correct answer is C.** Penile erection is mediated by the parasympathetic nervous system. The neurons involved are termed nonadrenergic, noncholinergic (NANC) autonomic neurons, and they may release nitric oxide (NO). NO binds to the iron in the heme molecule of guanylate cyclase, activating it to form cGMP. This results in a decrease in intracellular calcium and subsequent smooth muscle relaxation and vasodilatation in the corpus cavernosa, producing erection. Nitric oxide synthase (NOS) is the enzyme required for the formation of NO from circulating arginine, and androgens are necessary to maintain normal amounts of this enzyme. Inhibition of this enzyme could result in impotence (although most currently used drugs that have impotence as a side effect do not affect NOS).

Inhibition of the conversion of testosterone to DHT, not DHT to testosterone (**choice A**), would be accomplished by a 5-alpha-reductase inhibitor. This could cause impotence by its anti-androgen effect. In fact, finasteride, a clinically used 5-alpha-reductase inhibitor, produces drastic decreases in libido in some men.

Inhibition of forward motility factor (**choice B**) would hamper sperm motility and result in infertility, not impotence.

Inhibition of oxytocin (**choice D**) or prostaglandins (**choice E**) would result in failure to ejaculate (ejaculatory incompetence), not impotence.

15. **The correct answer is A.** The increase in muscle blood flow that occurs during exercise is caused by dilation of the arterioles (i.e., decreased arteriolar resistance). In normal skeletal muscles, the blood flow can increase as much as 20-fold during strenuous exercise. Most of this increase in blood flow can be attributed to the dilatory actions of metabolic factors (e.g., adenosine, lactic acid, carbon dioxide) produced by the exercising muscles.

Exercise causes the concentration of carbon dioxide (**choice B**) and lactic acid (**choice C**) to increase in the muscles.

Mass discharge of the sympathetic nervous system (**choice D**) occurs throughout the body during exercise, causing arterioles to constrict in most tissues. The arterioles in the exercising muscles, however, are strongly dilated by vasodilator substances released from the muscles.

A decrease in vascular conductance (**choice E**) occurs when the vasculature is constricted. Resistance and conductance are inversely related, so that a decrease in arteriolar resistance is associated with an increase in arteriolar conductance.

16. **The correct answer is E.** Red blood cells (and many other blood cells) contain the enzyme carbonic anhy-drase, which catalyzes the intracellular conversion of $CO_2$ to bicarbonate and $H^+$ ion. Most of the bicarbonate in the red cell is exchanged across the plasmalemma for chloride ion. This means that although the bulk of the production of bicarbonate occurs in the red cell (**choice D**), the bulk of the actual transport occurs in serum. Carbonic anhydrase is not present in serum. Bicarbonate can also be produced in serum by nonenzymatic means, but the process is slow.

$CO_2$ is also carried as carbaminohemoglobin (**choice A**), which forms when $CO_2$ binds to an $NH_2$ side group of the hemoglobin protein, rather than to the heme iron ($Fe^{2+}$), as with carbon monoxide and oxygen.

$CO_2$ is not transported in the form of bubbles (**choice B**), which is a good thing, because gas bubbles are effectively emboli, which can lead to considerable morbidity or death.

Some $CO_2$ is carried directly dissolved in blood (**choice C**). It is 20 times more soluble in blood than is $O_2$, but this is still only about 5% of the total $CO_2$ in the blood.

17. **The correct answer is C.** The various points on the volume-pressure diagram correspond to specific events of the cardiac cycle as follows:

**Choice A:** The mitral valve opens, and the *period of filling* begins.

**Choice B:** This is the *period of filling*.

**Choice C:** This marks the beginning of ventricular *systole*. The mitral valve closes, and S1 can be heard. The end-diastolic pressure (5 mm Hg) and end-diastolic volume (125 mL) can be determined on the *y*-axis and *x*-axis from this point.

**Choice D:** This is the period of *isovolumetric contraction*. Left ventricular pressure increases rapidly, but left ventricular volume remains constant. All heart valves are closed.

**Choice E:** The aortic valve opens, which marks the beginning of the *period of ejection*. The pressure at this point is equal to the aortic diastolic blood pressure, which is about 80 mm Hg on the diagram.

**Choice F:** This is the *period of ejection*. The pressure at the apex of the curve is the peak systolic pressure of the left ventricle.

**Choice G:** This marks the beginning of *diastole*. The aortic valve closes, and S2 can be heard. The end-systolic volume (50 mL) can be read from *x*-axis at this point.

**Choice H:** The is the period of *isovolumetric relaxation*. Left ventricular pressure is falling rapidly, but left ventricular volume remains constant. All heart valves are closed.

18. **The correct answer is B.** Gastrinomas are gastrin-secreting tumors usually present in the pancreas. Patients with gastrinoma have high serum gastrin levels, which lead to hypersecretion of gastric acid and consequent duodenal and jejunal ulcers. Injection of secretin is the most specific and easiest test for gastrinoma.

    Secretin inhibits antral release of gastrin (**choice A**), but it stimulates release of gastrin from gastrin tumors (gastrinoma) in almost all patients. A doubling of serum gastrin 5 to 10 minutes after administration of secretin (1 U/kg), coupled with acid hypersecretion and increased basal serum gastrin, strongly indicates the presence of gastrinoma. Secretin can inhibit gastric emptying (**choice C**), inhibit gastric secretion (**choice D**), and stimulate pancreatic $HCO_3^-$ secretion (**choice E**), but these effects are not diagnostic for gastrinoma.

19. **The correct answer is E.** Inulin is freely filtered, but is neither reabsorbed nor secreted. Since all inulin filtered in the glomerulus will appear in the urine, the amount of water in the urine will determine the concentration of the inulin. Therefore, (U/P) inulin will decrease if the urine flow rate increases.

    In the presence of adequate amounts of antidiuretic hormone (ADH; vasopressin), increased aldosterone (**choice A**) increases reabsorption of sodium in the collecting duct. Water will follow the sodium chloride, which will increase (U/P) inulin.

    Inulin clearance = glomerular filtration rate, which has not changed (**choice B**).

    Reabsorbing less water in the collecting duct represents either a decrease in negative free water clearance (if concentrated urine was being made), or an increase in positive free water clearance (**choice C**).

    Inulin is neither reabsorbed nor secreted (**choice D**).

20. **The correct answer is C.** This question requires you to know that bacterial infections are associated with an elevated neutrophil count. These leukocytes have 3 to 5 nuclear lobes and are filled with granules that contain bactericidal products, including lysozyme. Note that neutrophils normally constitute 54 to 62% of leukocytes, so if you were unsure of the percentages occurring in response to bacterial infections, **choice C** would still have been a good guess. Had the infection been viral, there would have been an increase in lymphocytes instead.

    Histamine (**choice A**) is released by basophils and mast cells, along with other vasoactive amines (**choice E**). Slow-reacting substance of anaphylaxis, which consists of leukotrienes LTC4, LTD4, and LTE4 (**choice B**), is also released by these cells, which possess large spheroidal granules. Basophils and mast cells are basophilic (thus their name) and metachromatic, because of the presence of heparin, a glycosaminoglycan.

    Eosinophils contain peroxidase (**choice D**). These white blood cells have a bilobed nucleus and possess acidophilic granules in their cytoplasm. They also contain hydrolytic enzymes. Note that an increased eosinophil count is associated with parasitic infections, allergies, asthma, and some neoplasms.

21. **The correct answer is B.** Normally, stretching of muscle results in a reflex contraction: the harder the stretch, the stronger the contraction. At a certain point, when the tension becomes too great, the contracting muscle suddenly relaxes. The reflex that underlies this sudden muscle relaxation is called the Golgi tendon organ (GTO) reflex, also known as the inverse stretch reflex or autogenic inhibition. The GTO is an extensive arborization of nerve endings (encapsulated by a connective tissue sheath and located near the muscle attachment) that is connected in series with the extrafusal skeletal muscle fibers. As a result, GTOs respond to muscle tension rather than muscle length. Increased tension leads to stimulation of Ib afferents, which inhibit the homonymous muscle via spinal interneurons.

    Free nerve endings (**choice A**) are unmyelinated, unencapsulated nerve endings that penetrate the epidermis. These types of receptors respond to pain and temperature.

    Merkel disks (**choice C**) are composed of specialized tactile epidermal cells and their associated nerve endings. They are located in the basal layer of the epithelium and are slowly adapting receptors that respond to touch and pressure.

    Muscle spindles (**choice D**) are spindle-shaped bundles of muscle fibers (intrafusal fibers) that are encapsulated by connective tissue. Muscle spindles are arranged in parallel with extrafusal skeletal muscle fibers, so they sense the length of the muscle. They are innervated by Group Ia and II sensory afferent neurons.

    Pacinian corpuscles (**choice E**) are unmyelinated nerve endings surrounded by thin, concentric layers of epithelioid fibroblasts. In transverse section, this receptor resembles a sliced onion. They are found primarily in the deep layer of the dermis, loose connective tissue, male and female genitalia, mesentery, and visceral ligaments. They are rapidly adapting receptors that respond to touch and pressure.

22. **The correct answer is A.** Gastric inhibitory peptide (GIP) is produced in the duodenal and jejunal mucosa by K cells and is released in response to intraluminal

glucose and fatty acids. GIP is sometimes called "glucose-dependent insulinotropic" peptide because it stimulates pancreatic insulin secretion in the presence of hyperglycemia. Note that although GIP release would be stimulated, the hormone would not have a pronounced effect in this type 1 diabetic, whose pancreatic islet cells do not produce adequate amounts of insulin.

Gastrin (**choice B**) is synthesized and stored primarily in the G cells of the stomach and TG cells of the stomach and small intestine. The stimuli for gastrin secretion include increased vagal discharge, digestive products, calcium salts, and gastric distention. Gastrin stimulates HCl secretion by parietal cells, histamine release from enterochromaffin cells, pepsinogen secretion by chief cells, gastric blood flow, and contraction of gastric circular smooth muscle. It has a trophic effect on gastric and small-intestinal mucosa and the pancreas, increases lower esophageal sphincter (LES) tone, and is a weak stimulus for the secretion of pancreatic enzymes and bicarbonate.

Motilin (**choice C**) is produced in the M and enterochromaffin cells of the duodenum and jejunum. Secretion occurs during fasting. Motilin acts to regulate the migrating myoelectric complex (MMC).

Secretin (**choice D**) is synthesized and stored in the S cells of the mucosa of the upper intestine. Acidification of the duodenal mucosa and the presence of fat and protein degradation products in the duodenum stimulate its secretion. The main role of secretin is to stimulate bicarbonate secretion from the pancreas and liver.

Somatostatin (**choice E**) is synthesized and stored in the D cells of the pancreatic islets, in the gastric antrum, and throughout the intestine. It is also present in the hypothalamus. It inhibits the release of gastrin, cholecystokinin (CCK), and most other gastrointestinal hormones. In brief, it "shuts off" the gut. Somatostatin inhibits the release of glucagon by pancreatic alpha cells, as well as the release of insulin by the pancreatic beta cells (of the islets of Langerhans).

Substance P (**choice F**) is synthesized in the enterochromaffin cells of the upper small intestine and colon and also in the CNS. The stimulus for release of the substance occurs through vagal efferent pathways. Substance P stimulates salivary flow and gastrointestinal motility and functions in the transmission of pain impulses in the nervous system.

Vasoactive intestinal polypeptide (VIP; **choice G**) is produced by cells in the parasympathetic ganglia of sphincters, the gallbladder, and the small intestine. Stimuli for its release include vagal stimulation and intestinal distention. VIP promotes water and electrolyte secretion by the jejunum, ileum, and colon (via

cAMP), relaxation of the smooth muscle and sphincters, stimulation of pancreatic bicarbonate secretion, and intestinal dilatation. It inhibits the secretion of gastric acid and gastrin.

23. **The correct answer is E.** Glucagon is released from the alpha cells of the pancreas in response to hypoglycemia and stimulates glycogenolysis to increase serum glucose.

Augmented calcium deposition in bone (**choice A**) is achieved by calcitonin (inhibits bone resorption), which is secreted by the C-cells in the thyroid gland. Glucagon plays no role in calcium metabolism.

Glucagon favors the conversion of amino acids to glucose (gluconeogenesis) rather than their storage in the liver (**choice B**).

Insulin (which generally has opposite effects of glucagon) promotes lipogenesis in the liver and in adipose tissue (**choice C**).

Glucagon stimulates gluconeogenesis (**choice D**).

24. **The correct answer is B.** At less than saturating concentrations, PAH is completely secreted into the proximal tubule and excreted into the urine. Therefore, the volume of plasma cleared of PAH is approximately equal to the volume of plasma flowing through the peritubular capillaries, also called the effective renal plasma flow, or ERPF.

$$ERPF = \frac{U_{PAH} \times V}{P_{PAH}}$$

At very high concentrations, the clearance of PAH would be less than ERPF and approaches GFR.

The ECF volume (**choice A**) can be calculated by measuring the volume of distribution of solutes that move freely across capillary walls but cannot permeate cell membranes (e.g., inulin and mannitol).

GFR (**choice C**) is best calculated using a substance that is freely filtered at the glomerulus, not reabsorbed, and only minimally secreted into the urine. Creatinine fits the bill and is used clinically to measure the GFR (inulin also works and is used experimentally). Whereas the creatinine excretion exceeds filtration by 10 to 20% (because of the secretion), creatinine clearance is still a good approximation for GFR because the error due to secretion is balanced by an overestimation of plasma creatinine inherent in the measurement technique.

$$GRF = \frac{U_{creatine} \times V}{P_{creatine}}$$

The plasma volume (**choice D**) can be measured by measuring the volume of distribution of radioactively labeled serum albumin or of Evans blue dye (binds to albumin).

Total body water (TBW; **choice E**) can be measured by measuring the volume of distribution of tritium, deuterium, or antipyrine.

25. **The correct answer is D.** Ascites often occurs in patients with cirrhosis and other forms of severe liver disease and is usually noticed by the patient because of abdominal swelling. Shortness of breath may occur because the diaphragm is elevated when the accumulation of fluid becomes more pronounced. A number of factors contribute to accumulation of fluid in the abdominal cavity. Portal hypertension plays an important role in the production of ascites by raising capillary hydrostatic pressure within the splanchnic bed.

Elevated serum levels of epinephrine and norepinephrine (compare with **choice A**), resulting from increased central sympathetic outflow, are found in patients with cirrhosis and ascites.

The increased sympathetic output leads to decreased natriuresis (compare with **choice E**) by activation of the renin-angiotensin system and diminished sensitivity to atrial natriuretic peptide.

Hypoalbuminemia (compare with **choice F**) and reduced plasma oncotic pressure (compare with **choice G**) promote extravasation of fluid into the peritoneal cavity, thereby contributing to the development of ascites.

Interstitial fluid often weeps freely from the surface of the cirrhotic liver because of distortion and obstruction of hepatic lymphatics (compare with **choice C**). This interstitial fluid has a high protein concentration because the endothelial lining of the hepatic sinusoids is discontinuous. The entry of protein-rich interstitial fluid into the peritoneal cavity may account for the high protein concentration present in the ascitic fluid of some patients.

26. **The correct answer is A.** Achalasia is a disorder of esophageal motility that affects the lower esophageal sphincter (LES) and lower two-thirds of the esophageal body. The LES remains tonically contracted and does not relax as food moves down the esophagus. Relaxation is via the release of vasoactive intestinal peptide (VIP) from nerve endings. Therefore, food cannot move easily from the esophagus into the stomach. The distal esophagus often becomes greatly dilated. Patients with achalasia most commonly complain of dysphagia (difficulty swallowing), chest pain, and regurgitation.

During swallowing, the bolus of food is propelled through the pharynx (**choice D**) by peristaltic contractions.

These contractions, along with relaxation of the upper esophageal sphincter (**choice E**), propel the bolus of food into the esophagus. Relaxation of the upper esophageal sphincter occurs normally in patients with achalasia.

The upper, middle, and lower esophagus (**choices B, C, and F**) propel the bolus toward the stomach by coordinated contractions of the muscle layers.

27. **The correct answer is C.** Because substance X is filtered, but not secreted or reabsorbed (like inulin), the clearance of substance X can be used to approximate GFR.

$GFR = [U]_X \times V / [P]_X$; therefore,

$GFR = (10 \text{ mg/mL}) \times (60 \text{ mL/hour}) / (0.1 \text{ mg/mL})$
$\quad\quad = (10 \text{ mg/mL}) \times (1 \text{ mL/min}) / (0.1 \text{ mg/mL})$
$\quad\quad = 100 \text{ mL/min}$

Note that you need to convert 60 mL/hour to 1 mL/min to get the correct answer in the correct units. Checking to make sure the units are correct will help make sure you are using the formula properly.

28. **The correct answer is A.** Sawtooth waves appearing in bursts are associated with REM sleep.

Stage 1 (**choice B**) is associated with 4-7-Hz theta waves.

Stage 2 (**choice C**) is associated with 12-14-Hz sleep spindles and K-complexes.

Stage 3 (**choice D**) is associated with <4-Hz, high-amplitude delta waves.

Stage 4 (**choice E**) is characterized by an EEG composed of about 50% delta waves.

Note that beta waves (15-18 Hz) occur during periods of more intense mental activity while awake. Alpha waves (8-12 Hz) occur during awake, relaxed states. REM is the stage of sleep that most resembles the awake state on the EEG.

29. **The correct answer is C.** This is a classic presentation of carpal tunnel syndrome, which typically affects women between the ages of 40 and 60 who chronically perform repetitive tasks that involve movement of the structures that pass through the carpal tunnel. One important structure that passes through the carpal tunnel is the median nerve. Patients often note tingling, loss of sensation, or diminished sensation in the digits. There is also often a loss of coordination and strength in the thumb, because the median nerve also sends fibers to the abductor pollicis brevis, flexor pollicis brevis, and the opponens pollicis. A final function of the median nerve distal to the carpal tunnel is control of the first and second lumbricals, which function to flex digits two and three at the metacarpophalangeal joints and extend interphalangeal joints of the same digits.

Abduction of the fifth digit (**choice A**) is a function controlled by the ulnar nerve, which does not pass through the carpal tunnel.

Adduction of the thumb (**choice B**) is a function of the adductor pollicis, which is the only short thumb muscle that is not innervated by the median nerve, but rather by the deep branch of the ulnar nerve.

Sensation of the lateral half of the dorsum of the hand (**choice D**) is mediated by the radial nerve, which also does not pass through the carpal tunnel.

Sensation over the lateral aspect of the palm (**choice E**) is mediated by the median nerve; however, the branch innervating the palm (palmar cutaneous branch of the median nerve) passes superficially to the carpal tunnel.

Sensation over the medial aspect of the dorsum of the hand (**choice F**) is mediated by the ulnar nerve.

Sensation over the medial aspect of the palm (**choice G**) is mediated by the ulnar nerve.

30. **The correct answer is E.** The parietal cells of the stomach produce intrinsic factor, a glycoprotein that binds vitamin $B_{12}$ in the lumen of the stomach and facilitates its absorption in the terminal ileum. Patients without a stomach and those with pernicious anemia (autoimmune destruction of parietal cells) require $B_{12}$ replacement therapy. Recall that $B_{12}$ deficiency will lead to megaloblastic anemia and the USMLE-favorite picture of a blood smear with hypersegmented neutrophils. Note that parietal cells also synthesize and secrete HCl.

Chief cells (**choice A**) are responsible for secreting pepsinogen, the precursor to pepsin.

G cells (**choice B**) secrete gastrin, which stimulates secretion of acid by the parietal cells found in the body and fundus of the stomach. Zollinger-Ellison syndrome is caused by a pancreatic or duodenal tumor that secretes gastrin (a gastrinoma). It is characterized by the development of severe peptic ulcer disease.

Goblet cells (**choice C**) are part of the mucosa of the small intestine, not the stomach. They produce glycoproteins (mucins) that protect and lubricate the lining of the intestine.

Mucous neck cells (**choice D**) secrete mucus and are located in the necks of the gastric glands.

31. **The correct answer is B.** Total body water (TBW) in liters equals approximately 60% of body weight in kilograms and therefore equals 45 L in a 75-kg person. Intracellular volume = 2/3 of TBW and is therefore 30 L in this case. Extracellular volume = 1/3 of TBW and is therefore 15 L in this case.

**Choices A, C, D,** and **E** do not satisfy these conditions.

32. **The correct answer is D.** This patient appears to be experiencing *mittelschmerz*, abdominal pain occurring at the time of ovulation that can mimic acute appendicitis (which is ruled out because of the patient's surgical history). If this information did not clue you into the stage of the menstrual cycle, you are told explicitly that the patient's last menstrual period was 14 days ago. Therefore, she is at the conclusion of the proliferative (estrogenic) phase. This stage begins during the latter period of menstrual flow and continues through the thirteenth-fourteenth day of a typical 28-day cycle; it is characterized by regrowth of the endometrium. The epithelial cells of the glandular structures remaining after menstruation migrate and proliferate to cover the new mucosal surface. Also, the spiral arteries grow into the regenerating endometrium (this process continues through the secretory stage as well). Significant edema develops by the end of the proliferative stage and continues to develop during the secretory phase.

Apical movement of secretions in the glandular cells (**choice A**) occurs during the secretory phase.

Degeneration of the glandular structures (**choice B**) occurs during the premenstrual stage of the cycle.

Glandular glycogen accumulation in the functionalis (**choice C**) occurs during the secretory phase (luteal phase).

Tissue expansion by cellular hypertrophy (**choice E**) occurs during the secretory phase since mitosis of the endometrial tissue has ceased at this point.

33. **The correct answer is A.** A scenario of postoperative oliguria raises the possibility of two potential diagnoses: fluid volume deficit and acute renal failure. The urinary sodium concentration provides a good indication of which of the two is present: If good kidneys are saving fluid because of a volume deficit, the amount of sodium in the urine is very small, with a concentration typically less than 20 mEq/L. When the sodium in the urine exceeds a concentration of 40 mEq/L in the same general scenario, renal failure is the answer.

She is not getting a lot of sodium (**choice B**). Half normal saline has 77 mEq/L, and she is getting 3 L per day—hardly an excessive amount and certainly not a reason to become oliguric.

As pointed out, if her problem was fluid deficit (**choice C**), she would have a low sodium concentration in the urine.

Surgical ligation of both ureters (**choice D**) is offered as an option because she had surgery in the vicinity of those structures, but had that calamity occurred, her urinary output would have been zero since the operation.

**KAPLAN**) MEDICAL

A ureteroenteric fistula (**choice E**) is a more intriguing choice, but nevertheless a wrong one. It is conceivable that damage to a ureter, sustained near a colonic suture line, would produce a fistula. But we have had extensive experience in the past with such situations because ureterosigmoidostomies were used at one time to reconstruct the urinary tract after cystectomy. The procedure was abandoned because it produced hyperchloremic metabolic acidosis with hypokalemia: The acids and the chloride were reabsorbed, whereas the potassium was "washed away." This patient has the more typical hyperkalemia that accompanies acidosis and renal failure.

34. **The correct answer is C.** On the left side of the body, the lymphatic fluid flows from the lymphatic capillaries, to the thin lymphatic vessels, and then to the thoracic duct, which empties into the junction of the left internal jugular and left subclavian veins. On the right side, lymphatic fluid flows from the lymphatic capillaries to the thin lymphatic vessels, to the right thoracic duct, which empties into the junction of the right internal jugular and the right subclavian veins.

35. **The correct answer is C.** Lithium inhibits the action of antidiuretic hormone (ADH; vasopressin) on the V2 receptors in the collecting duct that regulate the permeability to water. Therefore, lithium administration will decrease water permeability in the collecting duct, which will increase urine flow rate and decrease urine osmolarity. Because ADH has minimal effects on sodium reabsorption in humans, the fractional clearance of sodium and the osmolar clearance are unaffected. (Osmolar clearance refers to the clearance of all particles, including sodium and anions, from the plasma per minute.)

Furosemide (**choice A**) inhibits the active reabsorption of sodium, potassium, and chloride in the thick ascending limb. This will deplete the medullary gradient, which could result in a slightly hypotonic urine, but furosemide will significantly increase the fractional clearance of sodium and hence the osmolar clearance.

Hydrochlorothiazide (**choice B**) inhibits the active reabsorption of sodium chloride from the distal convoluted tubule. Since the distal tubule is in the renal cortex, it will not inhibit the ability of the kidney to concentrate urine and therefore will not decrease the urine osmolarity so dramatically. It will also increase the fractional clearance of sodium, and hence the osmolar clearance, but not as much as with furosemide.

High dietary intake of potassium (**choice D**) will increase plasma potassium levels, which will increase aldosterone secretion by direct action on the adrenal cortical cells. The aldosterone will decrease fractional clearance of sodium and will not increase urine flow rate.

Increased isotonic plasma volume (**choice E**) will increase atrial natriuretic factor (ANF), which will inhibit sodium reabsorption in the nephron and thus increase the fractional clearance of sodium as well as osmolar clearance.

36. **The correct answer is C.** This is a really simple definition question: What is the difference between serum and plasma? Essentially, serum is derived from plasma by the extraction of fibrinogen and coagulation factors II, V, and VIII. This can be achieved by allowing whole blood to clot, then removing the clot.

Albumin (**choice A**) is present in both serum and plasma.

Neither erythrocytes (**choice B**) nor granulocytes (**choice D**) are present in either serum or plasma.

Serotonin (**choice E**) levels may be increased in serum because of the platelet breakdown that occurs during the extraction process. Serotonin is normally found in the highest concentration in platelets, as well as in the enterochromaffin cells and myenteric plexus of the gastrointestinal tract. The brain and the retina contain smaller amounts.

37. **The correct answer is B.** Pressure in the left atrium can be approximated by wedging an arterial catheter into a small branch of the pulmonary artery. Remember that the pulmonary vascular tree abuts the left atrium anatomically. The pulmonary artery carries deoxygenated blood from the right ventricle into the pulmonary circulation, where it is oxygenated and then returned to the left atrium via the pulmonary veins.

Aortic (**choice A**) pressure is usually five times greater than pulmonary artery pressure.

Left ventricular (**choice C**) pressure is usually about six times greater than right ventricular pressure.

Right atrial (**choice D**) and systemic venous (**choice E**) pressures can be estimated on the basis of central venous pressure (CVP), which is the pressure present in the great veins as they enter the right atrium. CVP is measured by placing a catheter into the thoracic great veins.

38. **The correct answer is C.** This question requires use of the alveolar ventilation equation:

$$P_{A_{CO_2}} = \frac{\dot{V}_{CO_2}}{\dot{V}_A}, \text{ where}$$

$P_{A_{CO_2}}$ is the partial pressure of alveolar $CO_2$, $\dot{V}_{CO_2}$ is $CO_2$ production, and $\dot{V}_A$ is alveolar ventilation.

If $\dot{V}_{CO_2}$ remains constant and alveolar ventilation doubles, $P_{A_{CO_2}}$ must decrease to half its original value.

Therefore, $PA_{CO_2}$ equals 20 mm Hg after hyperventilation.

Memorizing the formula is not necessary if you think about this intuitively: If $CO_2$ production remains constant and alveolar ventilation doubles, the partial pressure of alveolar $CO_2$ must decrease to half its original value and would therefore equal 20 mm Hg after hyperventilation.

39. **The correct answer is E.** The maximum expiratory flow-volume (MEFV) curve is created when the patient inhales as much air as possible and then expires with maximal effort until no more air can be expired. The amount of air that remains in the lungs after maximal expiration is the residual volume, and is depicted by point E. Note that the absolute value of the residual volume cannot be determined from a MEFV curve alone. Additional studies, such as helium dilution, are needed to determine the absolute value.

    **Choice A** is the lung volume at the total lung capacity; however, absolute lung volumes cannot be determined from a MEFV curve without additional methods. The other points on the curve correspond to the following:

    At **choice B**, the patient has just begun to exhale with a maximal effort at this point.

    At **choice C**, the patient is exhaling with a maximal effort and the rate of air flow has reached its maximal value of nearly 400 L/minute at this high lung volume.

    The descending portion of the curve (**choice D**) represents the maximum expiratory flow at each lung volume along the curve. This portion of the curve is sometimes referred to as the "effort-independent" portion of the curve because the patient cannot increase expiratory flow rate further by expending greater effort.

40. **The correct answer is A.** This woman has a risk profile (female, fat, forties) and symptomatology consistent with gallstones (cholelithiasis). As would be expected, contraction of the gallbladder following a fatty meal often exacerbates the pain caused by gallstones. Cholecystokinin (CCK) is the hormone responsible for stimulation of gallbladder contraction; the release of CCK is stimulated by dietary fat. It is produced in I cells of the duodenum and jejunum. In addition to gallbladder contraction, CCK also stimulates pancreatic enzyme secretion and decreases the rate of gastric emptying.

    Gastrin (**choice B**) is produced by the G cells of the antrum and duodenum. Gastrin stimulates the secretion of HCl from the parietal cells and pepsinogen from the chief cells of the stomach. Gastrin secretion is stimulated by gastric distention, digestive products (e.g., amino acids), and vagal discharge.

Pepsin (**choice C**) is a protease produced by the chief cells of the stomach (as pepsinogen). It is involved in the digestion of proteins. Pepsinogen release is stimulated by vagal stimulation, gastrin, local acid production, secretin, CCK, and histamine.

Secretin (**choice D**) is produced by the S cells of the duodenum. It is secreted primarily in response to acidification of the duodenal mucosa. Secretin stimulates the secretion of bicarbonate-containing fluid from the pancreas and biliary ducts. This neutralization allows pancreatic enzymes to function. Secretin also inhibits gastric acid production and gastric emptying.

Somatostatin (**choice E**) is produced by the D cells of the pancreatic islets and in the gastric and intestinal mucosa. Somatostatin is an inhibitory hormone; it inhibits most gastrointestinal hormones, gallbladder contraction, gastric acid and pepsinogen secretion, pancreatic and small intestinal fluid secretion, and both glucagon and insulin release.

41. **The correct answer is B.** Renal blood flow = (renal artery pressure – renal vein pressure)/renal vascular resistance (RVR). Therefore, if RVR is decreased to half its original value, with no pressure changes, renal blood flow must double (not increase 50%). Increased blood flow to the kidney and pressure in the glomerular capillaries increase renal oxygen use by increasing glomerular filtration rate, which increases the filtered load of sodium and other solutes. Since active sodium reabsorption is load-dependent, increased tubular fluid sodium increases all active sodium reabsorption, which requires more ATP hydrolysis and synthesis (and hence more oxygen use). Renal artery oxygen concentration does not change, since it is dependent on normal lung function, not oxygen extraction by the kidney.

42. **The correct answer is C.** All of the choices listed are reactions that occur in the synthetic pathway from cholesterol to cortisol. ACTH stimulates the first reaction in the pathway: cholesterol to pregnenolone. This reaction is catalyzed by the enzyme cholesterol desmolase.

    The next step in the pathway is pregnenolone to progesterone (**choice D**); progesterone is then converted to 17-hydroxyprogesterone (**choice E**); 17-hydroxyprogesterone is converted to 11-deoxycortisol (**choice B**) by the enzyme 21 beta-hydroxylase; and the 11-deoxycortisol is then converted to cortisol (**choice A**).

43. **The correct answer is E.** The sequence of the auditory pathway is as follows: Organ of Corti → spiral ganglion in the cochlea → vestibulocochlear nerve (CN VIII) → cochlear nuclei (dorsal and ventral) → superior olivary nuclei → lateral lemniscus → inferior colliculus →

medial geniculate nucleus of the thalamus (MGN) → primary auditory cortex (Heschl's gyrus).

Each ear projects to both sides of the brainstem and cortex via multiple commissures, including the trapezoid body (which contains fibers crossing contralateral to the superior olivary nucleus), the commissure of the inferior colliculus (connecting the right and left inferior colliculi), and another commissure that connects the right and left nuclei of the lateral lemniscus. Therefore, a lesion of any structure up until the superior olivary nuclei will produce an ipsilateral deafness. The only structure listed that is proximal to the superior olivary nuclei is the organ of Corti (**choice E**).

The inferior colliculus (**choice A**), the lateral lemniscus (**choice B**), the medial geniculate body (**choice C**), and the superior olivary nucleus (**choice F**) all receive information from both ears, and unilateral hearing loss could not result from a lesion of any of these structures.

The medial lemniscus (**choice D**) is not a part of the auditory system. It is part of the somatosensory system, which conveys proprioception, discriminative touch, and vibration information. More specifically, neurons of the gracile and cuneate nuclei send projections that decussate as the internal arcuate fibers and ascend as the medial lemniscus to synapse in the ventroposterolateral nucleus (VPL) of the thalamus.

44.  **The correct answer is E.** Enteropeptidase, formerly called enterokinase, activates trypsinogen by limited proteolytic digestion to give trypsin. Trypsin is itself capable of activating trypsinogen, which produces a positive feedback effect. Trypsin also activates chymotrypsinogen (and several other proteolytic enzymes), so deficiency of enteropeptidase results in a severe deficiency of enzymes that digest protein.

Amylase (**choice A**) aids in the breakdown of starches to oligosaccharides, maltose, and maltotriose.

Colipase (**choice B**), along with other lipases, functions to digest fats.

Lactase (**choice C**) is a brush-border disaccharidase that hydrolyzes the bond between galactose and glucose in lactose.

Pepsin (**choice D**) is a proteolytic enzyme secreted in an inactive form (pepsinogen) by the chief cells of the stomach. Pepsinogen is activated by stomach acid, and so is not dependent on enteropeptidase. Pepsin alone will not replace the activities of other proteolytic enzymes, partly because food does not remain in the stomach for an extended period of time.

45.  **The correct answer is B.** Diagram P shows a normal heart with an end-diastolic volume (EDV) of 125 mL

and an end-systolic volume (ESV) of 50 mL. Stroke volume (SV) can be calculated as EDV – ESV = 75 mL, and ejection fraction can be calculated as SV/EDV = 0.6. The untreated failing heart (diagram R) has an EDV of ~188 mL, an ESV of ~156, an SV of ~32 mL, and an ejection fraction of only ~0.17. Note also that the peak systolic pressure of the failing heart (95 mm Hg) is lower than that of the control heart (100 mm Hg). Treatment with digitalis (diagram Q) has increased the contractility of the myocardium. This increase in contractility has increased stroke volume to 45 mm Hg and ejection fraction to 0.26. Note also on diagram Q that the peak systolic pressure has returned to a normal value of 100 mm Hg and is better maintained throughout systole.

46.  **The correct answer is C.** This question requires you to equate salt restriction with an increased synthesis of aldosterone (aldosterone promotes sodium reabsorption) and then to remember that aldosterone is produced in the zona glomerulosa of the adrenal cortex. The zona glomerulosa is the outermost layer of the adrenal cortex.

The adrenal medulla (**choice A**) secretes catecholamines.

The zona fasciculata (**choice B**) is the middle layer of the adrenal cortex. It primarily secretes glucocorticoids.

The zona reticularis (**choice D**) is the innermost layer of the adrenal cortex. It primarily secretes androgens such as dehydroepiandrosterone (DHEA).

47.  **The correct answer is D.** To calculate the direction and driving force for fluid movement, use the Starling equation [net filtration pressure = $(P_c - P_i) - (\pi_c - \pi_i)$]. The net pressure in this case is positive because fluid is being forced out of the capillary.

$P_c$ = capillary hydrostatic pressure = 18, $\pi_c$ = capillary colloid osmotic pressure = 25, and $\pi_i$ = interstitial osmotic pressure = 9. Substituting these values into the equation and solving for $P_i$, we get:

8 mm Hg = $(24 - 7) - (17 - \pi_i)$ mm Hg

$\pi_i$ = 8 mm Hg

48.  **The correct answer is E.** By the time of implantation, approximately 7 days after ovulation, the fertilized ovum has developed to the blastocyst stage. At this stage, the blastocyst typically contains 100 or more cells, which have differentiated into an inner cell mass (designed to become the embryo) and trophoblast (which surrounds both the outer edge of the inner cell mass and a large fluid-filled cavity). The blastocyst is able to burrow into the endometrium in less than 24 hours after touching the endometrial surface. During the next several days, a

primitive placenta begins to develop that penetrates the maternal capillary bed and begins circulating maternal blood by about day 11.

49.  **The correct answer is C.** Glycoprotein GPIb on the platelet membrane binds von Willebrand factor, a plasma protein that circulates in a complex with factor VIII.

ADP (**choice A**) is a powerful inducer of platelet aggregation and strengthens the platelet plug by the addition of more activated platelets.

Calcium (**choice B**) is essential for increasing the degree of platelet aggregation and for strengthening the platelet plug. It is also a necessary cofactor in the coagulation cascade [required for the conversion of factors IX to IXa, X to Xa, V to Va, and prothrombin (factor II) to thrombin (factor IIa)].

Platelet factor 3 (PF3; **choice D**) is involved in platelet plug formation.

Prostacyclin (**choice E**) is synthesized by blood vessel endothelial cells and inhibits platelet aggregation.

Serotonin (**choice F**), along with epinephrine and kinins, is a vasoactive amine that promotes vasoconstriction.

Thromboplastin (**choice G**) initiates a series of reactions resulting in the formation of a permanent clot.

Thromboxane $A_2$ (**choice H**) is synthesized by platelets and promotes aggregation.

50.  **The correct answer is C.** The decrease in blood pressure caused by hemorrhage activates the baroreceptor reflex, which tends to increase sympathetic nerve activity and decrease parasympathetic (vagal) nerve activity (**choice D**). The increase in sympathetic nerve activity constricts arterioles in skeletal muscle (**choice A**) and elsewhere in the body. The fact that the patient has lost 600 mL blood and yet her blood pressure has decreased only slightly from a normal value of about 120/80 mm Hg may be attributed to the following compensatory responses: baroreceptor reflex, chemoreceptor reflex, epinephrine and norepinephrine released from the adrenal medulla, formation of angiotensin II, formation of vasopressin, and the capillary fluid shift mechanism.

Activation of the renin-angiotensin system during hemorrhage also plays an important role in maintaining blood pressure. Angiotensin II increases blood pressure acutely by constricting arterioles throughout the body (**choice A**), and chronically by decreasing the renal excretion of both salt (**choice B**) and water (**choice E**). The decrease in salt and water excretion returns blood volume to a normal value.

# Physiology: **Test Two**

1. In a controlled experiment, radiolabeled ATP is injected into an isolated muscle. The muscle is stimulated and allowed to contract for 10 seconds. An autoradiogram from a biopsy of the muscle will show radiolabeled ATP bound to

   (A) actin

   (B) myosin

   (C) sarcoplasmic reticulum

   (D) tropomyosin

   (E) troponin C

2. A medical student decides to conduct a neurochemical experiment to measure extracellular neurotransmitter levels in the brain following electrical stimulation of the raphe nuclei. Which of the following neurotransmitter levels would be expected to rise?

   (A) Acetylcholine

   (B) Dopamine

   (C) Gamma-amino-butyric acid (GABA)

   (D) Norepinephrine

   (E) Serotonin

3. A 60-year-old man with heart disease is brought to the emergency department. Cardiovascular evaluation reveals a resting $O_2$ consumption of 200 mL/min, a systemic arterial $O_2$ content of 0.20 mL $O_2$/mL of blood, and a mixed venous $O_2$ content of 0.15 mL $O_2$/mL of blood. What is his cardiac output?

   (A) 2.5 L/min

   (B) 4 L/min

   (C) 10 L/min

   (D) 25 L/min

   (E) 100 L/min

4. A normal volunteer consents to an IV infusion of p-aminohippuric acid (PAH). After a short time, the plasma PAH is 0.02 mg/mL, the concentration of PAH in urine is 13 mg/mL, and the urine flow is 1.0 mL/min. What is the effective renal plasma flow (ERPF)?

   (A) 0.26 mL/min

   (B) 26 mL/min

   (C) 65 mL/min

   (D) 260 mL/min

   (E) 650 mL/min

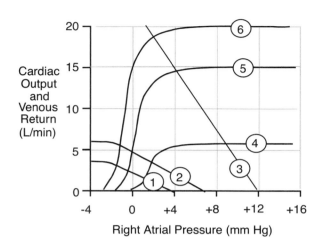

Right Atrial Pressure (mm Hg)

5.  A 25-year-old man has a cardiac output of 5 L/min, a right atrial pressure of 0 mm Hg, and a mean systemic filling pressure of 7 mm Hg during resting conditions. In the cardiac output-venous return curves above, his resting cardiac output function curve is depicted as curve 5, and his venous return curve is depicted as curve 2. Which of the following sets of values would represent his cardiac output (CO), right atrial pressure (RAP), and mean systemic filling pressure (MSFP) following moderate exercise?

| | CO | RAP | MSPF |
|---|---|---|---|
| (A) | 15 | 4 | 8 |
| (B) | 15 | 4 | 12 |
| (C) | 18 | 0 | 7 |
| (D) | 18 | 2 | 12 |
| (E) | 20 | 0 | 7 |
| (F) | 20 | 2 | 12 |

6.  Administration of an experimental drug that acts on peripheral nervous system (PNS) myelin is shown to increase the space constant (increase insulating effect of myelin) of an axon in a peripheral nerve. Action potentials traveling down the axon would be predicted to be

(A)  faster
(B)  larger
(C)  slower
(D)  smaller
(E)  unchanged

7.  A patient undergoes a total gastrectomy because of a proximally located gastric cancer. After the surgery, which of the following digestive enzymes will be produced in reduced amounts?

(A)  Amylase
(B)  Chymotrypsin
(C)  Lipase
(D)  Pepsin
(E)  Trypsin

8.  A 23-year-old woman gives blood to be a volunteer for bone-marrow donation. She is found to be a match for a 7-year-old boy with leukemia. Her bone marrow is harvested and examined for abnormalities. When the pathologist checks her marrow, what myeloid-to-erythroid ratio is she looking for to indicate that this young woman has a normal cell composition?

(A)  1:1
(B)  1:3
(C)  1:10
(D)  3:1
(E)  10:1

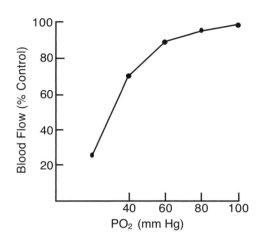

9. A research physiologist is studying the effects of hypoxia on vascular resistance. An anesthetized animal is ventilated with varying partial pressures of oxygen, and the venous outflow from different organs is measured using Doppler technology. The graph depicted above most likely represents data obtained from the

   (A) brain
   (B) kidney
   (C) liver
   (D) lungs
   (E) spleen

10. A boy-and-girl set of twins is beginning to undergo puberty at age 14. In the development of their reproductive systems, which of the following characteristics is similar for spermatogenesis and oogenesis?

   (A) Age at which meiosis begins
   (B) Amount of cytoplasm retained
   (C) DNA replication during meiosis
   (D) Length of prophase I
   (E) Transmission to fetus of mitochondrial DNA

11. A pathologist is looking at slides of a lung that were removed during autopsy of a woman who died of lung cancer. On examination of the slide, the doctor orients herself to the respiratory zone of the lung. She identifies this area by which structure?

   (A) Goblet cells
   (B) Main bronchi
   (C) Mucous cells
   (D) Terminal bronchioles
   (E) Type I epithelial cells

12. A 28-year-old man decides to donate a kidney to his brother, who is in chronic renal failure, after HLA typing suggests that he would be a suitable donor. He is admitted to the hospital, and his right kidney is removed and transplanted into his brother. Which of the following indices would be expected to be decreased in the donor after full recovery from the operation?

   (A) Creatinine clearance
   (B) Creatinine production
   (C) Daily excretion of sodium
   (D) Plasma creatinine concentration
   (E) Renal excretion of creatinine

13. A 49-year-old woman comes to the clinic complaining of fatigue. She denies fever, vomiting, or diarrhea, but physical examination shows dry mucous membranes. Her blood pressure is 90/60 mm Hg. Laboratory studies show a plasma sodium level of 129 mEq/L and a potassium level of 5.5 mEq/L. Which of the following is the most likely cause of her hyponatremia?

   (A) Addison disease
   (B) Diabetes insipidus
   (C) Hyperaldosteronism
   (D) Psychogenic polydipsia
   (E) Syndrome of inappropriate ADH secretion

14. A 32-year-old man is on a high-protein, low-carbohydrate diet because he has heard that this will help him build muscle. Which of the following peptides needs to be released to increase the secretion of pancreatic enzymes into the small intestine so that he can digest these types of meals?

   (A) Cholecystokinin
   (B) Gastrin
   (C) Motilin
   (D) Secretin
   (E) Somatostatin

15. In a study of renal function, the urine flow rate of an experimental animal is 2.0 mL/min, the glomerular filtration rate is 100 mL/min, and renal plasma flow is 500 mL/min. During this time, substance X is infused, and a steady state is achieved. The afferent arteriolar concentration of X is 100 mg/dL, the efferent arteriolar concentration is 120 mg/dL, and the renal vein concentration is 102 mg/dL. From these data, you can conclude that X is

    (A) freely filtered and reabsorbed
    (B) freely filtered and secreted
    (C) freely filtered, but neither reabsorbed nor secreted
    (D) not filtered, but secreted
    (E) not filtered or secreted

16. A medical student is studying pancreatic function on a computer-simulated patient. The student is specifically trying to understand the insulin secretion pattern in the pancreatic cells. The student is presented with a list of substances that affect insulin secretion. She clicks on a substance and finds that it directly inhibits the patient's insulin secretion. This response was most likely caused by which of the following substances?

    (A) Alpha$_2$-adrenergic agonist
    (B) Beta$_2$-adrenergic agonist
    (C) Cholecystokinin
    (D) Glucagon
    (E) Sugar water
    (F) Muscarinic agonists

17. A patient placed on a ventilator in the intensive care unit has an anatomic dead space of 150 mL. If the ventilator has a dead space of 350 mL and a rate of 20/min, which tidal volume should be selected for the ventilator to provide an alveolar ventilation of 6 L/min?

    (A) 1200 mL
    (B) 1000 mL
    (C) 800 mL
    (D) 600 mL
    (E) 400 mL

18. A 55-year-old woman stopped menstruating approximately 3 months ago. Worried that she may be pregnant, she decides to have a pregnancy test. The result is negative. Which of the following series of test results will confirm that the woman is postmenopausal?

    (A) Decreased LH, decreased FSH, increased estrogen
    (B) Decreased LH, increased FSH, decreased estrogen
    (C) Increased LH, decreased FSH, decreased estrogen
    (D) Increased LH, increased FSH, decreased estrogen
    (E) Increased LH, increased FSH, increased estrogen

19. A child falls and bumps her head on the floor. Tissue factor is exposed beneath the endothelium of traumatized blood vessels. Which of the following procoagulant proteins binds to tissue factor and initiates the clotting cascade?

    (A) Factor V
    (B) Factor VII
    (C) Factor X
    (D) Fibrinogen
    (E) Prothrombin

20. A 63-year-old man with essential hypertension has gone several weeks without taking his medications. He arrives at the emergency department after falling on his outstretched right hand. He has a heart rate of 90 min and a blood pressure of 170/115 mm Hg. Which of the following is most likely to be decreased in the skeletal muscles of his legs?

    (A) Adenosine levels
    (B) Arterial blood pressure
    (C) Arteriolar resistance
    (D) Blood flow
    (E) Venous oxygen concentration

21. A man with normal lungs overdoses on secobarbital, causing hypoventilation. He is brought to a hospital where the barometric pressure is 500 mm Hg. Alveolar $P_{CO_2}$ rises to 80 mm Hg, and the respiratory exchange ratio is 1.0. Assuming that the patient's condition remains unchanged, what percentage of inspired $O_2$ will return his alveolar $P_{O_2}$ to normal (100 mm Hg)?

    (A) 55
    (B) 40
    (C) 36
    (D) 28
    (E) 24

22. The clearance of several substances was measured at a constant glomerular filtration rate and constant urine flow rate, but at increasing plasma concentrations of the substance. Under these conditions, clearance will increase at high plasma concentrations for which of the following substances?

    (A) Creatinine

    (B) Mannitol

    (C) Penicillin

    (D) Phosphate

    (E) Urea

23. In the clotting process, as the hemostatic plug develops, fibrin polymerizes into monomeric threads that are held together by noncovalent bonds. Which clotting protein increases the strength of the clot by cross-linking the newly formed fibrin threads?

    (A) Factor XIII

    (B) High molecular weight kininogen (HMWK)

    (C) Plasminogen

    (D) Thrombin

    (E) von Willebrand Factor (vWF)

24. A 26-year-old man receives a concussion from a car accident. The brain edema that follows causes compression of the cerebral arteries to such an extent that he needs to be placed on mechanical ventilation to control his breathing. His respiratory drive is diminished mainly because of decreased

    (A) arterial $P_{CO_2}$ acting through central chemoreceptors

    (B) arterial $P_{CO_2}$ acting through peripheral chemoreceptors

    (C) arterial pH acting through central chemoreceptors

    (D) arterial pH acting through peripheral chemoreceptors

    (E) arterial $P_{O_2}$ acting through central chemoreceptors

    (F) arterial $P_{O_2}$ acting through peripheral chemoreceptors

25. A construction worker has a serious accident in which his rib cage and abdominal muscles become completely paralyzed. He is still able to breathe, however, because his diaphragm continues to contract. At which level might his spinal cord injury have occurred?

    (A) C2

    (B) C7

    (C) L3

    (D) T5

    (E) T12

26. A 49-year-old mildly obese man with no history of heart disease is prescribed a diet and aerobic exercise regimen. Which of the following is most important for maintaining adequate cardiac output during exercise?

    (A) Decreased cardiac index

    (B) Decreased diastolic blood pressure

    (C) Increased heart rate and stroke volume

    (D) Increased systemic vascular resistance

27. A woodworker operating a bandsaw accidently injures his wrist, severing his radial artery and producing severe hemorrhage. As he loses blood, his body tries to compensate for the developing hypotension by increasing sympathetic outflow. The postganglionic signals carrying the impulses to constrict his arterioles are transmitted along which of the following fiber types?

    (A) A-δ fibers

    (B) B fibers

    (C) C fibers

    (D) Ia fibers

    (E) Ib fibers

28. A 35-year-old man complains of difficulty eating food and drinking liquids. On history he reveals that he can swallow the food but feels as though what he eats and drinks does not "go anywhere" after he swallows. He has recently begun to vomit undigested food, and he has a cough that wakes him from sleep at nighttime. He has lost 5 lb within the past month without trying to lose weight. His laboratory studies are normal. A barium swallow shows dilation of the distal esophagus with a tapered end. Which of the following is the most likely cause of his disorder?

    (A) A defect in segmentation contraction

    (B) A defect in the migrating myoelectric complex

    (C) A defect in the neural network of the myenteric plexus

    (D) Damage to the vagus nerve

    (E) Increased amounts of vasoactive intestinal peptide

29. A 1-week-old infant has a coarctation of the aorta just distal to the subclavian arteries. The blood pressure distal to the constriction is 50% lower than normal. Which of the following is increased in this infant?

    (A) Blood flow in the lower body

    (B) Glomerular filtration rate

    (C) Plasma levels of angiotensin II

    (D) Renal excretion of sodium

    (E) Renal excretion of water

30. A research physiologist decides to use a marker to measure the volume of total body water in a volunteer medical student. Which of the following substances would he most likely use?

    (A) Tritium

    (B) Cresyl violet

    (C) Evans blue

    (D) $^{131}$I-albumin

    (E) Inulin

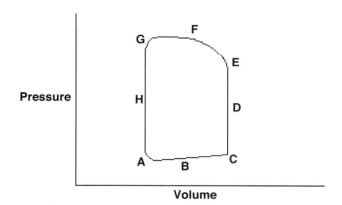

31. A 73-year-old woman has mild hemoptysis, dyspnea, orthopnea, and paroxysmal nocturnal dyspnea. She has a low-pitched, rumbling diastolic murmur, produced by a stenotic valve, that is accentuated by exercise. The murmur is heard best at the apex when she lies in the left lateral recumbent position. In normal patients, which of the following points on a left ventricular pressure volume loop (above) represents the opening of the affected valve?

    (A) A

    (B) B

    (C) C

    (D) D

    (E) E

    (F) F

    (G) G

    (H) H

32. A 65-year-old woman receives 3 liters of 0.9% saline following a minor surgical procedure. This results in increased right atrial filling and contraction. Which of the following is most likely to be secreted in response?

    (A) Aldosterone

    (B) Antidiuretic hormone (ADH)

    (C) Atrial natriuretic factor (ANF)

    (D) Norepinephrine

    (E) Renin

33. A 67-year-old woman goes to her primary care physician because of muscle weakness, frequent urination, and increased thirst. On examination, her blood pressure is 180/90 mm Hg. On prior visits she has been normotensive. Laboratory studies show that she is hypernatremic and hypokalemic. A CT scan of the abdomen shows a nodule on her left adrenal gland. What is the most likely mechanism for her disorder?

    (A) Decreased glomerular capillary filtration coefficient

    (B) Excessive tubular sodium reabsorption

    (C) Increased renal secretion of renin

    (D) Increased renal vascular resistance

    (E) Patchy renal damage

34. A medical-school professor is using tape-recorded heartbeats for a lecture on heart sounds. He draws an atrial pressure tracing on the board for correlation. The first tape played has normal first and second heart sounds. The second heart sound would correspond to which of the following points on an atrial pressure tracing?

    (A) a wave

    (B) c wave

    (C) v wave

    (D) x descent

    (E) y descent

35. A 65-year-old woman with renal failure presents for hemodialysis. She is found to be anemic and is given a dose of erythropoietin along with her usual vitamin and mineral supplements. Erythropoietin stimulates which of the following intermediates in hematopoiesis?

    (A) Basophilic erythroblasts

    (B) Colony forming units-erythroid (CFU-E)

    (C) Multipotential stem cells

    (D) Proerythroblasts

    (E) Reticulocytes

36. After an accident at work resulting in severe hemorrhage, a machinist is rushed to the emergency department. Which of the following sets of autonomic responses would be predicted in this patient?

| | Heart rate | Bowel sounds | Pupil diameter |
|---|---|---|---|
| (A) | Decreased | Decreased | Constricted |
| (B) | Decreased | Decreased | Dilated |
| (C) | Decreased | Increased | Constricted |
| (D) | Decreased | Increased | Dilated |
| (E) | Increased | Decreased | Constricted |
| (F) | Increased | Decreased | Dilated |
| (G) | Increased | Increased | Constricted |
| (H) | Increased | Increased | Dilated |

37. In a tissue capillary, the interstitial hydrostatic pressure is 2 mm Hg, the capillary hydrostatic pressure is 25 mm Hg, and the interstitial oncotic pressure is 7 mm Hg. If the net driving force across the capillary wall is 3 mm Hg favoring filtration, what is the capillary oncotic pressure?

    (A) 21 mm Hg

    (B) 23 mm Hg

    (C) 24 mm Hg

    (D) 25 mm Hg

    (E) 27 mm Hg

38. A medical student volunteers to have his lung volumes and capacities measured for his organ physiology laboratory class. He is connected at the end of a normal expiration to a spirometer containing a known concentration of helium. He is instructed to breathe several times until the helium has equilibrated between the spirometer and his lungs. Calculations are made to determine the amount of air in his lungs when he was connected to the spirometer, which is called the

    (A) expiratory reserve volume

    (B) functional residual capacity

    (C) inspiratory capacity

    (D) inspiratory reserve volume

    (E) residual volume

    (F) tidal volume

    (G) vital capacity

39. A 78-year-old woman has a mean arterial pressure of 120 mm Hg and a heart rate of 60/min. She has a stroke volume of 50 mL, cardiac output of 3000 mL/min, and a right atrial pressure of 0 mm Hg. What is the total peripheral resistance (in mm Hg/mL/min) in this woman?

    (A) 0.01

    (B) 0.02

    (C) 0.04

    (D) 0.08

    (E) 0.10

40. A 23-year-old man with diabetes mellitus has a glomerular filtration rate (GFR) significantly greater that normal, especially when he consumes excessive amounts of sweets. A decrease in which of the following parameters would tend to increase the glomerular capillary hydrostatic pressure?

    (A) Afferent arteriolar resistance

    (B) Bowman's capsular hydrostatic pressure

    (C) Capillary filtration coefficient

    (D) Efferent arteriolar resistance

    (E) Plasma colloid osmotic pressure

41. A woman goes to a restaurant for a friend's birthday and eats a large meal. After the meal, a certain hormone is stimulated by acid entering her duodenum. This hormone inhibits stomach motility and stimulates bicarbonate secretion from the pancreas. Which of the following hormones is structurally related to the hormone in question?

    (A) Cholecystokinin

    (B) Gastrin

    (C) Glucagon

    (D) Somatostatin

    (E) Substance P

42. With time, blood stored in a blood bank tends to become relatively depleted of 2,3-diphosphoglycerate (2,3-DPG). What effect does this have on the hemoglobin-oxygen dissociation curve?

    (A) Shifts the curve to the left, so that the hemoglobin has a decreased oxygen affinity

    (B) Shifts the curve to the left, so that the hemoglobin has an increased oxygen affinity

    (C) Shifts the curve to the right, so that the hemoglobin has a decreased oxygen affinity

    (D) Shifts the curve to the right, so that the hemoglobin has an increased oxygen affinity

    (E) Does not change the dissociation curve

43. A researcher attaches a video camera to his microscope so that he can observe all of the stages of spermatogenesis. He is specifically interested in observing the process of crossing over. This particular process occurs during the meiotic division of which of the following cells?

    (A) Primary spermatocytes

    (B) Secondary spermatocytes

    (C) Spermatids

    (D) Spermatogonia

    (E) Spermatozoa

44. To make extra money, a medical student participates in a study to determine hormone levels during the menstrual cycle. Her menarche was at age 13, and she has always had regular, 28-day cycles. When analyzing the results of her studies, it is correct to assume that the *dotted line* in the figure below represents the cyclic secretion pattern of

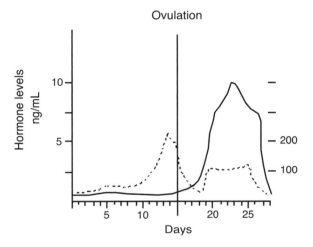

(A) Estrogen
(B) Follicle-stimulating hormone (FSH)
(C) Gonadotropin-releasing hormone (GnRH)
(D) Luteinizing hormone (LH)
(E) Progesterone

45. A 30-year-old woman with menorrhagia visits her gynecologist. She is evaluated for possible iron-deficiency anemia. Her hemoglobin is 10 g/dL, hematocrit is 36%, red blood cell count is 4.0 million/μL, and mean cell diameter is 7.5 μm. What is the patient's mean corpuscular volume (MCV)?

(A) 67.5 fL
(B) 75.0 fL
(C) 83.3 fL
(D) 90.0 fL
(E) 111.1 fL

46. To celebrate the end of the semester, a college student goes on an alcohol binge. She drinks day and night for 3 days straight. During this period, her urinary flow rate increased from 1 to 10 mL/min. This increase in urinary flow rate will significantly increase the clearance of

(A) creatinine
(B) inulin
(C) penicillin
(D) phosphate
(E) urea

47. A 66-year-old woman complains of fatigue to her physician. Her pulse is 80/min and her hematocrit is 32%. Ultrasound shows an end-systolic volume of 65 mL and an end-diastolic volume of 115 mL. Which of the following is the ejection fraction in this woman?

(A) 0.29
(B) 0.32
(C) 0.43
(D) 0.51
(E) 0.62

48. Under normal conditions virtually 100% of the filtered load of glucose is reabsorbed by the kidney tubules. Which part of the tubule shown below is expected to have the highest concentration of glucose under normal conditions?

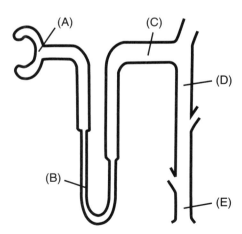

49. A 30-year-old woman is given 0.1 g inulin intravenously. One hour later the plasma inulin concentration is 1 mg/100 mL. Which of the following is the extracellular fluid volume (in liters) of this woman (assuming that urinary loss of inulin is insignificant)?

    (A) 8
    (B) 10
    (C) 12
    (D) 14
    (E) 16

50. A 62-year-old man has tingling in his feet and difficulty with balance. He has a mean corpuscular volume of 130 fl. A peripheral blood smear shows six-lobed neutrophils and macro-ovalocytes. Which of the following conditions is associated with a lifelong requirement for parenteral administration of the vitamin deficient in this patient?

    I.   Pernicious anemia
    II.  Removal of colon
    III. Removal of gallbladder
    IV.  Removal of ileum
    V.   Removal of jejunum
    VI.  Removal of stomach

    (A) I only
    (B) I and V
    (C) I, IV, and V
    (D) I, IV, and VI
    (E) I, V, and VI
    (F) III only
    (G) III and IV

# Physiology Test Two: **Answers and Explanations**

## ANSWER KEY

| | | | | |
|---|---|---|---|---|
| 1. | B | | 26. | C |
| 2. | E | | 27. | C |
| 3. | B | | 28. | C |
| 4. | E | | 29. | C |
| 5. | D | | 30. | A |
| 6. | A | | 31. | A |
| 7. | D | | 32. | C |
| 8. | D | | 33. | B |
| 9. | D | | 34. | C |
| 10. | C | | 35. | B |
| 11. | E | | 36. | F |
| 12. | A | | 37. | E |
| 13. | A | | 38. | B |
| 14. | A | | 39. | C |
| 15. | E | | 40. | A |
| 16. | A | | 41. | C |
| 17. | C | | 42. | B |
| 18. | D | | 43. | A |
| 19. | B | | 44. | A |
| 20. | A | | 45. | D |
| 21. | B | | 46. | E |
| 22. | D | | 47. | C |
| 23. | A | | 48. | A |
| 24. | A | | 49. | B |
| 25. | B | | 50. | D |

1. **The correct answer is B.** During the contraction cycle, ATP binds to myosin cross-bridge heads, causing the dissociation of myosin from actin.

   Actin (**choice A**) forms cross-bridges with myosin but does not bind to ATP.

   The sarcoplasmic reticulum (**choice C**) is involved in storing and releasing $Ca^{2+}$ for muscle contraction.

   Tropomyosin (**choice D**) is a thin filament that runs alongside actin. In the absence of calcium, tropomyosin lies in the groove of the actin filament and blocks actin's myosin-binding sites.

   Troponin C (**choice E**) is the calcium-binding subunit of the troponin complex. When troponin C binds calcium, a conformational change causes tropomyosin to shift, thereby exposing the myosin-binding sites on actin.

2. **The correct answer is E.** Serotonin is the primary neurotransmitter of the raphe nuclei. Ascending serotonin projections from the dorsal and median raphe nuclei distribute diffusely throughout the brain. Other raphe nuclei provide descending serotonin projections to the spinal cord and brainstem.

   Cell bodies that contain acetylcholine (**choice A**) are found in the basal nucleus of Meynert (which degenerates in Alzheimer disease), in the medial septum and diagonal band complex, and in the striatum.

   Dopamine- (**choice B**) containing cell bodies are found in the midbrain (in the substantia nigra pars compacta and in the ventral tegmental area). The cell bodies in the hypothalamus contribute to the tuberoinfundibular pathway.

   GABA (**choice C**) is the primary inhibitory neurotransmitter of the brain and is therefore located throughout the brain. Such areas include the cerebellar cortex, striatum, globus pallidus, and substantia nigra pars reticulata.

   Norepinephrine- (**choice D**) containing neurons are found predominantly in the locus ceruleus of the pons and midbrain.

3. **The correct answer is B.** Cardiac output can be measured by way of $O_2$ consumption using the Fick principle:

$$\text{Cardiac output} = \frac{O_2 \text{ consumption}}{([O_2] \text{ arterial} - [O_2] \text{ venous})}$$

   In this case, oxygen consumption was 200 mL/min, $(O_2)$ arterial was 0.20 mL $O_2$/mL of blood, and $(O_2)$ venous was 0.15 mL $O_2$/mL of blood:

$$\text{Cardiac output} =$$
$$\frac{200 \text{ mL/min}}{0.20 \text{ mL } O_2/\text{mL blood} - 0.15 \text{ mL } O_2/\text{mL blood}}$$
$$= 4000 \text{ mL/min}$$
$$= 4.0 \text{ L/min}$$

   **Choice A** corresponds to a very low cardiac output, as average cardiac output is approximately 5 L/min.

   **Choices C, D, and E** are illogical since the heart is virtually incapable of pumping so much blood in 1 minute, especially in a patient with heart disease.

   Instead of systemic arterial, pulmonary venous $O_2$ could be used, and instead of systemic venous, pulmonary arterial $O_2$ could be used.

4. **The correct answer is E.** Approximately 90% of a small dose of PAH is cleared by the kidney in a single pass. If it were 100%, then the amount of PAH in urine (concentration times urine flow rate) divided by the amount of PAH in plasma would exactly equal the renal plasma flow. Because the extraction ratio (arterial-venous PAH concentration divided by arterial concentration) is 0.9 (90%) instead of 100%, physiologists speak of the quantity $U_{PAH}V/P_{PAH}$ as the effective renal plasma flow, or ERPF. So, in this patient, we have (13 mg/mL x 1.0 mL/min)/0.02 mg/mL = 650 mL/min.

   0.26 mL/min (**choice A**) can be obtained by multiplying 13 by 0.02 and dividing by 1. This value is far too low to be a normal ERPF, which is typically around 625 mL/min.

   26 mL/min (**choice B**) is 100 times (13 × 0.02)/1. This value is far too low to be a normal ERPF, which is typically around 625 mL/min.

   65 mL/min (**choice C**) might indicate that you set the ratio up correctly, but dropped a power of 10 in your calculations. This value is far too low to be a normal ERPF, which is typically around 625 mL/min.

   260 mL/min (**choice D**) is 1000 times (13 3 0.02)/1, and is still too low to be a normal ERPF.

   Timesaving note: If you remember that the ERPF is approximately 625 mL/min, you do not really need to calculate anything in this question. Choice E is the only reasonable answer.

5. **The correct answer is D.** Following moderate exercise, the cardiac function curve is represented by curve 6, and the venous return curve is represented by curve 3 in the diagram. Note from the point where curves 6 and 3

intersect that (a) drawing a horizontal line to the *y*-axis gives a value of CO of about 18 L/min, (b) drawing a vertical line to the *x*-axis gives a RAP of about 2 mm Hg, and (c) the point where curve 3 (the venous return curve) intersects the *x*-axis is the MSFP, which is about +12 mm Hg.

The increased level of the cardiac function curve results almost entirely from sympathetic stimulation of the heart, which increases heart rate and myocardial contractility. Note on the diagram that, without the increased level of the cardiac function curve, the maximal level of cardiac output would be about 15 L/min (intersection of curves 3 and 5). Note also that the resting venous return curve (curve 2) would limit the maximal cardiac output to about 6 L/min, even with enhanced performance of the heart, depicted by curve 6.

The mean systemic filling pressure (MSFP) is the pressure that exists in all parts of the circulation when the heart has been stopped and the blood volume has become redistributed in the system until all pressures are at equilibrium. The MSFP is thus a measure of the "tightness" with which the circulatory system is filled with blood. The greater the system is filled (i.e., when MSFP increases), the easier it is for blood to flow into the heart, which tends to increase venous return. However, venous return also depends on the right atrial pressure because the pressure gradient for venous return is equal to MSFP − RAP. MSFP is increased during exercise because of venular constriction resulting from (a) sympathetic stimulation of veins and other capacitance vessels, and (b) compression of veins and other capacitance vessels by tensing the muscles in the abdomen. The venous return curve (curve 3) is also rotated upward (increased slope) because the resistance to venous return has decreased because the vessels in the exercising muscles have dilated greatly.

6. **The correct answer is A.** The space constant of an axon reflects the amount of passive or electrotonic spread of current within the axon. The larger the space constant, the further the current can spread, allowing action potentials to propagate faster. This is why myelin increases the conduction velocity of action potentials down an axon. Conversely, demyelination decreases the space constant and slows action potential conduction.

7. **The correct answer is D.** Pepsin is secreted (in an inactive or zymogen form as pepsinogen) by the chief cells of the stomach. Pepsinogen is activated by contact with stomach acid. Although protein digestion usually begins with the actions of hydrochloric acid and pepsin, pancreatic enzymes complete the job as the food passes into the small intestine.

Amylases (**choice A**) hydrolyze $1 \rightarrow 4$ glycosidic linkages of starches to produce oligosaccharides, maltose, maltotriose, and limit dextrins. These enzymes are produced by the pancreas and salivary glands.

Chymotrypsin (**choice B**) is a proteolytic enzyme released by the pancreas as the inactive proenzyme, chymotrypsinogen.

Lipases (**choice C**) are mostly released by the pancreas and serve to digest various lipids, including triacylglycerols.

Trypsin (**choice E**) is a proteolytic enzyme released by the pancreas as the inactive proenzyme trypsinogen.

8. **The correct answer is D.** The ratio of cells in bone marrow developing along myeloid lines to cells developing along erythroid lines is 3:1. An alternative way to remember the normal marrow composition is that it typically contains about 60% granulocytes and their precursors; 20% erythroid precursors; 10% lymphocytes, monocytes, and their precursors; and 10% unidentified or disintegrating cells. These numbers are worth remembering, because shifts away from normal values may be a subtle clue to marrow abnormalities.

9. **The correct answer is D.** The graph indicates that blood flow decreases with hypoxia. Only the lungs exhibit vasoconstriction in response to hypoxia (pulmonary hypoxic vasoconstriction). This is an adaptive mechanism that causes blood to shunt away from regions of the lung that are poorly ventilated (e.g., because of airway obstruction) to areas that are better ventilated. In other organs, vasodilation generally occurs in response to hypoxia.

10. **The correct answer is C.** The actual process of manipulation of DNA and chromosomes during meiosis is very similar in spermatogenesis and oogenesis. However, the processes also differ in many other respects:

In oogenesis, the process of meiosis begins before birth and arrests between birth and puberty in prophase I. In contrast, spermatogenesis does not begin until puberty (**see choice A**).

The egg retains a large volume of cytoplasm (**choice B**), whereas nearly all the cytoplasm is stripped during formation of a sperm.

As noted above, in oogenesis, meiosis is arrested in prophase I, which is consequently very prolonged in the female. In spermatogenesis, meiosis is completed in a much shorter time (**choice D**).

Both the egg and the sperm have mitochondria, but those of the sperm are left outside when the sperm nucleus enters the egg and consequently do not contribute to the mitochondrial genome of the fetus. Instead, the mitochondria are transmitted from the egg to the fetus (**choice E**). Traits coded for by mitochondrial DNA are therefore inherited in a matrilineal fashion.

11. **The correct answer is E.** There are two zones in the lung: the conducting zone (where there is no gas exchange) and the respiratory zone (where there is gas exchange). Of all of the structures listed, only type I epithelial cells are located in the respiratory zone. Type I epithelial cells are the primary structural cells of the alveolar wall. Type II epithelial cells, also located in the alveoli, produce surfactant.

    Goblet cells (**choice A**), which are mucus-secreting cells, are present in the conducting airways.

    The main bronchi (**choice B**) are part of the conducting airways.

    Mucous cells (**choice C**), which are mucus-secreting cells, are present in the conducting airways.

    Terminal bronchioles (**choice D**) are the most distal part of the conducting airways. Respiratory bronchioles, which are just distal to the terminal bronchioles, are part of the respiratory zone. These two types of bronchioles can be differentiated from each other by whether they have alveoli budding from their walls. Respiratory bronchioles have alveoli, terminal bronchioles do not.

12. **The correct answer is A.** Because creatinine is freely filtered by the glomerulus, but not secreted or reabsorbed to a significant extent, the renal clearance of creatinine is approximately equal to the glomerular filtration rate. In fact, creatinine clearance is commonly used to assess renal function in the clinical setting. When a kidney is removed, the total glomerular filtration rate decreases because 50% of the nephrons have been removed, which causes the creatinine clearance to decrease. In turn, the plasma creatinine concentration (**choice D**) increases until the rate of creatinine excretion by the kidneys (**choice E**) is equal to the rate of creatinine production by the body. Recall that creatinine excretion = GFR × plasma creatinine concentration. Therefore, creatinine excretion is normal when GFR is decreased following removal of a kidney because the plasma concentration of creatinine is elevated.

    Creatinine is a waste product of metabolism. Creatinine production (**choice B**) is directly related to the muscle mass of an individual, but is independent of renal function.

    The daily excretion of sodium (**choice C**) is unaffected by the removal of a kidney. The amount of sodium excreted each day by the remaining kidney exactly matches the amount of sodium entering the body in the diet.

13. **The correct answer is A.** Addison disease, or primary adrenal insufficiency, is caused by destruction of adrenal cortical tissue. As a consequence of the loss of mineralocorticoids, there is reduced ability to retain sodium and excrete potassium. (Recall that aldosterone acts on the renal collecting duct to promote resorption of $Na^+$ and secretion of $K^+$.) Hence, this patient has hyponatremia and hyperkalemia. Low plasma sodium is accompanied by hypovolemia, signs of dehydration, and hypotension.

    Hyperaldosteronism (**choice C**), in contrast with the hypoaldosteronism of Addison disease, is accompanied by *hypo*kalemia and *hyper*tension.

    Diabetes insipidus (**choice B**) is the consequence of a lack of sufficient ADH. The ensuing loss of urinary water also can result in *hyper*natremia.

    Psychogenic polydipsia (**choice D**) can produce hyponatremia. However, the outcome of excessive drinking of water would not be signs of dehydration or hypotension.

    In the syndrome of inappropriate ADH secretion (SIADH) (**choice E**), ADH is secreted and water is retained. SIADH also produces hyponatremia without signs of hypovolemia or dehydration.

14. **The correct answer A.** Release of cholecystokinin is stimulated by the presence of peptides, amino acids, or fatty acids in the small intestine. Cholecystokinin acts on the pancreas to stimulate secretion of pancreatic enzymes that aid in the digestion of these compounds.

    Gastrin (**choice B**) secretion, which is stimulated by the presence of peptides or amino acids in the lumen of the stomach, produces an increase in gastric $H^+$ secretion.

    Motilin (**choice C**) is a hormone that regulates the migrating myoelectric complex, a series of contractions that occur during fasting, clearing the stomach and small intestine of any residual food.

    Secretin (**choice D**) secretion, which is stimulated by the presence of $H^+$ and fatty acids in the duodenum, causes an increase in pancreatic and biliary $HCO_3^-$ release and a decrease in gastric $H^+$ release.

    Somatostatin (**choice E**) secretion, which is stimulated by the presence of $H^+$ in the lumen, results in decreased release of all gastrointestinal hormones and decreased $H^+$ secretion in the stomach.

15. **The correct answer is E.** If a substance is not filtered, its concentration in the efferent arteriole will be greater than the concentration in the afferent arteriole by an amount equal to the fraction of water filtered into the glomerulus. In this case, the filtration fraction (FF = glomerular filtration rate/renal plasma flow) = 100/500 = 20%, so efferent arteriolar concentration equals

120 mg/dL. All the filtered water except for that amount necessary to sustain urine flow is reabsorbed back into the peritubular capillaries, and so is present in the renal vein. In this case, the fractional excretion of water (= urine flow rate/glomerular filtration rate) = 2/100 = 2%, so renal vein concentration is 2% greater than afferent arteriolar concentration, giving a renal vein concentration of 102 mg/dL.

Note that answering this question did not require any calculations. The numbers are used in the discussion only to highlight the general concepts you should have recognized: the relationship between a substance's concentration in the afferent arteriole vs. the efferent arteriole provides information about filtration of the substance. The concentration of the substance in the afferent arteriole vs. the renal vein provides information about the secretion of that substance.

Filtration does not affect the concentration of freely filtered substances, so the afferent and efferent concentrations of any freely filtered substance will be the same (**choices A, B, and C**).

Secretion of a substance increases its excretion, which would decrease the renal vein concentration of the substance. Therefore, the renal vein concentration of a substance that is not filtered, but is secreted (to any significant degree), would be less than the afferent arteriolar concentration (**choice D**).

16.  **The correct answer is A.** Alpha$_2$-receptor agonists directly inhibit pancreatic insulin secretion.

Beta$_2$-adrenergic agonists (**choice B**) stimulate insulin secretion.

Cholecystokinin (**choice C**) is a hormone that causes not only gallbladder contraction, but also insulin secretion from the pancreas.

Pancreatic glucagon release (**choice D**) acts as a paracrine stimulus for insulin secretion.

Sugar water (**choice E**) is a stimulus for the secretion of insulin from the pancreas.

Muscarinic activity (**choice F**) in the gastrointestinal tract enhances secretion of insulin from the pancreas.

17.  **The correct answer is C.** Recall that total ventilation is equal to alveolar ventilation plus dead space ventilation. This can be expressed mathematically as:

$V_T \times n = V_A \times n + V_D \times n$, where

$V_T$ = tidal volume

$V_A$ = the volume of alveolar gas in the tidal volume

$V_D$ = dead space

n  = respiratory frequency

To calculate the answer, just plug the given values into this equation and solve for $V_T$. Realize also that the dead space is the combined dead space of the patient and the ventilator: 150 mL + 350 mL = 500 mL. Do not forget to check your units: you need to convert 6 L/min to 6000 mL/min.

$(V_T \times 20/\text{min}) = (6000 \text{ mL/min}) + (500 \text{ mL} \ 20/\text{min})$

$(V_T \times 20/\text{min}) = 16{,}000 \text{ mL/min}$

$V_T = 800 \text{ mL}$

18.  **The correct answer is D.** During menopause, there is a loss of functioning follicles in the ovaries such that GnRH-stimulated LH and FSH secretion do not result in normal estrogen secretion. The low estrogen levels cannot inhibit gonadotropin secretion in a negative-feedback fashion, resulting in very high levels of LH and FSH.

**Choices A, B, C, and E** do not accurately describe normal hormonal levels in menopause.

19.  **The correct answer is B.** The extrinsic pathway of clotting begins with tissue factor binding to Factor VII or Factor VIIa. All other clotting proteins require proteolytic cleavage to become active; however, Factor VII has a low level of activity in its inactive form and can act with tissue factor and phospholipids to initiate the clotting cascade. In the extrinsic pathway, Factor VII cleaves Factor X to Xa (**choice C**), which acts in concert with Factor V (**choice A**) to cleave prothrombin to thrombin (**choice E**). The final step in the coagulation pathway is the cleavage of fibrinogen to fibrin by thrombin (**choice D**). Fibrin polymerizes and cross-links, thereby forming a hemostatic net of insoluble protein.

20.  **The correct answer is A.** The skeletal muscles of the body have a normal blood flow even when blood pressure is chronically elevated. Organs and tissues in which the vasculature has primarily a nutritive function (e.g., brain, heart, and skeletal muscle) regulate their blood flow in accordance with the metabolic needs of the tissues. These tissues exhibit short-term autoregulation of blood flow such that the increase in flow caused by an elevated arterial pressure is minimized by constriction of the arterioles. The constriction is caused in part by decreased levels of adenosine (an endogenous vasodilator) in the tissues. The rate of adenosine production in a tissue is a function of its metabolic rate, which is not affected significantly by an increase in systemic pressure. When blood flow to the muscle increases, the adenosine is literally washed from the muscle, lowering the tissue levels of adenosine. The decrease in adenosine concentration causes small arteries and arterioles in the muscle to constrict, and this increase in resistance (**choice C**) maintains blood flow (**choice D**) at a normal

rate in the face of increased arterial pressure (**choice B**). The overall process is called autoregulation of blood flow.

Venous oxygen concentration (**choice E**) does not decrease in the skeletal muscles of hypertensives because blood flow is maintained at an adequate level to meet the nutritional demands of the muscles.

21. **The correct answer is B.** The patient is hypoventilating because of the effects of barbiturates on respiration. This question requires use of the alveolar gas equation:

$P_{A_{O_2}} = P_{I_{O_2}} - P_{A_{CO_2}}/R$, where

$P_{A_{O_2}}$ = the partial pressure of alveolar $O_2$

$P_{I_{O_2}}$ = the partial pressure of inspired $O_2$

$P_{A_{CO_2}}$ = the partial pressure of alveolar $CO_2$

R = respiratory exchange ratio

We know that $P_{A_{O_2}}$ = 100 mm Hg, $P_{A_{CO_2}}$ = 80 mm Hg, and R = 1, so we can solve for $P_{I_{O_2}}$:

100 mm Hg = $P_{I_{O_2}}$ – 80 mm Hg/1

$P_{I_{O_2}}$ = 180 mm Hg

$P_{I_{O_2}}$ = $F_{O_2} \times (P_B - P_{H_2O})$, where $F_{O_2}$ is the fraction of inspired $O_2$ and $P_B$ is the barometric pressure. $P_{H_2O}$ is the water vapor pressure in the airways and always remains constant at 47 mm Hg. Solving for $F_{O_2}$:

180 mm Hg = $F_{O_2} \times$ (500 mm Hg – 47 mm Hg)

$F_{O_2} \approx 0.40$

For this patient to re-establish a normal value for alveolar $P_{O_2}$, a 40% oxygen mixture must be inhaled. (The percent of oxygen present in the atmosphere is 21%.)

22. **The correct answer is D.** Clearance of a substance will change with increasing plasma concentration if that substance is secreted or reabsorbed by a facilitated mechanism. As the concentration of the substance increases, the transporter becomes saturated, and its contribution to excretion changes, changing the clearance. If the substance is reabsorbed by a facilitated mechanism, clearance will eventually increase with increasing plasma concentrations. Approximately 80% of filtered phosphate is reabsorbed in the proximal tubule by a sodium-phosphate cotransporter, which is a facilitated mechanism.

23. **The correct answer is A.** Fibrinogen is cleaved by thrombin twice as it is activated to form fibrin. The initial cleavage causes it to polymerize, and the second causes it to branch. Thrombin also activates Factor XIII to XIIIa, which cross-links the fibrin strands and strengthens the clot.

High molecular weight kininogen (HMWK; **choice B**) is a cofactor in the intrinsic pathway that converts Factor XI to XIa.

Plasminogen (**choice C**) is a central proenzyme in clot lysis. When plasminogen is converted to plasmin, it digests fibrin threads, as well as a number of protein factors including Factors V, VIII, XII, and prothrombin.

Thrombin (**choice D**) is an enzyme derived from pro-thrombin. It converts fibrinogen to fibrin and activates factor XIII.

von Willebrand Factor (vWF; **choice E**) is a tissue-bound protein that is exposed with vascular trauma and helps in the process of platelet adhesion.

24. **The correct answer is A.** The most important factor in the control of minute-to-minute ventilation is arterial $P_{CO_2}$, which influences chemoreceptors located near the ventral surface of the medulla. As arterial $P_{CO_2}$ rises, $CO_2$ diffuses from cerebral blood vessels into the CSF. Carbonic acid is formed and dissociates into bicarbonate and protons. Protons directly stimulate these central chemoreceptors, resulting in hyperventilation. Hyperventilating reduces the $P_{CO_2}$ in the arterial blood and subsequently in the CSF.

Peripheral chemoreceptors located in the carotid and aortic bodies respond to increases in $P_{CO_2}$ (**choice B**), but are less important than the central chemoreceptors. It is estimated that when a normal subject hyperventilates in response to inhalation of $CO_2$, less than 20% of the response can be attributed to the peripheral receptors. However, they respond more quickly than their central counterparts and are thought to play a role in regulating ventilation after abrupt changes in $P_{CO_2}$.

There are no known central chemoreceptors that respond to either arterial pH (**choice C**) or arterial $P_{O_2}$ (**choice E**).

Carotid chemoreceptors (**choice D**) cause hyperventilation in response to decreases in arterial pH; however, $CO_2$ acting through central chemoreceptors is the most important regulator of ventilation under normal conditions.

Peripheral chemoreceptors located in the carotid and aortic bodies respond to decreases in $P_{O_2}$ (**choice F**) and are solely responsible for the increase in ventilation due to arterial hypoxemia. Nonetheless, the $CO_2$ acting through central chemoreceptors is the most important regulator of ventilation under normal circumstances.

25. **The correct answer is B.** Trauma to the lower cervical cord (at C7, for example) can cause the pattern described in the question stem, since the lesion is below the origin of the phrenic nerve, but above the origin of the nerves innervating the muscles of the rib cage and abdomen.

Trauma high in the neck at C2 (**choice A**), above the origin of the phrenic nerve (C3-C5 nerve roots), would cause diaphragmatic paralysis as well.

A lesion at L3 (**choice C**) would spare all of the accessory respiratory muscles, as well as the diaphragm.

A lesion at T5 (**choice D**) would spare part of the accessory muscles of the rib cage.

A lesion at T12 (**choice E**) would spare the accessory muscles of the rib cage.

26. **The correct answer is C.** Both increased stroke volume and heart rate are important for maintaining an adequate cardiac output during exercise.

There is an increased, not decreased, cardiac index (**choice A**) during isotonic exercise.

Diastolic blood pressure usually remains unchanged during isotonic exercise; it is not decreased (**choice B**). In contrast, systolic blood pressure usually rises during isotonic exercise.

There is decreased, not increased, systemic vascular resistance (**choice D**) during isotonic exercise.

27. **The correct answer is C.** There are two systems currently used for classifying nerve fibers. The first system groups both sensory and motor fibers together, describing A-α, A-β, A-γ, A-δ, B, and C fibers. Another system relates only to sensory fibers, describing Ia, Ib, II, III, IV categories. Both classification schemes begin with large, myelinated fibers, progressing to finer, unmyelinated fibers.

The C fiber (or IV fibers) is the only type of fiber that is unmyelinated. Remember that preganglionic neurons are myelinated, but postganglionic neurons are unmyelinated. Neurons that carry slow pain and temperature information are also classified as C fibers. See the table below for more information.

| Sensory and Motor Fibers | Sensory Fibers | Function |
|---|---|---|
| A-α | Ia (**choice D**) | Alpha motor neurons, primary afferents of muscle spindles |
| A-α | Ib (**choice E**) | Golgi tendon organ afferents, touch and pressure |
| A-β | II | Secondary afferents of muscle spindles, touch and pressure |
| A-γ | | Gamma motor neurons |
| A-δ (**choice A**) | III | Touch, pressure; pain and temperature (fast) |
| B (**choice B**) | | Preganglionic autonomic, visceral afferents |
| C (**choice C**) | IV | Postganglionic autonomic; pain and temperature (slow) |

28. **The correct answer is C.** This patient has achalasia. Symptoms of this disorder include dysphagia for solids and liquids, chest pain, vomiting of undigested food, and weight loss. Symptoms of aspiration, such as coughing at nighttime, pneumonia, and dyspnea, can also be present. On barium swallow study, his esophagus has the classic "bird beak" appearance. This disorder is caused by the failure of the lower esophageal sphincter to relax during a swallow due to damage to the neural network of the myenteric plexus in the lower two thirds of the esophagus. The myenteric plexus cannot transmit a signal to cause relaxation of the lower esophageal sphincter as food approaches this area during the swallowing process. This causes the musculature of the lower esophagus to be spastically contracted, leading to the retention of swallowed food.

    **Choice A,** a defect in segmentation contraction, is incorrect because segmentation contraction is responsible for mixing of contents in the small intestine.

    The migrating myoelectric complex (**choice B**) begins in the stomach and starts during fasting. It moves undigested material from the stomach and small intestine into the colon.

    Damage to the vagus nerve (**choice D**) would cause problems with initially swallowing foods. This patient can swallow initially but the food cannot pass through the lower esophageal sphincter.

    Vasoactive intestinal peptide (**choice E**) relaxes the lower esophageal sphincter. An excess of this hormone would not cause achalasia.

29. **The correct answer is C.** The aorta is constricted at a point beyond the arterial branches to the head and arms but proximal to the kidneys. Collateral vessels in the body wall carry much of the blood flow to the lower body, and the arterial pressure in the lower body is about 50% lower compared with the pressure in the upper body. The lower-than-normal pressure at the level of the kidneys causes renin to be secreted and angiotensin to be formed. The angiotensin causes salt and water retention so that within a few days to weeks the arterial pressure in the lower body (at the level of the kidneys) increases to normal, but in doing so, the blood pressure in the upper body has increased to hypertensive levels. The kidneys are no longer ischemic when the blood pressure has increased; therefore, renin secretion decreases and the formation of angiotensin returns to normal levels.

    Blood flow in the lower body (**choice A**) is lower than normal at this early stage of aortic coarctation. However, blood flow can be normal above and below the constriction if the body is able to compensate fully.

The decrease in blood pressure at the level of the kidneys causes the glomerular filtration rate (**choice B**) to decrease.

Increase plasma levels of angiotensin II causes salt and water retention; thus, salt and water excretion (**choices D and E**) are decreased.

30. **The correct answer is A.** Antipyrine and tritium are both markers for total body water.

    Cresyl violet (**choice B**) is a histologic dye used to stain Nissl substance in neurons. It stains cell bodies.

    Evans blue (**choice C**) is used to measure the plasma compartment.

    $^{131}$I-albumin (**choice D**) is used to measure the plasma compartment.

    Inulin (**choice E**) is used to measure the extracellular fluid compartment.

31. **The correct answer is A.** The four corners of the pressure/volume loop represent points of aortic/mitral valve openings or closings. Aortic stenosis produces a dramatic systolic murmur, whereas a mitral stenosis produces a diastolic murmur. The mitral valve opens at the beginning of diastole, when the left ventricle is at its lowest pressure.

    **Point B** represents ventricular filling. Pressure in the left ventricle gradually increases as blood begins to enter it from the left atrium during diastolic ventricular filling.

    **Point C** represents the closing of the mitral valve.

    **Point D** represents isovolumetric contraction. It occurs when the left ventricle contracts in response to ventricular filling (**B**) but has not yet achieved enough pressure to force open the aortic valve (**E**).

    **Point F** represents systolic ejection. It occurs after the aortic valve opens (**E**), allowing the left ventricle to pump its blood volume into the aorta, consequently decreasing left ventricular volume.

    **Point G** represents the closing of the aortic valve at the end of systole.

    **Point H** is in the middle of isovolumetric relaxation.

32. **The correct answer is C.** Atrial stretch results in secretion of atrial natriuretic factor (ANF), a polypeptide hormone that increases urinary sodium excretion and therefore decreases intravascular volume to maintain homeostasis. None of the remaining answer choices are appropriate physiologic responses to increased atrial filling.

    Aldosterone (**choice A**) causes sodium retention by increasing sodium and water reabsorption in the distal convoluted tubule. This leads to an increased intravascular volume.

Activation of atrial baroreceptors results in increased secretion of ADH (**choice B**), a polypeptide hormone that decreases urine concentration and increases intravascular volume.

Norepinephrine (**choice D**) causes vasoconstriction and increased blood pressure, which can produce a reflex decrease in heart rate.

Renin (**choice E**) converts angiotensin I to angiotensin II, a potent vasoconstrictor that stimulates aldosterone secretion from the adrenal cortex, resulting in increased intravascular volume.

33. **The correct answer is B.** This patient has symptoms of primary hyperaldosteronism caused by an adrenal adenoma. Symptoms for this are hypertension, muscle weakness, polyuria, polydipsia, edema, hypokalemia, hypernatremia, and metabolic alkalosis. The adrenal adenoma is secreting excess aldosterone, leading to increased sodium reabsorption and increased potassium secretion in the cortical collecting tubules. This increases intravascular volume, thus causing hypertension.

**Choice A** is incorrect because a decreased glomerular capillary filtration coefficient decreases GFR, leading to hypertension. This occurs in chronic glomerulonephritis due to inflammation and thickening of the glomerular capillary membranes.

With an excess of aldosterone, renin amounts (**choice C**) are actually decreased due to negative feedback caused by excess aldosterone or by the excess extracellular fluid volume and increased arterial pressure.

Increased renal vascular resistance (**choice D**) occurs when one renal artery is severely constricted. The ischemic tissue secretes large amounts of renin, leading to the formation of angiotensin II, which can cause hypertension. This patient does not have a disorder of the renal arteries.

Patchy renal damage (**choice E**) causes the damaged renal cells to secrete large amounts of renin, causing hypertension as described earlier. In this patient, the adrenal adenoma is not causing renal damage.

34. **The correct answer is C.** The second heart sound and the v wave both occur during isovolumetric relaxation.

The onset of the a wave (**choice A**) occurs during atrial systole and coincides with the fourth heart sound, if present.

The onset of the c wave (**choice B**) coincides with the first heart sound and evolves into the x descent (**choice D**) during rapid ejection. It does not correspond to any heart sounds.

The y descent (**choice E**) occurs during rapid filling and does not correspond to any heart sounds.

35. **The correct answer is B.** The colony forming unit-erythroid (CFU-E) is a unipotential stem cell that develops from a burst forming unit-erythroid (BFU-E), which develops eventually from the multipotential stem cell. The BFU-E is somewhat responsive to erythropoietin, but the CFU-E is completely dependent on erythropoietin. Erythropoietin is normally released from the kidney in response to hypoxic or anemic conditions. Its half-life is about 3-6 hours. Clinically, it takes 5 days to see reticulocyte formation in the peripheral blood following erythropoietin administration.

The basophilic erythroblast (**choice A**) differentiates from the proerythroblast. It is recognizable by light microscopy and has a dark basophilic staining due to hemoglobin synthesis. It is not directly affected by erythropoietin, but is instead indirectly increased by the increase in precursor cells from the increase in CFU-E earlier in development.

The multipotential stem cell (**choice C**) appears earlier in development than CFU-E and does not increase with erythropoietin. The development of all major components of blood (RBC, WBC, and platelets) begins with the multipotential stem cell (CFU-S). This cell is non-committed and can self-renew. It is located in the bone marrow and is not recognizable by light microscopy.

The proerythroblast (**choice D**), which is the first recognizable cell in the red cell lineage, develops from the CFU-E cell. It is not affected directly by erythropoietin, but instead increases in number from the increased CFU-E cells.

The reticulocyte (**choice E**) is the enucleated cell just before the mature red blood cell. Reticulocytes enter the peripheral circulation but continue to synthesize hemoglobin. This cell is not directly stimulated by erythropoietin, but increases in number as a result of the increase in precursors.

36. **The correct answer is F.** This is simply a question about baroreceptor reflexes. The reflex response that would be anticipated after a decrease in blood pressure (e.g., after a hemorrhage) would be an increase in sympathetic outflow and a decrease in parasympathetic outflow. As a result, heart rate would increase, gastrointestinal motility would decrease, and the pupils would dilate.

37. **The correct answer is E.** The net driving force for fluid across a capillary wall is given by the following equation:

driving force =
$(\text{hydrostatic}_c - \text{hydrostatic}_i) - (\text{oncotic}_c - \text{oncotic}_i)$

where:

hydrostatic$_i$ = interstitial hydrostatic pressure

hydrostatic$_c$ = capillary hydrostatic pressure

oncotic$_i$ = interstitial oncotic pressure

oncotic$_c$ = capillary oncotic pressure

Substituting the values in the question stem: $3 = (25 - 2) - (x - 7)$. Simplifying, $3 = 23 - x + 7$; therefore, $x = 27$.

38. **The correct answer is B.** There are two ways to arrive at the correct answer to this question. The first is to simply remember the definition of functional residual capacity (FRC): the amount of air remaining in the lungs after a passive expiration. The second way is to recall that the helium dilution technique described above is used to measure FRC and residual volume (RV), which narrows the reasonable option choices to B and E only. All of the other volumes and capacities can be directly measured with spirometry because they are blown into the spirometer. Only FRC and RV represent amounts of air that remain in the lungs.

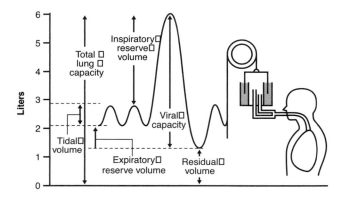

Expiratory reserve volume (**choice A**) is the volume expelled by an active expiratory effort after passive expiration.

Inspiratory capacity (**choice C**) is the maximal amount of air inspired after a passive expiration.

Inspiratory reserve volume (**choice D**) is the amount of air inspired with a maximal inspiratory effort over and above the tidal volume.

Residual volume (**choice E**) is the amount of air remaining in the lungs after maximal expiration.

Tidal volume (**choice F**) is the amount of air that is inspired (or expired) with each normal breath.

Vital capacity (**choice G**) is the largest amount of air that can be expired after a maximal inspiratory effort.

39. **The correct answer is C.** Total peripheral resistance (TPR) is equal to the pressure gradient across the circulation (mean arterial pressure − right atrial pressure) divided by the cardiac output. Thus, TPR = 120/3000 = 0.04 mm Hg/mL/min. The "ABC rule" is useful in remembering the relation between pressure (P), flow (Q), and resistance (R) because P = QR (note the alphabetical order). Note that knowledge of heart rate and stroke volume is not required to solve this problem because cardiac output is provided.

40. **The correct answer is A.** A decrease in the resistance of the afferent arteriole (i.e., arteriolar dilation) directly increases glomerular capillary hydrostatic pressure by lessening the drop in blood pressure that normally occurs along the vasculature proximal to the glomerulus. [Recall that the afferent arteriole is upstream from the glomerulus; the efferent arteriole is downstream from the glomerulus.] The glomerular capillary hydrostatic pressure is the determinant of glomerular filtration rate most subject to physiologic control.

Bowman's capsular hydrostatic pressure (**choice B**), capillary filtration coefficient (**choice C**), and plasma colloid osmotic pressure (**choice E**) are important determinants of GFR, but they do not have any direct effect to increase or decrease the glomerular capillary hydrostatic pressure.

A decrease in efferent arteriolar resistance (**choice D**) would tend to decrease the glomerular capillary hydrostatic pressure because the efferent arteriole is downstream from the glomerular capillaries.

41. **The correct answer is C.** The hormone in question is secretin. Acid entering the duodenum stimulates its secretion by the S cells in the duodenal lining. It inhibits stomach motility and stimulates bicarbonate secretion from the pancreas. Glucagon, secretin, and vasoactive peptide (VIP) are all structurally related.

Cholecystokinin (**choice A**) and gastrin (**choice B**) form another family of related hormones.

Neither somatostatin (**choice D**) nor substance P (**choice E**) are structurally related to secretin. In addition to their role in the gastrointestinal system, both hormones are also present in the brain.

42. **The correct answer is B.** 2,3-Diphosphoglycerate (2,3-DPG) is produced in red cells by a variation on the glycolytic pathway, and levels diminish when glycolysis by the red cells slows. The depletion of 2,3-DPG in stored blood causes a conformation change in the Hb molecule, which increases the affinity of the molecule for oxygen. This is expressed as a shift in the Hb-dissociation curve to the left. This is helpful in the picking up of oxygen by

hemoglobin in the lungs, but it can be very problematic in the release of oxygen from the blood in tissues. This is not just a theoretical point: considerable effort has been expended in developing improved solutions for storing packed red cells and methods for "restoring" older stored cells so that the 2,3-DPG levels are adequate. In practice, in otherwise reasonably healthy patients, older transfused blood will quickly regenerate 2,3-DPG when placed in the glucose-containing environment of the serum; however, even transiently decreased 2,3-DPG levels in a severely compromised patient can be dangerous.

43. **The correct answer is A.** Crossing over, a transposition of genetic information, occurs during the first meiotic (reduction) division, when the primary spermatocyte divides to form two secondary spermatocytes. This division does not consist of separation of sister chromatids after DNA replication, but rather involves the separation of previously paired, homologous chromosomes. Crossing over occurs during prophase of meiosis I.

The secondary spermatocyte (**choice B**) undergoes the second meiotic division, which results in four spermatids (**choice C**), each with the haploid number of chromosomes. The spermatids are located adjacent to the lumen of the seminiferous tubules and are distinguished by their small size. These cells undergo no further division, but become transformed into mature spermatozoa (**choice E**) through the process of spermiogenesis.

The spermatogonia (**choice D**) are the primitive germ cells. These cells give rise to the primary spermatocytes through repeated mitotic divisions.

Remember the sequence of spermatogenesis:

Spermatogonia (2n) → REPEATED MITOSES → Primary spermatocytes (2n) → FIRST MEIOTIC DIVISION → Secondary spermatocytes (n) → SECOND MEIOTIC DIVISION → Spermatids (n) → SPERMIOGENESIS → Spermatozoa (n)

44. **The correct answer is A.** Estrogen levels peak at the end of the follicular phase of the menstrual cycle, creating positive feedback to the hypothalamus and pituitary gland. This increases the number of GnRH spikes per 24 hours, causing a surge of both follicle-stimulating hormone (FSH) and luteinizing hormone (LH). It is the surge of LH, in combination with the high estrogen levels, that induces ovulation.

FSH levels (**choice B**) peak at ovulation.

Gonadotropin-releasing hormone (**choice C**) is released in pulses, not in a continuous pattern as is estrogen.

LH levels (**choice D**) peak at ovulation.

Progesterone (**choice E**) peaks during the premenstrual phase of the cycle. It is represented by the solid line on the graph.

45. **The correct answer is D.** MCV is calculated by the following formula:

$$(Hct \times 10)/\text{red blood cell count}$$

Hemoglobin and mean cell diameter are not needed for this calculation. The remaining answer choices are incorrect calculations based on the numbers given. Although patients with menorrhagia (excessive menstrual bleeding) are at risk for iron-deficiency anemia (which is associated with microcytosis [MCV <85]), this patient has not developed this complication. Her MCV is in the normal range.

Note that if you did not know the correct formula for calculating MCV, you should have at least been able to eliminate **choice E**, because macrocytosis (MCV >95) is characteristic of megaloblastic anemia (vitamin $B_{12}$ deficiency and folate deficiency), not of iron-deficiency anemia.

46. **The correct answer is E.** Urine flow rate is controlled primarily by antidiuretic hormone (ADH), which regulates the amount of pure water retained in the urine. ADH also controls the reabsorption of urea in the papillary collecting duct. High urine flow rates indicate low ADH, which would increase urea clearance. In contrast, low urine flow rates indicate high ADH, which would result in a greater reabsorption of urea and a lower urea clearance.

The concentration (and osmolarity) of all other solutes (**choices A, B, C, and D**) varies inversely with urine flow rate, resulting in no change in clearance. Recall that clearance = (urine concentration × urine flow rate)/ plasma concentration.

47. **The correct answer is C.** Ejection fraction is an index of contractility equal to the ratio of stroke volume to end-diastolic volume. The stroke volume is equal to the difference between the amount of blood in the ventricle prior to systole (end-diastolic volume) and the amount of blood in the ventricle at the end of systole (end-systolic volume). Because the end-diastolic volume is 115 mL and the end-systolic volume is 65 mL, the stroke volume is 115 − 65 = 50 mL. The ejection fraction is calculated as 50 mL/115 mL = 0.43. Ejection fraction (normal value = 0.65) can be estimated by radionuclide angiography or echocardiography and is frequently depressed in systolic heart failure, even when the stroke volume itself is normal.

**KAPLAN) MEDICAL**

**48.    The correct answer is A.** Glucose is freely filtered by the glomerular capillary membrane and totally reabsorbed in the proximal tubule under normal conditions. Therefore, the concentration of glucose is highest in the fluid leaving the Bowman capsule. The concentration of glucose is essentially zero in the thin descending limb of loop of Henle (**choice B**), distal convoluted tubule (**choice C**), cortical collecting tubule (**choice D**), and medullary collecting tubule (**choice E**).

**49.    The correct answer is B.** The volume of a fluid compartment can be measured by placing a substance into the compartment, allowing it to disperse evenly throughout the compartment, and then measuring the extent to which the indicator is diluted in the fluid. The volume of a compartment can be determined using the following formula:

Volume of Compartment =

$$\frac{\text{Quantity of Indicator Substance Administered}}{\text{Concentration of Indicator in Compartment}}$$

The extracellular fluid volume can be measured using inulin as the indicator: 0.1 g inulin was administered intravenously and the concentration of inulin in the compartment was 1 mg/100 mL an hour later (when the inulin had dispersed evenly in the extracellular fluid compartment). Therefore,

$$\text{Extracellular Fluid Volume} = \frac{0.1 \text{ g}}{1 \text{ mg/100 mL}}$$

$$= \frac{100 \text{ mg}}{1 \text{ mg/0.1 L}} = 10 \text{ L}$$

**50.    The correct answer is D.** This question tests your knowledge of how vitamin $B_{12}$ is normally absorbed. In summary, parietal cells in the gastric lining secrete a glycoprotein called intrinsic factor into the gastric lumen. This protein binds to vitamin $B_{12}$, protecting it from degradation and allowing for its eventual absorption. At the level of the ileum, $B_{12}$ bound to intrinsic factor is actively reabsorbed. Therefore, a loss of intrinsic factor or of its reabsorption site, the ileum, would lead to the need for lifelong injection of vitamin $B_{12}$. Removal of the stomach would obviously lead to loss of intrinsic factor. Pernicious anemia is actually an autoimmune disease that targets the gastric epithelium. In many cases, patients have autoantibodies against intrinsic factor, preventing the absorption of ingested vitamin $B_{12}$.

Removal of the colon, jejunum, or gallbladder would not affect reabsorption of intrinsic factor or $B_{12}$. A total absence of bile (which occurs with bile duct blockage, but not with cholecystectomy) may lead to malabsorption of fat-soluble vitamins such as A, D, E, and K, but not of $B_{12}$.

# Biochemistry: **Test One**

1.  A newborn presents with severe acidosis, vomiting, hypotonia, and neurologic deficits. Laboratory analysis reveals elevated levels of lactate and alanine. These observations suggest a deficiency of which of the following enzymes?

    (A) Alanine aminotransferase

    (B) Glutamate dehydrogenase

    (C) Lactate dehydrogenase

    (D) Phenylethanolamine N-methyltransferase

    (E) Pyruvate dehydrogenase

2.  Several members of a family have an autosomal recessive disease characterized by intellectual deterioration, weakness, ataxia, seizures, and death at a young age. Special studies demonstrate a deficiency of cytochrome C oxidase activity. Which of the following subcellular organelles is defective in affected members of this family?

    (A) Golgi apparatus

    (B) Lysosomes

    (C) Mitochondria

    (D) Ribosomes

    (E) Smooth endoplasmic reticulum

3.  A 17-year-old high-school student comes to the school health clinic. She has missed her last menstrual period and is worried about being pregnant. In the past history, it is noted that she has sickle-cell trait and mild asthma but is otherwise healthy. She has never been pregnant before and is sexually active with one boyfriend. They use barrier contraception on an irregular basis. She reports that her boyfriend once told her that he too had sickle-cell trait. She is determined to continue with the pregnancy if the urine pregnancy test turns out to be positive. Her main concern is whether her child will have sickle-cell anemia. At this stage, it is appropriate to counsel her that in cases where both parents have sickle-cell trait the risk of having a baby born with sickle-cell anemia is which of the following?

    (A) 5%

    (B) 25%

    (C) 50%

    (D) 75%

    (E) 100%

4.  A prokaryotic operon codes for two enzymes and one regulatory protein. The operon is expressed only in the presence of a particular sugar. Initial mapping of the operon has differentiated the nontranscribed sequences from the transcribed sequences. Deletion of 10 nucleotides from one of the nontranscribed sequences results in transcription of the operon in both the presence and absence of the sugar. Which of the following sequences was most likely affected?

    (A) Activator binding site

    (B) Activator gene

    (C) Operator

    (D) Promoter

    (E) Repressor gene

5. Genomic DNA from a child with pyruvate kinase deficiency identifies a mutation in the 3′-splice site of intron 3. The mRNA from the child's reticulocytes is used to produce cDNA. Primers flanking the exon 3/exon 4 border are used to amplify this region from the cDNA (RT-PCR). The products are separated by electrophoresis and compared to the RT-PCR products from normal reticulocytes (control). The results are shown below. Which of the following mechanisms best accounts for the results of the splice mutation?

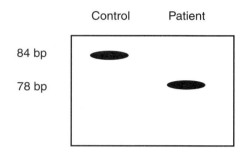

   (A) Exon skipping
   (B) Frameshift mutation
   (C) Missense mutation
   (D) Trinucleotide expansion
   (E) Two codon deletion

6. A 36-year-old Greek man with viral pneumonia has a self-limiting episode of hemolysis. Over the next week, he has an increased rate of reticulocytosis. Which of the following compounds serves as a precursor to heme in the reticulocytes?

   (A) α-Ketoglutarate
   (B) Fumarate
   (C) Isocitrate
   (D) Oxaloacetate
   (E) Succinyl-CoA *and Glycine*

7. A 22-year-old woman presents with a fusiform swelling of the Achilles tendon, which, when biopsied, shows cholesterol-laden macrophages (foam cells) dispersed among the collagen fibers. She had been troubled with joint pains for several years. Both her mother and father developed arthritis associated with production of xanthomas, but their first symptoms occurred in middle age. She was referred to a nutritionist and treated with an enzyme inhibitor. Which of the following is most likely elevated in the blood of this woman?

   (A) Chylomicron remnants
   (B) Chylomicrons
   (C) High density lipoproteins (HDL)
   (D) Low density lipoproteins (LDL)
   (E) Very low density lipoproteins (VLDL)

8. A 23-year-old, single, unemployed woman in her eighth month of pregnancy is seen in a volunteer-staffed obstetrics clinic. Her first child, born at home and exclusively breast-fed, had prolonged diarrhea and died from an intracranial hemorrhage at 1 month of age. To help prevent a similar problem in this pregnancy, the resident gives her a free prescription for a vitamin and advises her to take one 20-mg tablet each day. He also informs her that the infant should receive an injection of this vitamin soon after birth. The vitamin prescribed is required as a coenzyme by which of the following enzymes?

   (A) δ-Aminolevulinate synthase
   (B) γ-Glutamyl carboxylase *for Vit K*
   (C) Homocysteine methyltransferase
   (D) Prolyl hydroxylase
   (E) Thrombin

9. A 26-year-old pregnant woman complains of persistent, dry, ulcerated skin over her knees and elbows. Examination of her eyes reveals small, gray plaques on the conjunctiva. Which of the following is the most likely diagnosis?

   (A) Ascorbic acid deficiency
   (B) Excessive α-tocopherol intake
   (C) Excessive cholecalciferol intake
   (D) Retinol deficiency
   (E) Thiamine deficiency

10. The pregnant mother of a 6-year-old son with glucose-6-phosphate dehydrogenase deficiency is very worried that her female fetus will have the disease. The father and mother are clinically normal. Which of the following is true about her baby?

    (A) The baby has a 25% chance of clinical disease

    (B) The baby has a 50% chance of being a carrier

    (C) The baby has a 50% chance of clinical disease

    (D) The baby will be a carrier

    (E) The baby will have clinical disease

11. A genetics researcher is trying to identify a potential gene from a gene signature/motif that encodes a seven-helix transmembrane domain. Which of the following is an example of a glycosylated, integral membrane protein with seven transmembrane segments?

    (A) Adenylate cyclase

    (B) Beta-adrenergic receptor for epinephrine

    (C) Cystic fibrosis transmembrane conductance regulator channel

    (D) Glucose transporter

    (E) $Na^+/K^+$ ATPase

12. A previously normal child begins deteriorating developmentally at about 6 months of age. She is seen by an ophthalmologist because she no longer responds to visual stimuli. A cherry-red spot on the macula is noted on ophthalmologic examination. The enzyme that is deficient in this child normally carries out which of the following functions?

    (A) Degradation of glycogen in muscle

    (B) Degradation of glycolipids in the brain

    (C) Degradation of mucopolysaccharides in bone marrow

    (D) Synthesis of glycoproteins in the liver

    (E) Synthesis of peptides in the spleen

13. A 30-year-old vegetarian presents to his physician complaining of diminished sensation in his lower extremities. He has not eaten meat for the past 15 years. A complete blood count reveals hypersegmented neutrophils and elevated mean corpuscular volume. Which of the following findings would be expected on urinalysis?

    (A) Argininosuccinic aciduria

    (B) Cystinuria

    (C) Hemoglobinuria

    (D) Methylmalonic aciduria

    (E) Propionic aciduria

14. A 12-year-old boy has a particular genetic disease. His mother is a carrier of the mutated gene, but his father is not clinically affected and is not a carrier. The man has four siblings: a sister and a brother who are not clinically affected and are not carriers; a sister who is a carrier but is not clinically affected; and a brother who is clinically affected. This inheritance pattern is consistent with which of the following diseases?

    (A) Alpha$_1$-antitrypsin deficiency

    (B) Cystic fibrosis

    (C) Duchenne muscular dystrophy

    (D) Phenylketonuria

    (E) Tay-Sachs disease

15. A newborn vomits after each feeding of milk-based formula and does not gain weight. Biochemical testing reveals a severe deficiency of galactose-1-phosphate uridyltransferase, consistent with homozygosity. If this condition goes untreated, which of the following is the likely outcome for this patient?

    (A) Benign disease except for cataract formation

    (B) Chronic emphysema appearing in early adulthood

    (C) Chronic renal failure appearing in adolescence

    (D) Death in infancy

    (E) Gastrointestinal symptoms that remit with puberty

16. Following the ingestion of glyburide, a type 2 diabetic patient begins to experience anxiety, diaphoresis, and hunger. The patient subsequently ingests a health food bar containing glucose. The glycolytic degradation of the ingested glucose commences with the action of which of the following enzymes?

    (A) Aldolase
    (B) Hexokinase
    (C) Phosphofructokinase
    (D) Phosphoglucose isomerase
    (E) Pyruvate kinase

17. A 24-year-old woman with phenylketonuria (PKU) gives birth to her first child. Although there is no history of PKU in the father's family, the couple could not afford genetic testing of the father or consistent prenatal care. At birth, the child is small, microcephalic, and has elevated blood phenylalanine. What is the most likely explanation for this neonate's symptoms?

    (A) Father is a carrier of PKU
    (B) Maternal translocation with unbalanced segregation in meiosis I
    (C) Maternal translocation with unbalanced segregation in meiosis II
    (D) Maternal uniparental disomy
    (E) Phenylalanine was not adequately restricted from the mother's diet during pregnancy

18. A 26-year-old woman and her 29-year-old husband have been trying to have a child for the past 3 years. During this time the woman has had five spontaneous abortions. The karyotypes of the mother, father, and the most recently aborted fetus all contained 46 chromosomes, and all pairs were normal except for the pairs shown below.

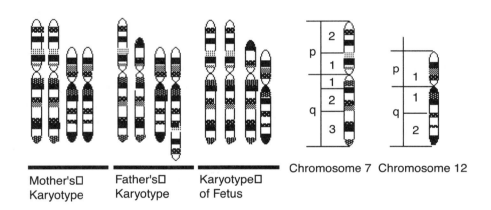

Mother's Karyotype    Father's Karyotype    Karyotype of Fetus    Chromosome 7    Chromosome 12

Which of the following events during spermatogenesis in the father is most likely to have produced the abdominal karyotype in the fetus?

(A) Adjacent segregation during meiosis
(B) Alternate segregation during meiosis
(C) A recombination event with paracentric inversion
(D) A reciprocal translocation
(E) A Robertsonian translocation

19. A 30-year-old man has been fasting for religious reasons for several days. His blood glucose level is now about 60% of its normal value, but he does not feel lightheaded because his brain has reduced its need for serum glucose by using which of the following substances as an alternate energy source?

    (A) Apoprotein B

    (B) Beta-carotene

    (C) Beta-hydroxybutyrate

    (D) C-reactive protein

    (E) Coenzyme A

20. A lethal mutation occurs in a bacterium, rendering it incapable of replicating its chromosome. Because of this mutation, DNA synthesis produces many short fragments of DNA that have RNA sequences at their 5′ ends. The mutation is most likely in a gene encoding which of the following?

    (A) DNA gyrase

    (B) DNA helicase

    (C) DNA ligase

    (D) DNA polymerase I

    (E) Primase

21. A 2-year-old boy has a past medical history significant for mental retardation, hepatosplenomegaly, foam cells in the bone marrow, and neurologic deficits. The boy dies by the age of 3. Which of the following enzymes was most likely deficient in this child?

    (A) Alpha-galactosidase

    (B) Beta-glucocerebrosidase

    (C) Ceramidase

    (D) HMG-CoA reductase

    (E) Sphingomyelinase

22. A 58-year-old woman is admitted to the hospital with fever, abdominal cramps, and severe watery diarrhea. The symptoms began one day after attending a banquet. She was treated with ciprofloxacin, but her condition did not improve. PCR amplification and analysis of a gene region in the bacteria isolated from the patient revealed a missense mutation that conferred resistance to ciprofloxacin. The missense mutation is most likely in the gene encoding an enzyme essential for which of the following functions?

    (A) DNA replication

    (B) Folate synthesis

    (C) mRNA translocation on a ribosome

    (D) Peptide bond formation

    (E) Reduction of folate to tetrahydrofolate

23. A 62-year-old man is prescribed a pharmaceutical agent that inhibits the activity of the enzyme HMG-CoA reductase. This patient most likely has which of the following conditions?

    (A) Chronic inflammation

    (B) Familial hypercholesterolemia

    (C) Hypertension

    (D) Hyperuricemia

    (E) Type 2 diabetes

24. A 5-year-old, mentally retarded boy is brought to the city from a rural community for evaluation. A careful history reveals mental retardation in a number of other family members, especially the males. Physical examination is remarkable for a long face with large ears, a large jaw, and bilateral enlargement of the testes. This presentation is suggestive of

    (A) Down syndrome

    (B) Edwards syndrome

    (C) Fragile X syndrome

    (D) Klinefelter syndrome

    (E) Turner syndrome

25. Liver cells in culture were kept at 0 C (32.0 F) and treated with trypsin to digest the receptors on the cell surface. The temperature was then raised to 37.0 C (98.6 F), and radioactive LDL was added to the culture media. Several hours later, the labeled LDL was found to be inside the cells. This specific process of LDL uptake is

    (A) active transport
    (B) facilitated diffusion
    (C) phagocytosis
    (D) pinocytosis
    (E) receptor-mediated endocytosis

26. On physical examination, a newborn is found to have micrognathia, a prominent occiput, low-set ears, and rocker-bottom feet. There is very little mental development during the first months of life, and the infant dies of cardiac complications after 8 months. A complete karyotype of this child would show which of the following?

    (A) XO
    (B) XXY
    (C) Trisomy 13
    (D) Trisomy 18
    (E) Trisomy 21

27. A college student goes to a fraternity party and consumes large quantities of beer. The alcohol in the beer is metabolized by the liver, with almost half the alcohol being oxidized to acetaldehyde. In which of the following sites does this reaction occur?

    (A) Golgi bodies
    (B) Lysosomes
    (C) Mitochondrial matrix
    (D) Peroxisomes
    (E) Ribosomes

28. A patient has an enlarged liver and kidneys, gout, and xanthomas. Studies show that he has a genetic deficiency of glucose 6-phosphatase. Additional studies would most likely show which of the following sets of laboratory results?

|  | Serum glucose | Serum lactate | Serum pyruvate |
|---|---|---|---|
| (A) | High | High | High |
| (B) | High | High | Low |
| (C) | High | Low | Low |
| (D) | Low | High | High |
| (E) | Low | Low | Low |

29. A neonate with ambiguous genitalia and microcephaly is suspected of having a genetic disease characterized by failure to metabolize 7-dehydrocholesterol to cholesterol. Which of the following is the most likely diagnosis?

    (A) Down syndrome
    (B) Edwards syndrome
    (C) Patau syndrome
    (D) Smith-Lemli-Opitz syndrome
    (E) WAGR syndrome

30. A researcher is trying to identify a specific protein within a mixture. He subjects the mixture to gel electrophoresis and then transfers the separation to nitrocellulose filters. The filters are incubated with antibody to the specific protein, and the excess antibody is washed off. The antibody-protein complex is then incubated with a radiolabeled protein that binds to the antibody. Autoradiography is performed to detect the presence of the protein. This technique represents

    (A) Northern blotting
    (B) Southern blotting
    (C) Southwestern blotting
    (D) Western blotting

31. A rapid way to purify proteins that are targeted to lysosomes would be to use affinity chromatography. An appropriate antibody to use on an affinity chromatography column would be one directed against

    (A) acid hydrolases
    (B) clathrin
    (C) glucose-6-phosphate
    (D) mannose-6-phosphate
    (E) sialic acid

32. When a cloned DNA fragment is used as a probe, a restriction fragment length polymorphism (RFLP) is revealed in the region adjacent to the centromere of chromosome 21. Four haplotypes exist: A, B, C, and D. An AB woman and a CD man have an ACC child with trisomy 21. Nondisjunction occurred in

    (A) the child during the first mitotic division
    (B) the father during meiosis I
    (C) the father during meiosis II
    (D) the mother during meiosis I
    (E) the mother during meiosis II

33. A 5-year-old boy has temporary weakness and cramping of skeletal muscle after exercise. He has normal mental development. This child most likely has a deficiency of which of the following enzymes?

    (A) α-1,4-Glucan transferase
    (B) Glycogen phosphorylase
    (C) Glycogen synthase
    (D) Phosphoglucomutase
    (E) UDP-glucose pyrophosphorylase

34. A patient with acute lymphocytic leukemia is treated appropriately with antineoplastic therapy. Inhibition of which of the following enzymes will help prevent side effects of this therapy?

    (A) Alpha-glucosidase
    (B) Angiotensin-converting enzyme
    (C) Beta-lactamase
    (D) Cyclooxygenase
    (E) Xanthine oxidase

35. A 4-year-old retarded child hurls himself into walls and bites his fingertips so severely that they must be heavily bandaged. This child most likely has a deficiency of which of the following enzymes?

    (A) Cystathionine synthase
    (B) Hexosaminidase A
    (C) Homogentisic acid oxidase
    (D) Hypoxanthine-guanine phosphoribosyltransferase
    (E) Phenylalanine hydroxylase

36. A gene product thought to be involved in the down-regulation of fetal hemoglobin expression is being investigated. Samples of primary tissue cultures of fetal, neonatal, and adult liver and bone marrow, as well as adequate amounts of a DNA probe believed to contain the studied gene, are provided. The best method for determining which of the tissue culture samples expresses the studied gene is

    (A) DNA sequencing
    (B) Northern blot
    (C) Polymerase chain reaction (PCR)
    (D) Southern blot
    (E) Western blot

37. A 28-year-old woman and a 25-year-old man present for genetic counseling. Both are white and have one sibling affected with cystic fibrosis. The most appropriate method to assess the risk of transmitting cystic fibrosis to a potential child would be

    (A) biochemical testing
    (B) fluorescence *in situ* hybridization (FISH)
    (C) karyotype analysis
    (D) polymerase chain reaction (PCR)
    (E) Western blot analysis

38. A 7-year-old girl is brought to the emergency department by her parents with a complaint of severe polyuria and polydipsia. Laboratory examination reveals ketones in her urine. Which of the following is the most likely source of the ketones?

    (A) Free fatty acid breakdown
    (B) Gluconeogenesis
    (C) Glycogenolysis
    (D) Protein breakdown
    (E) Triglyceride breakdown

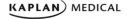

39. An infant receives an exchange blood transfusion due to severe neonatal jaundice. Red blood cell transfusion is required monthly, and at 6 months of age, a splenectomy is performed. Histologic examination of the spleen reveals marked hemosiderosis. Laboratory studies show:

| | Patient | Normal |
|---|---|---|
| RBC | $2.54 \times 10^6/mm^3$ | $3.5\text{-}5.5 \times 10^6/mm^3$ |
| Hemoglobin | 8.3 g/dL | 12-16 g/dL |
| Hematocrit | 23.4% | 34-46% |
| Reticulocytes | 27% | 0.5-1.5% |
| Indirect bilirubin (conjugated) | 6.1 mg/dL | 0.4-3.4 mg/dL |

Analysis of red cell glycolytic intermediates indicates markedly elevated concentrations of 2,3-bisphosphoglycerate, 3-phosphoglycerate, 2-phosphoglycerate, and phosphoenolpyruvate. Which of the following is the most likely diagnosis?

(A) Glucose 6-phosphate dehydrogenase (G6PD) deficiency

(B) Lead poisoning

(C) Pyruvate kinase (PK) deficiency

(D) Sickle cell anemia

(E) β-Thalassemia

40. Pseudogenes are homologues of functional genes that lack promoters and are therefore part of the unexpressed DNA. It is thought that at least some of these pseudogenes were produced by reverse transcription of mRNA and insertion of the resultant cDNA into a chromosome by a virus. In addition to lacking a promoter and other regulatory elements, a pseudogene produced in this manner will also differ from the authentic gene in which one of the following ways?

(A) It will contain an oncogenic mutation

(B) It will contain nested genes for antibiotic resistance

(C) It will have lost some coding regions

(D) It will lack introns

(E) It will require Shine-Dalgarno sequences

41. Methotrexate is used as therapy for rheumatoid arthritis, but has many side effects related to competitive inhibition of the enzyme dihydrofolate reductase. These side effects can be decreased without interfering with the efficacy of methotrexate by ingestion of additional folate. If patients treated with methotrexate are given sufficient folate, which of the following would most likely occur?

(A) Dihydrofolate reductase will have a higher apparent $K_m$ for dihydrofolate

(B) Dihydrofolate reductase will have a higher $V_{max}$ than it would in the absence of methotrexate

(C) Dihydrofolate reductase will have a lower apparent $K_m$ for dihydrofolate

(D) Dihydrofolate reductase will increase its affinity for methotrexate

(E) Dihydrofolate reductase will reach the same $V_{max}$ as it would in the absence of methotrexate

42. A 69-year-old edentulous alcoholic man, who lives alone, is admitted to the hospital for evaluation of a shoulder wound that is not healing well. On physical examination, numerous ecchymoses are noted on the posterior aspect of his legs and thighs. Careful examination of the man's skin reveals minute hemorrhages around hair follicles and splinter hemorrhages in the nail beds. Laboratory examination is remarkable for a hemoglobin of 10 g/dL; no other hematologic abnormalities are noted. Which of the following is the most appropriate therapy for this disorder?

(A) Factor VIII

(B) Iron

(C) Vitamin $B_{12}$

(D) Vitamin C

(E) Vitamin K

43. A 45-year-old man is diagnosed with cancer of the proximal portion of the colon. His father died of colon cancer at the age of 52. He has three siblings. His 55-year-old brother has not been diagnosed with cancer, but his 57-year-old sister has an endometrial carcinoma, and his other sister died of ovarian cancer. A diagnosis of hereditary nonpolyposis colorectal cancer (HNPCC) is made. Which of the following types of mutations most likely occurred in this family?

    (A) A mutation causing defects in the mismatch repair system

    (B) A point mutation in the gene coding for an excision exonuclease

    (C) A reciprocal translocation between chromosomes 8 and 14, associated with the Epstein-Barr virus

    (D) Loss of the retinoblastoma (RB) tumor suppressor gene

44. A 2-year-old boy is diagnosed with a biochemical defect involving hexosaminidase A. The patient's condition would be most appropriately categorized as belonging to which of the following general classes of defects?

    (A) Aminoacidopathy

    (B) Gangliosidosis

    (C) Lipid metabolism

    (D) Mucopolysaccharidosis

    (E) Porphyria

45. A 4-year-old boy is brought to the pediatrician because of gastroenteritis for three days, followed by a brief generalized seizure that left him semicomatose. The blood glucose level at admission is 18 mg/dL (0.10 mM) and urine is negative for glucose and ketones, but positive for a variety of organic dicarboxylic acids. Intravenous administration of glucose improves his condition within 10 minutes. Following diagnosis of an enzyme deficiency, his parents are cautioned to make sure he eats frequently. Which of the following is the most likely diagnosis?

    (A) Glucose-6-phosphatase deficiency

    (B) Hepatic glycogen phosphorylase deficiency

    (C) Medium chain acyl CoA dehydrogenase deficiency

    (D) Mitochondrial carbamoyl phosphate synthetase deficiency

    (E) Ornithine transcarbamoylase deficiency

46. A patient with short stature presents with hypoglycemia, hepatomegaly, bleeding diathesis, hepatic adenomas, and enlarged kidneys. Laboratory evaluation reveals the presence of increased lactate, cholesterol, triglyceride, and uric acid. This patient most likely has a deficiency of which of the following enzymes?

    (A) Brancher enzyme

    (B) Debrancher enzyme

    (C) Glucose-6-phosphatase

    (D) Hepatic phosphorylase

    (E) Muscle phosphorylase

47. A 50-year-old chronic alcoholic presents with dementia, paralysis of lateral gaze, and difficulty walking. The vitamin deficient in this patient is required as a cofactor for which of the following enzymes?

    (A) Aspartate aminotransferase

    (B) Methylmalonyl-CoA mutase

    (C) Prolyl hydroxylase

    (D) Pyruvate carboxylase

    (E) Pyruvate dehydrogenase

48. A 27-year-old medical student is unable to eat lunch and dinner during her clinical rotation. Which of the following enzymes is responsible for helping to maintain blood glucose levels by releasing glucose from its storage form in the liver?

    (A) Acetyl-CoA carboxylase

    (B) Glucose-6-phosphate dehydrogenase

    (C) Glycogen phosphorylase

    (D) Glycogen synthase

    (E) Thiolase

49. A family has a history of genetic disease with an autosomal dominant pattern of inheritance. DNA from the grandfather (who is heterozygous for the disease) is cloned and used to construct a restriction map of the gene region involved in the disease. He has a restriction site polymorphism at *Eco*HV site 2 (*HV-2*), which is useful as a marker. His abnormal chromosome lacks the HV-2 site. DNA from his affected grandson is digested with *Eco*HV, Southern blotted, and probed with $^{32}$P-cDNA complementary to exon 2. Which of the following options most likely represents the restriction fragment length polymorphism (RFLP) pattern obtained from the affected grandson?

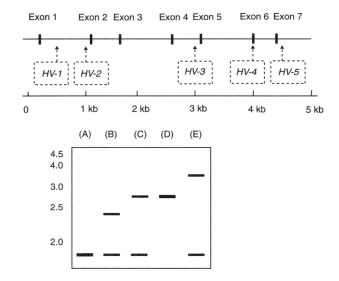

(A) A
(B) B
(C) C
(D) D
(E) E

50. In the family shown below, individuals affected with profound deafness are represented by a shaded symbol.

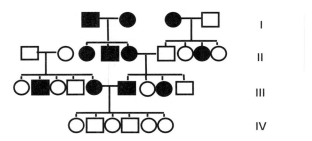

The phenotypes of individuals in the fourth generation can best be explained by

(A) autosomal dominant inheritance
(B) locus heterogeneity
(C) mitochondrial inheritance
(D) multifactorial inheritance
(E) X-linked dominant inheritance

# Biochemistry Test One: **Answers and Explanations**

## ANSWER KEY

| | | | |
|---|---|---|---|
| 1. | E | 26. | D |
| 2. | C | 27. | D |
| 3. | B | 28. | D |
| 4. | C | 29. | D |
| 5. | E | 30. | D |
| 6. | E | 31. | D |
| 7. | D | 32. | C |
| 8. | B | 33. | B |
| 9. | D | 34. | E |
| 10. | B | 35. | D |
| 11. | B | 36. | B |
| 12. | B | 37. | D |
| 13. | D | 38. | A |
| 14. | C | 39. | C |
| 15. | D | 40. | D |
| 16. | B | 41. | E |
| 17. | E | 42. | D |
| 18. | A | 43. | A |
| 19. | C | 44. | B |
| 20. | D | 45. | C |
| 21. | E | 46. | C |
| 22. | A | 47. | E |
| 23. | B | 48. | C |
| 24. | C | 49. | B |
| 25. | E | 50. | B |

1. **The correct answer is E.** Pyruvate dehydrogenase (PDH) catalyzes the irreversible conversion of pyruvate to acetyl-CoA. If PDH is absent, pyruvate will be used in other pathways instead. Pyruvate will be converted to alanine via alanine aminotransferase (**choice A**) and to lactate via lactate dehydrogenase (**choice C**).

   Glutamate dehydrogenase (**choice B**) is involved in oxidative deamination, releasing ammonium ion for urea synthesis. Deficiency of this enzyme would not cause the symptoms described.

   Phenylethanolamine N-methyltransferase (**choice D**) is an enzyme involved in the synthesis of epinephrine. Deficiency of this enzyme would not cause the symptoms described.

2. **The correct answer is C.** This is Leigh's disease, a rare condition also known as subacute necrotizing encephalomyelopathy. The underlying problem is a defective form of cytochrome C oxidase, an electron transport chain component, in the mitochondria of muscle and brain. Clinically, the features described in the question stem are seen. Pathologically, there is a symmetric necrosis that affects central areas of the nervous system from the thalamus to the spinal cord. No effective treatment exists at this time.

   The Golgi apparatus (**choice A**) is involved in packaging materials for secretion outside the cell. You should associate the mucolipidosis I-cell disease with Golgi apparatus problems.

   Lysosomes (**choice B**) are the organelles that degrade many cellular products. Defects can produce a wide variety of lysosomal storage diseases, including Hurler and Hunter syndromes.

   Ribosomes (**choice D**) are the organelles that translate mRNA into proteins. There are no known diseases of ribosomes, probably because their function is so crucial that any problems produce death in utero.

   Hypertrophy of the smooth endoplasmic reticulum (**choice E**) in the liver is associated with conditions that stimulate the cytochrome P450 detoxification systems (e.g., barbiturate use and alcoholism).

3. **The correct answer is B.** Sickle cell anemia arises due to the mutation in the beta-globin gene. Because both of the beta-globin genes have to be abnormal to produce the disease, it is an example of autosomal recessive inheritance. When both parents are carriers of the abnormal gene (sickle-cell trait), the risk of having a child with disease (two abnormal genes; sickle-cell anemia) is 25%. The probability of having a child who is a carrier (one abnormal gene; sickle-cell trait) is 50%, and the probability of having a child who is normal (no abnormal gene) is 25%.

   Certain congenital anomalies follow multigenic inheritance (non-Mendelian inheritance). Examples include Hirschsprung disease, pyloric stenosis, cleft lip, and other common congenital malformations. The recurrence risk in the second offspring after one affected child is in the range of 5% for such disorders (**choice A**).

   In diseases that follow autosomal dominant inheritance, the risk to the child where one parent is affected is 50% (**choice C**). Examples of such disorders include polycystic kidney disease and Huntington chorea.

   Under rare circumstances, the risk to the offspring can be higher than 50% in diseases with Mendelian inheritance. For example, if in the index case, both parents have sickle cell anemia (homozygous state), the risk to the offspring will be 100% because none of the beta-globin genes is normal (**choices D and E**).

4. **The correct answer is C.** The description of the operon expression pattern identifies it as an inducible operon; after the deletion, the operon is expressed constitutively. This pattern can occur only if the deletion removes a negative regulator; i.e., a repressor protein, or the DNA sequence to which it binds, called an operator. Since the question stipulates a nontranscribed DNA sequence, the operator must have been affected.

   The activator binding site (**choice A**) is incorrect since deletion of an activator binding site would result in a noninducible phenotype.

   Disruption of an activator gene (**choice B**) would also result in a noninducible phenotype. In addition, the activator gene is a transcribed DNA sequence.

   Deletion of the promoter (**choice D**) would result in a noninducible phenotype.

   A repressor gene (**choice E**) is a transcribed sequence.

5. **The correct answer is E.** The RT-PCR product from the patient's reticulocytes is 6 nucleotides shorter than the RT-PCR product from normal reticulocytes. This six-base pair deletion would be consistent with removing two codons from the mRNA.

   Exon skipping (**choice A**) would have removed a much larger section of the mRNA.

   A frameshift mutation (**choice B**) would have resulted if the number of base pairs deleted had not been a multiple of 3.

   A missense mutation (**choice C**) would not have affected the length, only the sequence.

   A trinucleotide expansion (**choice D**) would have introduced nucleotides into the patient's mRNA.

6. **The correct answer is E.** The porphyrin ring of heme is derived from the citric acid cycle intermediate

succinyl-CoA and the amino acid glycine. The initial synthetic step, which is rate-limiting, is catalyzed by aminolevulinic acid synthase (ALA synthase).

The other answer choices do not play a role in heme synthesis.

7. **The correct answer is D.** Deposition of xanthomas around the Achilles tendon is characteristic of familial type IIa hyperlipidemia, an autosomal dominant deficiency of the LDL receptor. The resultant reduced rate of LDL clearance leads to elevated LDL levels and hypercholesterolemia. For some poorly understood reason, arthritic pain in various joints, often prior to any appearance of xanthomas, is a characteristic of familial type IIa hyperlipidemia manifestation. Although Achilles tendonitis with associated xanthomas is common, other tendons may be involved. Symptoms in the heterozygous patient usually do not occur until the third or fourth decade, but homozygotes are affected much earlier, often in childhood. The patient was most likely treated with an HMG CoA reductase inhibitor such as simvastatin. Her condition carries a strong risk for cardiovascular disease. Although xanthomas are common in other familial hyperlipemias, such as type III and hepatic lipase deficiency, these are not associated with Achilles tendonitis.

Chylomicron remnants (**choice A**) accumulate in familial type III hyperlipidemia (also known as familial dysbetalipoproteinemia) due to a lack of functional apolipoprotein E.

Chylomicronemia (**choice B**) is associated with familial lipoprotein lipase deficiency (type I hyperlipoproteinemia). This rare autosomal recessive disease inhibits the clearance of the chylomicrons.

HDLs (**choice C**) are the "good" lipoproteins; they have a protective effect against atherosclerosis. Their role is to take up free cholesterol from cell surfaces and circulating apolipoproteins.

There is a tendency of VLDL (**choice E**) to be increased in several of the hyperlipoproteinemias, none of which produce the symptoms described. Familial type IV hyperlipidemia is probably the most significant, as it is associated with the hyperinsulinemia commonly observed in insulin-resistant, type 2 diabetes. The resultant concomitant increase in cholesterol and decrease in HDL lead to vascular disease, a critically important part of the insulin resistance syndrome.

8. **The correct answer is B.** Late-onset vitamin K deficiency bleeding can occur between 1 and 6 months after birth. Risk factors include exclusive breast-feeding because human milk is low in vitamin K. In hospital settings, infants are given injections of vitamin K after birth, but the first child of this patient was born at home. Additional factors contributing to vitamin K deficiency in infants include poor transfer of vitamin K from maternal to fetal blood and sterile intestines (in this case exacerbated by prolonged diarrhea). In addition, hepatic storage of vitamin K is about 1 month. This is the time when late-onset vitamin K deficiency may manifest in infants.

Vitamin K is an important coenzyme for γ-glutamyl carboxylase, an enzyme that catalyses a post-translational modification of a group of calcium-binding proteins. Important examples include factors II, VII, IX, and X, as well as proteins C and S. Vitamin K deficiencies in infants may manifest as gastrointestinal bleeding, skin hemorrhages, and intracranial hemorrhage.

δ-Aminolevulinate synthase (**choice A**) catalyses the first step in heme synthesis from glycine and succinyl CoA. It requires pyridoxine (vitamin $B_6$). Deficiency of pyridoxine does not present with hemorrhages but rather as a microcytic anemia and neuropathy. There is nothing specific about this case, other than the possibility of malnutrition that indicates a pyridoxine deficiency.

Homocysteine methyltransferase (**choice C**) requires cobalamin (vitamin $B_{12}$) and folate. Deficiency of folate during pregnancy would present in the infant as a neural tube defect. Later deficiency of folate or cobalamin may result in megaloblastic anemia. Deficiency of $B_{12}$ may also produce a progressive neuropathy.

Prolyl hydroxylase (**choice D**) requires ascorbate (vitamin C). The enzyme, which adds a hydroxyl group to the pro-α chains during their synthesis, is important for the stability of collagen molecules and therefore collagen fibers. Vitamin C deficiency may result in poor wound healing, easy bruising, inflamed and bleeding gums, petechiae, and perifollicular hyperkeratosis (an accumulation of epithelial cells around hair follicles)—all symptoms of scurvy. In infants, hemorrhages under the periosteum may occur. Intracranial hemorrhages are not typical.

Thrombin (**choice E**) is an enzyme that cleaves and activates factor VIII, and deficiency of active factor VIII could result in hemorrhage. Thrombin itself does not, however, require a vitamin-derived coenzyme for this activity. Synthesis of prothrombin in hepatocytes requires vitamin K for the γ-glutamyl carboxylase activity.

9. **The correct answer is D.** This patient has vitamin A (retinol) deficiency, which typically occurs in people with increased requirements for the nutrient, e.g., pregnant women and patients with chronic diseases. Night blindness is usually the earliest manifestation of this deficiency and may be followed by retinal degeneration and blindness in untreated patients. Drying of the bulbar

conjunctiva (xerosis) and Bitot spots (small, gray plaques on the conjunctiva) may also occur. Keratomalacia (corneal necrosis) is a serious potential complication of this deficiency.

Ascorbic acid (vitamin C) deficiency (**choice A**) leads to scurvy, which is characterized by poor wound healing, poor bone formation, gingival changes, and petechiae. Vitamin C excess can lead to decreased absorption of vitamin $B_{12}$, increased estrogen levels in women on estrogen replacement therapy, uricosuria, and oxalate kidney stones. Interestingly, small doses of the vitamin (200 mg daily) may effectively treat leukocyte abnormalities associated with Chédiak-Higashi syndrome.

Excessive α-tocopherol (vitamin E) intake (**choice B**) can lead to vitamin E excess, which is characterized by malaise, headaches, gastrointestinal complaints, and, sometimes, hypertension. Vitamin E deficiency is characterized by areflexia, decreased proprioception and vibratory sense, gait disturbances, and paresis of gaze.

Excessive cholecalciferol (vitamin D) intake (**choice C**) can lead to vitamin D excess, resulting in hypercalcemia and widespread calcification of soft tissues. A deficiency of vitamin D occurs with lack of sunshine or renal failure and leads to rickets in children and osteomalacia in adults.

Mild thiamine (vitamin $B_1$) deficiency (**choice E**) leads to peripheral neuropathy (dry beriberi). More severe vitamin depletion leads to high-output cardiac failure (wet beriberi) and the dementia, ataxia, and ophthalmoplegia of the Wernicke-Korsakoff syndrome frequently seen in chronic alcoholics. Thiamine excess is not common.

10. **The correct answer is B.** Glucose-6-phosphate dehydrogenase disease is an X-linked condition. The father has a normal X chromosome since he does not have clinical disease. The mother has one normal X chromosome and one defective X chromosome, since her 6-year-old son has the disease and she does not. Therefore, the baby has a 50% chance of having two normal X chromosomes and a 50% chance of having one normal and one abnormal X chromosome, making her a carrier.

    Glucose-6-phosphate dehydrogenase deficiency is a defect in the pentose phosphate pathway of glucose metabolism, leading to defective production of reduced NADPH. Reduced NADPH is used in many biochemical pathways and is specifically used to regenerate the reduced form of glutathione that protects the body against oxidant drugs.

11. **The correct answer is B.** This question requires that you recognize the family of receptors that interact with G proteins to initiate a signal transduction cascade. These receptors are all glycosylated integral membrane proteins that have seven transmembrane segments. Beta-adrenergic receptors for epinephrine are an example.

    Adenylate cyclase (**choice A**) is an intracellular effector protein involved in signal transduction. It is not an integral membrane protein.

    The cystic fibrosis transmembrane conductance regulator channel (**choice C**) is a cyclic AMP-activated chloride channel.

    Glucose transporters (**choice D**) are integral membrane proteins with 12 membrane-spanning domains.

    $Na^+/K^+$ ATPase (**choice E**) pumps sodium into and potassium out of the cell. It provides energy for active transport by hydrolyzing ATP.

12. **The correct answer is B.** Tay-Sachs disease is a severe autosomal recessive disease characterized clinically by mental retardation, blindness, muscular weakness, and death by 3 years of age. The cherry-red spot is a classic clue for Tay-Sachs disease. The disease is prevalent in Ashkenazi (East European) Jews. Hexosaminidase A normally functions to hydrolyze a bond between N-acetylglucosamine and galactose in the polar head of the ganglioside $GM_2$, an N-acetylneuraminic acid-containing glycolipid found in high concentration in the brain. Without hexosaminidase A activity, this ganglioside accumulates, leading to degenerative CNS changes.

13. **The correct answer is D.** This patient has vitamin $B_{12}$ deficiency (a USMLE favorite). Absence of vitamin $B_{12}$ as a cofactor in the conversion of methylmalonyl-CoA to succinyl-CoA results in the accumulation of methylmalonyl-CoA, which is subsequently excreted in the urine. Methylmalonyl-CoA mutase deficiency can also cause this type of aciduria.

    *Vitamin $B_{12}$*

    Methylmalonyl-CoA $\longrightarrow$ Succinyl-CoA

    *Methylmalonyl-CoA mutase*

    Argininosuccinic aciduria (**choice A**) can result from argininosuccinate lyase deficiency.

    Cystinuria (**choice B**) is the most common amino aciduria. It is an autosomal recessive disease, caused by a defect in the transport protein for lysine, arginine, cystine, and ornithine, that results in the excretion of these amino acids in the urine.

    Hemoglobinuria (**choice C**) occurs with hemolytic anemias, not with megaloblastic anemia caused by vitamin $B_{12}$ deficiency.

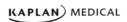

Propionic aciduria (**choice E**) can result from deficiency of biotin, propionyl-CoA carboxylase, or the enzyme that covalently attaches biotin to all carboxylases. In the latter case, additional organic acids accumulate as well.

14. **The correct answer is C.** Duchenne-type muscular dystrophy is the only disease listed that is X-linked; the other diseases are autosomal recessive. Remembering the genetics of myriad diseases is very problematic, but here are some imperfect rules of thumb that can help you out if you encounter an unfamiliar disease on an examination. Deficiencies of most enzymes are recessive (either autosomal or X-linked), since each person has at least two copies (from each of the parents) of each enzyme, and one working gene is usually enough (although careful evaluation of heterozygotes often shows mildly altered physiology). In contrast, alterations in structural proteins are often autosomal dominant, since having any amount of abnormal protein in structures such as basement membranes or in collagen tends to perturb their function. The number of common X-linked diseases (almost all recessive) is small and can be memorized: Duchenne muscular dystrophy, hemophilia A and B, chronic granulomatous disease, glucose-6-phosphate dehydrogenase deficiency, agammaglobulinemia, Wiskott-Aldrich syndrome, diabetes insipidus, Lesch-Nyhan syndrome, fragile X-syndrome, and color blindness.

Alpha$_1$-antitrypsin deficiency (**choice A**) is a deficiency of an enzyme (alpha$_1$-antitrypsin) that inhibits the action of various proteolytic enzymes. The two autosomal alleles for alpha$_1$-antitrypsin are codominantly expressed, such that they both contribute to the levels of circulating alpha$_1$-antitrypsin.

Cystic fibrosis (**choice B**) is an autosomal recessive disorder. The gene for cystic fibrosis has been localized to chromosome 7.

Phenylketonuria (**choice D**), in its classic form, is an autosomal recessive deficiency of phenylalanine hydroxylase.

Tay-Sachs disease (**choice E**) is caused by an autosomal recessive deficiency of the enzyme hexosaminidase A.

15. **The correct answer is D.** Galactosemia occurs in two very different clinical forms. Deficiency of galactokinase produces very mild disease; the only significant complication is cataract formation. In contrast, homozygous deficiency of galactose-1-phosphate uridyltransferase produces severe disease, culminating in death in infancy. In addition to galactosemia and galactosuria, these patients have impaired renal tubular resorption leading to aminoaciduria, gastrointestinal symptoms, hepatosplenomegaly, cataracts, bleeding diatheses, hypoglycemia, and mental retardation. Pathologically, the CNS shows neuronal loss and gliosis, and the liver shows fatty change progressing to cirrhosis.

Benign disease with cataract formation (**choice A**) is characteristic of galactokinase deficiency.

Chronic emphysema (**choice B**) is not associated with homozygous galactose-1-phosphate uridyltransferase deficiency, but rather with alpha$_1$-antitrypsin deficiency.

Impaired tubular reabsorption (producing aminoaciduria) is seen within a few days or weeks of feeding milk to an infant with severe galactosemia, as opposed to chronic renal failure appearing in adolescence (**choice C**).

Gastrointestinal symptoms (**choice E**) certainly occur in homozygous galactose-1-phosphate uridyltransferase deficiency, but they would not be expected to remit with puberty. Instead, most untreated infants with this disorder show failure to thrive and die in infancy from wasting and inanition.

16. **The correct answer is B.** The process of glycolysis is defined as the sequence of reactions that converts glucose into pyruvate with the concomitant production of ATP.

Glycolysis begins when glucose is converted by hexokinase to glucose-6-phosphate. When this compound interacts with the enzyme phosphoglucose isomerase (**choice D**), fructose-6-phosphate is formed. Fructose-6-phosphate is then converted by phosphofructokinase (**choice C**) to form fructose 1,6-bisphosphate, which is subsequently converted to glyceraldehyde 3-phosphate by aldolase (**choice A**). After a number of enzymatic reactions, phosphoenolpyruvate is formed.

Phosphoenolpyruvate is converted to pyruvate by pyruvate kinase (**choice E**), and the glycolytic pathway is then completed.

17. **The correct answer is E.** The child is affected at birth, indicating in utero exposure to high levels of maternally derived phenylalanine. Women with PKU must strictly adhere to their special diet during pregnancy to avoid adversely affecting the fetus.

Even if the father is a carrier of PKU (**choice A**) and the child is homozygous for the PKU allele (phenylalanine hydroxylase gene), there would have been no symptoms in the infant until 4-5 days after birth, providing the maternal blood phenylalanine level was in the normal range throughout pregnancy.

Maternal translocation with unbalanced segregation in meiosis I (**choice B**) and maternal translocation with unbalanced segregation in meiosis II (**choice C**) would likely have no effect on phenylalanine levels but might lead to trisomy.

Maternal uniparental disomy (**choice D**) simply means that two copies of a chromosome are derived from the mother and implies paternal nullisomy. Although there are rare occurrences of uniparental disomy, this mechanism is not known to be involved in any case of PKU. If maternal uniparental disomy occurred, the child would be expected to have PKU, and as in **choice A**, symptoms would not occur until 4-5 days after birth.

18.  **The correct answer is A.** The father is a carrier of a reciprocal translocation between 7p and 12q. Although this has no described phenotypic effect on the father, it is likely to increase the rate of spontaneous pregnancy loss as described in this question. The most recently aborted fetus has a partial but extensive trisomy 7 and a small partial monosomy 12. All autosomal trisomies except 21, 18, and 13 are incompatible with life, as are autosomal monosomies. The cause of the fetal karyotype was adjacent segregation during spermatogenesis in the father. Alternate segregation (**choice B**) in a reciprocal translocation carrier during gametogenesis produces a normal karyotype or another balanced translocation carrier.

An inversion is the result of two breaks on a chromosome with subsequent reinsertion of the fragment at its original site but in an inverted order. A paracentric inversion (**choice C**) does not involve the centromere. There is usually no effect on the carrier of the inversion, but acentric or dicentric chromosomes with deletions or duplications can be produced during gametogenesis. The father's karyogram does not show an inversion.

The reciprocal translocation (**choice D**) did not occur during spermatogenesis in the father. He is already a translocation carrier, indicating the translocation occurred in one of his parents or further back in his family.

A Robertsonian translocation (**choice E**) occurs when the q arms of two acrocentric chromosomes fuse with loss of the tiny p arms. The karyogram is not consistent with this definition, and the chromosomes involved are acrocentric.

19.  **The correct answer is C.** Ketone bodies, which include acetoacetate, beta-hydroxybutyrate, and acetone, are produced by the liver in the fasting state by beta-oxidation of fatty acids. They are then released into the blood stream, where they can be used as alternative energy sources for other organs, such as muscle, kidney, and brain. The brain specifically still requires a small amount of circulating glucose to function, but the amount required is reduced when ketone bodies are available.

Apoprotein B (**choice A**) is one of the proteins that hold lipoproteins together.

Beta-carotene (**choice B**) is a vitamin with antioxidant properties.

C-reactive protein (**choice D**) is a serum protein produced by the liver that rises during infections and in inflammatory states.

Coenzyme A (**choice E**) is found in mitochondria and carries acetyl groups into the citric acid, or tricarboxylic acid, cycle.

20.  **The correct answer is D.** DNA polymerase I in bacteria digests the RNA primers from the 5′ ends of the short Okazaki fragments and extends the adjacent fragment into the digested area.

DNA gyrase (**choice A**) is a type II topoisomerase found in *E. coli*. A deficiency would result in no DNA synthesis. The topoisomerases make transient breaks in DNA supercoils, permitting them to unwind and get ready for replication.

DNA helicase (**choice B**) deficiency would result in no DNA synthesis. The helicases bind to single-stranded DNA near the replication fork and force the double strand apart, making room for the synthetic enzymes to start their work.

If DNA ligase (**choice C**) had been defective, the short pieces accumulating would have consisted only of DNA because this enzyme functions after the RNA primer has been removed.

Primase (**choice E**) deficiency would result in no DNA synthesis. Primase works to attach short RNA sequences at the replication fork. If it were defective, there would be no RNA.

21.  **The correct answer is E.** The patient has characteristics of Niemann-Pick disease, an autosomal-recessive condition caused by a deficiency of the enzyme sphingomyelinase. This condition is associated with mental retardation, hepatosplenomegaly, foam cells in the bone marrow, cherry red spots on the maculae in 40% of cases, and neurologic deficits. Furthermore, death by 3 years of age is common.

A deficiency of alpha-galactosidase (**choice A**) is associated with the X-linked disorder known as Fabry disease. This condition is characterized by renal failure, telangiectasia, skin rash, and pain in the lower extremities.

A deficiency of beta-glucocerebrosidase (**choice B**) is associated with the autosomal recessive disorder known as Gaucher disease. This condition is characterized by hepatosplenomegaly, neurologic deficits, and mental retardation.

Individuals with a deficiency of ceramidase (**choice C**) have Farber disease, which is associated with hoarseness, dermatitis, skeletal deformations, mental retardation, and hepatomegaly.

HMG-CoA reductase (**choice D**) is the enzyme that carries out the rate limiting step of cholesterol synthesis. Several agents used in the treatment of hyperlipidemia block the activity of this enzyme, resulting in a decrease in LDL and total cholesterol.

22. **The correct answer is A.** Ciprofloxacin, a quinolone derivative, inhibits DNA gyrase (prokaryotic topoisomerase II) essential for DNA replication. A mutation in the gene for DNA gyrase has made the enzyme insensitive to the effects of ciprofloxacin.

Folate synthesis (**choice B**) is inhibited by sulfamethoxazole, not ciprofloxacin.

mRNA translocation on a ribosome (**choice C**) is inhibited by erythromycin, not ciprofloxacin.

Peptide bond formation (**choice D**) is inhibited by chloramphenicol, not ciprofloxacin.

Reduction of folate to tetrahydrofolate (**choice E**) is inhibited by trimethoprim, not ciprofloxacin.

23. **The correct answer is B.** The "statins" are a class of medications that inhibit the activity of the enzyme HMG-CoA reductase. Medications such as pravastatin and simvastatin produce a reversible inhibition of this enzyme, which subsequently leads to a reduction in LDL, total cholesterol, and triglycerides in patients with familial hypercholesterolemia.

Chronic inflammation (**choice A**) can be effectively treated with cyclooxygenase inhibitors, including nonsteroidal antiinflammatory drugs (NSAIDs), such as naproxen and ibuprofen, and cyclooxygenase-2 (COX-2) inhibitors, such as rofecoxib and celecoxib.

Essential hypertension (**choice C**) can be treated with angiotensin-converting enzyme (ACE) inhibitors, such as captopril. These agents decrease angiotensin production and reduce systolic and diastolic blood pressure.

Hyperuricemia (**choice D**) can be treated with allopurinol, which inhibits the activity of xanthine oxidase, leading to decreased production of uric acid.

One of the treatment measures for type 2 diabetes (**choice E**) is to inhibit the activity of the enzyme alpha-glucosidase. Acarbose, an alpha-glucosidase inhibitor, helps prevent postprandial surges in blood glucose levels.

24. **The correct answer is C.** Enlarged testes are the most specific phenotypic feature to suggest Fragile X syndrome in an individual who appears to have a hereditary mental retardation. The condition has unusual genetics, as it is related to expansion of a CGG repeat sequence located on the X chromosome. The larger the number of repeats, the higher the probability of significant retardation; hence, the retardation tends to become more severe in successive generations, as more CGG repeats accumulate. Sisters of affected males tend to show milder retardation than their brothers.

Features of Down syndrome (**choice A**), or trisomy 21, include mental retardation, epicanthal folds, dysplastic ears, hypotonia, a horizontal palmar crease (simian crease), redundant neck skin, and a short trunk.

Edwards syndrome (**choice B**), or trisomy 18, causes death in infancy. Characteristics include rocker-bottom feet, low-set ears, micrognathia, congenital heart disease, and mental retardation.

Klinefelter syndrome (47,XXY; **choice D**) is associated with testicular atrophy, a eunuchoid body shape, long extremities, and a small penis.

Turner syndrome (45,X; **choice E**) produces a female phenotype with short stature, ovarian dysgenesis, and webbing of the neck.

25. **The correct answer is E.** Even though the surface LDL receptors were digested by the trypsin, the recycling of unoccupied receptors to the cell surface provides a continual supply of new receptors to bind the labeled LDL. The LDL-receptor complex is internalized by receptor-mediated endocytosis.

Active transport (**choice A**) is the energy-dependent movement of molecules across a membrane and against a concentration gradient.

Facilitated diffusion (**choice B**) is the transport of low-permeability molecules with the aid of a carrier protein.

Phagocytosis (**choice C**) is the process by which cells such as macrophages and neutrophils engulf large particles.

Pinocytosis (**choice D**), which is the uptake of small molecules in solution, is receptor-independent.

26. **The correct answer is D.** This chromosomal aberration is known as Edwards syndrome, or trisomy 18. It is characterized by mental deficiency, growth retardation, prominent occiput, micrognathia, low-set ears, rocker-bottom feet, and ventricular septal defect.

XO (**choice A**) is the karyotype of Turner syndrome. It is characterized by short stature, webbed neck, and hypogonadism.

XXY (**choice B**) represents Klinefelter syndrome. It is usually undetected at birth but is characterized by tall stature, male hypogonadism, and sometimes mental retardation.

Trisomy 13 (Patau syndrome; **choice C**) is characterized by mental retardation, nervous system malformations, rocker-bottom feet, polydactyly, and cleft lip and palate.

Trisomy 21 (Down syndrome; **choice E**) is characterized by mental retardation, protruding tongue, simian crease, congenital heart defects, and a flat nasal bridge.

27. **The correct answer is D.** Peroxisomes are interesting cell organelles that were historically neglected because they are present in only small numbers in most mammalian cells. In the liver, however, these single membrane-bound organelles are present in large numbers and are important in detoxification and long chain fatty acid metabolism. The clinically important degradation of ethanol to (potentially toxic) acetaldehyde occurs in humans in both peroxisomes and the smooth endoplasmic reticulum (P450 system). Disulfiram (Antabuse), used to discourage alcoholics from drinking, blocks the next reaction, in which acetaldehyde is oxidized to (nontoxic) acetate. This reaction, catalyzed by aldehyde dehydrogenase, occurs in the mitochondria.

    Golgi bodies (**choice A**) are involved with packaging substances that are transported out of the cell.

    Lysosomes (**choice B**) are sites of degradation of intracellular waste products.

    The mitochondria (**choice C**) are involved with ATP production and contain both the electron transport chain and the citric acid (Krebs) cycle.

    Ribosomes (**choice E**) are the sites of protein synthesis.

28. **The correct answer is D.** This is von Gierke disease, one of the glycogen storage diseases. The defect in glucose-6-phosphatase prevents release of glucose from glycogen across the liver cell membrane. The glucose-6-phosphate trapped in the liver cell is degraded to lactate and pyruvate, which are then released into the serum.

29. **The correct answer is D.** Smith-Lemli-Opitz syndrome is a recently described recessive genetic disease. It is the first single-gene (as opposed to trisomy or other gross chromosomal alterations) disease to be associated with multiple malformations. It presents with combinations of the following: microcephaly, mental retardation, hypotonia, incomplete development of the genitalia, high forehead, pyloric stenosis, and syndactyly of the second and third toes. The disease appears to have a carrier rate comparable to sickle cell disease or cystic fibrosis in selected populations (which are not yet well defined). Experiments reveal that nutritional therapies (such as the administration of vegetable oil supplemented by large amounts of cholesterol) begun within the first few weeks of life may markedly alter the course of this disease (unlike other devastating neurologic diseases that lack effective treatments).

Down syndrome (**choice A**), or trisomy 21, is a common cause of mental retardation, congenital heart disease, and premature aging.

Edwards syndrome (**choice B**), or trisomy 18, is a genetic defect that results in severely retarded infants who typically die within the first year of life. Characteristic features include micrognathia, a prominent occiput, congenital heart and kidney malformations, and low-set ears.

Patau syndrome (**choice C**), or trisomy 13, is characterized by severe mental retardation, microcephaly, microphthalmia, polydactyly, cleft lip and palate, renal defects, and cardiac abnormalities. Affected infants typically die before 1 year of age.

WAGR syndrome (**choice E**; for **W**ilms tumor, **A**niridia, **G**enital anomalies, and mental **R**etardation) is associated with defects in several closely linked genes on chromosome 11.

30. **The correct answer is D.** The technique described is Western blotting. Western blots are used to identify a specific protein that may be present in very small concentrations in a complex protein mixture. This technique is used to confirm the presence of anti-HIV antibodies in the serum of infected patients. Note that ELISA (enzyme-linked immunoabsorbent assay), which measures the amount of HIV antibody present, is used initially to detect the presence of anti-HIV antibody. All patients with positive ELISAs are further evaluated with the Western blot to rule out false-positive results. Because the Western blot is based on an initial electrophoretic separation, it gives additional information about the molecular weight of the suspected HIV protein that makes the identification more accurate.

    Northern blotting (**choice A**) utilizes DNA-RNA hybridization to determine the size and abundance of RNA for a specific gene. An RNA sample is subjected to electrophoresis and transferred to a nitrocellulose filter. The filter's RNA is exposed to a labeled DNA probe that will bind to its RNA complement. The labeled DNA-RNA hybrid can be visualized upon exposure to film.

    Southern blotting (**choice B**) utilizes DNA-DNA hybridization. This test can be used to determine the epidemiologic relatedness of different bacterial biotypes, such as the strains of *Staphylococcus aureus* that produce toxic-shock syndrome.

    Southwestern blotting (**choice C**) involves DNA-protein interactions. A protein sample is subjected to electrophoresis, transferred to a filter, and exposed to labeled DNA.

31. **The correct answer is D.** Proteins that are targeted for lysosomes have mannose-6-phosphate on their sugar chains. The mannose-6-phosphate is on an external site on the protein so that it can be recognized by the mannose-6-phosphate receptor on the lysosomal surface, and would be easily accessible to an antibody directed against it.

    Acid hydrolases (**choice A**) are enzymes found inside the lysosomes.

    Coated pits (the cellular site for receptor-mediated endocytosis) contain clathrin (**choice B**).

    Production of glucose-6-phosphate (**choice C**) from glucose is the first step in the process of glycolysis.

    Sialic acid (**choice E**) is a terminal glycosylation product added to proteins (usually those destined for secretion) in the Golgi apparatus.

32. **The correct answer is C.** The RFLP detects a region near the centromere of chromosome 21. The region around the centromere exhibits a phenomenon called crossover suppression. Since genetic exchange cannot happen in this area, the probe is a reliable marker for the individual chromosomes. During meiosis II, sister chromatids, which are two identical copies of the same chromosome, should separate. If a nondisjunction event occurs in this division, two copies of the same chromosome are passed to the progeny. In this case, both parents are heterozygous for the RFLP. The child received an A from the mother and two Cs from the father, leading us to conclude that the problem occurred in the father during meiosis II.

    If a nondisjunction event of chromosome 21 occurs early in development, the result is a child who is a mosaic for trisomy 21 (**choice A**). This accounts for approximately 1% of children with trisomy 21. Since some of their cells are normal, these individuals show only a mild expression of the trisomy 21 phenotype.

    During meiosis I, homologues that carry similar, but not identical, information separate. If a failure occurred in this division, we would expect the man to pass CD (**choice B**), and the woman to pass A or B, producing a child that was ACD or BCD.

    If an AB woman had a failure in meiosis I (**choice D**), an AB gamete would be produced. When fertilized by the man's C or D sperm, a child that was ABC or ABD would result.

    If an AB woman's sister chromatids failed to disjoin during meiosis II (**choice E**), AA or BB gametes would result. When fertilized by the CD male's sperm, a child that was AAC, AAD, BBC, or BBD would result.

33. **The correct answer is B.** The key to excelling in biochemistry on the USMLE is to master the most clinically

important elements of metabolic pathways, e.g., rate-limiting steps, irreversible steps, and steps involving enzymes affected by genetic diseases. In this case, glycogen phosphorylase is the enzyme involved in the rate-limiting step of glycogenolysis:

*Glycogen phosphorylase*

$$(Glucose)_n + P_i \longrightarrow (Glucose)_{n-1} + Glucose\text{-}1\text{-}P$$

Note that this enzyme is activated in response to the binding of glucagon to liver cell receptors or the binding of epinephrine to muscle receptors, via signal transduction.

α-1,4-Glucan transferase (**choice A**) is a debranching enzyme that removes three or four glucose units from a branch point and transfers them to the end of another chain. In this reaction, one α-1,4 bond is cleaved and another is formed. The elongated chain then becomes a substrate for glycogen phosphorylase.

Glycogen synthase (**choice C**) is the enzyme involved in the rate-limiting step of glycogen synthesis:

*Glycogen synthase*

$$(Glucose)_n + UDP\text{-}glucose \rightarrow (Glucose)_{n+1} + UDP$$

Note that this enzyme is inactivated in response to the binding of glucagon to liver cell receptors or the binding of epinephrine to muscle receptors.

Phosphoglucomutase (**choice D**) is a key enzyme in glycogen synthesis that reversibly converts glucose-6-phosphate to glucose-1-phosphate.

UDP-glucose pyrophosphorylase (**choice E**) is another key enzyme in glycogen synthesis:

*UDP-glucose pyrophosphorylase*

$$Glu\text{-}1\text{-}P + Uridine\text{-}P\text{-}P\text{-}P \longrightarrow UDP\text{-}Glu + PP_i$$

Note that the linkage formed between UDP and glucose is a high-energy bond that can provide energy to many biosynthetic reactions.

34. **The correct answer is E.** Following antineoplastic therapy for treatment of acute lymphocytic leukemia, patients often have a high level of urate secondary to the breakdown of nucleic acids. Therefore, patients are often given allopurinol to decrease plasma urate levels. Allopurinol prevents uric acid formation by inhibiting the enzyme xanthine oxidase. Decreasing uric acid levels will help prevent the formation of kidney stones as well as block the appearance of other deleterious effects of hyperuricemia.

    Acarbose is an agent used in the treatment of type 2 diabetes. It inhibits the activity of alpha-glucosidase (**choice A**) in the intestinal tract, thereby helping to prevent postprandial hyperglycemia.

**KAPLAN) MEDICAL**

Inhibition of angiotensin-converting enzyme (**choice B**) will lower blood pressure and help prevent the "ventricular remodeling" that occurs secondary to congestive heart failure.

Beta-lactamase (**choice C**) inhibitors are combined with penicillin antibiotics to help improve their activity against bacteria that produce the enzyme beta-lactamase.

Nonsteroidal antiinflammatory drugs (NSAIDs) inhibit the activity of the enzyme cyclooxygenase (**choice D**), thereby decreasing the production of prostaglandins.

35. **The correct answer is D.** The combination of retardation and self-mutilation should lead you immediately to the diagnosis of Lesch-Nyhan disease. The hard part is remembering which enzyme is deficient in this disease. Hypoxanthine-guanine phosphoribosyltransferase (HGPRT) is part of the purine salvage pathway. A deficiency of this enzyme results in the inability to recycle purines and an overproduction of uric acid. Affected children are mentally retarded, have hyperuricemia and gout, and engage in compulsive self-destructive behaviors.

Deficiency of cystathionine synthase (**choice A**) results in homocystinuria, a disease characterized by elevated urinary homocystine. Afflicted children typically present with failure to thrive and visual problems due to lens displacement. In addition to cystathionine synthase deficiency, other causes of homocystinuria include methionine synthase deficiency and deficiency of pyridoxine, folate, or vitamin $B_{12}$.

Deficiency of hexosaminidase A (**choice B**) causes Tay-Sachs disease. This enzymatic deficiency results in the accumulation of $GM_2$ ganglioside. Clinical characteristics include mental retardation, blindness, and muscular weakness. A characteristic feature is the presence of a cherry-red spot on the macula. Remember that this disease is more common in Ashkenazi Jews and typically results in death by 3 years of age.

Deficiency of homogentisic acid oxidase (**choice C**), an enzyme involved in the degradation of tyrosine, results in a condition known as alkaptonuria. The classic finding of this typically benign disease is dark urine. There can also be darkening of connective tissue (e.g., ear cartilage may appear bluish).

Deficiency of phenylalanine hydroxylase (**choice E**) is one cause of phenylketonuria (PKU). Phenylalanine hydroxylase catalyzes the conversion of phenylalanine to tyrosine. In patients with PKU, tyrosine becomes an essential amino acid. Children with PKU have mental retardation, fair skin, and a characteristically musty body odor. (Note: if you see the adjective "musty" on the USMLE, the answer is usually PKU.)

36. **The correct answer is B.** In a Northern blot, all the mRNA from a cell type (isolated through the presence of its polyadenosine tails) is electrophoresed on a gel; since all mRNA is negatively charged, the electrophoresis separates it by size. The gel is then blotted onto nitrocellulose, the probe is applied and hybridized, and the excess is washed off; the resultant blot is autoradiographed. Bands on the autoradiograph film indicate the mRNAs that contain sequences complementary to the probe; this indicates that the gene on the probe has been expressed in the mRNA of that cell. This is the best technique for determining whether a gene is expressed in a particular cell type.

DNA sequencing (**choice A**) and Southern blot (**choice D**) are both incorrect, since they examine the DNA of the cell, and the DNA of all the cells involved is identical.

Polymerase chain reaction (PCR; **choice C**) is used to amplify DNA and could not alone determine which tissue culture expressed the gene being studied. PCR can be used to amplify the DNA probe necessary for Northern blotting. Note that in this case, however, the DNA probe was supplied in adequate amounts, making PCR unnecessary.

A Western blot (**choice E**) is used to characterize the expression of a particular protein or to assay the serum for antibodies against a specific protein. Total protein is extracted, then electrophoresed on a gel and blotted to nitrocellulose. The nitrocellulose blot is incubated with a patient's serum to identify the presence of antibodies that can bind to the protein.

37. **The correct answer is D.** Cystic fibrosis is an autosomal recessive disease caused by point mutations or small deletions in the gene encoding an integral membrane protein that functions as a chloride transporter. Although many mutations within the gene cause the phenotype, it is not practical or cost-effective to sequence the entire region to screen for a carrier. In the white population, however, the most frequent mutant allele causing cystic fibrosis is due to a small deletion at phenylalanine 508 in exon 10 on chromosome 7. This mutation accounts for greater than 50% of mutant cystic fibrosis alleles in white populations. An amplification of this region using the polymerase chain reaction (PCR) can be done, and the PCR products are sequenced and compared against the normal sequence for this region. If comparison reveals the deletion, the donor of that template DNA would be classified as a carrier. If the mutation is not present, the probability that the DNA donor is a carrier of cystic fibrosis is greatly reduced, but still exists. Most diagnostic laboratories will use this method to screen for between 4 and 10 of the most common

mutations. Note that if a person belongs to a different ethnic group, PCR must be used to amplify the exons that contain the majority of cystic fibrosis mutations within that particular ethnic group.

Biochemical testing (**choice A**) is usually used to detect a defective enzyme or a reduced amount of the normal enzyme. It is more economical than DNA testing for detecting carriers or affected individuals. It is used in the detection of carriers of autosomal recessive diseases, such as Tay-Sachs disease, sickle cell anemia, and the thalassemias.

Fluorescence *in situ* hybridization (FISH; **choice B**) uses a DNA probe that has been labeled with a fluorescent compound to visualize locations on the chromosomes that have homology to the probe. It can be used to detect microdeletions in a gene of interest.

Karyotype analysis (**choice C**) is used to determine whether an individual's chromosomes are grossly normal in their number and structure. It can be used to detect trisomies, monosomies, and translocations, as well as large inversions and deletions.

Western blot analysis (**choice E**) is a technique commonly used to detect the presence of antibody against specific proteins in serum. It is primarily used as a confirmatory test for HIV infection.

38. **The correct answer is A.** The patient is presenting with signs and symptoms highly suggestive of type 1 diabetes. The primary source of ketones in the urine is free fatty acid breakdown. Ketone body formation occurs as follows: insulin deficiency → activated lipolysis → increased plasma free fatty acids → increased hepatic fatty acids → accelerated ketogenesis. In summary, as fatty acids break down, acetyl-CoA is generated. As acetyl-CoA levels increase, ketone bodies begin to form. When excessive amounts of ketone bodies are formed, the pathologic state known as ketosis can occur.

Gluconeogenesis (**choice B**) and glycogenolysis (**choice C**) occur when glucose is needed for the production of ATP in various cells in the body.

Protein breakdown (**choice D**) results in the formation of amino acids.

Triglyceride breakdown (**choice E**) results in the release of free fatty acids.

39. **The correct answer is C.** Taken together, severe neonatal jaundice, elevated indirect bilirubin, and exchange blood transfusion strongly suggest hemolysis. The hemoglobin and hematocrit values are low and reticulocytosis is present, indicating an anemia. Thus, this infant has a hemolytic anemia. Increased levels of 2,3-BPG, 3-PG, 2-PG, and PEP (all distal glycolysis intermediates) are consistent with a block in glycolysis below phospho-

enolpyruvate. Only a hemolytic anemia induced by a PK deficiency meets all these criteria. Hemolytic anemias have been reported in association with deficiencies of most of the enzymes of glycolysis. Most are quite rare, but PK deficiency is the most common. There are many variant forms of PK deficiency, some affecting $K_m$, some $V_{max}$, and some allosteric regulation. Most have a relatively mild clinical symptomology limited to the red cell. The tissue specificity is a consequence of the fact that there is a red-cell-specific PK isozyme. The relative lack of severe symptoms is a consequence of the fact that many of the aberrations affect kinetic parameters rather than total activity and because the body compensates with accelerated RBC production and the high 2,3 DPG level. The latter causes the hemoglobin to dump oxygen at a lower partial oxygen pressure.

G6PD deficiency (**choice A**) is the most common enzymatic effect causing hemolytic anemia. Over 300 different mutant forms of G6PD have been described, but only the "African" and the "Mediterranean" are common. Patients with either of these have few symptoms under normal conditions but can go into a hemolytic crisis when stressed by certain oxidizing drugs and infections, and in the case of the Mediterranean variant, by fava beans. In none of these variants do glycolytic intermediates accumulate.

Lead is a heavy metal that tends to bind to enzymes with multiple sulfhydryl groups, for example, pyruvate dehydrogenase and α-ketoglutarate dehydrogenase. Because of the key role these enzymes have in energy metabolism, lead poisoning (**choice B**) has multiple organ effects. The brain in particular is vulnerable because of its dependency on glucose. In this organ, lead poisoning causes delayed or inhibited development, permanent learning disabilities, and in acute cases, seizures, coma, and even death. Lead also lowers the hemoglobin level by interfering with the dehydration of aminolevulinic acid and the incorporation of iron into the protoporphyrin molecule. Thus, chronic lead poisoning will cause an anemia, but it will not be a hemolytic one.

Sickle cell anemia (**choice D**) is the most common hemoglobinopathy. It, like the common forms of glucose 6-phosphate dehydrogenase deficiency, provides a partial protection against malaria. The molecular defect is a substitution of glutamate by valine on position six of the beta-chain. The resultant product can form a tetramer with the alpha chains and is called hemoglobin-S (HbS). HbS has a low solubility in the deoxy form, and it precipitates when subjected to a low oxygen partial pressure. This causes red cells to sickle. These sickled cells can then block small vessels and cause a myriad of problems. Glycolytic intermediates do not accumulate.

β-Thalassemia (**choice E**) results from reduced synthesis of the hemoglobin β-chain. This leads to an excess of α-globin chains, which precipitate and prevent nascent red cells from maturing. Since there are two copies of the β-globin gene, some individuals only have one affected gene (β-thalassemia minor), whereas others have defects in both genes (β-thalassemia major). Individuals with β-thalassemia minor are essentially asymptomatic while those with β-thalassemia major require transfusions on a regular basis after their first or second year. Symptoms of anemia are delayed because the β-globin gene is not expressed until shortly before birth and fetal hemoglobin continues to be produced in the neonate. There is no accumulation of glycolytic intermediates.

40. **The correct answer is D.** DNA sequences produced by reverse transcription from mRNA templates would lack introns because the intron sequences are removed from RNA in the nucleus prior to its release as mRNA into the cytoplasm.

Oncogenic mutations (**choice A**) alter proto-oncogenes in such a way that expression of the oncogene causes cancer. By definition, pseudogenes are not expressed; therefore, a pseudogene cannot be an oncogene.

Because this is a nonfunctional gene sequence, it is unlikely to contain nested genes (**choice B**) or to provide antibiotic resistance.

Having lost some coding regions (**choice C**) is not the best answer because if completely transcribed, it should have all the coding regions found within the true gene. However, some pseudogenes, while maintaining a high degree of homology with their true gene counterpart, are further mutated. This further mutation may alter a coding region.

Shine-Dalgarno sequences (**choice E**) help prokaryotic mRNA bind to the 30s ribosomal subunit. This sequence would not be present in human (eukaryotic) mRNAs.

41. **The correct answer is E.** Folate (as 7,8-dihydrofolate) is converted to tetrahydrofolate by dihydrofolate reductase. Methotrexate is a competitive inhibitor of dihydrofolate reductase. Therefore, providing sufficiently high concentrations of folate will allow the enzyme to reach the same $V_{max}$ as obtained in the absence of inhibitor.

Increasing substrate concentration would not increase (**choice A**) or decrease (**choice C**) the affinity ($K_m$) for the substrate dihydrofolate.

The $V_{max}$ would not increase above the uninhibited $V_{max}$ (compare with **choice B**) in the absence of methotrexate.

Increasing substrate concentration would not increase the affinity for methotrexate (**choice D**).

42. **The correct answer is D.** The patient described has scurvy, resulting from a deficiency of dietary vitamin C. Absence of vitamin C leads to impaired hydroxylation of proline residues in the nascent procollagen chains, leading to weakness of blood vessel walls. Clinically, the deficiency syndrome is characterized by perifollicular hemorrhages, fragmentation of hairs, purpura, ecchymoses, splinter hemorrhages, and hemorrhages into muscle. In patients with normal dentition, gum changes (swelling, bleeding, loosening of teeth) are also noted. Without vitamin C supplementation, death may eventually occur.

Administration of factor VIII (**choice A**) would be indicated for factor VIII deficiency. This deficiency would also lead to a prolonged partial thromboplastin time (PTT), which was not noted.

Administration of iron (**choice B**) would be of benefit in iron-deficiency anemia, but there is no indication of a hypochromic, microcytic anemia in this patient. The anemia of scurvy is typically normochromic and normocytic because of bleeding.

Administration of vitamin $B_{12}$ (**choice C**) would be indicated for a megaloblastic anemia. Although a macrocytic anemia may be observed in scurvy (because of concomitant dietary folate deficiency or perturbations in the folate pool), this patient did not show macrocytosis.

Administration of vitamin K (**choice E**) would be appropriate in the setting of vitamin K deficiency, which would produce a prolonged prothrombin time (PT), followed eventually by a prolonged PTT as the vitamin K-dependent factors (II, VII, IX, X, protein C, and protein S) are depleted.

43. **The correct answer is A.** Hereditary nonpolyposis colorectal cancer (HNPCC) is an autosomal dominant condition causing early colorectal cancer, often before the age of 50. Female relatives are also at high risk for endometrial and ovarian cancer. Nearly 90% of cases of HNPCC are linked to mutations in mismatch repair genes such as hMLH1 and hMSH2. The proteins encoded by these genes function during G2 of the cell cycle to repair areas of DNA with mismatched bases introduced during DNA replication. Dinucleotide (microsatellite) repeat instability is characteristic of tumor cells in HNPCC.

A point mutation in the gene coding for an excision exonuclease (**choice B**) is characteristic of xeroderma pigmentosum.

A reciprocal translocation between chromosomes 8 and 14 (**choice C**) is characteristic of Burkitt lymphoma. This translocation occurs near the *myc* gene and results in transcriptional activation of *myc*. There is a strong association between Burkitt lymphoma and infection with the Epstein-Barr virus.

Loss of the RB tumor suppressor gene (**choice D**) causes retinoblastoma. The RB gene products normally regulate the G1 to S transition, thereby promoting differentiation and inhibiting unrestricted cellular division. Mutations causing loss of RB gene function are usually inherited as a dominant trait. This also is true of tumor suppressor genes in general. The sequence of events follows: A defective allele is inherited, and then the second allele becomes mutated as an early somatic event. This leads to a high incidence of that cancer at an early age. Sporadic nonfamilial retinoblastomas are also reported. These usually occur at a later age and only affect one eye.

44.  **The correct answer is B.** Deficiencies of the enzyme hexosaminidase A result in Tay-Sachs disease, an autosomal-recessive disorder characterized by mental retardation, blindness, muscular weakness, and the appearance of a cherry red spot on the macula. Death by 3 years of age is common. This condition is most commonly seen in Ashkenazi Jews. Tay-Sachs can best be described as a gangliosidosis, since ganglioside $GM_2$ accumulates.

An example of an aminoacidopathy (**choice A**) would be the autosomal recessive phenylalanine hydroxylase deficiency associated with phenylketonuria.

Lipid metabolism (**choice C**) disorders often involve a defect at the LDL receptor. These types of disorders can be seen in patients with the autosomal dominant disorder familial hypercholesterolemia.

An example of a mucopolysaccharidosis (**choice D**) is an X-linked recessive deficiency of iduronate sulfatase, or Hunter syndrome.

Acute intermittent porphyria (**choice E**) is an autosomal dominant disorder involving a biochemical defect of porphobilinogen deaminase.

45.  **The correct answer is C.** Hypoglycemia with hypoketosis after fasting suggests a block in fatty acid oxidation. Accumulation of organic dicarboxylic acids further indicates a fatty acyl-CoA dehydrogenase deficiency; most commonly this will be a medium chain acyl CoA dehydrogenase (MCAD) deficiency. MCAD deficiency is an autosomal recessive disease expressed with high frequency among people of Northern European descent. Homozygous individuals are unable to break down fatty acids, and so cannot use fat for energy production when glucose supplies are limited. This blockage may also lead

to a secondary carnitine deficiency because the accumulated acyl-CoA is transesterified to produce acyl carnitine. Because carnitine is required to transport fatty acids into mitochondria for oxidation, this also will increase tissue dependence on glucose metabolism. Because ketogenesis also depends on fatty acid catabolism, the brain has no source of ketones to use as an alternative fuel. Whether due to the primary block, the induced carnitine deficiency, or a combination of the two, the net result is acute hypoglycemia whenever glucose is not readily available. Symptoms most commonly appear between two months and two years, but they may be noted as early as two days or as late as six years, and on occasion, asymptomatic parents have first been diagnosed after one of their children have an episode. Generally, symptoms appear after a period of dietary carbohydrate deficiency; presumably, this is what happened in this boy due to his gastroenteritis. It has been estimated that MCAD accounts for about 1% of deaths due to sudden infant death syndrome (SIDS), and about 20% of children with MCAD die after the first episode. The hypoglycemia can occur quickly, and CNS symptoms become marked when venous blood glucose levels drop to about 20 mg/dL (0.11 mM). The mainstay of treatment is to remain well fed on a high carbohydrate diet. Some physicians also prescribe L-carnitine, which is claimed to help maintain blood glucose levels during sickness or other forms of stress.

Glucose 6-phosphatase deficiency (**choice A**) is a glycogen storage disease that will also lead to a fasting hypoglycemia, but ketone bodies would accumulate, and there would be no accumulation of organic dicarboxylic acids.

Hepatic glycogen phosphorylase deficiency (**choice B**) is a glycogen storage disease that will also lead to a mild fasting hypoglycemia with formation of ketone bodies, but without accumulation of organic dicarboxylic acids.

Mitochondrial carbamoyl phosphate synthetase deficiency (**choice D**) is a urea cycle enzyme deficiency disease that will cause hyperammonemia, not hypoglycemia, and accumulation of organic dicarboxylic acids.

Ornithine transcarbamoylase deficiency (**choice E**) is also a urea cycle enzyme deficiency disease that will cause hyperammonemia, rather than hypoglycemia, and accumulation of organic dicarboxylic acids.

46.  **The correct answer is C.** The patient is presenting with the classic signs and symptoms of von Gierke disease, which is an autosomal recessive genetic disorder that usually manifests in the first 12 months of life. Laboratory evaluation often reveals the presence of increased lactate, cholesterol, triglyceride, and uric acid

levels. This condition is caused by a basic enzyme defect involving glucose-6-phosphatase deficiency.

Brancher enzyme deficiency (**choice A**), otherwise known as Anderson disease, is associated with infantile failure to thrive, cirrhosis, liver failure, and extreme hypotonia.

Debrancher enzyme deficiency (**choice B**), also known as Cori disease, is characterized by hypoglycemia, hepatomegaly, short-stature, and myopathy. Laboratory evaluation often reveals the presence of normal lactate and uric acid and increased cholesterol and triglyceride levels.

Hepatic phosphorylase deficiency (**choice D**), otherwise known as Hers disease, is associated with hepatomegaly and variable hypoglycemia.

Muscle phosphorylase deficiency (**choice E**), or McArdle disease, causes pain, cramps, and myoglobinuria on strenuous exercise. It is associated with episodes of increased creatine kinase and deficient lactate production.

47. **The correct answer is E.** This question is a "two-step" item, which is common on the USMLE. First, you need to figure out from the clinical clues which vitamin deficiency you are dealing with. Next, you need to remember which enzymes utilize the deficient vitamin as a cofactor.

This patient has all the signs of Wernicke encephalopathy—a favorite Step 1 disease characterized by dementia, ataxia, and ophthalmoplegia. This disease typically occurs in alcoholics and is the result of thiamine deficiency. Thiamine pyrophosphate (TPP), the activated form of thiamine, is a cofactor in the oxidative decarboxylation of $\alpha$-ketoacids. The four major enzymes requiring TPP are pyruvate dehydrogenase (pyruvate to acetyl-CoA; links glycolysis to TCA cycle), $\alpha$-ketoglutarate dehydrogenase (TCA cycle), branched-chain ketoacid dehydrogenase (involved in metabolism of branched-chain amino acids; deficiency results in maple syrup urine disease), and transketolase (hexose monophosphate shunt).

Aspartate aminotransferase (**choice A**) is a transaminase involved in the transfer of the $\alpha$-amino group from aspartate. The transaminases are a family of enzymes involved in amino acid degradation; they transfer the $\alpha$-amino group from an amino acid to an $\alpha$-ketoacid receptor (usually $\alpha$-ketoglutarate). The transaminases require pyridoxal phosphate, a derivative of pyridoxine (vitamin $B_6$), as a cofactor.

Methylmalonyl-CoA mutase (**choice B**) catalyzes the conversion of methylmalonyl-CoA (a product of fatty acid oxidation and branched-chain amino acid catabolism) to succinyl-CoA, which can then enter the TCA cycle. This enzyme is one of two reactions in

humans that requires deoxyadenosylcobalamin, the activated form of vitamin $B_{12}$, as a cofactor. The other is methionine synthase, which converts homocysteine to methionine. Recall that vitamin $B_{12}$ is absorbed in the stomach and that absorption requires intrinsic factor produced by gastric parietal cells. The classic finding of $B_{12}$ deficiency is megaloblastic anemia. Peripheral neuropathy may also occur.

Prolyl hydroxylase (**choice C**) catalyzes the hydroxylation of prolyl residues in collagen biosynthesis. Along with lysyl hydroxylase, it requires vitamin C as a cofactor. Deficiency of vitamin C inhibits the cross-linking of collagen fibers, resulting in a condition known as scurvy. Scurvy is characterized by poor wound healing, fragile blood vessels, bleeding gums, and loose teeth.

Pyruvate carboxylase (**choice D**) catalyzes the first step in gluconeogenesis—the carboxylation of pyruvate to oxaloacetate. Biotin serves as the carrier of the "activated carboxyl" group in this reaction, as well as in the carboxylation reactions catalyzed by acetyl-CoA carboxylase (fatty acid synthesis) and propionyl-CoA carboxylase (branched-chain amino acid catabolism and odd-chain fatty acid oxidation).

48. **The correct answer is C.** Glycogen is the storage form of glucose and a readily mobilizable fuel store. When individuals do not consume adequate quantities of carbohydrates, the body responds by breaking down glycogen stores in the liver to maintain normal blood glucose levels. The two enzymes involved in the degradation and synthesis of glycogen are glycogen phosphorylase (**choice C**) and glycogen synthase (**choice D**), respectively. The processes of glycogen synthesis and degradation are coordinated by a hormone-triggered cascade that ensures that when one enzyme is active, the other enzyme is inactive.

Acetyl-CoA carboxylase (**choice A**) is the key enzyme involved in fatty acid synthesis.

Glucose-6-phosphate dehydrogenase (**choice B**) is involved in the pentose phosphate pathway.

Thiolase (**choice E**) converts acetoacetyl-CoA into acetyl-CoA.

49. **The correct answer is B.** The $^{32}$P-cDNA probe will mark the fragment containing exon 2. On the grandfather's abnormal chromosome that lacks HV-2, the fragment will be about 2.5 kb long. An affected descendent would necessarily have inherited this chromosome, and the RFLP pattern should show a 2.5-kb band. Note that the affected grandson has an additional restriction fragment (2.5 kb) in his pattern that must have originated from the chromosome of his other parent. Because that parent is

from outside the family, the additional restriction fragment can be a variety of sizes. In this particular case, the chromosomes must have all the *HV-1* sites present.

**Choices A, C, D,** and **E** lack a 2.5-kb fragment, and therefore, the DNA being studied was not derived from the affected grandson.

50. **The correct answer is B.** Locus heterogeneity refers to the situation in which the same phenotype is caused by defects in different genes. It is commonly seen in syndromes resulting from failures in a complex pathway, such as hearing. In this example, locus heterogeneity is indicated because of complementation. In generations I through III, deafness appears to be due to a single autosomal recessive trait. In generation IV, deaf parents produce normal hearing children, suggesting that the parents have defects in different genes. The children are heterozygous at both loci and so have normal hearing (complementation).

Autosomal dominant inheritance (**choice A**) would require multiple assumptions. In generation IV, the parents produce six normal children, although at best they are both heterozygous for the trait. The probability of that event, given that they are both heterozygous, is $(1/4)^6$. Even more troublesome is the mating between II-1 and II-2, in which normal parents produce affected children. Although it is possible that the gene is an autosomal dominant with incomplete penetrance, no data about this frequency are given, and this hypothesis still requires many more assumptions than the correct answer. Penetrance is the frequency at which the phenotype is expressed in a person who carries a particular genotype. It can complicate pedigree analysis.

Mitochondrial inheritance (**choice C**) would show a completely different pattern. Genetic information is transmitted to progeny on nuclear chromosomes, as well as on mitochondrial chromosomes. Since mitochondria are inherited only from the mother, if affected, she will give the trait to all of her progeny. A male with the trait will never transmit it to his progeny.

Multifactorial inheritance (**choice D**) is a non-mendelian inheritance pattern that depends on the incremental contributions of multiple loci to a single phenotype, as well as on contributions from environmental factors. Characteristics that exhibit a broad range of values, like height or eye color, are inherited in this manner.

X-linked dominant inheritance (**choice E**) affects either sex, but which of the children are affected depends on the sex of the affected parent. If the male parent is affected, he will produce only affected daughters and normal sons, because he gives his X chromosome to all of his daughters and none of his sons. If the female parent is affected, she contributes an X chromosome to both daughters and sons; hence, both can be affected. However, since she is almost always heterozygous for the trait, the probability is 50% that her children will receive a normal X chromosome. Remember that human females randomly inactivate one of their X chromosomes (Lyon hypothesis). Because of this inactivation, a female who is heterozygous for an X-linked dominant trait will tend to be both more mildly and more variably affected then a male with the same trait.

# Biochemistry: **Test Two**

1. A 3-year-old girl who is small for her age has had multiple hypoglycemic episodes associated with moderate fasting during periods of illness. In her most recent episode associated with influenza, her parents slept late, and at 10 AM were unable to rouse the child from sleep. Blood and urine samples collected at the emergency department reveal marked hypoglycemia, ketonuria, and ketonemia along with an appropriately low insulin level. The blood alanine level is abnormally low; however, infusion of alanine produces a rapid rise in blood glucose. The defect most likely responsible for these symptoms is found in which of the following pathways?

   (A) Gluconeogenesis

   (B) Glycogenolysis

   (C) Protein catabolism in muscle

   (D) Triglyceride hydrolysis in adipose tissue

   (E) β-Oxidation of fatty acids

2. A large family has multiple members affected with a form of colorectal cancer. The locus involved is mapped to chromosome 3p. A single nucleotide polymorphism (D3S1298) at 3p21 is informative in this family. The recombination frequency is calculated, and LOD scores for linkage distance between the gene and marker D3S1298 are calculated and displayed in the table below. What is the best conclusion from the data shown?

**LOD Scores for Recombination Frequencies with D3S1298**

| 0.00 | 0.0001 | 0.001 | 0.01 | 0.05 | 0.10 | 0.20 | 0.30 | 0.40 |
|------|--------|-------|------|------|------|------|------|------|
| 1.40 | 1.53 | 1.69 | 1.80 | 1.62 | 1.52 | 1.27 | 0.93 | 0.50 |

   (A) D3S1298 is not linked to the disease-producing gene in this family

   (B) Significant linkage is demonstrated at a distance of 0.01 cM

   (C) Significant linkage is demonstrated at a distance of 1 cM

   (D) Significant linkage is demonstrated at a distance of 40 cM

   (E) The data are suggestive of linkage, but more families will need to be tested before significant linkage can be demonstrated

3. During her internal medicine rotation, a third-year medical student is asked to evaluate a patient with known pyruvate kinase deficiency. While interviewing the patient, the medical student remembers learning about another disease with similar characteristics. This patient's disease is most clinically similar to which of the following diseases?

   (A) α-Thalassemia

   (B) β-Thalassemia

   (C) Glucose-6-phosphate dehydrogenase deficiency

   (D) Hereditary spherocytosis

   (E) Iron deficiency anemia

4. A 32-year-old pregnant woman with a history of deep venous thrombosis associated with oral contraceptive use is seen for her first prenatal visit. Her mother also had an episode of deep vein thrombosis during pregnancy. DNA from the woman is tested for a potential mutation in the factor V gene known to cause this condition. The DNA sequence to be amplified by PCR is shown below. The *dashed line* indicates the internal sequence where the potential mutation is located. Which answer choice represents the pair of primers that should be used in the PCR?

   TCCTGAGC--------------AAATGTGT

   (A) AGGACTCG and TTTACACA

   (B) GCTCAGGA and AAATGTGT

   (C) GCTCAGGA and ACACATTT

   (D) TCCTGAGC and ACACATTT

   (E) TCCTGAGC and TTTACACA

5. A 40-year-old, formerly obese woman presents to her physician. She was very proud of having lost 80 lb during the previous 2 years, but has now noticed that her "hair is falling out." On questioning, she reports having followed a strict, fat-free diet. Her alopecia is probably related to a deficiency of which of the following vitamins?

   (A) A

   (B) C

   (C) D

   (D) E

   (E) K

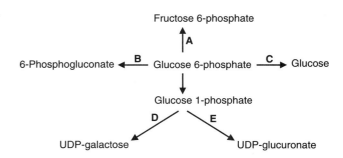

6. Which reaction or pathway in the diagram shown above would most likely be stimulated by a decrease in hepatic [NADPH]/[NADP$^+$]?

   (A) A

   (B) B

   (C) C

   (D) D

   (E) E

7. An amino-terminal leader sequence is part of a nascent protein being translated on the rough endoplasmic reticulum (RER). Which of the following proteins is being synthesized?

   (A) Acetyl CoA carboxylase

   (B) Coagulation factor VIII

   (C) Cytochrome oxidase

   (D) Myosin

   (E) Phosphofructokinase

8. A 25-year old woman with type 1 diabetes mellitus has maintained good glycemic control for several years. Recently she has gained 10 pounds and joined a group exercise program. By the end of her first 1-hour aerobics session, she is dizzy, nauseated, and feels faint. Which underlying mechanism is the most likely explanation for this episode?

   (A) Inadequate delivery of oxygen to the muscle

   (B) Stimulation of gluconeogenesis in the liver

   (C) Stimulation of glycogenolysis in liver

   (D) Stimulation of glycogenolysis in muscle

   (E) Translocation of GLUT4 to the cell membranes of myocytes

9. A 10-year-old boy with short stature is being evaluated for progressive neuropathy. Deep tendon reflexes are decreased, and vibratory sensation and proprioception are impaired. He has ataxia and a spastic gait. Ophthalmologic examination reveals decreased vision in dim light and pigmentary retinal degeneration. He has a history of frequent diarrhea with fatty stools. A serum lipid profile shows:

| | | |
|---|---|---|
| Cholesterol | 33 mg/dL | (normal: 132-220 mg/dL) |
| Triglyceride | 0 mg/dL | (normal: 32-150 mg/dL) |
| HDL cholesterol | 28 mg/dL | (normal: 34-86 mg/dL) |

Genetic testing reveals a mutation in a gene encoding a protein necessary for normal lipoprotein metabolism. In which of the following genes is this mutation most likely?

(A) ApoB gene

(B) ApoB100 receptor gene

(C) ApoC2 gene

(D) ApoE gene

(E) Lecithin acyl cholesterol transferase (LCAT) gene

10. An infant diagnosed with phenylketonuria would be expected to be deficient in which of the following nonessential amino acids, assuming that it is not obtained from dietary sources?

(A) Asparagine

(B) Cysteine

(C) Glutamine

(D) Proline

(E) Tyrosine

11. A 2-year-old obese girl with difficulty breathing is admitted to the hospital and given oxygen. She shows signs of developmental delay and has just taken her first steps. At birth, she had generalized hypotonia and fed poorly, although she now has a voracious appetite. Her older brother and sister are both normal. A probe for 15q11-13 reveals a deletion from one of her chromosomes. Prader-Willi syndrome is diagnosed. To confirm the diagnosis, a DNA methylation assay is performed. A sample of her DNA is first cut with *Eco*RI, releasing a 12-kb fragment, shown below, which is detected by the probe for the involved region on chromosome 15.

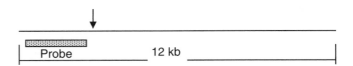

This fragment is then treated with a second restriction endonuclease that cuts within a CGCGCG sequence located at the position indicated by the arrow. If the CGCGCG sequence is methylated, the restriction endonuclease will not cut it. Assuming that the results confirm the diagnosis of Prader-Willi, which pattern below represents the girl's DNA?

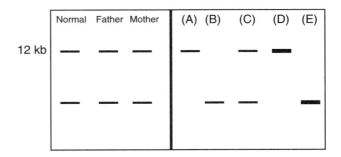

12. A cardiovascular researcher is conducting a study to evaluate the relationship between folate levels and cardiovascular disease. The results of the study show that persons with lower folate levels have twice the risk of cardiovascular disease mortality than do those with higher folate levels. Which of the following enzymes is most closely related to the role of folate in lowering the risk of cardiovascular disease?

   (A) Dihydrofolate reductase

   (B) Glycinamide ribonucleotide transformylase

   (C) Homocysteine methyltransferase

   (D) Ribonucleotide reductase

   (E) Thymidylate synthase

13. A 9-year-old girl with mild mental retardation was healthy at birth but presented during the first week of life with vomiting, lethargy, seizures, and hypertonia. An amino acid screen revealed elevated levels of leucine, isoleucine, and valine, so the child was put on a special diet restricted in these amino acids. She has had no medical problems related to her disease since that time. Which of the following enzymes is most likely deficient in this child?

   (A) Branched chain ketoacid dehydrogenase

   (B) Cystathionine synthase

   (C) Methylmalonyl CoA mutase

   (D) Ornithine transcarbamoylase

   (E) Propionyl CoA carboxylase

14. A 2-month-old boy is evaluated for failure to thrive. As the pediatrician is examining the patient, she witnesses a seizure. Physical examination is remarkable for hepatomegaly, a finding later confirmed by CT scan, which also reveals renomegaly. Serum chemistries demonstrate severe hypoglycemia, hyperlipidemia, and lactic acidosis. Which of the following enzyme deficiencies best accounts for this clinical presentation?

   (A) Glucocerebrosidase

   (B) Glycogen phosphorylase

   (C) Sphingomyelinase

   (D) α-1,4-Glucosidase (acid maltase)

   (E) Glucose 6-phosphatase

15. A 52-year-old woman is diagnosed with breast cancer. After discussing treatment options with her oncologist, she decides to turn to the Internet for advice. In a cancer survival chat room, she learns about laetrile, which is metabolized to cyanide. She begins taking laetrile, against medical advice, and develops progressive neuromuscular weakness of the upper and lower extremities, bilateral ptosis, and hypotension. The toxic effects of this unconventional anticancer agent are probably due to an inhibition of which of the following enzymes?

   (A) 2,3-Bisphosphoglycerate mutase

   (B) Cytochrome oxidase

   (C) Guanylate cyclase

   (D) $Na^+/K^+$-ATPase

   (E) Phosphofructokinase-2

16. A 2-year-old child is brought to the pediatrician because of hematuria. Examination reveals hypertension and an abdominal mass. A tumor is localized to the right kidney, and biopsy reveals a stroma containing smooth and striated muscle, bone, cartilage, and fat, with areas of necrosis. The gene for this disorder has been localized to which of the following chromosomes?

    (A) 5

    (B) 11

    (C) 13

    (D) 17

    (E) 22

17. A jealous husband is concerned that his wife had an affair with her best friend's husband and that he is not the biologic father of their 7-month-old child. Restriction fragment length polymorphism (RFLP) analysis is performed on DNA samples from the two couples and from their two children (each couple has one child). The ethidium bromide-stained agarose gel used to separate the fragments is shown below. Which conclusion can be drawn from these results?

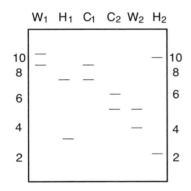

    $W_1$ = wife 1; $H_1$ = husband 1; $C_1$ = child 1
    $W_2$ = wife 2; $H_2$ = husband 2; $C_2$ = child 2

    (A) Husband 1 is the father of both children

    (B) Husband 1 is the father of child 1

    (C) Husband 1 is the father of child 2

    (D) Husband 2 is the father of both children

    (E) Husband 2 is the father of child 1

    (F) Husband 2 is the father of child 2

18. The enzyme hypoxanthine guanine phosphoribosyl transferase (HGPRT) isolated from a child with Lesch-Nyhan syndrome is compared with HGPRT isolated from a healthy control individual. The results are shown in the graph below. Which of the following is the best conclusion about the HGPRT from the child with Lesch-Nyhan disease?

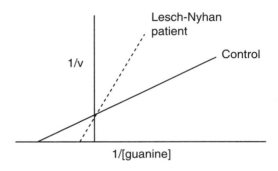

    (A) A competitive inhibitor was added to the enzyme from the Lesch-Nyhan patient.

    (B) The enzyme has a lower affinity for guanine than the control enzyme.

    (C) The gene for HGPRT is repressed in the Lesch-Nyhan patient.

    (D) There is an activating mutation in the HGPRT from the Lesch-Nyhan patient.

    (E) There is more HGPRT in the Lesch-Nyhan cells.

19. A 25-year-old man and his wife go to a fertility clinic for evaluation. His wife has no significant past medical history and is given a "clean bill of health." He has had bronchiectasis and a history of recurrent sinusitis, and was diagnosed with situs inversus as a child. He is found to be sterile. What is the most likely cause of his infertility?

    (A) Abnormal levels of sphingomyelinase

    (B) Abnormal structure of cilia

    (C) Fibrillin deficiency

    (D) 47,XXY karyotype

    (E) Hexosaminidase A deficiency

20. RNA is isolated from the rough endoplasmic reticulum of several tissues, subjected to electrophoresis, blotted, and probed with a $^{32}$P-cDNA. The results from the autoradiogram are shown below. The $^{32}$P-cDNA probe used on the blot most likely is specific for which of the following genes?

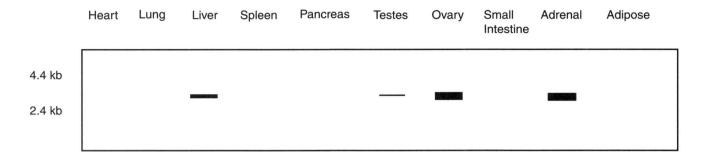

(A) Apoprotein B48

(B) Apoprotein B100

(C) Apoprotein CII

(D) Lipoprotein lipase

(E) Scavenger receptor SR-B1

21. A 57-year-old alcoholic man is brought to the emergency department in a state of global confusion, psychosis, and ataxia. On examination, ophthalmoplegia and polyneuropathy are also noted. Administration of which of the following would be the most appropriate treatment for this patient?

(A) Biotin

(B) Niacin

(C) Pyridoxine

(D) Riboflavin

(E) Thiamine

22. A pathologist is examining microscope slides of a skin biopsy from a patient with malignant melanoma. The pathologist notes in the microscopic description of the report that almost all of the melanoma cells have very large, visible nucleoli. This finding specifically suggests that these cells are making large amounts of which of the following?

(A) Cell surface markers

(B) Golgi apparatus

(C) Immunoglobulins

(D) New DNA

(E) Ribosomes

23. A 57-year-old sales representative for a biotechnology firm has a history of alcohol abuse and hyperuricemia. He attends an out-of-town conference and gorges himself on appetizers, including liver pâté, caviar, and sweetbreads before dinner. Early the following morning he develops a painful swelling in his big toe. In addition to the alcohol consumed with his meals, which other component may have contributed to this episode?

(A) Carbohydrate

(B) Cholesterol

(C) Nucleic acid

(D) Protein

(E) Triglyceride

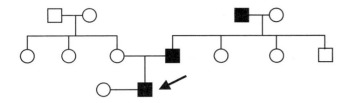

24. The condition shown in the family above is known to have a prevalence of 1/40,000 in the general population. Assuming the most likely interpretation of the pedigree shown, what is the probability that the proband's first daughter will be affected?

    (A) 1/40,000

    (B) 1/200

    (C) 1/100

    (D) 1/4

    (E) 1/2

25. A neonate who initially appears healthy develops vomiting, diarrhea, abdominal pain, and hypoglycemia when weaning is attempted. Other features include a generalized metabolic disturbance with lactic acidosis, hyperuricemia, and hyperphosphatemia. Hereditary fructose intolerance is confirmed with an IV fructose tolerance test, and strict dietary restriction of fructose is ordered to prevent the long-term complications of the condition. In addition to fructose, dietary intake of which of the following substances should also be restricted?

    (A) Galactitol

    (B) Galactose

    (C) Glucose

    (D) Lactose

    (E) Sucrose

26. A 10-year-old girl is admitted to the hospital because of a recurrent neurologic disorder. Her right arm and leg have become limp, and she is found to have lactic acidosis. Two months earlier, the girl had a grand mal seizure followed by cortical blindness with slow resolution. Muscle biopsy revealed ragged red muscle fibers and abnormal mitochondria. Which of the following pedigrees is most likely related to her disease?

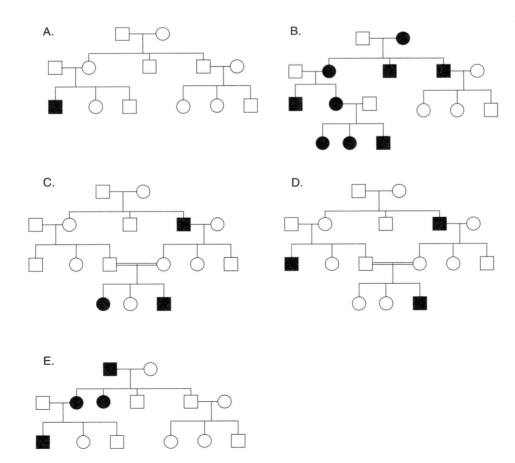

27. In the citric acid cycle, succinate thiokinase (succinyl-CoA synthetase) catalyzes the cleavage of the succinyl-CoA thioester bond with formation of a high-energy compound. This compound can then be used by the body in which of the following biochemical pathways?

    (A) Cysteine degradation
    (B) Elongation of the polypeptide chain
    (C) Epinephrine synthesis from tyrosine
    (D) Isopentyl pyrophosphate synthesis
    (E) Oxidative phosphorylation

28. A 5-year-old boy with growth retardation and mild mental retardation has an enlarged thyroid. His serum thyroid-stimulating hormone (TSH) level is 4.3 mU/L (normal: 0.1-4.0 mU/L), and his serum thyroglobulin level is <15 pmol/L (normal: 15-50 pmol/L). A biopsy of the thyroid stained with antithyroglobulin antibodies reveals accumulation of thyroglobulin in the rough endoplasmic reticulum. Which of the following underlying defects is most likely in this boy?

    (A) A TSH receptor defect
    (B) Failure to phosphorylate mannose attached to thyroglobulin
    (C) Loss of function mutation in the DNA encoding the hydrophobic signal sequence on thyroglobulin
    (D) Loss of function mutation in the ubiquitin gene
    (E) Thyroglobulin monomer misfolding and failure of subunit assembly

29. A 72-year-old man presents to the hospital with a several week history of fatigue. Physical examination is remarkable for severe pallor. Neurologic examination reveals poor short-term memory and decreased vibration sense in his legs. An ECG shows changes consistent with the presence of cardiac ischemia. The hemoglobin level is 4.1 g/dL, with a mean corpuscular volume of 105 $\mu m^3$, a white-cell count of 3100 per $mm^3$, and a platelet count of 55,000 per $mm^3$. The peripheral blood smear shows hypersegmentation of neutrophils, marked anisocytosis, poikilocytosis with some large oval erythrocytes, and basophilic stippling. Which of the following metabolic responses is most specific for the vitamin deficiency affecting this patient?

    (A) Decreased blood δ-aminolevulinic acid (ALA)
    (B) Decreased transketolase activity in erythrocytes
    (C) Decreased urinary homocysteine
    (D) Increased urinary methylmalonate (MMA)
    (E) Lactic acidosis

30. A 22-year-old woman with anorexia nervosa is seen in a specialty clinic that deals with eating disorders. A nutritional nurse estimates the content of the woman's regular diet. She is consuming about 125 g carbohydrate, 15 g protein, and 10 g fat daily. Her daily caloric intake is roughly equal to which of the following values?

    (A) 450 kcal/day
    (B) 650 kcal/day
    (C) 850 kcal/day
    (D) 1050 kcal/day
    (E) 1250 kcal/day

31. A scientist exposes a culture of a bacterium with minimal nutritional requirements to a chemical mutagen, then streaks out the bacteria on plates filled with a complex medium supplemented with all necessary nutrients. When the bacteria begin growing, she isolates individual colonies and tests each one for the ability to grow on a minimal medium. Cells derived from colonies unable to grow on a minimal medium are considered mutants, and their genome is sequenced. In one case, she finds that a two-nucleotide segment of DNA has been deleted. This event would most likely give rise to a

    (A) conservative mutation

    (B) frameshift mutation

    (C) missense mutation

    (D) nonsense mutation

    (E) silent mutation

32. An 8-year-old girl with a history of progressive hepatosplenomegaly and epistaxis was admitted to the hospital with severe pain in her right thigh of 3 days' duration. A similar episode occurred 5 months earlier. There is no family history of these symptoms, and her two siblings are unaffected. A CT scan reveals flaring of the right distal femur. Results of a neurologic examination are normal. A bone marrow biopsy demonstrates the cells characteristic of her disease (shown below). What is the material accumulating abnormally in these cells most likely to be?

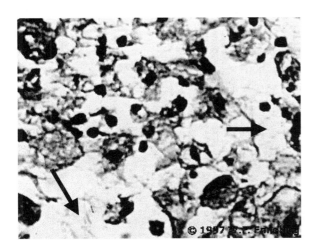

    (A) Cholesterol esters

    (B) Dermatan sulfate

    (C) Fatty acyl carnitines

    (D) Glucocerebroside

    (E) Sphingomyelin

33. A female infant (46,XX) with ambiguous genitalia and hyperkalemia is diagnosed with 21-hydroxylase deficiency. The adrenal hormones that cannot be synthesized in this patient normally bind to receptors with which of the following characteristics?

    (A) Guanylate cyclase activity

    (B) Helix-loop-helix motif with dyad symmetry

    (C) Seven transmembrane helices

    (D) Tyrosine kinase activity

    (E) Zinc finger motif

34. An 83-year-old man is brought to the physician because of diarrhea and vomiting for the past month. He is unable to give a clear history, but his daughter reports that he has been "quite sad" lately and often seems very confused. His diet consists of dried cereal and maize; he never eats milk or eggs. Physical examination shows sharply demarcated plaques on his hands, feet, and around his neck. Which of the following amino acids can substitute for a portion of the vitamin deficient in this patient?

    (A) Alanine

    (B) Asparagine

    (C) Methionine

    (D) Proline

    (E) Tryptophan

35. Examination of a late aborted fetus reveals a small head, small eyes, prominent cleft lip and palate, six fingers on each hand, and dextrocardia. The developmental abnormalities noted in this fetus were probably due to

    (A) 5p-

    (B) 45, XO

    (C) trisomy 13

    (D) trisomy 18

    (E) trisomy 21

36. A patient has a past medical history significant for multiple infections involving the lungs, liver, and bones, as well as excessive inflammation with granulomas, gingivitis, aphthous ulcers, and seborrheic dermatitis. This patient most likely has a deficiency of which of the following enzymes?

    (A) Muscle glycogen phosphorylase

    (B) Myeloperoxidase

    (C) NADPH oxidase

    (D) Transketolase

    (E) Xanthine oxidase

37. A 50-year-old man was admitted into the hospital of a leading research university with a diagnosis of hepatitis and early cirrhosis of the liver. His past medical history is significant for heavy smoking and only occasional consumption of alcohol. He did not use any drugs, and he had no viral infections. DNA studies showed that he was homozygous for the Z allele of $\alpha_1$-antitrypsin, produced by a missense mutation that prevents the proper folding of the protein. A liver biopsy would most likely show accumulation of a proteinaceous substance in which of the following subcellular sites?

    (A) Endoplasmic reticulum

    (B) Extracellular matrix

    (C) Golgi apparatus

    (D) Inclusion bodies

    (E) Lysosomes

38. A 20-year-old develops weakness accompanied by difficulty in relaxation that is most pronounced in the hands and feet. Muscle biopsy demonstrates prominent ring fibers, centrally located nuclei, chains of nuclei, and disorganized sarcoplasmic masses. This condition has been associated with a mutation on which of the following chromosomes?

    (A) X

    (B) Y

    (C) 4

    (D) 5

    (E) 19

39. A woman whose brother has cystic fibrosis seeks genetic counseling. She is told that she, her brother, and other family members can be tested for the common mutations known to cause this disease. DNA is obtained from her brother, and the relevant regions of the *CFTR* gene are amplified using a polymerase chain reaction (PCR). The DNA polymerase used in the PCR is highly resistant to which of the following?

    (A) Acid

    (B) Base

    (C) Heat

    (D) High $Na^+$ concentration

    (E) Low $Ca^{2+}$ concentration

40. In a certain population, the frequency of color-blind males is 1 in 100. Assuming that the population is in Hardy-Weinberg equilibrium at this locus, the frequency of color-blind females is approximately

    (A) 0.0001

    (B) 0.0005

    (C) 0.01

    (D) 0.02

    (E) 0.025

41. A young woman is doing intense aerobic exercise. Aerobic glycolysis is being used for the source of energy for the muscle activity. In which of the following forms will the carbons derived from glucose enter the citric acid cycle?

    (A) Acetyl-CoA

    (B) Citrate

    (C) Oxaloacetate

    (D) Pyruvate

    (E) Succinate

42. An X-linked genetic disease affects a cation-transporting P-type ATPase, resulting in accumulation of copper in the intestinal epithelium because of failure to transport it normally into the blood. Infants with this disease have only 10% of normal blood copper levels. Arteriograms show elongation and tortuosity of major arteries. Bladder diverticula and subdural hematomas are also characteristic findings. These symptoms would most likely be caused by decreased activity of which of the following enzymes?

    (A) Cytochrome aa$_3$

    (B) Lysyl oxidase

    (C) Prolyl hydroxylase

    (D) Tyrosinase

    (E) γ-Glutamyl carboxylase

43. An Olympic runner participates in a 100-meter race. During this race, it is estimated that only ½ L oxygen will be consumed by the runner. However, more than 10 L oxygen would be consumed if the metabolism in this interval were entirely aerobic. The majority of ATP generated during this 100-meter race is derived from which of the following?

    (A) ATP stores

    (B) Creatine phosphate

    (C) Gluconeogenesis

    (D) Glycolysis

    (E) Lipolysis

44. A 57-year-old man with type 1 diabetes mellitus has progressive retinopathy. Ophthalmoscopic examination reveals macular edema and retinal thickening with hard exudates of yellow-white lipid deposits. Which of the following contributes to hyperlipidemia in type 1 diabetes, and thus the risk for lipid deposition in the retina?

    (A) Glucose conversion to sorbitol in the lens

    (B) Overactive GLUT-2 in liver

    (C) Overactive GLUT-4 in adipose

    (D) Overactive hormone-sensitive lipase

    (E) Overactive lipoprotein lipase

45. A 34-year old woman presents to her physician complaining of oral ulcers. A careful history reveals that she is a strict vegetarian and does not eat meat, fish, poultry, eggs, or dairy products. She is found to have a severe riboflavin deficiency. The function of which of the following enzymes in the citric acid cycle would be most directly affected by the riboflavin deficiency?

    (A) Aconitase

    (B) Citrate synthase

    (C) Isocitrate dehydrogenase

    (D) Malate dehydrogenase

    (E) Succinate dehydrogenase

46. A 23-year-old, HIV-positive woman is treated with dideoxycytidine as part of her antiviral therapy. This drug works by preventing which of the following?

    (A) Addition of nucleotides to RNA during transcription of proviral cDNA

    (B) Formation of a peptide bond during translation of viral proteins

    (C) Formation of a phosphodiester bond during viral DNA synthesis

    (D) Hydrolysis of a peptide bond during post-translational modification of viral proteins

    (E) Viral RNA processing by nucleases

47. A 35-year-old woman and her husband seek genetic counseling before attempting to conceive. The woman suffers from a particular condition and wants to know the chances that her child will be affected. The pedigree is shown below. Based on the mode of inheritance, this patient most likely suffers from which of the following diseases?

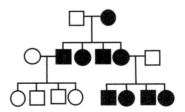

    (A) Glucose-6-phosphate dehydrogenase deficiency

    (B) Leber hereditary optic neuropathy

    (C) Neurofibromatosis

    (D) Sickle cell anemia

    (E) Tay-Sachs disease

48. A mother is informed that her daughter has an inherited disorder in which the administration of a "sugar-free" product that contains aspartame could be detrimental to her health. This patient most likely has which of the following genetic disorders?

    (A) Hyperornithinemia

    (B) Hyperuricemia

    (C) Hypervalinemia

    (D) Phenylketonuria

    (E) Wilson disease

49. A 45-year-old man with a confirmed diagnosis of hemachromatosis tests negative for the two most common mutations in the *HFE* gene known to cause this disease. The patient and several family members, including an affected brother and uncle, are tested for 5 single nucleotide polymorphisms (SNPs) closely linked to the *HFE* gene on chromosome 6. No linkage is found in this family to any of these markers. What is the most likely explanation for these results?

    (A) Heteroplasmy

    (B) Incomplete penetrance

    (C) Locus heterogeneity

    (D) Recombination between the SNPs and the *HFE* gene

    (E) A rare *HFE* allele

50. Concerned parents bring their 3-month-old boy to the physician because of a "white dot" on his left eye that they noticed in pictures. Examination reveals a white pupillary reflex in the left eye. A CT scan of the orbits reveals a tumor in the left eye that does not involve the optic nerve. This condition is associated with an abnormality in which of the following chromosomes?

    (A) 5

    (B) 8

    (C) 13

    (D) 21

    (E) X

# Biochemistry Test Two: **Answers and Explanations**

## ANSWER KEY

| | | | |
|---|---|---|---|
| 1. | C | 26. | B |
| 2. | E | 27. | B |
| 3. | C | 28. | E |
| 4. | D | 29. | D |
| 5. | A | 30. | B |
| 6. | B | 31. | B |
| 7. | B | 32. | D |
| 8. | E | 33. | E |
| 9. | A | 34. | E |
| 10. | E | 35. | C |
| 11. | A | 36. | C |
| 12. | C | 37. | A |
| 13. | A | 38. | E |
| 14. | E | 39. | C |
| 15. | B | 40. | A |
| 16. | B | 41. | A |
| 17. | B | 42. | B |
| 18. | B | 43. | D |
| 19. | B | 44. | D |
| 20. | E | 45. | E |
| 21. | E | 46. | C |
| 22. | E | 47. | B |
| 23. | C | 48. | D |
| 24. | E | 49. | C |
| 25. | E | 50. | C |

1. **The correct answer is C.** A child with ketotic hypoglycemia following a period of fasting most likely has a defect in gluconeogenesis or in a pathway providing substrates for gluconeogenesis. Under fasting conditions, the primary substrate for gluconeogenesis is alanine derived from muscle protein. As muscle proteins are catabolized, the amino acid skeletons are used as fuel in the muscle, while the amino groups are transaminated to pyruvate, forming alanine, which is then transported to the liver and kidney cortex to be used in gluconeogenesis (Cahill cycle). In this child, alanine levels are abnormally low and infusion of alanine rapidly increases blood glucose. These findings rule out a defect in gluconeogenesis and are most consistent with a defect in protein catabolism in muscle.

   Gluconeogenesis (**choice A**) was shown to be intact by the response to alanine infusion.

   Glycogenolysis (**choice B**) is not involved, since liver glycogen stores would have been exhausted by this time. Moreover, defects in glycogenolysis should not produce such a severe hypoglycemia because they would be mitigated by gluconeogenesis and ketone body formation.

   The ketosis indicates that triglyceride hydrolysis in adipose tissue (**choice D**) and β-oxidation of fatty acids (**choice E**) are functional, i.e., acetate is being formed and is being converted to ketones. However, the acetyl-CoA formed cannot contribute to net production of glucose because it cannot be converted to pyruvate.

2. **The correct answer is E.** By convention, a LOD score of 3.00 or higher is required to establish linkage between two loci. This value indicates the odds favoring linkage are 1000 to 1. A LOD score of −2.00 or less is the standard to rule out linkage between two loci, indicating that the odds of linkage are 1 in 100 or less. If, as in this case, the LOD score falls between these two values (−2.00 and 3.00), more data must be obtained and added to the data from this family until the cumulative LOD score goes above 3.00 or below −2.00.

   The highest LOD score in the present data is at a recombination frequency of 0.01 (equivalent to 1 cM or approximately $1 \times 10^6$ base pairs). The LOD score of 1.80 indicates that the odds favoring linkage at this distance are about 67 to 1, suggestive of linkage but not yet conventionally significant. Note that one does not have to calculate the actual odds to deduce this from the table.

   One cannot rule out linkage (**choice A**) based on the data shown either, because none of the values are −2.00 or less.

   There is no significant linkage at any recombination frequency in this table (**choices B, C, and D**) because none of the LOD scores are 3.00 or greater.

3. **The correct answer is C.** Both pyruvate kinase deficiency and glucose-6-phosphate dehydrogenase deficiency are red cell enzyme deficiencies characterized clinically by long "normal" periods interspersed with episodes of hemolytic anemia triggered by infections and oxidant drug injury (antimalarial drugs, sulfonamides, nitrofurans). In both of these conditions, the cell morphology between hemolytic episodes is usually normal or close to normal.

   The α (**choice A**) and β (**choice B**) thalassemias, in their major forms, are characterized by persistent severe anemia. In the trait forms, they are characterized by mild anemia.

   Hereditary spherocytosis (**choice D**) is characterized by intermittent hemolysis. Unlike pyruvate kinase deficiency and glucose-6-phosphate dehydrogenase deficiency, however, oxidant drugs are not a specific trigger for hemolysis.

   Iron deficiency anemia (**choice E**) is characterized by chronic anemia with hypochromic, microcytic erythrocytes.

4. **The correct answer is D.** The dsDNA sequence (only one strand is shown in the diagram) to be amplified would be:

   5′ TCCTGAGC---------------AAATGTGT 3′

   3′ AGGACTCG---------------TTTACACA 5′

   The primers must pair with the 3′ sequences of the two strands. The sequence of the left primer would be identical to that of the top strand, TCCTGAGC. The sequence of the right primer would be identical to the bottom strand, written 5′ to 3′: ACACATTT.

   **Choices A, C, and E** all represent primer pairs that would bind to only one of the 3′ flanking regions (**choices C and E**) or neither of them (**choice A**).

   **Choice B** represents primers that would bind to the 5′ flanking sequences. In that case, DNA synthesis during the amplification step would proceed away from the desired sequence.

5. **The correct answer is A.** This question is based on a real case. Although it is hard to develop a deficiency in oil-soluble vitamins (A, D, E, K) because the liver stores these substances, deficiency states can be seen in chronic malnutrition (specifically chronic fat deprivation) and chronic malabsorption. Vitamin A is necessary for formation of retinal pigments (deficiency can cause night blindness) and for appropriate differentiation of epithelial tissues (including hair follicles, mucous membranes, skin, bone, and adrenal cortex).

Vitamin C (**choice B**), which is water soluble rather than oil soluble, is necessary for collagen synthesis.

Vitamin D (**choice C**) is important in calcium absorption and metabolism.

Vitamin E (**choice D**) is a lipid antioxidant that is important in the stabilization of cell membranes.

Vitamin K (**choice E**) is necessary for normal blood coagulation.

6.   **The correct answer is B.** Conversion of glucose-6-phosphate to 6-phosphogluconate begins the hexose monophosphate shunt, a pathway that increases the $[NADPH]/[NADP^+]$. The reaction shown is catalyzed by glucose-6-phosphate dehydrogenase, an enzyme inhibited by NADPH.

Conversion of glucose-6-phosphate to fructose-6-phosphate (**choice A**) leads into glycolysis. This pathway serves several functions but is not controlled by the $[NADPH]/[NADP^+]$. Glycolysis increases NADH and ATP levels.

Hydrolysis of glucose-6-phosphate to glucose (**choice C**) is an important reaction in hepatocytes for releasing glucose into the peripheral circulation. The enzyme glucose-6-phosphatase that catalyzes this reaction is associated with the endoplasmic reticulum in hepatocytes but is not found in brain or muscle. NADPH levels do not influence its activity.

Conversion of glucose-6-phosphate to UDP-galactose (**choice D**) occurs in breast tissue during lactation as part of lactose production.

Conversion of glucose-6-phosphate to UDP-glucuronate (**choice E**) occurs in hepatocytes for conjugation with bilirubin, some steroids, and a variety of drugs. Conjugation renders the structures more water soluble for excretion by the kidneys (drugs, steroids) or secretion into the bile (bilirubin).

7.   **The correct answer is B.** This question requires you to know that proteins destined for the cytosol and several organelles are synthesized on "free" ribosomes, while those destined to be secreted are synthesized on the ribosomes associated with the RER. Of the choices offered, only coagulation factor VIII is secreted; the remainder are cytosolic or mitochondrial proteins. Proteins destined to be secreted are directed to the RER by an $NH_2$-terminal leader sequence signal. A signal recognition particle (SRP) recognizes this leader sequence as it leaves the 5′ end of the mRNA. This SRP then binds to both the ribosome and the leading signal peptide and thereby interrupts the translation process. During this period of translation arrest, the SRP binds to an SRP receptor, a protein integral to the endoplasmic

reticulum (ER) membrane. This "docking" event allows translation to continue, and now as the protein is synthesized, the hydrophobic leading signaling peptide is "threaded" through the ER membrane. As the protein continues to be synthesized on the RER, it follows the leading peptide and is itself threaded through the membrane. As it pokes through the membrane into the ER lumen, the leading hydrophobic signal sequence is removed and, unless destined for the RER itself, the protein continues its trip and enters the Golgi apparatus. Its final destination is determined in the Golgi apparatus as follows:

| **Destination** | **Addition** |
| --- | --- |
| Lysosomes | Mannose 6-phosphate |
| Cell surface and exocytosis via a constitutive secretory vesicle | No addition |

Similarly, proteins that are synthesized on free ribosomes and are not destined to remain in the cytosol are also provided with signaling sequences that direct them to their proper destination.

Acetyl CoA carboxylase (**choice A**) is a cytosolic enzyme.

Cytochrome oxidase (**choice C**) is a mitochondrial enzyme.

Myosin (**choice D**) is a cytosolic protein.

Phosphofructokinase (**choice E**) is a cytosolic enzyme.

8.   **The correct answer is E.** The woman is having an exercise-induced hypoglycemic episode. Exercise stimulates the uptake of glucose from the blood, thus lowering blood glucose levels. The normal response to this is to decrease blood insulin levels and increase glucagon levels, thereby stimulating glycogenolysis and restoring blood glucose. However, this person has type 1 diabetes mellitus and her insulin levels are determined largely by injection. Therefore, the insulin/glucagon ratio remained high, glycogenolysis could not be stimulated, and hypoglycemia resulted. It is time for her to ingest glucose in some readily absorbed form that should be carried by all type 1 diabetics.

This question requires you to associate translocation of GLUT4 with increased glucose uptake by muscle. Because glucose is a water-soluble molecule and cell membranes are lipid bilayers, specific transport proteins are required to get glucose into cells. This family of transporters is called GLUT, and there are five members, plus a sodium-dependent glucose transporter (SGLT1). Their properties are summarized in the following table.

| Transporter | Location | Characteristics | Function |
|---|---|---|---|
| GLUT1 | Brain, red cells, kidney, placenta, colon | Facilitative, bidirectional Insulin-independent | Uptake of glucose |
| GLUT2 | Liver, pancreatic β cells Small intestine, kidney | Facilitative, bidirectional Insulin-independent | Rapid uptake and release of glucose Glucose sensor in pancreatic β cells |
| GLUT3 | Brain, kidney, placenta | Facilitative, bidirectional Insulin-independent | Uptake of glucose |
| GLUT4 | Cardiac and skeletal muscle, adipocytes | Facilitative, bidirectional **Insulin-dependent in adipose and muscle** **Exercise (AMP)–dependent in skeletal muscle** | Uptake of glucose by muscle and by adipocytes when glucose and insulin levels are high Uptake of glucose in skeletal muscle during exercise |
| GLUT5 | Small intestine | Facilitative, bidirectional Insulin-independent | Lowers Km for fructose but also transports glucose |
| SGLT1 | Small intestine and kidney | Na$^+$ cotransport system driven by the Na/K ATPase Only one that works against a concentration gradient | Uptake of glucose from the intestinal lumen and in the kidney proximal tubule |

During fasting, much of the GLUT4 in skeletal muscle and adipose resides in the membranes of cytoplasmic vesicles. Increased insulin following a meal induces the translocation of these vesicles to the cell membrane, thus increasing glucose uptake (and lowering the peripheral blood glucose). In skeletal muscle, GLUT4 translocation is also stimulated by increased AMP associated with exercising muscle. This AMP-stimulated increase in GLUT4 and glucose uptake is independent of insulin. In this patient, the insulin dose has been adequate to maintain glycemic control. When she began the new exercise program, the additional AMP-stimulated glucose uptake was sufficient to cause hypoglycemia and the symptoms described. If the woman continues this exercise program, her physician should consider lowering the amount of insulin she takes.

Inadequate delivery of oxygen to the muscle (**choice A**) would produce different symptoms, such as pain and/or cramping.

Stimulation of gluconeogenesis in the liver (**choice B**) would increase blood glucose levels. However, gluconeogenesis would not be relevant even in a normal individual who had eaten recently (as long as hepatic glycogen levels were adequate).

Stimulation of glycogenolysis in liver (**choice C**) would increase blood glucose levels.

Stimulation of glycogenolysis in muscle (**choice D**) would occur in response to the lowering of intracellular glucose levels due to the exercise, but to the extent it maintained glucose levels near normal, this would prevent, not induce, symptoms of hypoglycemia.

9. **The correct answer is A.** Abetalipoproteinemia is a rare autosomal recessive disorder characterized by very low levels of serum cholesterol and triglyceride and the absence of ApoB-containing lipoproteins (chylomicrons, VLDL, and LDL). ApoB48 (chylomicrons) and apoB100 (VLDL and LDL) are encoded by the same gene. Absence of chylomicron formation produces a deficiency of essential fatty acids (linolenic and linoleic acids) and the fat-soluble vitamins. Symptoms include malabsorption, spinocerebellar dysfunction, retinopathy that causes impaired night and color vision, and acanthocytosis (thorny-appearing red cells).

Deficiency of the apoB100 receptor (**choice B**) results in hypercholesterolemia associated with high levels of LDL cholesterol. Although the value of LDL cholesterol is not given directly in the laboratory data, one can deduce by comparing the total serum cholesterol and the HDL cholesterol that the LDL cholesterol is extremely low, not high. Symptoms of LDL-receptor deficiency include xanthomas, xanthemias, corneal arcus, and a high risk for coronary artery disease.

Deficiency of apoC2 (**choice C**) produces hypertriglyc-eridemia because apoC2 is an activator of lipoprotein lipase. This enzyme is required for metabolism of VLDL and chylomicrons in the capillaries of adipose and muscle. Symptoms include pancreatitis, pain after a fatty meal, and xanthomas.

Mutations in the apoE gene (**choice D**) create a variety of alleles ($\epsilon2$, $\epsilon3$ $\epsilon4$), and each allele is associated with different clinical phenotypes. In the United States, the most common allele (allele frequency averages 75%) is $\epsilon3$, and the most common genotype is $\epsilon3/\epsilon3$. It is not associated with clinical abnormalities and is considered normal. Individuals with the $\epsilon2/\epsilon2$ genotype may be clinically normal or may have higher than normal levels of chylomicron and VLDL remnants. Those clinically affected have high triglyceride and cholesterol levels, although the cholesterol is mainly associated with VLDL and IDL rather than with LDL. Xanthomas are charac-teristic of cholesterol deposits (tuberous xanthomas on elbows, around tendons, xanthelasmas, and occasional-ly, corneal arcus). Although these deposits are also symptoms of an LDL-receptor deficiency, there are two characteristics that distinguish them. In the $\epsilon2/\epsilon2$, LDL cholesterol is normal or often below normal, and xan-thomas in the palmar creases are often seen.

The $\epsilon4/\epsilon4$ genotype is associated with high total choles-terol and an increased risk of coronary artery disease. It may also be seen with higher frequency in Alzheimer patients, although the relation to underlying pathology, if any, is unclear.

LCAT (**choice E**) is a plasma enzyme that catalyzes for-mation of plasma lipoprotein cholesterol esters (a cholesterol ester is cholesterol with a fatty acid attached). The classic triad of symptoms includes corneal opacities due to diffuse lipid deposition, renal failure with proteinuria, and anemia often character-ized by target cells. Foam cells are found in the glomerular tufts of the kidney and in bone marrow. They may also accumulate in the intimal lining of blood vessels but, surprisingly, there is often no increased incidence of atherosclerosis or coronary artery disease.

10. **The correct answer is E.** The human body is able to synthesize roughly half the amino acids necessary to build protein. These amino acids, termed nonessential, include alanine, arginine, asparagine, aspartate, cys-teine, glutamate, glutamine, glycine, proline, serine, and tyrosine. The amino acids that must be supplied in the diet are termed essential; these include histidine, isoleucine, leucine, lysine, methionine, phenylalanine, threonine, tryptophan, and valine. Phenylalanine undergoes hydroxylation to tyrosine, catalyzed by the enzyme phenylalanine hydroxylase. It is noteworthy that tyrosine becomes an essential amino acid in indi-viduals lacking this enzyme. The hyperphenylalanine-mias, which include phenylketonuria, result from impaired conversion of phenylalanine to tyrosine, and are also associated with mental retardation. This con-dition is associated with increased phenylalanine in blood and increased phenylalanine and its by-products (e.g., phenylpyruvate, phenylacetate, and phenyllac-tate) in urine.

Asparagine (**choice A**) is a member of the "oxaloacetate family"; its immediate precursor is aspartate.

The immediate precursor of cysteine (**choice B**) is ser-ine. Serine is also the precursor of the nonessential amino acid glycine.

Glutamine (**choice C**), proline (**choice D**), and arginine are produced from glutamate. The synthesis of glutamate occurs by the reductive amination of alpha-ketoglutarate.

11. **The correct answer is A.** This pattern shows only one fragment 12 kb long corresponding to the methylated 15q11-13. The majority of Prader-Willi cases are caused by an inherited deletion in 15q11-13 from the paternal chromosome. Because this region on the maternally inherited 15q is imprinted and inactivated by methyla-tion, loss from the paternal 15q deletes the only active copy the child would inherit. Symptoms include (at birth) low birth weight and hypotonia, and, in the first years, hyperphagia, obesity, developmental delay, some-what lower IQ, behavioral problems, and hypogonadism.

The normal control and both parents have two fragments in their patterns. The 12-kb fragment corresponds to the methylated (therefore inactive and imprinted) 15q. The short fragment corresponds to the unmethylated (active) fragment cut from the other 15q. **Choice B** shows only one shorter fragment corresponding to the unmethylated (active) sequence. **Choice C** shows the expected pattern from a normal individual.

**Choice D** shows two fragments that are methylated. This is the pattern one might expect in a case of Prader-Willi caused by maternal uniparental disomy of chromosome 15.

**Choice E** shows two fragments that are unmethylated. This would correspond to paternal uniparental disomy of chromosome 15 and would not be associated with Prader-Willi.

12. **The correct answer is C.** The conversion of homo cysteine to methionine is catalyzed by homocysteine methyltransferase. An essential cofactor is the methylated form of vitamin $B_{12}$ (methylcobalamin); the methyl group is obtained from $N^5$-methylenetetrahydrofolate.

Thus, a deficiency of either vitamin increases the homocysteine concentration in the blood. Several different inborn errors of metabolism affecting this reaction cause homocystinuria, characterized by a marked increase in homocysteine levels. However, recent clinical studies have shown that a modest increase in homocysteine levels in "normal" individuals is a significant risk factor for cardiovascular disease and deep vein thrombosis. Moreover, these increased levels can be lowered by appropriate vitamin therapy.

Dihydrofolate reductase (**choice A**) is required to convert the folate to its active form, but it is not as closely related to the role of folate in lowering the risk of cardiovascular disease as is the cofactor for homocysteine methyltransferase.

Glycinamide ribonucleotide transformylase (**choice B**) catalyzes the transfer of a formyl group from $N^{10}$-formyltetrahydrofolate to the amino group of glycinamide ribonucleotide. Although it requires folate, it has no known role in lowering the risk of cardiovascular disease.

Ribonucleotide reductase (**choice D**) catalyzes the reduction of nucleoside diphosphates to their deoxy forms. Neither vitamin influences its activity, nor is its activity linked to cardiovascular disease

Thymidylate synthase (**choice E**) converts dUMP to dTMP. Although folate is required for its activity, it is not related to the role of folate in lowering the risk of cardiovascular disease.

13. **The correct answer is A.** Valine, leucine, and isoleucine are the branched chain amino acids. Deficiency of the branched chain ketoacid dehydrogenase causes maple syrup urine disease, in which branched chain ketoacids build up in blood, urine, and tissues. The urine has the odor of maple syrup and a metabolic acidosis is produced. Early diagnosis is essential to limit an irreversible mental retardation. Treatment consists of a special diet with limited amounts of these amino acids. If untreated, death occurs within a year.

Cystathionine synthase (**choice B**) converts homocysteine to cystathionine. A deficiency of this enzyme causes a form of homocystinuria (homocystinuria I).

Methylmalonyl CoA mutase (**choice C**) catalyzes a vitamin $B_{12}$–requiring step in the conversion of propionate from the amino acids threonine, valine, isoleucine, and methionine, and from odd numbered fatty acids to succinyl-CoA. Note that these are not the same set of amino acids involved in maple syrup urine disease, although the symptoms of the condition are somewhat similar. Deficiency of the methylmalonyl CoA mutase results most commonly in neonatal ketosis and metabolic acidosis with lethargy, vomiting, diarrhea, muscle hypotonia, and if not treated, coma and death. Some cases can be treated by restricting protein and supplementing with extra cobalamin.

Ornithine transcarbamoylase deficiency (**choice D**) is a urea cycle enzyme deficiency disease associated with hyperammonemia.

Propionyl CoA carboxylase (**choice E**) catalyzes a reaction analogous to that of acetyl-CoA carboxylase. Both form a malonyl derivative and require biotin as a cofactor. The carboxylation is a step in the conversion of propionate and odd numbered fatty acids to succinyl-CoA.

14. **The correct answer is E.** Von Gierke disease is a glycogen storage disease caused by a deficiency of glucose-6-phosphatase. It typically presents with neonatal hypoglycemia, hyperlipidemia, and lactic acidosis. Failure to thrive is common in early life; convulsions may occur because of profound hypoglycemia. The glycogen accumulation in von Gierke disease occurs primarily in the liver and kidneys, accounting for the enlargement of these organs. Gout may develop later because of the derangement of glucose metabolism.

Even if you do not remember all of the details of the presentation of these genetic diseases, you should be able to narrow the choices:

Glucocerebrosidase deficiency (Gaucher disease; **choice A**) and sphingomyelinase deficiency (Niemann-Pick disease; **choice C**) are lipid storage diseases and would not be expected to produce hypoglycemia.

The other diseases are glycogen storage diseases, but McArdle (**choice B**) and Pompe (**choice D**) diseases affect muscle, rather than liver, and would not be expected to produce profound hypoglycemia, since the liver is the major source for blood glucose. In McArdle disease, glycogen phosphorylase is deficient, and in Pompe disease, $\alpha$-1, 4-glucosidase (acid maltase) is deficient.

15. **The correct answer is B.** The byproduct cyanide strongly inhibits cytochrome oxidase (complex IV of the electron transport chain), causing loss of all ATP production associated with oxidative phosphorylation. Therefore, in a manner similar to the effects of hypoxia, cyanide poisoning causes rapid cell death. Highly aerobic tissues (nerves, muscle) are affected first.

2,3-Bisphosphoglycerate mutase (**choice A**) catalyzes the formation of 2,3-bisphosphoglycerate from 1,3-bisphosphoglycerate and is not inhibited by cyanide. 2,3-Bisphosphoglycerate is found in all cells in small quantities and is found in high concentrations in red cells.

Guanylate cyclase (**choice C**) catalyzes the formation of cGMP from GTP and is not inhibited by cyanide.

$Na^+/K^+$-ATPase (**choice D**) is coupled to the transport of various substances across cell membranes and accounts for the majority of the basal metabolic energy (BMR) utilization. It is not inhibited by cyanide.

Phosphofructokinase-2 (**choice E**) catalyzes the formation of fructose 2,6-bisphosphate from ATP and fructose 6-phosphate and is not inhibited by cyanide.

16. **The correct answer is B.** This is a two-step question. You first need to make the diagnosis, and you then need to recall the localization of this particular disease to a specific chromosome. In this case, everything in the vignette leads you to a diagnosis of Wilms tumor. Wilms tumor occurs in children and typically presents with an abdominal mass, as well as with hypertension, hematuria, nausea, and intestinal obstruction. Because the tumor is derived from mesonephric mesoderm, it can include mesodermal derivatives such as bone, cartilage, and muscle. The Wilms tumor suppressor gene (WT-1) has been localized to chromosome 11 (11p).

The remaining answer choices provide us the opportunity to discuss some other known relationships between genes and disease. This is a topic of intense research that is likely to be increasingly emphasized on the USMLE examinations.

Chromosome 5 (**choice A**) is the site of the tumor suppressor gene APC, which is involved in the pathogenesis of colon cancer and familial adenomatous polyposis.

Chromosome 13 (**choice C**) is the site of the tumor suppressor gene for retinoblastoma and osteosarcoma (Rb), as well as the BRCA-2 gene for breast cancer.

Chromosome 17 (**choice D**) is the site of p53 (involved in most human cancers), NF-1 (neurofibromatosis type I), and BRCA-1 (breast and ovarian cancer).

Chromosome 22 (**choice E**) is home to the NF-2 gene, which is involved in neurofibromatosis type II.

17. **The correct answer is B.** Restriction length fragment polymorphism (RFLP) is a powerful tool that is used to compare DNA samples from several different sources. This technique has been used to convict or acquit criminals and has utility in the determination of paternity. Basically, total DNA is extracted (usually from a blood sample) and then digested with restriction enzymes. Restriction enzymes cut DNA at specific points (often palindromic sequences) called restriction sites. Differences in the DNA between two individuals will, with a very high probability, produce differences in the number and position of restriction sites, and so will produce differences in the length of the fragments made by digestion with restriction enzymes. The digested samples are then subjected to electrophoresis, and the fragments separated according to size. In the pattern shown, child 1 has a fragment approximately 7 kilobases (kb) in length that matches a similar fragment in the DNA of husband 1, verifying that he is the biologic father. No 7-kb fragment is found in husband 2, implying that he could not be the father. Interestingly, child 2 shows a 6-kb fragment that neither wife 2 nor husband 2 (nor husband 1) exhibit. An unexpected conclusion of this RFLP is that child 2 may not be the child of husband 2.

18. **The correct answer is B.** The graph shows that the patient's HGPRT has a higher $K_m$ value than the HGPRT from the control cells; a higher $K_m$ value means a lower affinity.

Although the resultant pattern would look like competitive inhibition (**choice A**), it would be a comparison between two different enzymes, not one enzyme with and without an inhibitor as described.

Since the $V_{max}$ is the same, there is no evidence that there is less HGPRT (i.e., repression of the HGPRT gene; **choice C**) in the child's cells.

If a mutation activated the Lesch-Nyhan enzyme (**choice D**), either the $V_{max}$ value would be higher or the $K_m$ value lower. Neither is true.

Since the $V_{max}$ is the same, there is no evidence that there is more HGPRT in the Lesch-Nyhan child's cells (**choice E**).

19. **The correct answer is B.** Kartagener syndrome, an autosomal recessive disorder characterized by bronchiectasis, sinusitis, and situs inversus, is classified as an "immotile cilia syndrome." It is associated with the absence of inner or outer dynein arms in the cilia. This leads to abnormal ciliary mobility of the sperm, producing infertility. Ciliary abnormalities in the respiratory tract lead to sinusitis and bronchiectasis.

Sphingomyelinase deficiency (**choice A**) occurs in Niemann-Pick disease (autosomal recessive transmission). Sphingomyelin accumulates in the phagocytes. "Foamy histiocytes" appear in the liver, spleen, lymph nodes, and skin. Clinical manifestations include hepatosplenomegaly and, in some cases, neurologic deterioration. Patients usually do not survive beyond 3 years of age.

Fibrillin deficiency (**choice C**) occurs in Marfan syndrome (autosomal dominant). Patients are characteristically tall and thin, and their fingers are spider-like (arachnodactyly). Anatomic abnormalities include ectopia lentis (displaced lens of the eye) and aortic dilatation predisposing to aortic aneurysm.

**KAPLAN**) MEDICAL

47,XXY karyotype (**choice D**), also known as Klinefelter syndrome, is characterized by male hypogonadism. It can cause male infertility, but nothing else in the question suggests this is the case. One would expect to see atrophic testes, tall stature, and gynecomastia. Mental retardation is sometimes present.

Hexosaminidase A deficiency (**choice E**) causes Tay-Sachs disease (autosomal recessive), which occurs most commonly in Ashkenazi Jews. The disease causes CNS degeneration and blindness, and patients exhibit motor and mental deterioration (e.g., loss of developmental milestones). A classic clue is a macular "cherry-red spot" on ophthalmoscopic examination. Patients usually do not survive beyond 3 years of age.

20. **The correct answer is E.** The Northern blot identifies a gene expressed in liver, adrenal, ovaries, and testes, but not in the other tissues tested. Liver and steroidogenic tissues have a scavenger receptor SR-B1 that recognizes HDL and mediates transfer of cholesterol into these tissues.

Apoprotein B48 (**choice A**), apoprotein B100 (**choice B**), and apoprotein CII (**choice C**), are synthesized primarily in liver and intestine.

Lipoprotein lipase (**choice D**) RNA should be seen primarily in adipose and muscle tissue.

21. **The correct answer is E.** The patient is presenting with the signs and symptoms of Wernicke encephalopathy, which consists of the classic triad of ophthalmoplegia, ataxia, and global confusion. This syndrome is considered a medical emergency and necessitates immediate administration of thiamine, or vitamin $B_1$.

Biotin (**choice A**) acts as a carrier of "activated carboxyl" groups for three key enzymes that catalyze carboxylation reactions. Symptoms of biotin deficiency include alopecia, skin and bowel inflammation, and muscle pain.

Niacin (**choice B**), or vitamin $B_3$, is converted to nicotinamide, which is then incorporated into the coenzymes $NAD^+$ and $NADP^+$. Pellagra, a condition associated with niacin deficiency, leads to diarrhea, dermatitis, and dementia.

Pyridoxine (**choice C**), or vitamin $B_6$, is utilized as the coenzyme pyridoxal phosphate. A deficiency in pyridoxine can lead to peripheral neuropathy and dermatitis.

Riboflavin (**choice D**), or vitamin $B_2$, is responsible for maintaining proper levels of both FMN and FAD. Individuals with riboflavin deficiency are likely to present with lesions of the lips, mouth, skin, and genitalia.

22. **The correct answer is E.** The nucleolus is the site of manufacture of ribosomal RNA with its subsequent packaging into ribosomes. Consequently, very large nucleoli indicate an increased rate of ribosome production, which, in turn, suggests an increased rate of production of proteins. Large nucleoli are seen in many active cancers but can also be prominent in benign conditions characterized by high metabolic rate, such as tissue repair after trauma.

Depending on the cells involved, the increased protein production associated with more ribosomes might produce more cell surface markers (**choice A**), but it is impossible to predict this simply from the presence of a large nucleolus.

You should associate a large Golgi apparatus (**choice B**) with transport of material to the cell surface.

Plasma cells that produce large amounts of immunoglobulins (**choice C**) may have large nucleoli, but more specifically have a very large endoplasmic reticulum and Golgi apparatus.

The nucleolus is not involved with new DNA (**choice D**) synthesis; this is done elsewhere in the nucleus.

23. **The correct answer is C.** Purines from ingested nucleic acids are converted to uric acid by intestinal epithelial cells and released into the blood for potential excretion by the kidney. Foods rich in DNA (caviar) or RNA (liver pâté and sweetbreads [pancreas], derived from organs with active protein synthesis) are particularly rich sources of purines, and their ingestion coupled with excess alcohol consumption presumably increased his plasma urate levels to the point at which uric acid crystallized in a susceptible joint. The resultant painful swelling is gout. The pain is caused by precipitation of uric acid crystals in the joints with attendant inflammation.

Carbohydrate (**choice A**), cholesterol (**choice B**), protein (**choice D**), and triglyceride (**choice E**) by themselves do not contain purines, and their metabolism does not contribute to the uric acid pool. To the extent that protein-rich foods are cellular, they will, however, contain nucleic acids that will be catabolized to uric acid.

24. **The correct answer is E.** The most likely mode of inheritance is autosomal dominant. Male-to-male transmission occurs (autosomal), and all affected individuals have an affected parent. Because the proband is heterozygous (his mother does not carry the disease-producing allele), he has a 1/2 chance of passing the disease to his children irrespective of their sex.

A cursory glance at the pedigree might have suggested X-linked recessive because only males are affected. In an X-recessive, an affected male always passes the disease-producing allele to his daughters. There would be a 1/20,000 chance of the mother being a carrier, and a 1/2 chance of passing that allele to her daughter. Thus, the risk would be 1/40,000 (**choice A**).

If the mode of inheritance had been autosomal recessive and the father homozygous for the disease allele, the chance of his daughter being affected would depend on the probability that his wife also carried the same disease allele. In that case, the carrier prevalence (2q) would have to be calculated from the disease prevalence ($q^2$) given in the stem (1/40,000). Calculated in this way, the mother would have a 1/100 chance of being a carrier and then a 1/2 chance of passing along the disease allele. The chance of having an affected daughter would then be 1/200 (**choice B**).

25. **The correct answer is E.** Several forms of genetic abnormalities of fructose can occur. The mildest, virtually asymptomatic, condition is essential (benign) fructosuria, due to a lack of fructokinase, which phosphorylates fructose. In marked contrast, the genetic abnormality of fructose metabolism described in the question stem is hereditary fructose intolerance (fructosemia), the most severe of these conditions. It is due to a deficiency of the enzyme aldolase B, which is found in liver, small intestine, and kidney. Aldolase B normally cleaves fructose-1-phosphate, and the severe abnormalities seen are related to a disastrous depletion of intracellular phosphate, which is needed for making ATP and other phosphorylated compounds. Hereditary fructose intolerance requires very strict dietary control of fructose, which in practice means that not only fructose (fruit sugar) itself must be controlled, but the much more prevalent sucrose (table sugar) must also be controlled, since it is a disaccharide composed of fructose and glucose. The sugar alcohol sorbitol (an artificial sweetener) is also restricted, since this compound can also be converted to fructose.

    Galactitol (**choice A**) is a sugar alcohol related to galactose, which need not be restricted in this condition.

    Galactose (**choice B**) is a monosaccharide that is metabolized normally in this condition. Metabolic disorders associated with galactose metabolism, analogous to those of fructose, occur because of genetic defects in the kinase enzyme (galactokinase deficiency) and a transfer enzyme (galactose-1-phosphate uridyl transferase deficiency).

    Glucose (**choice C**) is metabolized normally in this condition.

    Lactose (**choice D**), a disaccharide composed of galactose and glucose, should be restricted in severe genetic diseases of galactose, as well as in lactose intolerance.

26. **The correct answer is B.** The condition described is MELAS (mitochondrial encephalomyopathy, lactic acidosis, and stroke-like episodes). Ragged red muscle fibers and disrupted mitochondria are seen on muscle biopsy. Two major features characterize mitochondrial patterns of transmission: no inheritance from an affected male, and usually all children of an affected female are affected. However, expression among siblings can vary to a considerable extent because there are so many mitochondria, each with their own set of genes, which are distributed into the eggs in a random fashion.

    The pedigree in **choice A** is most likely a new mutation, but could be a recessive trait that has skipped several generations.

    The pedigree in **choice C** is most likely autosomal recessive.

    The pedigree in **choice D** is most likely X-linked recessive.

    The pedigree in **choice E** is most likely X-linked dominant.

27. **The correct answer is B.** In this question, you need to know that GTP is synthesized when CoASH is cleaved from succinyl-CoA to form succinate in the citric acid cycle. You also need to know that GTP, rather than ATP, is used as the energy source in protein synthesis, specifically in the formation of the activated elongation factor to which tRNA binds, and in the transfer of the elongating chain from the P to the A site in the ribosome.

    Cysteine degradation (**choice A**) requires $O_2$ and produces sulfite and then sulfate, which is secreted in urine.

    Epinephrine synthesis from tyrosine (**choice C**) requires tetrahydrobiopterin, pyridoxal phosphate, oxygen, copper, and S-adenosylmethionine.

    Isopentyl pyrophosphate synthesis from HMG CoA (**choice D**) requires NADPH and ATP, and releases $CO_2$.

    Oxidative phosphorylation (**choice E**) uses NADH, $FADH_2$, coenzyme Q, oxygen, and a variety of cytochromes to produce ATP.

28. **The correct answer is E.** Proper folding and subunit assembly of proteins are required for transport from the rough endoplasmic reticulum (RER) to the Golgi. Proteins that fail to achieve normal tertiary and quaternary structures are retained in the RER.

    A defect in the TSH receptor (**choice A**) would decrease thyroglobulin synthesis, not cause accumulation in the RER.

    Phosphorylation of mannose in the Golgi (**choice B**) would prevent transfer of a protein to lysosomes. Thyroglobulin is not a lysosomal protein, and this modification would not be part of its synthesis.

    Loss of function mutation in the DNA encoding the hydrophobic signal sequence on thyroglobulin (**choice C**) would prevent attachment of the ribosome to the endoplasmic reticulum. Thyroglobulin would not accumulate in the RER, if that were the case in this boy.

Loss of function mutation in the ubiquitin gene (**choice D**) would decrease recognition and therefore digestion of proteins by proteasomes. Although this defect could cause accumulation of defective proteins in RER, it would not be specific to thyroglobulin, as is the case with this boy. **Choice E** is a much more likely explanation.

29. **The correct answer is D.** The combination of neurologic symptoms and megaloblastic anemia is characteristic of a vitamin $B_{12}$ (cyanocobalamin) deficiency, which will also cause an increase in urinary methylmalonate (MMA) due to low activity of methylmalonyl CoA mutase. Megaloblastic anemia is caused by impaired DNA synthesis, which slows cell division, thus decreasing the count for cells with a rapid turnover. In the surviving cells, synthesis of cytoplasmic components proceeds unabated, while cellular division is slowed. Thus, these cells tend to be oversized, misshapen, and have various cytoplasmic inclusions. The direct cause of the decreased rate of DNA synthesis is the unavailability of folate, needed most acutely for conversion of dUMP to dTMP. Therefore, supplementation with folate will cause a rapid reversal of these symptoms. In the case described, there are also symptoms of neuropathy, a characteristic of vitamin $B_{12}$ deficiency not associated with folate deficiency. In addition to causing neuropathy, a vitamin $B_{12}$ deficiency will produce a secondary folate deficiency by preventing the regeneration of tetrahydrofolate.

Cofactors derived from vitamin $B_{12}$ carry out only two functions. One is in the conversion of homocysteine to methionine. $N^5$-methyltetrahydrofolate is a cosubstrate in this reaction and simultaneously loses its methyl moiety and is converted to tetrahydrofolate. $N^5$-methyltetrahydrofolate has no other function, and unless it is converted to a form that can be recycled, it serves as a folate sink, making tetrahydrofolate unavailable for any other reaction. The other reaction requiring a vitamin $B_{12}$ cofactor is catalyzed by methylmalonyl CoA mutase, in which methylmalonyl CoA is converted to succinyl CoA. This is the last step in the breakdown of odd carbon fatty acids, and inhibition of this reaction leads to odd carbon fatty acid accumulation in neuronal sheaths and, as a result, neuropathy.

Decreased blood δ-aminolevulinic acid (ALA; **choice A**) would occur with pyridoxine deficiency.

Decreased transketolase activity in erythrocytes (**choice B**) would occur with thiamine deficiency.

Because both cofactors are required to convert homocysteine to methionine, homocysteine levels would increase (compare with **choice C**) in the urine of either a folate- or vitamin $B_{12}$-deficient person.

Lactic acidosis (**choice E**) would occur in any condition in which lactate accumulates. These could involve many of the reactions in carbohydrate or oxidative metabolism, none of which are relevant to this question.

30. **The correct answer is B.** You may be asked to make this type of calculation on the Step 1 exam. You should know that 1 g of either protein or carbohydrate produces about 4 kcal = 4 calories (kcal) of energy, and 1 g of fat produces 9 kcal = 9 calories of energy. The calculation is then straightforward. The calories from carbohydrates are $125 \times 4 = 500$; from protein are $15 \times 4 = 60$; and from fat are $10 \times 9 = 90$. The total is $500 + 60 + 90 = 650$ kcal/day.

31. **The correct answer is B.** Deletion of two nucleotides will lead to a reading frame shift. The genetic code will be read differently from that point on until the end of the genome, or until another alteration in the DNA (e.g., the addition of two base pairs or the deletion of another base pair) restores the original reading frame. Often, this results in a truncated protein.

A conservative mutation (**choice A**) is a missense mutation (see below) that leads to the substitution of a given amino acid with a chemically similar amino acid. For example, one codon for leucine is CUC. Replacement of the 5′ cytosine with an adenosine produces AUC, which codes for isoleucine.

A missense mutation (**choice C**) is one that leads to the replacement of a given amino acid with a different amino acid.

A nonsense mutation (**choice D**) introduces a stop codon instead of a codon specifying an amino acid, leading to premature chain termination.

A silent mutation (**choice E**) is a mutation to a codon that specifies the same amino acid as the original codon, e.g., if ACU is mutated to ACC, threonine is still the amino acid specified by the code, and the protein is unchanged. Mutations in the third position (the wobble position) are generally the cause of silent mutations because of the degeneracy of the genetic code.

32. **The correct answer is D.** This child has symptoms of type 1 Gaucher disease due to the genetic deficiency (auto-somal recessive) of lysosomal glucocerebrosidase. Children with this condition are generally healthy at birth and for the first few years of life. They develop progressive hepatosplenomegaly with accumulation of glucocerebroside in macrophages. Later, the presence of these macrophages in bone marrow can cause bone infarctions and remodeling. Flaring of the distal femur is common and may be described as having an "Erlenmeyer flask" appearance. There are no neurologic symptoms.

Cholesterol esters (**choice A**) accumulate in macrophages (foamy macrophages) found in plaques of coronary artery disease. They may also accumulate in a variant form of Niemann Pick disease (Niemann Pick type C).

Dermatan sulfate (**choice B**) and heparan sulfate are mucopolysaccharides that accumulate in Hurler (deficiency of lysosomal α-L-iduronidase) and Hunter (deficiency of lysosomal iduronate sulfatase) syndromes. Both are usually severe diseases characterized by corneal clouding, organomegaly, mental retardation, and death in childhood.

Fatty acyl carnitines (**choice C**) accumulate in defects of fatty acid oxidation or carnitine transport. One important disease, medium chain acyl CoA dehydrogenase deficiency (MCAD), is characterized by fasting hypoglycemia and hypoketosis and can range from mild to severe and fatal in affected individuals. MCAD is the most commonly seen defect of β-oxidation.

Sphingomyelin (**choice E**) accumulates in macrophages (foamy macrophages) in the more common forms of Niemann Pick disease, causing hepatosplenomegaly and, frequently, neurologic symptoms but without the characteristic bone involvement of Gaucher disease. Some children with Niemann Pick have cherry red macula and most die in childhood.

33. **The correct answer is E.** Steroid 21-hydroxylase is required for the formation of cortisol and aldosterone. These hormones, like other steroid hormones, bind to intracellular receptors with zinc finger motifs. The hormone receptor complexes bind to DNA, altering the transcription of specific genes.

Guanylate cyclase activity (**choice A**) is associated with the receptor for atrial natriuretic peptide on vascular smooth muscles. The resultant increase in cGMP causes contraction of the smooth muscle and constriction of the arterioles.

Receptors for certain water-soluble hormones, including glucagon and epinephrine, have seven transmembrane helices (**choice C**). Receptors with this motif always transduce signals via trimeric GTP-binding proteins (G proteins) associated with the membrane. In the retina, rhodopsin (the light receptor) also has the seven-transmembrane helix motif.

Tyrosine kinase activity (**choice D**) is characteristic of the insulin receptor and several growth-factor receptors (PDGF-R, EGF-R).

34. **The correct answer is E.** Tryptophan is an aromatic amino acid that contains an indole group. By a very complex series of minor enzymatic reactions, a small amount (~2%) of the tryptophan can be converted to

quinolinate, which can then be used in place of niacin (nicotinic acid) in NAD (nicotinamide adenine dinucleotide) synthesis. Very high tryptophan levels can replace a portion of the dietary requirements for niacin. The nutritional disease pellagra (characterized by swollen tongue, dermatitis, neurologic dysfunction, and gastrointestinal dysfunction) usually occurs in the setting of combined tryptophan and niacin deficiency.

Alanine (**choice A**), the amino acid with a methyl R group, is a substrate of the liver enzyme alanine amino transferase (ALT, formerly called SGPT).

Asparagine (**choice B**) is one of the sources of ammonia for the urea cycle.

Methionine (**choice C**) is a sulfur-containing amino acid that is associated with associate with methyl group transfers.

Proline (**choice D**) is technically an imino acid, rather than an amino acid, with a ring structure. You should remember collagen has high proline concentration.

35. **The correct answer is C.** Chromosomal aberrations are common in spontaneously aborted fetuses. This fetus has Patau syndrome (trisomy 13). A convenient way to remember trisomy 13 is to think of polydactyly remembered as 13 fingers) and midline defects, including microphthalmia (just one central "eye"); cleft lip, palate, or face; arrhinencephaly (failure of development of olfactory nerves and related brain); and dextrocardia or ventricular septal defect. The head is usually small, with profound mental retardation. In fetuses that survive until birth, death usually occurs in the neonatal period. Patau syndrome has an incidence of 1 in 6,000 births.

Features of *cri du chat* syndrome (5p-; **choice A**) include a catlike cry, severe mental retardation, microcephaly, and epicanthal folds.

Features of Turner syndrome (45, XO; **choice B**) include webbed neck, short stature, broad chest, low hairline, primary amenorrhea, coarctation of aorta, and streak ovaries.

Features of Edwards syndrome, or trisomy 18 (**choice D**), include severe mental retardation, ventricular septal defect, micrognathia, rocker-bottom feet, low-set ears, prominent occiput, and hypotonia.

Features of Down syndrome, or trisomy 21 (**choice E**), include mental retardation, flat nasal bridge, epicanthal folds, oblique palpebral fissures, dysplastic ears, horizontal palmar crease, redundant neck skin, short trunk, ventricular septal defect, acute lymphoblastic leukemia, and neurologic changes similar to those of Alzheimer disease.

36. **The correct answer is C.** The patient is presenting with signs and symptoms of chronic granulomatous disease of childhood. Patients with this condition usually present with a past medical history as described in the question stem. This pathologic condition is caused by a defect in the NADPH oxidase complex, resulting in neutrophils and other phagocytic cells that do not produce superoxides. Affected individuals therefore present with an inability to kill invading microbes that are engulfed by these phagocytic cells.

Muscle glycogen phosphorylase (**choice A**) deficiency is seen in patients with McArdle disease. These patients often experience muscle cramps and weakness on exercise.

Myeloperoxidase (**choice B**) deficiency usually is not associated with clinical abnormalities, except in patients with an underlying disease, such as diabetes. These patients may experience an increased frequency of fungal infections.

Transketolase (**choice D**) is an enzyme used to diagnose thiamine deficiency by measuring erythrocyte transketolase activity on addition of thiamine pyrophosphate.

Xanthine oxidase (**choice E**) is an enzyme responsible for the production of uric acid. Deficiency of this enzyme would result in the development of hypouricemia.

37. **The correct answer is A.** The patient has liver disease secondary to homozygosity for the Z allele of $\alpha_1$-antitrypsin. $\alpha_1$-Antitrypsin, more properly $\alpha_1$-antiproteinase, is synthesized and secreted into the blood by the liver and macrophages. It is the principle serine protease of the human plasma, and it inhibits trypsin, elastin, and other proteases. It exists in several isoforms. Proteins such as $\alpha_1$-antitrypsin that are normally secreted must fold properly in the endoplasmic reticulum in order to be transferred to the Golgi apparatus. Sporadic misfolded proteins will be escorted into the cytoplasm for degradation in proteasomes, but if the cell is accumulating large quantities, they accumulate in the endoplasmic reticulum. ZZ individuals produce large amounts of misfolded protein, which accumulates in the cisternae of the endoplasmic reticulum and causes hepatitis and cirrhosis.

Extracellular matrix (**choice B**) could not be a possibility because these misfolded proteins could not get into the Golgi apparatus, which is a necessary step on their way to being excreted.

The misfolded proteins would be unable to proceed to the Golgi apparatus (**choice C**).

"Inclusion bodies" (**choice D**) is a nonspecific term describing aggregate material accumulating in cells.

The lysosomal storage diseases, including I-cell disease itself, result in inclusion bodies of material from endocytosis, phagocytosis, or autophagy that cannot be digested due to a lysosomal enzyme deficiency.

Misfolded proteins would accumulate in the ER, not in lysosomes (**choice E**).

38. **The correct answer is E.** The disease is myotonic dystrophy, which is an autosomal dominant disease; the affected gene has been localized to chromosome 19. Myotonic dystrophy is relatively common and is best thought of as a systemic disease, since it causes cataracts, testicular atrophy, heart disease, dementia, and baldness, in addition to muscular weakness.

A mutation on the X chromosome (**choice A**) causes Duchenne muscular dystrophy.

None of the muscle diseases are known to be related to defects on the Y chromosome (**choice B**).

Facioscapulohumeral dystrophy is associated with a defective gene on chromosome 4 (**choice C**).

Infantile hypotonia has been related to defective genes on chromosome 5 (**choice D**).

39. **The correct answer is C.** Polymerase chain reaction (PCR) technologies use heat to separate the DNA strands so that they can be used as templates for new DNA synthesis. The usual forms of the enzyme DNA polymerase cannot withstand the needed temperatures for the DNA separation; however, the DNA polymerase of bacteria that grow in hot springs (*Thermus aquaticus*) is sufficiently stable at high temperatures to be used for PCR reactions.

Stability in acid (**choice A**) or base (**choice B**) is not a limiting problem in PCR technologies.

Resistance to high $Na^+$ concentration (**choice D**) or low $Ca^{2+}$ concentration (**choice E**) is not a limiting problem in PCR technologies.

40. **The correct answer is A.** Color-blindness is an X-linked recessive trait. A male is hemizygous for the X chromosome and thus has only one copy of each trait. The frequency of an X-linked recessive in males is thus equal to the frequency of the allele in the population. From this, we know that $q = 0.01$ and $p = 0.99$. A female has two copies of each gene on the X chromosome, so the equation for Hardy-Weinberg equilibrium is the same as for the autosomal traits. In this case, a homozygous recessive female would occur at a frequency of $q^2$ or 0.0001.

**Choice B**, 0.0005, is incorrect. If you remembered that color-blindness was more frequent in males, but did not know how to use the equations to get the true estimate, you might have guessed this answer.

Choice C, 0.01, makes the assumption that the trait is autosomal, and so the frequencies of affected males and affected females are equal.

Choice D, 0.02, assumes that q = 0.01, and then calculates the frequency of carrier females (2pq).

Choice E, 0.025 is also incorrect; it is a distracter.

41. **The correct answer is A.** In aerobic glycolysis, glucose is degraded to pyruvate, which is then converted to acetyl-CoA, the form in which it actually enters the citric acid cycle. Two acetyl-CoAs, each containing two of the glucose's carbons, are produced from each glucose molecule. In addition, a total of two carbons from glucose are released as $CO_2$ when each of the two pyruvates are converted to acetyl-CoA.

Citrate (**choice B**) is the product formed in the citric acid cycle when acetyl-CoA condenses with oxaloacetate.

Oxaloacetate (**choice C**) is the citric acid cycle intermediate that condenses with acetyl-CoA to form citrate.

Two pyruvates (**choice D**) are produced from degradation of glucose. These are then converted to the two acetyl-CoAs that enter the citric acid cycle.

Succinate (**choice E**) is another citric acid cycle intermediate that forms when coenzyme A is removed from succinyl-CoA.

42. **The correct answer is B.** This infant has Menkes syndrome, also known as Ehlers-Danlos syndrome type IX or "kinky hair" disease. It is due to a defect in a copper transporting P-type ATPase, and in common with all of the Ehlers-Danlos diseases, it has a symptomology caused primarily by weak collagen. Most, if not all, copper-requiring enzymes are adversely affected by the associated copper deficiency. However, lysyl oxidase both requires copper and plays a direct role in collagen formation by catalyzing the cross-linking of collagen fibrils. A deficiency of this enzyme would thus be directly responsible for the described symptoms.

Cytochrome $aa_3$ (**choice A**) does require copper, but has no direct role in collagen formation. Deficient cytochrome $aa_3$ activity would principally affect muscles and nerves. The fact that these tissues appear to not be significantly affected may be a reflection of the fact that there is much more cytochrome $aa_3$ present than required for normal function. Thus, a loss of some activity would only reduce reserve capacity and have a minimal effect.

Prolyl hydroxylase (**choice C**) catalyzes the hydroxylation of proline on the nascent collagen fiber. Although clearly important for collagen synthesis, it does not require copper.

Tyrosinase (**choice D**) also is a copper-requiring enzyme. It plays an important role in the production of melanin, and the hypopigmentation associated with Menkes syndrome is undoubtedly due to hypoactivity of this enzyme. However, this is a relatively minor symptom and is not one of the ones described in the vignette.

γ-Glutamyl carboxylase (**choice E**) is a vitamin K-dependent enzyme that catalyzes the formation of γ-carboxyglutamate required for chelation of calcium ion by the clotting factors. It does not require copper, and it does not have a role in collagen formation.

43. **The correct answer is D.** The key to this question is understanding how and when the body utilizes fuel stores. The stores of ATP (**choice A**) will be used up in less than 1 second once the race has started. Creatine phosphate (**choice B**) will be the primary source of energy for the next 3 or 4 seconds. After the creatine phosphate stores are depleted, the majority of ATP needed to complete the race will be derived from glycolysis. If the race were to last for an extended period of time, then the processes of gluconeogenesis (**choice C**) and lipolysis (**choice E**) might be utilized. Gluconeogenesis is the process of synthesizing glucose in the liver from non-carbohydrate sources, such as amino and fatty acids. Lipolysis is the splitting up or decomposition of fat in the body.

44. **The correct answer is D.** In the absence of sufficient insulin or if there is decreased sensitivity to insulin, hormone-sensitive lipase in adipose tissue will be overactive. This will degrade stored triacylglycerols and release fatty acids into the blood.

Glucose conversion to sorbitol in the lens (**choice A**) will be enhanced due to the hyperglycemia of diabetes. This sorbitol will tend to accumulate in the lens, causing cataracts and probably contributing to other degenerative changes associated with diabetes. The reaction does not contribute to hyperlipidemia.

The GLUT-2 of liver (**choice B**) is insulin-independent and would not be affected.

The adipose and muscle glucose transporter, GLUT-4, will not be recruited maximally and will thus be underactive rather than overactive (**choice C**).

Lipoprotein lipase will be underactive rather than overactive (**choice E**). Underactive lipoprotein lipase will produce an increase in circulating triacylglycerol-rich lipoproteins by inhibiting their uptake into cells and will contribute to the hyperlipidemia.

45. **The correct answer is E.** To answer this question, you need two separate pieces of information. First, riboflavin (one of the B vitamins) is used to make the flavin part of FAD (flavin adenine dinucleotide).

Second, of the citric acid cycle enzymes listed, only succinate dehydrogenase (which catalyzes the conversion of succinate to fumarate) uses FAD (which is converted to $FADH_2$) as a cofactor.

Aconitase (**choice A**) converts citrate to isocitrate and does not require a cofactor.

Citrate synthetase (**choice B**) combines acetyl-CoA and oxaloacetate to make citrate with the release of coenzyme A (which requires pantothenic acid for synthesis).

Isocitrate dehydrogenase (**choice C**) converts isocitrate to alpha-ketoglutarate and uses $NAD^+$ (which is converted to $NADH + H^+$). The $NAD^+$ requires the vitamin niacin for synthesis.

Malate dehydrogenase (**choice D**) converts malate to oxaloacetate and uses $NAD^+$ (which is converted to $NADH + H^+$). The $NAD^+$ requires the vitamin niacin for synthesis.

46. **The correct answer is C.** Dideoxycytidine (DDC) can be incorporated into viral DNA during reverse transcription and cause chain termination. Because DDC lacks a 3′ hydroxyl group, once incorporated into DNA, it prevents further phosphodiester bond formation and thus cDNA elongation.

DDC is an analog of a deoxyribonucleotide and would not affect RNA synthesis, which uses ribonucleotides (**choice A**), RNA processing (**choice E**), or protein synthesis (**choice B**), which uses amino acids.

Hydrolysis of peptide bonds during post-translational modification of viral proteins (**choice D**) is inhibited by protease inhibitors, such as indinavir.

47. **The correct answer is B.** Leber hereditary optic neuropathy is a relatively common cause of acute or subacute vision loss, especially in young men. It exhibits a mitochondrial inheritance pattern. The hallmark of this pattern is matrilineal inheritance. All the children of an affected woman will be affected since they receive mitochondrial genes only from the female parent. Affected males do not contribute mitochondria to progeny, so their children will not receive the trait.

Glucose-6-phosphate dehydrogenase (G6PD) deficiency (**choice A**) is an X-linked recessive disorder that affects the pentose phosphate pathway. The hallmark of X-linked recessive inheritance is an abundance of affected males and an absence of affected females. Males are hemi-zygous for the X chromosome, so the phenotype is expressed with only one dose of the gene. Females have two copies of the X chromosome, so they appear phenotypically normal although they may carry the recessive allele. Since a male inherits his X chromosome from his mother, if he is affected, she must carry

the trait. Other X-linked recessive disorders include Lesch-Nyhan disease, hemophilia A, and Duchenne muscular dystrophy.

Neurofibromatosis (**choice C**) shows an autosomal dominant inheritance pattern, so the phenotype will be expressed if the allele is present in one dose. Deleterious autosomal dominants occur at very low frequencies, so affected individuals are almost always heterozygous for the trait. Since the gene is located on an autosome, both male and female progeny can be affected. Other autosomal dominant disorders include Ehlers-Danlos syndrome, Huntington disease, and osteogenesis imperfecta.

Sickle cell anemia (**choice D**) and Tay-Sachs disease (**choice E**) are both inherited in an autosomal recessive pattern. For the phenotype of the autosomal recessive to be expressed, the recessive allele must be present in two doses. Both male and female children can be affected. The hallmark feature is that unaffected parents have affected children of both sexes.

48. **The correct answer is D.** The administration of any product that contains phenylalanine, such as aspartame, to an individual with any of the hyperphenylalaninemias could be detrimental to his or her general health. The hyperphenylalaninemias result from an impaired conversion of phenylalanine to tyrosine. The most common and clinically important of these is phenylketonuria, which is characterized by an increased concentration of phenylalanine in blood, increased concentration of phenylalanine and its by-products (such as phenylpyruvate, phenylacetate, and phenyllactate) in urine, and mental retardation. Phenylketonuria is caused by a deficiency of phenylalanine hydrolase.

Hyperornithinemia (**choice A**) is an inherited disorder of amino acid metabolism that results from a defect of the enzyme ornithine decarboxylase. This condition is associated with mental retardation, neuropsychiatric dysfunction, and protein intolerance.

Hyperuricemia (**choice B**) is a condition associated with higher than normal blood levels of uric acid. Gout may be produced if the hyperuricemia persists.

Hypervalinemia (**choice C**) is an inherited disorder of amino acid metabolism that results from a defect of the enzyme valine aminotransferase. This condition is associated with mental retardation, neuropsychiatric dysfunction, and protein intolerance.

Wilson disease (**choice E**) is an autosomal recessive disorder associated with an abnormality of the hepatic excretion of copper, resulting in toxic accumulations of the metal in the brain, liver, and other organs.

49. **The correct answer is C.** The most likely explanation is that this family carries a mutation in a different gene that also causes hemochromatosis. This is locus heterogeneity.

   Heteroplasmy (**choice A**) is often the basis for variable expression in a mitochondrial pedigree. Some affected individuals may have a higher percentage of mitochondria with the mutation than others have, and thus more severe symptoms are produced. This is not the issue in this question.

   Hemochromatosis is a disease that has incomplete penetrance (**choice B**), but this is not the explanation for this genetic testing issue. The proband has symptoms—he just doesn't have a mutation in the *HFE* gene involved in most cases of hemochromatosis.

   Because the SNPs are "closely linked" to the *HFE* gene, recombination between them (**choice D**) in several family members would be very unlikely.

   The mutation is unlikely to be in the *HFE* gene (**choice E**) because 5 SNPs known to be closely linked to the *HFE* gene show no linkage to the disease-causing gene in this family.

50. **The correct answer is C.** About 20% of patients with a chromosome 13 abnormality (13q-syndrome) develop retinoblastoma. There is also a genetic dominant form of retinoblastoma that has an 80% penetrance rate. Retinoblastomas that have a genetic basis are more likely to be bilateral than the spontaneous lesions. Microscopically, retinoblastomas are composed of masses of small hyperchromatic cells that may form small rosettes composed of radially arranged cells surrounding a central lumen.

# Microbiology/Immunology: **Test One**

1. A 19-year-old man presents to the emergency department with pneumonia. Since the age of 6 months, he has had recurrent pneumonia and sinusitis due to *Streptococcus pneumoniae* and *Haemophilus influenzae.* Careful assessment of his immune function would likely reveal abnormal function of the

   (A) B lymphocytes
   (B) macrophages
   (C) natural killer cells
   (D) platelets
   (E) T lymphocytes

2. A 20-year-old woman presents with a 2-day history of dysuria and increased urinary frequency. She states that she was recently married and was not sexually active prior to the marriage. Physical examination reveals a temperature of 100.7 F with normal vital signs. Gynecologic examination reveals no evidence of discharge, vaginitis, or cervicitis. Urinalysis reveals 14 white blood cells per high-powered field with many gram-negative rods. Which of the following is the most appropriate pharmacotherapy?

   (A) Ampicillin
   (B) Ceftriaxone
   (C) Fluconazole
   (D) Gentamicin
   (E) Metronidazole

3. A 60-year-old woman comes to the physician because of fever, chills, and a cough for the past 2 weeks. She lives at home with her husband, has no chronic medical conditions, and has not traveled recently. She does not smoke cigarettes or drink alcohol. Her temperature is 38.2 C (100.8 F). Physical examination reveals altered breath sounds. Chest x-ray is abnormal. Which of the following is the most likely causal organism?

   (A) *Chlamydia pneumoniae*
   (B) *Haemophilus influenzae*
   (C) *Mycoplasma pneumoniae*
   (D) *Staphylococcus aureus*
   (E) *Streptococcus pneumoniae*

4. A 3-week-old boy develops focal seizures, lethargy, and vomiting. Examination shows a bulging fontanelle and nuchal rigidity. Which of the following organisms should be suspected?

   (A) *Escherichia coli* and *Streptococcus agalactiae*
   (B) *Haemophilus influenzae* and *Neisseria meningitidis*
   (C) *Haemophilus influenzae* and *Streptococcus pneumoniae*
   (D) *Listeria monocytogenes* and *Neisseria meningitidis*
   (E) *Staphylococcus aureus* and *Staphylococcus epidermidis*

5. A 24-year-old woman with a history of allergic rhinitis is involved in an automobile accident and sustains a splenic laceration. She undergoes abdominal surgery and is then transfused with 4 units of blood of the appropriate ABO and Rh type. As the transfusion progresses, she becomes rapidly hypotensive and develops airway edema, consistent with anaphylaxis. Which of the following pre-existing conditions best accounts for these symptoms?

    (A) AIDS

    (B) C1 esterase inhibitor deficiency

    (C) DiGeorge syndrome

    (D) Selective IgA deficiency

    (E) Wiskott-Aldrich syndrome

6. A 24-year-old woman in her third trimester of pregnancy presents with urinary frequency and burning for the past few days. She denies fever, nausea, vomiting, or chills. She takes no medications besides prenatal vitamins and is generally in good health. Physical examination is remarkable for mild suprapubic tenderness, and a urine dipstick is positive for white blood cells, protein, and a small amount of blood. Culture produces greater than 100,000 colonies of gram-negative bacilli. Which of the following attributes of this uropathogenic organism is most strongly associated with its virulence?

    (A) Bundle-forming pili

    (B) GVVPQ fimbriae

    (C) Heat labile toxins

    (D) Heat stable toxins

    (E) P pili

    (F) Type 1 pili

7. Which of the following cell surface markers is required for lysis of IgG-coated target cells (antibody-dependent, cell-mediated cytotoxicity, or ADCC) by natural killer cells?

    (A) CD3

    (B) CD16

    (C) CD19

    (D) CD21

    (E) CD56

8. A 35-year-old man presents to the emergency department with intense back pain. He is hydrated and given pain medication. After several hours he passes a kidney stone. Laboratory analysis of the stone reveals that it is composed of struvite (magnesium ammonium phosphate). Infection with which of the following organisms promotes the production of such stones?

    (A) *Escherichia coli*

    (B) *Proteus mirabilis*

    (C) *Pseudomonas aeruginosa*

    (D) *Staphylococcus saprophyticus*

    (E) *Ureaplasma urealyticum*

9. A 21-year-old man presents with cough, fever, and hemoptysis. Blood tests show significantly elevated BUN and creatinine. Immunofluorescent microscopy reveals a diffuse linear pattern of fluorescence along the basement membranes of alveolar septa and glomerular capillaries. Which type of hypersensitivity is associated with this disease?

    (A) I

    (B) II

    (C) III

    (D) IV

10. A 47-year-old man with a history of sickle cell disease has had numerous hospitalizations requiring the placement of IV lines. The patient has poor peripheral venous access, and a catheter is placed in right subclavian vein. The patient subsequently develops right arm discomfort and swelling and a temperature of 40.1 C with chills. Multiple blood cultures are taken, and gram-positive cocci are isolated. The organism is catalase-positive and produces whitish colonies on mannitol salt agar. The colonies are gamma-hemolytic on sheep blood agar. Which of the following organisms is the most likely cause of this patient's symptoms?

    (A) *Enterococcus faecalis*

    (B) *Staphylococcus aureus*

    (C) *Staphylococcus epidermidis*

    (D) *Streptococcus agalactiae*

    (E) *Streptococcus pyogenes*

11. A 58-year-old alcoholic man with multiple dental caries develops a pulmonary abscess and is treated with antibiotics. Several days later, he develops nausea, vomiting, abdominal pain, and voluminous green diarrhea. Which of the following antibiotics is most likely responsible for this patient's symptoms?

    (A) Chloramphenicol

    (B) Clindamycin

    (C) Gentamicin

    (D) Metronidazole

    (E) Vancomycin

12. A 54-year-old man with chronic renal failure receives a kidney transplant and is given immunosuppressive therapy with cyclosporine. Over the next 6 months, the patient's creatinine levels progressively rise, and a needle biopsy of the kidney is performed. What is the biopsy most likely to show?

    (A) Intimal fibrosis, interstitial fibrosis, and tubular atrophy

    (B) Linear deposition of immunoglobulin and complement in glomeruli

    (C) Neutrophils, immunoglobulin, and complement in vessel walls

    (D) T-cell interstitial infiltrate and edema

    (E) Thickening of the blood vessel intima due to cellular proliferation

13. A 69-year-old alcoholic man comes to the emergency department because of high fever, chills, and a cough. He says that he has been producing "lots of thick, bloody, gelatinous mucus" over the past 2 days. Gram staining of the sputum reveals pinkish-red bacilli. Chest x-ray shows consolidation of the upper lobes. Which of the following is found only in microorganisms with this color Gram-staining?

    (A) Cell envelope

    (B) Exotoxin

    (C) Peptidoglycan

    (D) Periplasmic space

    (E) Teichoic acids

14. A 7-year-old boy presents to the pediatrician because his mother noticed a "smoky" color to his urine. On questioning the mother, it is revealed that the child had a sore throat several weeks ago that was left untreated. Physical examination reveals hypertension and mild generalized edema. Urinalysis is significant for red blood cell casts. Which of the following accurately describes the microorganism responsible for this child's illness?

    (A) It causes alpha-hemolysis on blood agar

    (B) It is catalase-positive

    (C) It is coagulase-positive

    (D) It is sensitive to bacitracin

    (E) It is sensitive to optochin

15. A 34-year-old primigravid woman at 32 weeks' gestation comes to the emergency department complaining of fever, chills, dysuria, and back pain. The symptoms started 6 days ago with burning on urination and have progressively worsened. Her temperature is 39.1 C (102.4 F). Physical examination shows left costovertebral angle tenderness. Urinalysis is positive for leukocytes and nitrites. Which of the following interleukins is being produced by macrophages and is stimulating fever production by its action on this patient's hypothalamic cells?

    (A) IL-1

    (B) IL-2

    (C) IL-3

    (D) IL-4

    (E) IL-5

    (F) IL-6

    (G) IL-7

    (H) IL-8

    (I) IL-10

    (J) IL-12

16. A baby born at 32 weeks' gestation with Apgar scores of 2 and 7 was placed in the neonatal intensive care unit. She developed a fever and leukocytosis; lumbar puncture revealed pleocytosis with increased protein, decreased glucose, and gram-positive rods. Which of the following organisms was most likely isolated from the CSF?

    (A) *Escherichia coli*

    (B) *Listeria monocytogenes*

    (C) *Neisseria meningitidis*

    (D) *Streptococcus agalactiae*

    (E) *Streptococcus pneumoniae*

17. A young mother takes her infant to the pediatrician for the first time. The pediatrician notices the infant's teeth are yellow. The antibiotic this mother most likely took during pregnancy

    (A) inhibits aminoacyl-tRNA binding

    (B) inhibits peptidyl transferase

    (C) interferes with cell wall synthesis

    (D) is a large, cyclic, lactone-ring structure

18. A culture of smooth *Streptococcus agalactiae* bacteria is grown in nutrient broth and allowed to incubate until the culture enters the decline phase of the growth curve. Purified streptococcal DNAse is added to the flask, and the culture is agitated gently for 2 hours at 37° C. An extract of this process is added to a culture of rough *S. agalactiae* in the logarithmic phase of the growth curve and incubated for 24 hours under appropriate culture conditions. Which of the following processes would be necessary to achieve the production of encapsulated *S. agalactiae* in this system?

    (A) Conjugation

    (B) Lysogeny

    (C) Site-specific recombination

    (D) Transduction

    (E) Transformation

19. A 5-year-old child who has not had routine pediatric care develops a febrile disease with cough and a blotchy rash, and is brought to the emergency department. On physical examination, there is cervical and axillary lymphadenopathy. Also noted is an erythematous, maculopapular rash behind the ears and along the hairline, involving the neck and, to a lesser extent, the trunk. Examination of this patient's oropharynx would likely reveal which of the following lesions?

    (A) Adherent thin, whitish patch on gingiva

    (B) Cold sores on the lips

    (C) Curdy white material overlying an erythematous base on the oral mucosa

    (D) Large shallow ulcers on the oral mucosa

    (E) Multiple small white spots on the buccal mucosa

20. A 35-year-old man undergoes an appendectomy. Several days later, an abscess has formed at the surgical site. It does not improve with administration of a cephalosporin but does respond to nafcillin. The infecting organism most likely produced an enzyme that would hydrolyze which bond in the following molecule?

    (A) A

    (B) B

    (C) C

    (D) D

21. A 53-year-old engineer with diabetes mellitus comes to the employee health center for an annual examination. She has no complaints at this time. A review of her chart reveals that she is due for a few vaccinations, including the influenza A vaccine. She questions the physician about the necessity of the vaccine because she just received one a year ago. The physician should respond that last year's influenza vaccine may be ineffective today because influenza A

    (A) has a heavy polysaccharide coat

    (B) immunosuppresses the patient

    (C) kills lymphocytes

    (D) resists inactivation by complement

    (E) undergoes genetic reassortment

22. After eating a dinner of leftovers that included rewarmed vegetable fried rice, a 17-year-old boy develops diarrhea and stomach pain. Which of the following is the most likely pathogen?

    (A) *Bacillus cereus*

    (B) *Campylobacter jejuni*

    (C) *Clostridium botulinum*

    (D) *Clostridium difficile*

    (E) *Escherichia coli*

    (F) Norwalk agent

    (G) Rotavirus

    (H) *Salmonella typhi*

    (I) *Shigella dysenteriae*

    (J) *Vibrio parahaemolyticus*

    (K) *Yersinia pestis*

23. A 23-year-old woman with a history of sickle cell disease presents with fever and severe bone pain localized to her left tibia. An x-ray film reveals a lytic lesion, and blood cultures reveal infection. A bone culture grows gram-negative rods. Which of the following best describes the infecting organism?

    (A) It is comma-shaped and sensitive to acidic pH

    (B) It is an obligate intracellular parasite

    (C) It is motile and does not ferment lactose

    (D) It is motile and oxidase positive

    (E) It is a nonmotile facultative anaerobe

24. A 33-year-old HIV-positive man complains of headache and blurred vision. Physical examination reveals papilledema and ataxia. Head CT is normal but CSF obtained by lumbar puncture reveals encapsulated organisms observable with India ink. Which of the following is true concerning this organism?

    (A) It can also be identified with methenamine silver stain

    (B) It consists of branching septate hyphae

    (C) It exists as a mycelial form at room temperature and as yeast at 37.0 C

    (D) It is an encapsulated nondimorphic yeast found worldwide

    (E) It is a nonencapsulated dimorphic yeast that reproduces by budding

25. A French exchange student in a town near the Ohio River presents to the local hospital with headache, fever, malaise, and nonproductive cough. He became ill several days after cleaning and moving a chicken coop where hundreds of chickens had roosted for many years. Which of the following microorganisms is most likely responsible for his illness?

    (A) *Actinomyces israelii*

    (B) *Aspergillus fumigatus*

    (C) *Candida albicans*

    (D) *Coccidioides immitis*

    (E) *Cryptococcus neoformans*

    (F) *Histoplasma capsulatum*

    (G) *Nocardia asteroides*

    (H) *Sporothrix schenckii*

26. A 3-year-old girl presents with recurrent subcutaneous abscesses and furuncles. She has a history of pneumonia due to *Serratia marcescens*. Which of the following enzymes is most likely deficient in her neutrophils?

    (A) Aldolase B

    (B) Galactokinase

    (C) Glucokinase

    (D) Glucose-6-phosphate dehydrogenase

    (E) NADPH oxidase

27. An otherwise healthy patient who has just received a prosthetic aortic valve develops postoperative fever. Blood cultures are done, and she is given broad-spectrum antibiotics. Two days later she is still febrile and clinically deteriorating. Which of the following is the most likely pathogen?

    (A) *Actinomyces israelii*

    (B) *Candida albicans*

    (C) *Histoplasma capsulatum*

    (D) *Nocardia asteroides*

    (E) *Trichophyton rubrum*

28. After high-dose chemotherapy and irradiation, a 35-year-old woman with acute myeloid leukemia in remission receives a bone marrow transplant from her HLA-matched brother. One week after the graft, the patient develops a fever and a maculopapular rash over her upper extremities and back. She also notes abdominal pain and diarrhea. Laboratory examination is remarkable for elevation of alkaline phosphatase and bilirubin. Which of the following is the most likely cause of this patient's symptoms?

    (A) Bacterial infection from the graft

    (B) Blast crisis

    (C) Graft-versus-host disease

    (D) Hyperacute graft rejection

    (E) Radiation toxicity

29. A 16-year-old boy with sickle cell disease is hospitalized for a severe infection. His spleen has autosplenectomized, and he has had other minor infections in the past. His symptoms include fever, chills, cough, and chest pain. Bacteria from the patient's sputum are optochin-sensitive organisms with a positive Quellung reaction. Which of the following is the most likely pathogen?

    (A) *Escherichia coli*

    (B) *Haemophilus influenzae*

    (C) *Klebsiella pneumoniae*

    (D) *Neisseria gonorrhoeae*

    (E) *Streptococcus pneumoniae*

The figure below represents an Ouchterlony radial immunodiffusion test.

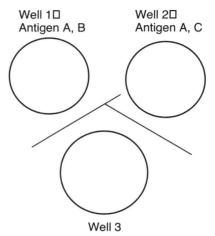

Well 1
Antigen A, B

Well 2
Antigen A, C

Well 3

30. The antigen in Well 1 has two different epitopes (antigenic determinant groups), A and B; the antigen in Well 2 also has two epitopes, A and C. Well 3 contains which of the following?

    (A) Antibody to A only

    (B) Antibodies to A and B

    (C) Antibodies to A and C

    (D) Antibodies to B and C

    (E) Antibodies to A, B, and C

31. A 3-year-old boy presents with a 1-day history of loose stools, fever, abdominal cramping, headache, and myalgia. He has no blood in the stool. A careful history reveals that he has several pet turtles. Which of the following is the most likely pathogen?

    (A) *Chlamydia psittaci*

    (B) *Entamoeba histolytica*

    (C) *Salmonella* spp.

    (D) *Staphylococcus aureus*

    (E) *Yersinia enterocolitica*

32. A 3-week-old infant is found to have a particular virus. The family practitioner is especially concerned because the virus produces disease or sequelae that is/are more severe if the infection occurs at a very young age. This infant is most likely infected with which of the following viruses?

    (A) Epstein-Barr virus
    (B) Hepatitis B virus
    (C) Measles virus
    (D) Poliovirus
    (E) Varicella zoster virus

33. A 20-year-old man with stridor is brought to the emergency department by his girlfriend. He had been complaining of abdominal pain earlier in the day. Physical examination is significant for well demarcated regions of subcutaneous edema. He has had similar episodes before, and his mother and sister have the same condition. Which of the following substances is most likely deficient in this patient?

    (A) C1 esterase inhibitor
    (B) C3b inactivator
    (C) Factor H
    (D) Carboxypeptidase
    (E) Properdin

34. About a month after being bitten by a bat, a man develops an influenza-like illness. He subsequently develops striking mood changes, pharyngeal spasms with drooling, and seizures, and he falls into a coma. He eventually dies of his illness. This patient's deterioration was most likely caused by a virus from which of the following groups?

    (A) Bunyaviruses
    (B) Caliciviruses
    (C) Flaviviruses
    (D) Rhabdoviruses
    (E) Togaviruses

35. A 23-year-old woman suffers from a condition in which her antibodies react with antigens present on the surface of cells. The mechanism of action involves complement fixation by the antibody-antigen complex, which causes lysis or phagocytosis of the affected cell. Which of the following conditions is an example of this type of hypersensitivity?

    (A) Allergic rhinitis
    (B) Agranulocytosis
    (C) Food allergy
    (D) Serum sickness
    (E) Tuberculosis

36. A 24-year-old woman has fever, malaise, and a dry, nonproductive cough. She also complains of headache, muscle aches, and leg pain. Laboratory values are significant for elevated cold agglutinins. Which of the following microorganisms is responsible for her symptoms?

    (A) *Haemophilus influenzae*
    (B) *Klebsiella pneumoniae*
    (C) *Legionella pneumophila*
    (D) *Mycoplasma pneumoniae*
    (E) *Streptococcus pneumoniae*

37. A 25-year-old Afghani immigrant presents with a confluent maculopapular rash that began on her face then spread downward over her trunk. She states that 3 days ago she started having a fever and headache, with bilateral pain associated with the front and back of her neck. She also complains of joint pain. Which of the following diseases does she most likely have?

    (A) Infectious mononucleosis
    (B) Lyme disease
    (C) Roseola
    (D) Rubella
    (E) Rubeola

**KAPLAN**) MEDICAL

38. An 18-year-old, previously healthy woman presents to the student health service with fever, vomiting, and diarrhea. On physical examination, she is hypotensive and has an erythematous, red, sunburn-like skin rash. She is currently menstruating and has been using super-absorbent tampons. Which of the following findings from a positive blood culture would confirm the suspected diagnosis?

    (A) Organisms are acid-fast

    (B) Organisms are coagulase-positive

    (C) Organisms grow on EMB (eosin-methylene blue) agar

    (D) Organisms grow on Thayer-Martin medium

    (E) Organisms have positive Quellung reaction

39. A culture of *Staphylococcus aureus* bacteria is selected over many months for its ability to grow in increasing concentrations of penicillin. When colonies of this original culture are capable of growth on blood agar containing 400,000 IU penicillin, the colonies are picked from the agar, placed in a nutrient broth, and a lytic phage is added. The bacteria and phage are cocultured until viral maturation is complete. The culture is centrifuged, and the supernatant liquid is added to culture tubes containing clones of penicillin-sensitive *S. aureus*. After 4 hours of incubation at 37.0 C, these broth cultures are dumped onto blood agar Petri dishes containing 400,000 IU penicillin and incubated for 24 hours. Out of 100 Petri dishes, 4 grow colonies. What process has taken place in this experiment?

    (A) Generalized transduction

    (B) Mobilization of transposons

    (C) Site-specific recombination

    (D) Specialized transduction

    (E) Transformation

40. A 27-year-old woman comes to the physician because of a 4-week history of lethargy and fatigue. She is generally healthy and, except for a red, annular lesion on her right buttock 4 weeks ago, she has no other complaints. She does not smoke cigarettes and does not drink alcohol. She proudly says that she goes for an afternoon jog 5 days a week in the woods by her home. Physical examination shows diffuse muscle tenderness and stiffness of the joints. Global eradication of this disease is unlikely in the foreseeable future because the causative organism

    (A) can be maintained in nature indefinitely by a tick vector

    (B) has a tough outer coat that is resistant to environmental stresses

    (C) has humans as its primary reservoir

    (D) is resistant to antibiotics and disinfectants

    (E) may reactivate and cause Brill-Zinsser disease

41. A 7-month-old child presents with a 4-day history of fever, deepening cough, and dyspnea. A chest x-ray film shows multiple interstitial infiltrates and hyperinflation of the lungs. Multinucleated giant cells with cytoplasmic inclusion bodies are seen when a nasal wash is inoculated into tissue culture. The most appropriate therapy includes administration of which of the following drugs?

    (A) Acyclovir

    (B) Ganciclovir

    (C) Ribavirin

    (D) Trifluorothymidine

    (E) Zidovudine

42. A formula-fed, 1-month-old boy is exposed to his sister, who has chickenpox. He does not develop signs of varicella. His mother had the infection 5 years ago. Which class of immunoglobulins did he acquire from his mother in utero that protected him from this virus?

    (A) IgA

    (B) IgD

    (C) IgE

    (D) IgG

    (E) IgM

43. After passing his physical examination, a 19-year-old army recruit gives urine and blood samples for further testing. Serum analysis yields elevated ALT, HBsAg, Anti-HBc, HBeAg, and bilirubin. All other values are normal. What is the hepatitis B status of this recruit?

    (A) Asymptomatic carrier

    (B) Active carrier

    (C) Fulminant hepatitis B

    (D) Recovered from acute self-limited HBV

    (E) Vaccinated against HBV

44. A 65-year-old man undergoes coronary artery bypass surgery that entails grafting the left internal mammary artery to the left main coronary artery to form an alternative conduit for blood flow. This patient received a(n)

    (A) allograft

    (B) autograft

    (C) homograft

    (D) isograft

    (E) xenograft

45. Following a barbecue hosted by a hunter who served "bear hamburgers," several guests develop abdominal pain and diarrhea; their condition progresses about a week later to fever, myalgia, periorbital edema, and petechial hemorrhages in the conjunctiva. A peripheral blood smear shows an increased eosinophil count. Which of the following is the most likely cause of these symptoms?

    (A) Anthrax

    (B) *Bacillus cereus* food poisoning

    (C) Botulism

    (D) *Escherichia coli* gastroenteritis

    (E) Trichinosis

46. A patient presents with right lower-quadrant pain, fever, and diarrhea. Physical examination reveals diffuse abdominal tenderness; laboratory examination shows a moderate leukocytosis, leading to a presumptive diagnosis of acute appendicitis. Surgical exploration of the abdomen reveals mesenteric adenitis, but the appendix is normal. Which of the following organisms is most likely responsible for these signs and symptoms?

    (A) *Clostridium difficile*

    (B) Enterohemorrhagic *Escherichia coli*

    (C) Enteroinvasive *E. coli*

    (D) Enteropathogenic *E. coli*

    (E) Enterotoxigenic *E. coli*

    (F) *Mycobacterium tuberculosis*

    (G) *Salmonella*

    (H) *Shigella*

    (I) *Vibrio cholerae*

    (J) *Yersinia enterocolitica*

47. A 68-year-old patient with alcoholic cirrhosis is hospitalized with ascites and esophageal varices. The patient's temperature is 38.3 C (101.0 F). Paracentesis reveals a polymorphonuclear cell count of $300/mm^3$. Which of the following is the most likely infecting organism?

    (A) *Bacillus cereus*

    (B) *Clostridium difficile*

    (C) *Escherichia coli*

    (D) *Entamoeba histolytica*

    (E) *Giardia lamblia*

48. A 4-year-old child who has had repeated infections with staphylococci and streptococci has normal phagocytic function and delayed hypersensitivity responses. Lymph node biopsy would most likely reveal

    (A) absence of postcapillary venules

    (B) absence of germinal centers

    (C) defective chemotactic response of neutrophils

    (D) depletion of paracortical areas

    (E) depletion of thymus-dependent areas

49. A 47-year-old man presents with a nonproductive cough and rales on his chest examination. A chest x-ray film suggests atypical pneumonia. The pneumonia resolves after treatment with azithromycin. A diagnosis of psittacosis is established by the presence of complement fixing antibodies against *Chlamydia psittaci* in the convalescent serum. Which of the following is the most likely occupation of this patient?

    (A) Cat breeder

    (B) Florist

    (C) Homeless shelter worker

    (D) Poultry farmer

    (E) Slaughterhouse worker

50. A 20-year-old college student presents to the university health clinic with sore throat, fever, and fatigue. Physical exam is significant for cervical lymphadenopathy and mild hepatomegaly. Heterophile antibody tests are negative. Microscopic examination of fibroblasts would be expected to reveal

    (A) an enlarged nucleus with peripherally displaced chromatin

    (B) conidia and septate hyphae

    (C) a giant nucleus surrounded by a clear zone

    (D) a multinucleated giant cell

    (E) staining with India ink

# Microbiology/Immunology Test One: **Answers and Explanations**

## ANSWER KEY

| | | | |
|---|---|---|---|
| 1. | A | 26. | E |
| 2. | A | 27. | B |
| 3. | E | 28. | C |
| 4. | A | 29. | E |
| 5. | D | 30. | B |
| 6. | E | 31. | C |
| 7. | B | 32. | B |
| 8. | B | 33. | A |
| 9. | B | 34. | D |
| 10. | C | 35. | B |
| 11. | B | 36. | D |
| 12. | A | 37. | D |
| 13. | D | 38. | B |
| 14. | D | 39. | A |
| 15. | A | 40. | A |
| 16. | B | 41. | C |
| 17. | A | 42. | D |
| 18. | E | 43. | B |
| 19. | E | 44. | B |
| 20. | D | 45. | E |
| 21. | E | 46. | J |
| 22. | A | 47. | C |
| 23. | C | 48. | B |
| 24. | D | 49. | D |
| 25. | F | 50. | C |

1. **The correct answer is A.** The symptoms in the question suggest a deficiency known as common variable hypogammaglobulinemia, characterized by very low serum levels of IgG. In this congenital disease, the number of B cells is normal, but their ability to synthesize IgG and the other immunoglobulins is severely compromised, leading to recurrent streptococcal and *Haemophilus* infections. The onset of the recurrent infections usually begins between 6 and 12 months of age—concurrent with the decreasing levels of maternal IgG in the newborn. Treatment often involves giving IV gamma globulin to reduce the number of infections.

   Abnormal function of macrophages (**choice B**) such as that seen in chronic granulomatous disease results in recurrent infections with catalase-positive organisms. *Streptococcus* is a catalase-negative genus.

   Abnormal function of NK cells (**choice C**) is unlikely to present as recurrent bacterial infections, because these cells are primarily involved in cellular, rather than humoral, immunity.

   Platelets (**choice D**) are not directly involved in the immune response. Deficiencies in platelets lead to problems in clotting and produce bleeding disorders.

   T-cell deficiencies (**choice E**) result in severe viral, fungal, and protozoal infections, rather than recurrent bacterial infections.

2. **The correct answer is A.** The patient's presentation is consistent with a simple urinary tract infection; there is a short history of dysuria, increased urinary frequency, and the appearance of white blood cells and gram-negative rods in the urine. Urinary tract infections are common in women after they become sexually active. The infection is likely caused by urethral trauma during intercourse, which leads to bacterial contamination of the bladder. Since most of these infections are caused by *Escherichia coli* (a gram-negative rod), the most appropriate therapy would be ampicillin for around 10 days.

   Ceftriaxone (**choice B**) is the treatment of choice for uncomplicated infections with *Neisseria gonorrhoeae*, now that most strains are resistant to penicillin. IV ceftriaxone is a regimen reserved for the treatment of life-threatening infections.

   Fluconazole (**choice C**) is indicated for the treatment of vaginal candidiasis. Since there is no vaginal discharge and the patient has gram-negative rods in the urine, a diagnosis of vaginal candidiasis can be excluded.

   Gentamicin (**choice D**) would be an inappropriate choice. Most urinary tract infections caused by gram-negative rods are sensitive to ampicillin, and the potential for toxicity secondary to gentamicin is great.

   Metronidazole (**choice E**) is an antibiotic typically used in the treatment of vaginal *Trichomonas* and *Gardnerella* infections, as well as serious infections believed to be caused by anaerobic bacteria. Since there is no vaginal discharge and the patient has gram-negative rods in the urine, this is not the best choice for treatment.

3. **The correct answer is E.** The most common bacterium implicated in community-acquired pneumonia is the pneumococcus *Streptococcus pneumoniae*. Other organisms frequently implicated in patients younger than 60 without comorbidity include *Mycoplasma pneumoniae*, respiratory viruses, *Chlamydia pneumoniae*, and *Haemophilus influenzae*. When community-acquired pneumonia occurs in elderly patients or patients with comorbidity, aerobic gram-negative bacilli and *Staphylococcus aureus* are added to the list.

   The organisms listed in **choices A, B, and C** are important causes of community-acquired pneumonia but are not the most frequent causes.

   *Staphylococcus aureus* (**choice D**) is an important cause of community-acquired pneumonia (particularly in the elderly and in patients with comorbidity) but is not the most frequent cause.

4. **The correct answer is A.** The pattern of microbial causes of meningitis varies with the patient's age and clinical setting. The most common organisms encountered in neonatal meningitis are *Streptococcus agalactiae* (a group B *Streptococcus*) and *Escherichia coli*.

   **Choice B:** *Haemophilus influenzae* type B was the most common agent isolated in children aged 1 to 5 years (before 1990), but is much less common today because of the introduction of an effective vaccine. It is uncommon in neonates. *Neisseria meningitidis* is the most common agent isolated in patients aged 5 to 40 years (35% of children aged 5 to 15 years, and 20% of adults).

   **Choice C:** *Haemophilus influenzae* type B was the most common agent isolated in children aged 1 to 5 years (before 1990), but is much less common today because of the introduction of an effective vaccine. *Streptococcus pneumoniae* occurs in all ages (40% of adult cases, 15% of childhood cases) but is uncommon in neonates (only 5% of cases).

   **Choice D:** *Neisseria meningitidis* is the most common agent isolated in patients aged 5 to 40 years (35% of children aged 5 to 15 years, and 20% of adults). *Listeria monocytogenes* accounts for only 1% of all cases of bacterial meningitis, and is seen in infants, the elderly, and immunosuppressed patients.

   **Choice E:** *Staphylococcus aureus* is seen in postsurgical and post-traumatic meningitis. *Staphylococcus epidermidis* accounts for 75% of shunt-related meningitis.

5. **The correct answer is D.** Patients with selective IgA deficiency may have circulating antibodies to IgA. Fatal anaphylaxis may ensue if they are transfused with blood products with serum containing IgA, although many patients with selective IgA deficiency are asymptomatic and never diagnosed. Symptomatic patients may have recurrent sinopulmonary infections and diarrhea, and also have an increased incidence of autoimmune and allergic diseases.

AIDS (**choice A**) predisposes for infections and neoplasms, but not anaphylaxis.

C1 esterase inhibitor deficiency (**choice B**) is an autosomal dominant disease characterized by recurrent attacks of colic and episodes of laryngeal edema, without pruritus or urticarial lesions. This disorder is also known as hereditary angioedema. It would not be expected to be associated with a blood transfusion but would occur throughout life.

DiGeorge syndrome (**choice C**) is characterized by thymic aplasia and sometimes, hypoparathyroidism. The disorder is due to abnormal development of the third and fourth pharyngeal pouches.

Wiskott-Aldrich syndrome (**choice E**) is a form of immunodeficiency associated with thrombocytopenia and eczema.

6. **The correct answer is E.** Urinary tract infections are the most common bacterial infections encountered during pregnancy, and *Escherichia coli* is the most commonly isolated organism. 70% of cases in the U.S. are caused by P pili-positive strains. Pili are believed to be important mediators of attachment to the epithelium.

Bundle-forming pili (**choice A**) are found in enteroaggregative *E. coli* (EAEC).

GVVPQ fimbriae (**choice B**) are found in EAEC.

Heat labile toxins (**choice C**) are pathogenic factors in enterotoxigenic strains (ETEC).

Heat stable toxins (**choice D**) are pathogenic factors in ETEC or EAEC.

Type 1 pili (**choice F**) are a major pathogenic factor in ETEC.

7. **The correct answer is B.** CD16 is a cell surface marker used to identify natural killer (NK) cells (lymphocytes lacking T- and B-cell markers). CD16 is an Fc receptor for IgG, allowing the NK cells to bind to the coated target cell during ADCC, facilitating lysis.

CD3 (**choice A**) is a five-polypeptide cluster that represents the nonvariable part of the T-cell receptor complex. NK cells are CD3-negative.

CD19 (**choice C**) is a B-cell marker. It is a signal-transducing molecule that is expressed in early B-cell differentiation. NK cells are negative for CD19.

C21 (**choice D**) is also a B-cell marker. It is a complement receptor, and is also the same receptor the Epstein-Barr virus uses to bind to cells during infection.

CD56 (**choice E**) is an NK cell marker, but is not involved with ADCC.

8. **The correct answer is B.** *Proteus* species produce urease, which raises the urinary pH and promotes the production of struvite stones.

*Escherichia coli* (**choice A**) is by far the most common cause of urinary tract infections but is not responsible for the development of struvite stones.

*Pseudomonas aeruginosa* (**choice C**) can also cause urinary tract infections, most commonly in hospitalized or immunocompromised patients (especially burn patients, patients on immunosuppressives/antimicrobials, and cystic fibrosis patients). It does not predispose to struvite stones.

*Staphylococcus saprophyticus* (**choice D**) is a common cause of urinary tract infections in sexually active young women.

*Ureaplasma urealyticum* (**choice E**) can produce urease (like *Proteus*), but it is responsible for urethritis, not stones.

9. **The correct answer is B.** This patient has a USMLE-favorite disease: Goodpasture syndrome, which affects both the renal and pulmonary systems. In the kidney, it causes a rapidly progressive glomerulonephritis associated with antibodies directed against a collagen component of the glomerular basement membrane (anti-GBM antibody—a classic clue to this diagnosis). These antibodies create a linear pattern on immunofluorescence. Note that they are also active against the basement membrane of respiratory alveoli, accounting for the pulmonary component of the disease.

Autoimmune reactions such as those found in Goodpasture syndrome, certain drug allergies, blood transfusion reactions, and hemolytic disease of the newborn, are classified as Type II hypersensitivities (antibody-mediated cytotoxicity). IgG or IgM antibody reacts with membrane-associated antigen on the surface of cells, causing activation of the complement cascade and, ultimately, cell destruction.

Type I (**choice A**) reactions (immediate, atopic, or anaphylactic) require an initial (sensitizing) exposure to an antigen. On re-exposure to the antigen, cross-linking of IgE receptors occurs on the surface of basophils and mast cells. The mast cells then release a variety of mediators, including histamine. Clinical syndromes include asthma, atopic dermatitis, eczema, and allergic rhinitis. Hives are characteristic of Type I hypersensitivity.

Type III (**choice C**) hypersensitivity (immune complex-mediated hypersensitivity) is caused by formation of antibody antigen complexes, which are filtered from the blood and activate complement. This results in the generation of C3b, which promotes neutrophil adherence to blood vessel walls. The complexes also generate C3a and C5a (anaphylatoxins), which lead to inflammation and tissue destruction. The hallmark signs of Type III sickness, which occur 7 to 14 days after exposure to the offending antigen, include urticaria, angioedema, fever, chills, malaise, and glomerulonephritis. Clinical syndromes include serum sickness (e.g., penicillin, streptomycin, sulfonamide, phenylbutazone hypersensitivity) and the Arthus reaction. Immune complexes are also observed in systemic lupus erythematosus (SLE). Type III glomerulonephritis (e.g., poststreptococcal glomerulonephritis) is characterized by a "lumpy bumpy" appearance on immunofluorescence using labeled antibody specific for immunoglobulin or complement.

Type IV (**choice D**) is also known as delayed-type hypersensitivity (DTH). Unlike the other types, which are mediated by antibody, DTH depends on T helper cells that have been sensitized to a particular antigen. T cells react with antigen in association with MHC class I gene products and release lymphokines. Examples include tuberculin skin testing and contact dermatitis (e.g., poison ivy rash).

10. **The correct answer is C.** The patient has developed bacteremia; the description of the causative agent is consistent with a staphylococcal organism (catalase-positive, gram-positive cocci that grow on mannitol salt agar). The organism is most likely *Staphylococcus epidermidis* as it was not able to ferment mannitol and was not hemolytic. Both of those characteristics tend to rule out *Staphylococcus aureus.* (**choice B**). Two other tests that are commonly used are coagulase production and excretion of DNAse from colonies. *S. aureus* is positive in both tests, *S. epidermidis* is negative. *S. aureus* produces golden yellow colonies.

*Enterococcus faecalis* (**choice A**) might grow on the mannitol salt agar as it is relatively haloduric, but these organisms are catalase-negative. The enterococci are extremely variable in hemolytic ability so this characteristic is not useful in species identification.

Both streptococcal organisms (**choices D and E**) are catalase negative and beta-hemolytic on sheep blood agar plates. Also, neither would grow on the mannitol salt agar. *Staphylococcus pyogenes* is sensitive to growth inhibition by bacitracin whereas *Staphylococcus agalactiae* (group B streptococci) is not.

11. **The correct answer is B.** Any time you see the development of diarrhea in the same question stem with "treated with antibiotics," you should immediately think of pseudomembranous colitis. This condition is caused by *Clostridium difficile* and typically occurs as a result of treatment with clindamycin or ampicillin. You would confirm your suspicion by sending a stool culture to be tested for the presence of the *C. difficile* toxin.

The most test-worthy side effect of chloramphenicol (**choice A**) is aplastic anemia, not diarrhea. In addition, you might have been able to eliminate this choice simply because of the extremely low probability that this patient would receive this antibiotic in the U.S.

The key side effects of gentamicin (**choice C**) include ototoxicity and nephrotoxicity.

Metronidazole (**choice D**) and vancomycin (**choice E**) do not cause pseudomembranous colitis; they are used to *treat* it.

12. **The correct answer is A.** Transplant rejection can be hyperacute (within minutes to hours), acute (usually within days, although it may appear later), or chronic (appearing 4-6 months after transplantation). Most acute rejection reactions are controlled, to some extent, by immunosuppressive therapy, so chronic rejection is more commonly seen. The patient described in this question is experiencing gradual renal failure over months, suggesting chronic rejection of the renal allograft. A renal biopsy from a patient experiencing chronic rejection typically shows intimal fibrosis in the vessels with fibrosis and tubular atrophy in the renal interstitium. Glomeruli may show ischemic changes, or may appear normal.

Linear deposition of immunoglobulin and complement in glomeruli (**choice B**) is a feature of Goodpasture syndrome (not a transplant rejection syndrome).

Neutrophils, immunoglobulin, and complement in blood vessels walls (**choice C**) are typical of hyperacute rejection, due to previous sensitization to an antigen found in the transplant.

A T-cell infiltrate (both CD4- and CD8-positive T cells) with interstitial edema (**choice D**) and hemorrhage characterizes acute cell-mediated rejection of an allograft. It would occur in a shorter time than that mentioned in this vignette.

Intimal thickening of vessels (**choice E**) due to proliferation of fibroblasts, myocytes, and foamy macrophages is a feature of subacute vasculitis, a common form of acute rejection generally seen in the first few months after transplantation.

13. **The correct answer is D.** This patient has *Klebsiella* pneumonia, caused by a gram-negative bacillus. Gram-negative organisms stain pinkish red, whereas gram-positive organisms stain a bluish color. This question requires you to appreciate the key structural difference between gram-positive and gram-negative microorganisms. Gram-negatives have a more complex cell envelope than gram-positive microorganisms. It includes both a cytoplasmic membrane and an outer membrane. Between these two membranes is the periplasmic space, which contains enzymes such as phosphatase and penicillinase, binding proteins for the transport of various nutrients, and peptidoglycan, as well as a portion of the lipoprotein that firmly anchors the outer membrane to the peptidoglycan. Gram-positives do not have outer membranes.

Choice A, the cell envelope, is incorrect because both gram-positive and gram-negative microorganisms have this structure, which is defined as all the layers that enclose the cytosol of the bacterium. It is the composition of the envelope that differs between gram-positive and gram-negative micro-organisms.

Choice B, exotoxins, are not exclusively produced by gram-negative microorganisms, but are also produced by some gram-positives. By contrast, endotoxin (lipopolysaccharide; LPS) is found exclusively in gram-negatives; it is an integral constituent of the outer membrane.

Choice C, peptidoglycan, is found in the cell walls of both gram-positive and gram-negative microorganisms. Note that there is a larger amount of peptidoglycan in gram-positive microorganisms.

Choice E, teichoic acids, are found exclusively in gram-positive organisms.

14. **The correct answer is D.** This is one of the "higher order" questions the USMLE favors. In this case, you need to figure out which disease the child has, which organism causes the disease, and which of the listed features is true of the microorganism. The disease in question is post-streptococcal glomerulonephritis, as evidenced by the smoky urine, hypertension, edema, and red blood cell casts in the urine sediment. The history of the prior sore throat is a tip-off that this is a nonsuppurative sequela of an infection due to *Streptococcus pyogenes* (group A β-hemolytic streptococci). *S. pyogenes* can be differentiated from *Streptococcus pneumoniae* and viridans streptococci by its hemolytic pattern; it is beta-hemolytic, whereas the

others are alpha-hemolytic (**choice A**). It can be distinguished from the other beta-hemolytic streptococci by its sensitivity to the antibiotic bacitracin. Other important things to remember about *S. pyogenes* are its many virulence factors, including M protein, antiphagocytic capsule, hyaluronidase, streptolysins O and S, and erythrogenic toxins.

Choice B is incorrect because streptococci are catalase-negative, whereas staphylococci are catalase-positive.

Choice C is incorrect because *S. pyogenes* is coagulase-negative. (In fact, there is no reason to perform a coagulase test on a catalase-negative organism.) The coagulase test is an important means of differentiating *Staphylococcus aureus*, which is coagulase-positive, from all other species of *Staphylococcus*, which are coagulase-negative. The only other medically important coagulase-positive organism is *Yersinia pestis*.

Choice E is incorrect because optochin is used to differentiate the viridans streptococci (resistant) from *S. pneumoniae* (sensitive).

15. **The correct answer is A.** IL-1 is produced by macrophages and other antigen-presenting cells. It is frequently called the endogenous pyrogen because of its direct effect on the hypothalamus. Other actions include stimulation of T cells to secrete IL-2, chemotactic activity for neutrophils and monocytes, increased expression of intercellular adhesion molecules (ICAMs) on vascular endothelial cells, and activation of macrophages and natural killer (NK) cells.

IL-2 (**choice B**) is produced by activated T helper cells. It stimulates the proliferation of other T cells as well as activated B cells. It also activates NK cells and stimulates lymphokine secretion.

IL-3 (**choice C**) stimulates all stem cells to produce hematopoietic cells; it is also know as multilineage colony stimulating factor (CSF).

IL-4 (**choice D**) is produced by T helper 2 (Th2) cells and mast cells. It has several functions, including inducing cells to express class II major histocompatibility complex (MHC) antigens and stimulation of B-cell proliferation. It is involved in the induction of atopic allergies by its mitogenic activity for mast cells and its enhancement of immunoglobulin class switching to IgG and IgE. (Note that IL-5 is involved in class switching to IgA.)

IL-5 (**choice E**) is secreted by activated T helper cells. It promotes B-cell proliferation and stimulates B-cell class switching to IgA.

IL-6 (**choice F**) is produced by T helper cells and macrophages. It stimulates the production of immunoglobulins and acute-phase reactants.

IL-7 (**choice G**) is produced in the bone marrow and secreted by thymic stromal cells. It stimulates pre-B cells, thymocytes, and mature T cells.

IL-8 (**choice H**) is produced by macrophages. It stimulates chemotaxis and adhesion of neutrophils.

IL-10 (**choice I**) is produced by a subset of T helper cells (Th2). It stimulates Th2 cells while inhibiting the growth of Th1 cells (which synthesize interferon and TNF-β).

IL-12 (**choice J**) is produced by B cells and macrophages. It activates NK cells and induces the differentiation of T helper (Th) cells into Th1 cells that can secrete IL-2 and interferon.

16. **The correct answer is B.** The three major causes of neonatal meningitis are group B streptococci (*Streptococcus agalactiae*; **choice D**), *Escherichia coli* (**choice A**), and *Listeria monocytogenes*. All can be found in the vaginal tract of normal women and may contaminate the infant during passage through the birth canal. They colonize the upper respiratory tract and can cause pneumonia, septicemia, and/or meningitis in the neonate. They are readily distinguished on morphologic grounds; the streptococci are gram-positive cocci in chains, *E. coli* is a gram-negative rod, and *L. monocytogenes* is a gram-positive pleomorphic rod. There are other gram-positive rods that resemble *Listeria* (e.g., the diphtheroid bacilli found in the upper respiratory tract and on the skin); hence, a motility test is done to confirm the identification. *L. monocytogenes* is motile at room temperature but not when grown at 37.0 C. *L. monocytogenes* is also associated with drinking unpasteurized milk.

    *Neisseria meningitidis* (**choice C**) is the most common cause of meningitis in school-aged children and young adults. It is a fastidious, nonmotile, gram-negative diplococcus that would be a very rare cause of meningeal disease in very young patients, such as this one.

    *Streptococcus pneumoniae* (**choice E**) is a gram-positive coccus that grows in pairs and short chains. It is the number one cause of pneumonia, septicemia, and meningitis in the elderly. It would not be a common cause of neonatal meningitis.

17. **The correct answer is A.** This question relates to a USMLE favorite side effect—the teeth mottling that occurs when a child is exposed to tetracycline *in utero*. You should remember that tetracycline is contraindicated in pregnancy and early childhood. Tetracycline is a bacteriostatic drug that binds to the 30s subunit of ribosomes, preventing aminoacyl-tRNA from binding with complementary mRNA. This inhibits peptide bond synthesis. Resistance is plasmid-mediated.

Inhibition of peptidyl transferase (**choice B**) occurs with chloramphenicol, a broad-spectrum bacteriostatic agent that binds to the 50s subunit of ribosomes. Resistance is plasmid mediated. It has high toxicity (gastrointestinal disturbances, aplastic anemia, and gray baby syndrome), so it is used mainly in severe infections or as a topical agent.

Interference with cell wall synthesis (**choice C**) occurs with penicillins and cephalosporins, the beta-lactam antibiotics. Resistance to these drugs appears in organisms that have developed beta-lactamases (penicillinases), enzymes that destroy the beta-lactam ring of these medications. The wider spectrum ampicillin, amoxicillin, ticarcillin, and carbenicillin are particularly penicillinase-susceptible.

Large, cyclic, lactone-ring structures (**choice D**) describe the macrolides: erythromycin, azithromycin, and clarithromycin. They inhibit bacterial protein synthesis by reacting with the 50s ribosomal subunit and preventing the release of the uncharged tRNA. Resistance is plasmid-mediated. Common side effects include gastrointestinal irritation, skin rashes, and eosinophilia. Erythromycin is a popular choice for patients with penicillin hypersensitivity. It is a cytochrome P450 inhibitor and therefore must be used with caution in patients taking other drugs.

18. **The correct answer is E.** Transformation is the process by which free DNA may be taken up and incorporated into the genome of competent bacteria. Because the original culture obviously had the genetic coding for capsule production when it was allowed to progress into the decline or death phase of the growth curve and subjected to treatment with a DNAse, those bacteria served as the source of free DNA. If "competent" bacteria (those capable of binding free DNA to their surface and importing it) are exposed to free DNA, and if it can be incorporated into the genome by homologous recombination, then the recipient bacteria may become capable of expressing new genetic traits; in this case, capsule production.

Conjugation (**choice A**) is a process of genetic exchange that requires cell-to-cell contact between living bacteria. Because the question stem refers to the death of the original encapsulated culture followed by the use of an "extract" from that culture to treat the second, nonencapsulated culture, it is unlikely that conjugation is being described. In addition, conjugation is the most common means of genetic exchange in the gram-negative bacilli, and the bacteria described in the question stem are gram-positive cocci.

Lysogeny (**choice B**) would not achieve the transfer of a genetic trait from a dead and disrupted bacterial culture extract to a living bacterium. Lysogeny is the state of stable association between bacterial and phage DNA that occurs in the life cycle of a temperate phage. Lysogeny is a necessary first step in the process of specialized transduction, and lysogenic conversion of bacteria gives bacteria the capacity to produce the O antigen (*Salmonella*), the botulinum toxin (*Clostridium botulinum*), the erythrogenic exotoxins (*Streptococcus pyogenes*), and the diphtheria toxin (*Corynebacterium diphtheriae*).

Site-specific recombination (**choice C**) is an intracellular process that allows the incorporation of foreign, circular DNA into the bacterial chromosome. It occurs when plasmids are recombined into the chromosome to form episomes (as in the Hfr cell), when transposons move from one location to another inside a cell, and when temperate phages infect bacterial chromosomes during the process of lysogeny. It is the bacterial analogy of the mechanism by which the human immunodeficiency virus infects the chromosomes of the human host. Because the DNA in this question stem was disrupted by DNAse, it is in linear, not circular form, and because it is from encapsulated *S. agalactiae*, it is not foreign, but homologous, DNA. Thus, in the process described, homologous recombination would be the final step to stabilize the new DNA, not site-specific recombination.

Transduction (**choice D**) is the process by which genetic information is transferred from one bacterium to another by a virus vector. There are two types of transduction: generalized (an accident of the life cycle of a lytic phage) and specialized (a DNA excision error in the life cycle of a temperate phage). Because the question stem does not mention the presence of any viruses, transduction can be ruled out as a possible mechanism.

19. **The correct answer is E.** The disease described is measles (rubeola), which has the typical presentation described in the question stem. Measles is caused by a Morbillivirus, an RNA virus belonging to the Paramyxovirus family. Koplik's spots, which are pathognomonic for measles, are small, bluish-white spots on the buccal mucosa in the early stages of measles. These lesions appear just before the onset of the characteristic rash (which can also involve the extremities) and fade as the rash develops.

Leukoplakia is a premalignant condition characterized by adherent whitish patches on the gingiva (**choice A**) and other sites in the oral cavity.

Cold sores of the lips (**choice B**) are due to infection with herpesviruses.

*Candida* infection (thrush) produces curdy white material loosely attached to an erythematous base (**choice C**).

Aphthous ulcers are large shallow ulcers of the oral mucosa (**choice D**), commonly known as canker sores.

20. **The correct answer is D.** Abscesses are often caused by *Staphylococcus aureus.* This organism may produce a penicillinase, an enzyme that cleaves the amide bond of beta-lactam antibiotics (the molecule shown is penicillin). The enzyme thus confers resistance to the beta-lactam antibiotics (penicillins and cephalosporins). Nafcillin (a semisynthetic penicillin) is very effective against penicillinase-producing *S. aureus.*

You should be familiar with other important enzymes and toxins produced by this organism, including heat-resistant enterotoxin, toxic shock syndrome toxin, exfoliatin (causes scalded-skin syndrome in children), alpha toxin (kills leukocytes), and coagulase.

21. **The correct answer is E.** The difficulty with developing a vaccine against influenza A arises because the influenza virus genome is composed of eight segments of single-stranded RNA. Minor shifts (antigenic drift) in surface antigens occur as point mutations in the genes accumulate. However, influenza A can also undergo larger, abrupt changes in antigen expression (antigenic shift) as a consequence of reassortment of some of the RNA fragments between human and non-human hosts. Thus, last year's vaccine does not necessarily work against this year's virus.

Polysaccharide coats (**choice A**) are a virulence factor of some bacteria, not of viruses.

Influenza A can compromise the lungs sufficiently to predispose to secondary infections, producing a functional immunosuppression (**choice B**), but this attribute does not make it difficult to produce vaccines against the virus.

Unlike AIDS, influenza virus does not selectively target lymphocytes (**choice C**).

Influenza A, coated with antibody and complement, can be effectively phagocytized (compare with **choice D**).

22. **The correct answer is A.** *Bacillus cereus* contaminates grains, such as rice, and produces spores resistant to quick frying and steaming. If you see the words "fried rice" on the USMLE, the odds are that the correct answer is *B. cereus.* The other most important clue for this etiology would be an onset of symptoms 1 to 2 hours after eating.

*Campylobacter jejuni* (**choice B**) causes enterocolitis with bloody diarrhea, crampy abdominal pain, malaise, and fever.

*Clostridium botulinum* (**choice C**) produces a constellation of signs and symptoms, including bulbar palsy, descending weakness or paralysis, progressive respiratory weakness, absence of fever, dry mucous membranes, and autonomic dysfunction.

*Clostridium difficile* (**choice D**) causes pseudomembranous colitis, classically resulting from clindamycin use.

*Escherichia coli* (**choice E**) comes in a variety of forms. The enterotoxigenic type is the most common cause of traveler's diarrhea.

Norwalk agent (**choice F**) is a common cause of epidemic viral diarrhea in adults.

Rotavirus (**choice G**) is the most common cause of diarrhea in children.

*Salmonella typhi* (**choice H**) causes typhoid fever.

*Shigella dysenteriae* (**choice I**) causes bacillary dysentery, characterized by abdominal cramps and bloody diarrhea. The feces contain polymorphonuclear leukocytes and mucus.

*Vibrio parahaemolyticus* (**choice J**) commonly causes food poisoning after ingestion of raw or improperly handled seafood.

*Yersinia pestis* (**choice K**) causes several forms of plague (bubonic, septicemic, and pneumonic).

23. **The correct answer is C.** The presence of sickle cell disease in a question stem is usually a significant clue. This question tests whether you know that patients with sickle cell anemia are more susceptible to osteomyelitis caused by *Salmonella*. (The patient's fever, bone pain, and x-ray results indicate osteomyelitis). *Staphylococcus aureus* (gram-positive coccus) is the most common cause of osteomyelitis overall, but 80% of osteomyelitis cases in sickle cell patients are caused by *Salmonella*. If *Staphylococcus aureus* had not been ruled out on bone culture, you should have looked for it in the answer choices. Notice that you were required to know more than just the organism's name; you needed to know its distinguishing features. **Choice C** describes *Salmonella* (a gram-negative rod) accurately. *Salmonella* exists in more than 1800 serotypes and is known to contaminate poultry.

A comma-shaped organism that is sensitive to acidic pH (**choice A**) is *Vibrio cholerae*, a gram-negative rod that causes severe enterotoxin-induced diarrhea, with "rice-water" stools and dehydration. The toxin acts by stimulating adenylyl cyclase to overproduce cAMP in the brush border of the small intestine.

A facultative intracellular parasite (**choice B**) could be any one of a number of organisms. Facultative intracellular organisms survive inside cells when endocytosed but are capable of being grown on cell-free media. Examples include *Legionella* and *Listeria*.

A motile and oxidase positive organism (**choice D**) is *Pseudomonas*, a gram-negative rod that produces a polysaccharide slime layer. *P. aeruginosa* is the prototype and commonly colonizes the lungs of patients with cystic fibrosis. It is associated with production of blue-green pus because of its production of blue-green pigments.

A nonmotile, facultative anaerobe (**choice E**) could also be any of a number of organisms. The great majority of bacteria are facultative anaerobes, and of the gram-negative bacilli, *Shigella* and *Yersinia* would be examples of nonmotile genera.

24. **The correct answer is D.** This patient has cryptococcal meningitis, as evidenced by the "encapsulated organisms observable with India ink" in the CSF (a classic clue). *Cryptococcus* is a nondimorphic yeast, i.e., it exists only in the yeast form. Its capsule can be highlighted with India ink, and it reproduces by budding. It is found worldwide in bird droppings. It can also cause transient pulmonary illness in otherwise healthy individuals exposed to massive environmental doses.

The methenamine silver stain (**choice A**) is used primarily to demonstrate *Pneumocystis carinii* in tissues.

Branching septate hyphae (**choice B**) are characteristic of *Aspergillus fumigatus*, among other fungi.

Mycoses that exist in mycelial and yeast forms (dimorphic, diphasic; **choice C**) are *Histoplasma capsulatum*, *Coccidioides immitis*, *Blastomyces dermatitidis*, and *Sporothrix schenckii*.

*Cryptococcus neoformans* is not dimorphic and has a capsule (**choice E**).

25. **The correct answer is F.** *Histoplasma capsulatum* is a fungus common in soil contaminated with bird or bat droppings, especially in the Mississippi and Ohio River Valleys. Infection is usually asymptomatic or is associated with only mild symptoms; however, both the quantity inhaled and the immune status of the host determine the degree of symptoms.

*Actinomyces israelii* (**choice A**) is a branching, gram-positive rod that is part of the normal flora of the oral cavity. It can invade across fascial planes to produce abscesses with draining sinus tracts.

*Aspergillus fumigatus* (**choice B**) is a monomorphic fungus that is an opportunistic pathogen, especially in neutropenics.

*Candida albicans* (**choice C**) is part of the normal flora in humans and can be an opportunistic pathogen if there is a defect in cell-mediated immunity.

*Coccidioides immitis* (**choice D**) is a pathogenic fungus that can cause pneumonia if inhaled. Resolution occurs with the development of T-cell-mediated immunity. If this response is not raised, persistent or disseminated infection can occur. Pregnant women and individuals of African and Asian descent are at increased risk of disseminated infection. *C. immitis* is limited to the southwestern U.S. and northern Mexico.

*Cryptococcus neoformans* (**choice E**) is a fungal pathogen that causes meningitis.

*Nocardia asteroides* (**choice G**) is an aerobic, gram-positive rod that primarily causes infections in immunosuppressed patients.

*Sporothrix schenckii* (**choice H**) is a fungal pathogen that causes subcutaneous abscesses following direct inoculation from a plant source.

26. **The correct answer is E.** The child most likely has chronic granulomatous disease (CGD), which results in recurrent staphylococcal infections (such as abscesses and furuncles) and an increased incidence of pneumonia due to *Serratia marcescens*. Organisms that cause recurrent infections in CGD patients are those that are catalase-positive. Neutrophils are unable to generate bacteria-killing superoxide radicals because of a lack of NADPH oxidase. Patients with CGD are susceptible to chronic infections with catalase-positive organisms.

Aldolase B (**choice A**) cleaves fructose-1-phosphate to glyceraldehyde and dihydroxyacetone. Deficiency of aldolase B can produce hereditary fructose intolerance.

Galactokinase (**choice B**) phosphorylates galactose prior to the sugar's entry into the glycolytic pathway; deficiency of this enzyme can produce galactosemia.

Glucokinase (**choice C**) and hexokinase catalyze the first reaction in glycolysis. Their deficiency is not usually described, probably because these enzymes are so necessary that a significant deficiency would be incompatible with life.

Glucose-6-phosphate dehydrogenase (**choice D**) is the enzyme that starts the hexose monophosphate shunt; its deficiency causes a hemolytic anemia.

27. **The correct answer is B.** The patient likely has a candidal infection of the prosthetic aortic valve. That is why she did not respond favorably to antibacterial therapy, which is known to promote fungal infection. Note that *Candida* tends to colonize foreign bodies, such as IV and Foley catheters, prosthetic valves, and ventricular shunts.

*Actinomyces israelii* (**choice A**) is known to cause cervicofacial infections in patients undergoing dental work. It is an anaerobe and would not favor an infection site in the bloodstream. It is the only bacterium on the list and is therefore least likely to be encouraged by a regimen of antibiotic therapy.

*Histoplasma capsulatum* (**choice C**) causes histoplasmosis, a pulmonary infection common in the midwestern river valleys. Multi-organ involvement is usually seen only in the immunocompromised. Transmission of the organism occurs through the inhalation of airborne microconidia (infectious spores). The organism is found in bird and bat droppings and in the soil.

*Nocardia asteroides* (**choice D**) is an aerobic filamentous bacterium that causes a chronic lobar pneumonia that may metastasize to the brain. It is more common in immunocompromised patients. It is found in soil and aquatic environments.

*Trichophyton rubrum* (**choice E**) is one of the organisms that commonly produce a variety of cutaneous mycoses, including tinea corporis (ringworm), tinea cruris (jock itch), and tinea pedis (athlete's foot).

28. **The correct answer is C.** Graft-versus-host disease is a feared complication of transplants of immunocompetent tissues from nonidentical (allogeneic) donors. It is thought to be caused by the transplantation of immuno-competent T cells, which attack the host tissues. Elevation of alkaline phosphatase and bilirubin commonly occurs in this disorder. The fever and rash are also characteristic, as is the diarrhea observed in this patient.

Bacterial infection (**choice A**) might produce fever and diarrhea but would be unlikely to produce isolated elevations of alkaline phosphatase and bilirubin.

A blast crisis (**choice B**) would be unlikely, since high-dose whole body irradiation generally destroys the viable stem cells in the bone marrow.

Hyperacute graft rejection (**choice D**) is generally due to the presence of preformed antibody or prior exposure to an antigen (e.g., a prior transfusion or transplant from the donor), which is not suggested by the history in this case.

The symptoms described are not consistent with whole-body radiation toxicity (**choice E**), although diarrhea and skin changes would likely occur.

29. **The correct answer is E.** The combination of optochin sensitivity and positive Quellung reaction is characteristic of a single organism, *Streptococcus pneumoniae*. The other encapsulated organisms that have Quellung-positive reactions are *Haemophilus influenzae* (**choice B**), *Neisseria meningitidis*, and *Klebsiella pneumoniae* (**choice C**). However, none of these organisms are optochin-sensitive.

The other choices, *Escherichia coli* (**choice A**) and *Neisseria gonorrhoeae* (**choice D**), are not encapsulated.

30. **The correct answer is B.** The precipitation lines joined between Wells 1 and 2 are called a chevron, which is formed by anti-A antibody in Well 3 reacting with epitope A in Wells 1 and 2. The "spur" on the precipitation line at Well 1 that is pointing toward Well 2 is formed by anti-B antibody reacting with epitope B in Well 1. Anti-B antibody migrates right through the precipitation line formed by anti-A antibody because there is no epitope B in Well 2 for the anti-B antibody to react with.

31. **The correct answer is C.** *Salmonella* spp., including *S. enteritidis* and *S. typhimurium*, produce a gastroenteritis or enterocolitis. Patients with decreased gastric acidity, sickle cell disease, or defects in immunity, and children younger than 4 years have a more severe course of disease. *Salmonella* spp. are carried in nature by animal reservoirs such as poultry, turtles, cattle, pigs, and sheep. The incubation period is 8 to 48 hours after ingestion of contaminated food or water.

*Chlamydia psittaci* (**choice A**) produces an interstitial pneumonitis accompanied by headache, backache, and a dry, hacking cough. A pale, macular rash is also found on the trunk (Horder's spots). Patients at risk include pet shop workers, pigeon handlers, and poultry workers.

*Entamoeba histolytica* (**choice B**) produces a diarrhea (frequently bloody or heme-positive), right lower quadrant crampy abdominal pain, and fever. Patients frequently have weight loss and anorexia. There is usually a history of travel outside the U.S. Most cases are chronic. Complications include liver abscesses.

*Staphylococcus aureus* (**choice D**) produces a self-limited gastroenteritis due to the production of preformed, heat-stable enterotoxins. The incubation period is 2 to 16 hours. The toxins enhance intestinal peristalsis and induce vomiting by a direct effect on the CNS.

*Yersinia enterocolitica* (**choice E**) usually produces a chronic enteritis in children. These patients have diarrhea, failure to thrive, hypoalbuminemia, and hypokalemia. Other findings include acute right lower quadrant abdominal pain, tenderness, nausea, and vomiting. The infection mimics appendicitis or Crohn disease.

32. **The correct answer is B.** Infection with hepatitis B virus (HBV) at birth or a very young age is associated with chronic HBV infection and the development of hepatocellular carcinoma later in life. In fact, infants born to hepatitis B surface antigen (HBsAg)-positive mothers are commonly infected, and approximately 90% become chronic carriers of the virus. In chronic carriers, hepatocellular carcinoma develops at an incidence more than 200 times higher than in noncarriers. The current recommendation for infants born of HBsAg-positive mothers is administration of hepatitis B immunoglobulin (HBIg) in the delivery room, with the first dose of the hepatitis B vaccine given at the same time or within 1 week. The second and third doses of the vaccine are then given at 1 and 6 months. With this protocol, 94% protection is achieved.

The Epstein-Barr virus (EBV; **choice A**) is the agent of heterophile-positive infectious mononucleosis. In children, primary EBV infection is often asymptomatic.

The measles virus (**choice C**) often causes a more severe disease in adults. The incidence of complications, including pneumonia, bacterial superinfection of the respiratory tract, bronchospasm, and hepatitis, is much higher in adults older than 20 than in children.

Poliovirus (**choice D**) causes asymptomatic or inapparent infections 95% of the time. Frank paralysis occurs in approximately 0.1% of all poliovirus infections. However, the probability of paralysis increases with increasing age.

Varicella zoster virus (**choice E**) is the agent of chickenpox and shingles. In immunocompetent children, it is a benign illness with a mortality of less than 2 per 100,000 cases. This risk is increased more than 15-fold in adults. Much of the increase is due to varicella pneumonitis, a complication that occurs more frequently in adults.

33. **The correct answer is A.** This patient has hereditary angioedema, which is caused by deficiency of C1 esterase inhibitor. Patients experience acute episodes of localized edema and colic. Stridor may occur because of airway obstruction due to laryngeal edema, the most dreaded complication of this condition. The disease is inherited as an autosomal dominant trait, explaining this patient's positive family history. Administration of epsilon-aminocaproate, an inhibitor of plasmin activation of C1, reduces the frequency of the episodes.

C3b inactivator (**choice B**) inhibits enzymes of the complement system.

Factor H (**choice C**) binds to C3b and C3b-containing convertases, precluding the binding of C3b to B. This interrupts the alternative pathway. Factor H also results in the dissociation of C3b from the Bb in the C3 and C5 convertases.

Carboxypeptidase (**choice D**) is a hydrolase that removes amino acids from the free carboxyl group at the end of a polypeptide chain.

Properdin (**choice E**) functions in the alternative pathway and recognizes a large range of microorganisms. Properdin places C3b on the microbial membrane, even in the absence of a specific antibody.

| RNA viruses | Examples |
|---|---|
| Picornaviruses | Polioviruses, echoviruses, coxsackie viruses, rhinoviruses, hepatitis A |
| Orthomyxoviruses | Influenza viruses |
| Paramyxoviruses | Rubeola virus, mumps virus, respiratory syncytial virus, parainfluenza viruses |
| Togaviruses | Equine encephalitis, rubella |
| Flaviviruses | Yellow fever, Dengue fever, hepatitis C, St. Louis encephalitis, Japanese encephalitis |
| Bunyaviruses | California encephalitis, hantavirus |
| Rhabdoviruses | Rabies |
| Coronaviruses | Common cold |
| Caliciviruses | Norwalk agent, hepatitis E |
| Arenaviruses | Lymphocytic choriomeningitis, Lassa fever |
| Filoviruses | Marburg, Ebola |
| Reoviruses | Rotaviruses, orbiviruses |
| Retroviruses | HIV, HTLV |

| DNA viruses | Examples |
|---|---|
| Hepadnavirus | Hepatitis B |
| Adenoviruses | Colds, diarrhea, conjunctivitis, pneumonia, flu-like syndromes |
| Papovaviruses | Human papillomavirus, BK, JC, SV40 |
| Herpesviruses | Herpes simplex I and II, Epstein-Barr, varicella-zoster, cytomegalovirus |
| Poxviruses | Smallpox, molluscum contagiosum |
| Parvoviruses | Erythema infectiosum |

34. **The correct answer is D.** The patient died of rabies, caused by a rhabdovirus. Rabies infects the nervous system, causing extraordinary excitability, extreme thirst, pharyngeal spasms, and eventually death due to respiratory failure. Negri bodies (intracytoplasmic eosinophilic inclusions) are considered pathognomonic. It's a challenge to remember all the different viruses, but the tables on this page should help.

35. **The correct answer is B.** Type II hypersensitivity occurs when antibodies react with antigens present on the surface of cells or other tissue components. It is conveniently subclassified into diseases produced by distinct mechanisms. One mechanism involves complement fixation by the antibody-antigen complex, which causes lysis or phagocytosis of the affected cell. This mechanism occurs in transfusion reactions, erythroblastosis fetalis, autoimmune hemolytic anemia, agranulocytosis, or thrombocytopenia. In some cases, target cells coated with low levels of IgG are lysed (extracellularly) by monocytes, neutrophils, eosinophils, or natural killer cells; this mechanism is thought to operate in the destruction of large parasites, and possibly some tumor cells, and in graft rejection. Another mechanism involves antibody-mediated cellular dysfunction, such as occurs in Graves disease or myasthenia gravis.

Allergic rhinitis (**choice A**) is an example of type I (allergic or anaphylactic) hypersensitivity.

Food allergy (**choice C**) is an example of type I (anaphylactic) hypersensitivity.

Serum sickness (**choice D**) is an example of type III (immune complex diseases) hypersensitivity.

Tuberculosis (**choice E**) is an example of type IV (cell-mediated or delayed) hypersensitivity.

36. **The correct answer is D.** *Mycoplasma pneumoniae* is a wall-less bacterium that causes interstitial pneumonia in young adults. Elevated cold agglutinins (a classic clue) are found in about half the patients. The cold agglutinins are IgM antibodies. *M. pneumoniae* may be diagnosed by sputum or complement fixation.

    *Haemophilus* (**choice A**) causes bronchopneumonia in infants and children and may occur in debilitated adults.

    *Klebsiella* (**choice B**) causes a bronchopneumonia with patchy infiltrates involving one or more lobes. The cough is productive, and the sputum is bright red and gelatinous. It frequently occurs in debilitated patients, diabetics, and alcoholics. Note that these organisms are highly encapsulated and produce mucoid colonies on laboratory media.

    *Legionella* (**choice C**) lives in contaminated water sources such as air conditioning systems. It causes an atypical pneumonia, most serious in elderly male smokers with high alcohol intake. It is not associated with cold agglutinin production.

    *Streptococcus pneumoniae* (**choice E**) is the most common cause of pneumonia in the elderly population and in those with poor nutrition. It causes abscesses, productive cough, and rusty-colored sputum.

37. **The correct answer is D.** Rubella, also called German measles or 3-day measles, is a disease caused by a Togavirus, which is a small, enveloped, single-stranded, (+) linear RNA virus. Approximately 40% of patients are asymptomatic or have mild symptoms. In symptomatic patients, the clinical presentation typically consists of an erythematous rash that begins on the head and spreads downward to involve the trunk, and lasts for approximately 3 days. In addition to a transient rash, symptoms include fever, posterior cervical lymphadenopathy, and arthralgias. The greatest danger from rubella is to the fetus. If clinical rubella develops or seroconversion is demonstrated, there is a high risk of congenital abnormalities or spontaneous abortion. The risk varies from 40 to 60% if infection occurs during the first 2 months of gestation to 10% by the 4th month. Women of childbearing age should be warned not to become pregnant within 2 to 3 months from the time of immunization. Mild arthralgias and other symptoms may develop in 25% of immunized women. Enteroviral rashes may mimic rubella and rubeola.

    Infectious mononucleosis (**choice A**) is caused by the Epstein-Barr virus, a herpesvirus. Classic findings include fever, exudative pharyngitis, generalized lymphadenopathy, severe malaise (most common complaint), and hepatosplenomegaly. A rash is not a characteristic feature unless the patient has been treated with ampicillin.

    Lyme disease (**choice B**) is caused by the spirochete *Borrelia burgdorferi*. The disease is transmitted by the bite of the tick *Ixodes dammini*. Reservoirs in nature include the white-tailed deer and the white-footed mouse. The initial lesion is an annular rash with central clearing and a raised red border (erythema chronicum migrans) at the bite site. The rash is warm, but not painful or itchy. Patients also have fever, malaise, myalgias, arthralgias, headache, generalized lymphadenopathy, and, occasionally, neurologic findings.

    Roseola (**choice C**) is caused by human herpesvirus 6. Other names include exanthem subitum or sixth disease. Children have a febrile period of 3 to 5 days with rapid defervescence followed by an erythematous maculopapular rash lasting 1 to 3 days.

    Rubeola (**choice E**), or regular measles, is a disease caused by a paramyxovirus. Patients present with an upper respiratory prodrome and characteristic oral lesions (Koplik's spots) that precede the rash. The nonpruritic maculopapular rash begins on the face and spreads to the trunk and extremities, including palms and soles. The incubation period is 10 to 14 days. Patients also have a posterior cervical lymphadenopathy. The virus is not associated with risk to a fetus.

38. **The correct answer is B.** This is a multistep microbiology question that requires you to diagnose the illness, identify the microorganism, and remember its key feature. The first part should be easy: everything about this vignette suggests toxic shock syndrome. The organism in question is therefore *Staphylococcus aureus*, which is coagulase-positive. All the other choices are classic features of other important pathogenic microorganisms:

    Acid-fast organisms (**choice A**) are associated with mycobacteria. (In addition, *Nocardia* species are partially acid-fast.)

    EMB agar (**choice C**) refers to a selective and differential medium used to isolate and identify enteric gram-negative bacteria. Gram-positive bacteria will not grow on EMB agar because the addition of eosin inhibits their growth. Nonlactose fermenters will have colorless colonies; fermentation of this sugar will cause the colonies to appear pink or purple.

    Thayer-Martin media (**choice D**) can be used for pathogenic *Neisseria* species. This growth medium contains the antibiotic vancomycin, which kills gram-positive organisms such as *Staphylococcus aureus*.

    The Quellung reaction (**choice E**) can be used to identify the capsule type of a microorganism. Encapsulated microorganisms, like the pneumococci and *Haemophilus*, are mixed with specific antisera. If the antibodies recognize the microorganism's capsule type, the capsule will swell.

39. **The correct answer is A.** Generalized transduction is the process by which a phage (bacterial virus) with a lytic life cycle can mistakenly incorporate pieces of the genomic DNA of a bacterium into its capsid and transfer that trait to a new bacterium it infects. The virus "delivers" the bacterial DNA from one bacterium to another, and the newly transferred DNA must be stabilized by the process of homologous recombination. In this way, DNA that had encoded a mutant penicillin-binding protein from the chromosome of the penicillin-resistant strain was accidentally picked up by the lytic phage and delivered to the penicillin-sensitive bacteria. Those that successfully incorporated the mutant DNA were transduced to become penicillin-resistant.

Mobilization of transposons (**choice B**) is a process of movement of segments of mobile DNA within a bacterial cell. Transposons require no presence of virus and do not mediate the transfer of traits from one bacterium to another. Transposons can only be moved from cell to cell if the DNA they inhabit is transferred by conjugation, transformation, or transduction.

Site-specific recombination (**choice C**) is the process by which circular, foreign DNA molecules can be joined into the chromosome of the bacterial cell. It is a requirement of the process of specialized transduction, but does not occur in generalized transduction, as described in this question stem.

Specialized transduction (**choice D**) is the process by which a phage with a temperate life cycle accidentally carries a portion of the bacterial genome with it as it excises its DNA from the chromosome prior to leaving the cell. This accidentally excised bacterial DNA can then be delivered to another bacterium that the specialized transducing phage infects. In this case, the experiment stipulates that a lytic, not a temperate phage is added; so specialized transduction is not a possibility.

Transformation (**choice E**) is the process by which free DNA can be taken up and incorporated by bacteria competent to do so. In this experiment, free DNA is not mentioned, and addition of a phage is mentioned, so the process has to be either specialized or generalized transduction.

40. **The correct answer is A.** *Borrelia burgdorferi*, the tick-transmitted spirochete that causes Lyme disease, can be maintained in nature indefinitely by a tick vector. The tick, *Ixodes dammini*, or *I. pacificus* can infect both white-footed mice and large mammals, such as deer, during their life cycle, making these animals reservoirs.

However, the tick itself is a reservoir since it can acquire the disease through transovarial passage of the organism. Together, these factors make Lyme disease an endemic infection with little hope for eradication.

*B. burgdorferi* is a delicate spirochete that is vulnerable to a number of chemical and physical agents. It does not have a tough outer coat (unlike **choice B**).

Humans are incidental hosts, not primary reservoirs (**choice C**), for *B. burgdorferi*. The primary reservoirs are ticks, mice, and large mammals.

*B. burgdorferi* can be successfully treated with penicillins, tetracycline, and ceftriaxone (unlike **choice D**).

Brill-Zinsser disease (**choice E**) is actually the reactivation of epidemic typhus infection caused by *Rickettsia prowazekii*. It can occur many years after an infection that was not treated with antibiotics.

41. **The correct answer is C.** Ribavirin is an antiviral drug approved for the treatment of severe respiratory syncytial virus infection, the most common cause of pneumonia and bronchiolitis in children younger than 1 year. It should be given by aerosol.

Acyclovir (**choice A**) is a guanosine analog that is useful for the treatment of primary and recurrent herpes infections and herpes simplex virus encephalitis.

Ganciclovir (**choice B**) is a guanosine analog used in the treatment of cytomegalovirus retinitis and cytomegalovirus infections in AIDS patients.

Trifluorothymidine (**choice D**) is a thymidine analog used topically for the treatment of recurrent epithelial keratitis and primary keratoconjunctivitis due to herpes simplex viruses.

Zidovudine (**choice E**) is a thymidine analog that inhibits reverse transcriptase. It is active against human retroviruses, including HIV-1, HIV-2, and HTLV-I.

42. **The correct answer is D.** This infant is exhibiting passive immunity acquired from his mother *in utero*. IgG is the only class of immunoglobulins that can cross the placenta. As such, IgG molecules diffuse into the fetal circulation, providing immunity. This circulating maternal IgG protects the newborn during the first 4 to 6 months of life. Note that IgG is also capable of complement activation (a feature shared with IgM) and opsonization (unique to IgG).

IgA (**choice A**) functions in the secretory immune response. The secretory form of this immunoglobulin (sIgA) is found in tears, colostrum, saliva, breast milk, and other secretions. It is produced by the plasma cells in the lamina propria of the gastrointestinal, respiratory, and reproductive tracts.

IgD (**choice B**) functions as a cell surface antigen receptor, along with IgM monomers, on undifferentiated B cells. It does not reach appreciable plasma concentrations.

IgE (**choice C**) is involved in the allergic response and immediate hypersensitivity reactions. The Fc region of IgE binds to the surface of basophils and mast cells. Antigen cross-linking of two IgE molecules leads to mast cell degranulation and the release of leukotrienes, histamine, eosinophil chemotactic factors, and heparin.

IgM (**choice E**) is the first antibody detected in serum after exposure to antigen. IgM circulates as a pentamer and thus has five complement binding regions and ten antigen combining sites.

43. **The correct choice is B.** The presence of elevated ALT, HBsAg, anti-HBc, HBeAg, and bilirubin all point to active hepatitis B.

    An asymptomatic carrier (**choice A**) would not have elevated ALT and bilirubin.

    The absence of findings on physical examination rules out fulminant hepatitis B (**choice C**).

    Recovery from acute self-limited HBV (**choice D**) is associated with the presence of anti-HBs and absence of HBsAg and HBeAg.

    Someone who is vaccinated against HBV (**choice E**) has only anti-HBs in serum.

44. **The correct answer is B.** Tissue grafts in which the same individual acts as both the donor and recipient are termed autografts.

    Allografts (**choice A**) refer to tissue transplants from one person to another genetically different individual.

    Homograft (**choice C**) is not a word used in transplant medicine.

    Isografts (**choice D**) refer to tissue transplants between genetically identical individuals (e.g., an identical twin donates her kidney to her twin sister).

    Xenografts (**choice E**) refer to tissue transplants between species (e.g., baboon heart transplanted into a human).

45. **The correct answer is E.** While the commonly remembered association is that of inadequately cooked pork and trichinosis, the quality of purchased pork and the degree of cooking in this country are sufficiently high that pork-related trichinosis is quite uncommon. The more common scenario is actually the one described in the question stem, for two reasons. First, bear meat is not inspected, and it may often be served "rare," or relatively uncooked. The infected meat contains larvae that are released in the gastrointestinal tract after ingestion. The *Trichinella spiralis* larvae penetrate the intestinal mucosa and develop into adult worms in 30 to 40 hours.

After reaching adulthood, they mate, and the females produce larvae that grow to maturity and seek out muscle in which to encyst (often in the orbital muscles) within approximately 5 to 8 days. The intestinal production of larvae may last up to 2 months, but may be shorter. Treatment to remove adults from the intestine is with mebendazole, but most patients are unaware of infection at this point. There is no suitable larvicide. (If you didn't know the answer to this question, you still might have noticed the presence of eosinophilia, which should have clued you in to the presence of a parasitic infection, making trichinosis the only plausible answer.)

Anthrax (**choice A**) after eating bear meat is very unlikely. In addition, anthrax would not produce the described symptoms; instead, cutaneous lesions (95% of cases) or respiratory disease culminating in death (5% of cases; wool sorters disease) would occur.

*Bacillus cereus* food poisoning (**choice B**) and *Escherichia coli* gastroenteritis (**choice D**) might lead to similar gastrointestinal symptoms but would not cause the eye findings nor eosinophilia.

Botulism (**choice C**) causes flaccid paralysis, not the symptoms described here.

46. **The correct answer is J.** Many patients with *Yersinia enterocolitica* infection present with symptoms suggesting appendicitis (although constipation, rather than diarrhea, is common in appendicitis). Surgical exploration of the abdomen reveals mesenteric adenitis (involvement of the lymph nodes located in the mesentery), along with a normal appendix. Mesenteric adenitis is the tip-off that the patient has a *Y. enterocolitica* infection, and culture of the involved lymph nodes or of the stool is generally diagnostic.

    Following antibiotic use (e.g., clindamycin, ampicillin, or a third-generation cephalosporin), *Clostridium difficile* (**choice A**) may cause bloody diarrhea due to pseudomembranous colitis.

    Enterohemorrhagic *Escherichia coli* (EHEC; **choice B**) is the causative organism to suspect in a patient who develops severe, hemorrhagic, traveler's diarrhea with bleeding manifestations, hematuria, oliguria, and a microangiopathic hemolytic anemia. This bacteria produces verocytotoxin, which is responsible for the symptoms.

    Enteroinvasive *E. coli* (EIEC; **choice C**) causes fever, pain, diarrhea, and dysentery, usually following ingestion of contaminated cheese or water.

    Enteropathogenic *E. coli* (EPEC; **choice D**) causes a watery diarrhea in infants and toddlers secondary to ingestion of contaminated food or water.

Enterotoxigenic *E. coli* (ETEC; **choice E**) causes traveler's diarrhea, a watery diarrhea due to ingestion of contaminated food or water (**T**raveler's diarrhea = **ETEC** = **T**oxigenic *E. coli*).

Gastrointestinal tuberculosis (**choice F**) can be due either to ingestion of contaminated milk (normally prevented by pasteurization) or to swallowing of coughed-up organisms. It presents with cough, chronic abdominal pain, malabsorption, stricture, perforation, fistulas, and hemorrhage.

*Salmonella* (**choice G**) causes fever, pain, diarrhea, dysentery, bacteremia, and extraintestinal infections. It is commonly found in outbreaks due to a common contaminated food source (e.g., milk, beef, eggs, poultry).

*Shigella* (**choice H**) causes fever, pain, diarrhea, and dysentery in epidemics usually due to person-to-person spread.

*Vibrio cholerae* (**choice I**) causes cholera, characterized by watery, life-threatening diarrhea. It tends to spread in epidemics through third-world countries via contaminated water or shellfish.

47.  **The correct answer is C.** This patient has primary subacute bacterial peritonitis, which commonly occurs in patients with alcoholic cirrhosis and ascites. Gram-negative bacilli in the normal flora, such as *Escherichia coli*, are the most likely causative agents.

*Bacillus cereus* (**choice A**) is a spore-forming, gram-positive rod. Its spores may germinate in rewarmed rice, causing food poisoning. It is not a normal flora organism.

*Clostridium difficile* (**choice B**) is a gram-positive rod that causes antibiotic-associated colitis (pseudomembranous colitis). It exists as normal flora in 2 to 10% of humans and is not likely to be a *common* cause of this presentation.

*Entamoeba histolytica* (**choice D**) is an intestinal protozoan that is frequent in the tropics and is prevalent in homosexual men. The liver is the most common site of systemic infection. It is not a normal flora organism.

*Giardia lamblia* (**choice E**) causes giardiasis, which presents with diarrhea, cramps, bloating, flatulence, malaise, weight loss, and occasional steatorrhea. It is not a normal flora organism.

48.  **The correct answer is B.** The combination of repeated staphylococcal and streptococcal infections, normal phagocytic function, and normal delayed hypersensitivity responses is suggestive of Bruton hypogammaglobulinemia. The disease is characterized by an IgG level less than 100 mg/dL, other immunoglobulins deficient or absent, B cells deficient or absent, intact cellular (T-cell) immunity, and onset of infections after the 6th

month of life, when maternal antibodies are no longer present. Therefore, B-cell-dependent areas, such as germinal centers, would be absent or greatly diminished in size and number.

Postcapillary venules (**choice A**) are not depleted in this disease.

The chemotactic response of neutrophils (**choice C**) is part of the phagocytic function assay, which was normal in the case presented.

Because T-cell functions are intact, the architecture of the portions of lymphoid tissues where T cells reside (e.g., paracortical areas, **choice D**; thymus-dependent areas, **choice E**) should be normal.

49.  **The correct answer is D.** When you see *Chlamydia psittaci*, one word should come to mind—birds! Infection with this organism is an occupational hazard for anyone who works with birds (e.g., veterinarians, pet store employees), including poultry farmers.

Individuals who work with cats (**choice A**) would be at an increased risk for infection with *Pasteurella multocida* (which is acquired primarily through cat bites), *Bartonella henselae* (cat-scratch fever), and the protozoan *Toxoplasma gondii* (which can be acquired from ingestion of food contaminated with cat feces).

Florists (**choice B**) are at increased risk for infection with the fungus *Sporothrix schenckii*, a primary pathogenic fungus acquired by inoculation (e.g., a rose thorn puncturing the skin).

A person who works at a homeless shelter (**choice C**) would be at increased risk for infection with *Mycobacterium tuberculosis*, since this organism is spread through the air and is prevalent in the homeless community.

Slaughterhouse workers (**choice E**) are at an increased risk for infection with *Brucella*, a bacterium that is acquired by handling infected animals.

50.  **The correct answer is C.** This patient has infectious mononucleosis due to cytomegalovirus (CMV). Patients present with symptoms similar to Epstein-Barr virus (EBV) infection (sore throat, fever, fatigue, cervical lymphadenopathy, and hepatomegaly), but their diagnostic workup (heterophile antibody, Epstein-Barr titer) is negative for EBV. Though diagnosis of CMV depends on virus isolation in secretions, microscopic exam of epithelial cells reveals giant nuclei surrounded by clear zones (owl's eye nuclei), which are pathognomonic. Cytoplasmic inclusions also appear.

An enlarged nucleus with peripherally displaced chromatin (**choice A**) is seen in cells infected with human parvovirus B19, which causes Fifth disease (erythema infectiosum) in children. A classic clue to the diagnosis is the presence of a "slapped cheek" rash.

Conidia and septate hyphae (**choice B**) appear in aspergillosis, a lung disease that occurs mostly in the immunocompromised. A classic clue is the appearance of a "fungus ball" (aspergilloma) on chest x-ray, which appears as a large, round mass surrounded by air.

Multinucleated giant cells (**choice D**) appear in several viral infections, including measles (rubeola), chicken-pox (varicella), RSV, herpes, and HIV.

Staining with India ink (**choice E**) is used on the CSF of patients with *Cryptococcus neoformans* CNS infection to highlight the yeast capsule.

# Microbiology/Immunology: **Test Two**

1. Patients with the HLA-B27 antigen are known to have an increased risk of developing certain pathologic conditions. Which of the following infectious agents may cause a syndrome characterized by arthritis, conjunctivitis, and urethritis in an HLA-B27 positive patient?

   (A) *Borrelia burgdorferi*

   (B) *Chlamydia trachomatis*

   (C) Enterotoxigenic *Escherichia coli*

   (D) Group A β-hemolytic streptococci

   (E) *Trichomonas vaginalis*

2. Five weeks after a trip to Africa, a 32-year-old woman develops fever, chills, malaise, and a dry cough. She is treated with erythromycin for a suspected *Mycoplasma* pneumonia. Six months later she has burning on urination, increased urination, and lower abdominal pain. She has also noticed that her urinary stream is visibly clear until the end of voiding, at which time the last part of the urine becomes grossly bloody. Examination of her urine shows elongated ova with rounded anterior ends and terminal spines at the posterior end. She is given a prescription for praziquantel. This patient is at increased risk for which of the following diseases?

   (A) Adenocarcinoma of the bladder

   (B) Adenocarcinoma of the renal pelvis

   (C) Squamous cell carcinoma of the bladder

   (D) Transitional cell carcinoma of the bladder

   (E) Transitional cell carcinoma of the renal pelvis

3. A 29-year-old woman diagnosed with AIDS has had a progressive blurring of vision in her right eye. On funduscopic examination, a small white opaque lesion is noted on the retina of her right eye. Which of the following is the most appropriate therapy for this patient?

   (A) Acyclovir

   (B) Amantadine

   (C) Flucytosine

   (D) Ganciclovir

   (E) Zidovudine

4. A 45-year-old homeless man has a chronic cough and a cavitary lesion of the lung. His sputum is positive for acid-fast bacilli. Which of the following is the principal form of defense by which the patient's body fights this infection?

   (A) Antibody-mediated phagocytosis

   (B) Cell-mediated immunity

   (C) IgA-mediated hypersensitivity

   (D) IgE-mediated hypersensitivity

   (E) Neutrophil ingestion of bacteria

5. A 10-year-old girl presents with sore throat and fever. She denies any cough or rhinorrhea. A throat culture grows bacitracin-sensitive bacterial colonies. The infecting organism would be protected from the lytic action of detergents by its

   (A) keratin-like proteins in the spore coat

   (B) lipopolysaccharide in the outer membrane

   (C) peptidoglycan layer

   (D) periplasmic space

   (E) $Ca^{2+}$ chelators

6. A hospitalized patient with dysuria and suprapubic pain is treated with ciprofloxacin. What is the mechanism of action of this antibiotic?

   (A) It inhibits dihydrofolate reductase

   (B) It inhibits DNA-dependent RNA polymerase

   (C) It inhibits protein synthesis by binding to the 30S ribosomal subunit

   (D) It inhibits protein synthesis by binding to the 50S ribosomal subunit

   (E) It inhibits topoisomerase II (DNA gyrase)

7. Two weeks after returning from a trip to New Delhi, India, a 35-year-old man presents to the emergency department complaining of daily fevers, headache, chills, and malaise. He recalls getting a number of flea bites on his ankles and calves during his trip. Physical examination reveals a maculopapular rash on his trunk, arms, and thighs. Which of the following is the most likely cause of this patient's condition?

   (A) *Bartonella henselae*

   (B) *Borrelia recurrentis*

   (C) *Coxiella burnetii*

   (D) *Ehrlichia chaffeensis*

   (E) *Rickettsia typhi*

8. A child in a developing country develops repeated eye infections with an organism that causes chronic conjunctivitis, scarring, eyelid deformities, pannus formation, and eventual blindness. Which of the following is a distinctive feature of the causative organism?

   (A) Also causes cat scratch fever

   (B) Antigen cross-reactivity with antibodies to *Proteus vulgaris*

   (C) Arthropod transmission

   (D) Bird reservoir

   (E) Reticulate body

9. A 34-year-old woman presents with fatigue, malaise, and swollen, tender joints. Physical examination is significant for a maculopapular eruption over sun-exposed areas, including the face. Examination of a peripheral blood smear reveals mild thrombocytopenia. Which of the following autoantibodies, if present, would be most specific for the diagnosis of the patient's disorder?

   (A) Anti-centromere antibody

   (B) Anti-IgG antibody

   (C) Antinuclear antibody

   (D) Anti-Sm (Smith antigen) antibody

   (E) Anti-SS-A (Ro) antibody

10. A 4-year-old girl presents with a maculopapular rash on her hands and feet and painful ulcers distributed anteriorly on her lips, palate, tongue, and buccal mucosa. Systemic features and lymphadenopathy are absent. Which of the following viruses is most likely to have caused this disorder?

    (A) Coronavirus

    (B) Coxsackievirus type A16

    (C) Herpes simplex virus type 1

    (D) Parainfluenza type 3

    (E) Rhinovirus

11. A patient with nuchal rigidity and headache undergoes lumbar puncture. The CSF contains markedly increased numbers of lymphocytes, leading to a presumptive diagnosis of viral meningitis. Which of the following groups of viruses is most likely to be involved?

    (A) Adenoviruses

    (B) Enteroviruses

    (C) Human papillomaviruses

    (D) Poxviruses

    (E) Reoviruses

12. A clone of F⁺ *Escherichia coli*, which possesses a *Thr⁺* marker on its fertility plasmid, was produced in the laboratory. These bacteria were mixed with wild-type F⁻ *E. coli*, which were *Thr⁻* under conditions that prevented binary fission but encouraged cell-to-cell contact. After 24 hours, the cultures were plated on threonine-deficient and threonine-enriched media, and the colonies were counted. What would be the expected result?

    (A) All clones would be F⁺ and grow on threonine-free medium

    (B) All clones would be F⁺ but would require threonine in their growth medium

    (C) Half of the clones would be F⁻ and would grow on threonine-free medium

    (D) Half of the clones would be F⁺ and would grow on threonine-free medium

    (E) Half of the clones would be F⁺ but would require threonine in their growth medium

13. A 6-year-old boy presents to the pediatric clinic with fever and earache. He has just finished an unsuccessful course of amoxicillin. On physical examination, his right tympanic membrane appears injected. Which of the following is the most appropriate pharmacotherapy?

    (A) Amphotericin B

    (B) Bacitracin

    (C) Cefaclor

    (D) Erythromycin

    (E) Sulfamethoxazole

14. A 4-year-old boy presents to the emergency department with muscle spasms. His past medical history is significant for recurrent infections and neonatal seizures. Evaluation of his serum electrolytes reveals hypocalcemia. This patient would be most susceptible to which of the following diseases?

    (A) Chickenpox

    (B) Diphtheria

    (C) Gas gangrene

    (D) Gonorrhea

    (E) Tetanus

15. A patient develops fever and shortness of breath, and appears to be quite ill. An x-ray film demonstrates bilateral interstitial lung infiltrates, and bronchial washings demonstrate small "hat-shaped" organisms visible on silver stain within the foamy alveolar exudate. Which predisposing condition is most likely present in this patient?

    (A) AIDS

    (B) Congestive heart failure

    (C) Pulmonary embolus

    (D) Rheumatoid arthritis

    (E) Systemic lupus erythematosus

16. A 30-year-old veterinarian visits her obstetrician for a first-trimester prenatal checkup. She has no complaints. Routine physical examination is significant only for mild cervical lymphadenopathy. She is prescribed spiramycin but is noncompliant. Her child is born with hydrocephalus and cerebral calcifications. Which of the following organisms is most likely responsible?

    (A) *Isospora belli*

    (B) *Leishmania donovani*

    (C) *Plasmodium vivax*

    (D) *Toxoplasma gondii*

    (E) *Trypanosoma cruzi*

17. A 38-year-old woman complains of cold and painful fingertips, as well as difficulty swallowing and indigestion. Physical examination is remarkable for a thickened, shiny epidermis over the entire body, with restricted movement of the extremities, particularly the fingers, which appear claw-like. Which of the following autoantibodies will likely be found in this patient's serum?

    (A) Anti-DNA topoisomerase I (anti-Scl-70)

    (B) Anti-double-stranded DNA (ds DNA)

    (C) Anti-IgG

    (D) Anti-Sm

    (E) Anti-SS-A

18. A 24-year-old AIDS patient develops chronic abdominal pain, low-grade fever, diarrhea, and malabsorption. Acid-fast oocysts are demonstrated in the stool. Which of the following organisms is most likely the cause of the patient's diarrhea?

    (A) *Diphyllobothrium latum*

    (B) *Entamoeba histolytica*

    (C) *Giardia lamblia*

    (D) *Isospora belli*

    (E) Microsporidia

19. An African child develops massive unilateral enlargement of his lower face in the vicinity of the mandible. Biopsy demonstrates sheets of medium-sized blast cells with admixed larger macrophages. This type of tumor has been associated with which of the following?

    (A) Epstein-Barr virus and t(8;14)

    (B) Hepatitis B and t(9;22)

    (C) Herpesvirus and CD5

    (D) HIV and CD4

    (E) Human papillomavirus and t(2;5)

20. A 1-week-old girl with symptoms of vomiting and anorexia has a temperature of 102.0 F. A bulging fontanel is noted on physical examination. Which of the following is the most likely causative agent?

    (A) *Haemophilus influenzae* type b

    (B) *Listeria monocytogenes*

    (C) *Neisseria meningitidis*

    (D) *Staphylococcus aureus*

    (E) *Streptococcus agalactiae*

21. A mailman gets a severe bite wound from a pit bull guarding a junkyard. The wound is cleansed and he receives a booster injection of tetanus toxoid and an injection of penicillin G. Several days later, the wound is inflamed and purulent. The exudate is cultured on blood agar and yields gram-negative rods. Antibiotic sensitivity tests are pending. Which of the following is the most likely pathogen?

    (A) *Bartonella henselae*

    (B) *Brucella canis*

    (C) *Clostridium tetani*

    (D) *Pasteurella multocida*

    (E) *Toxocara canis*

22. A 1-year-old girl presents with a 2-day history of fever, vomiting, and watery, nonbloody diarrhea. On physical examination, she appears dehydrated. Which of the following best describes the most likely infecting organism?

    (A) It has a complex double-stranded DNA genome

    (B) It has a partially double-stranded circular DNA genome

    (C) It has a segmented, double-stranded RNA genome

    (D) It has a single-stranded circular RNA genome

    (E) It has a single-stranded RNA genome

23. A 37-year-old woman who has rheumatoid arthritis and is on long-term corticosteroid therapy is brought to the physician because of nausea, vomiting, headache, and confusion. Examination reveals a temperature of 39.7 C (103.4 F) and nuchal rigidity. Cerebrospinal fluid analysis shows pleocytosis, increased protein, decreased glucose, and budding, encapsulated organisms. An India ink mount of the cerebrospinal fluid sediment shows budding yeasts surrounded by a wide, clear zone. Which of the following is the most appropriate pharmacotherapy?

    (A) Amphotericin B

    (B) Isoniazid

    (C) Ketoconazole

    (D) Metronidazole

    (E) Nystatin

24. A female *Anopheles* mosquito injects a single sporozoite of *Plasmodium vivax* into the bloodstream of a susceptible human host. Schizogony in the liver requires ten days and produces 100 merozoites per hepatocyte. Schizogony in the bloodstream produces 10 merozoites per erythrocyte. How many merozoites will be produced in 22 days of infection?

    (A) $1 \times 10^2$

    (B) $2 \times 10^2$

    (C) $1 \times 10^3$

    (D) $1 \times 10^5$

    (E) $1 \times 10^8$

25. A 78-year-old woman with a history of renal calculi and recurrent urinary tract infections presents with fever, chills, leukocytosis, and cloudy urine that has a pH of 8.2. A urine culture grows a lactose-negative, urease-positive, gram-negative rod. Which of the following microorganisms is most likely responsible for her infection?

    (A) *Candida albicans*

    (B) *Enterococcus faecalis*

    (C) *Escherichia coli*

    (D) *Klebsiella pneumoniae*

    (E) *Proteus mirabilis*

    (F) *Pseudomonas aeruginosa*

    (G) *Staphylococcus saprophyticus*

26. A 25-year-old woman presents with pain and tenosynovitis of the wrists and ankles, and arthralgias of other joints. She notes two prior episodes similar to the present one. She just had her menstrual period during the previous week. Physical examination reveals ulcerated lesions overlying the wrists and ankles. These symptoms are likely due to deficiency of which of the following?

    (A) C1 esterase inhibitor

    (B) Ciliary function

    (C) Complement (C6-C8) components

    (D) Endothelial adhesion molecules

    (E) Eosinophils

27. An 8-month-old infant presents to the emergency department with a 1-day history of poor feeding and generalized weakness. The mother states that she often feeds the infant honey to pacify her. The toxin responsible for this presentation works by which of the following mechanisms?

    (A) It blocks the release of acetylcholine from the nerve terminal

    (B) It blocks the release of inhibitory neurotransmitters such as glycine and GABA

    (C) It has a subunit that inactivates an elongation factor by ADP-ribosylation

    (D) It is a lecithinase

    (E) It stimulates guanylate cyclase

28. A 36-year-old, HIV-positive, white man presents with a fever and progressive headache. He complains of recent forgetfulness and "spells," during which he smells a "harsh, bitter smell." An MRI of the brain shows multiple, spherical, ring-enhancing lesions in the left temporal lobe. Laboratory analysis of CSF is normal. Which of the following microorganisms is most likely responsible for his illness?

    (A) Coxsackievirus

    (B) *Cryptococcus neoformans*

    (C) Cytomegalovirus

    (D) *Diphyllobothrium latum*

    (E) Herpes simplex virus

    (F) *Mycobacterium leprae*

    (G) *Pasteurella multocida*

    (H) *Pneumocystis carinii*

    (I) *Taenia solium*

    (J) *Toxoplasma gondii*

29. A 57-year-old woman with a history of hypertension and arthritis is referred to a rheumatologist for evaluation. A complete blood count (CBC) is normal, and a mini-chem panel shows no electrolyte abnormalities. Her erythrocyte sedimentation rate (ESR) is elevated, and an antinuclear antibody test (ANA) is positive. Further antibody studies are performed, and the results are shown below.

    | | |
    |---|---|
    | Anti-histones | high titer |
    | Anti-double-stranded DNA | not detected |
    | Anti-single-stranded DNA | not detected |
    | Anti-SSA | not detected |
    | Anti-SSB | not detected |
    | Anti-SCI-70 | not detected |
    | Anti-Smith | not detected |
    | Anti-centromere | not detected |
    | Anti-RNP | not detected |

    Which of the following diseases is suggested by these results?

    (A) CREST syndrome

    (B) Diffuse form of scleroderma

    (C) Drug-induced lupus

    (D) Sjögren syndrome

    (E) Systemic lupus erythematosus (SLE)

30. An otherwise healthy patient who wears contact lenses develops a small ulceration of the eye. Of the following organisms, which is most likely to have been introduced into her contact lens solution?

    (A) *Acanthamoeba*

    (B) Cytomegalovirus

    (C) Herpes simplex

    (D) *Toxocara*

    (E) *Toxoplasma*

31. A 32-year-old woman with increased frequency of urination, suprapubic pain, and dysuria for the past 3 days comes to the emergency department. She has no fever, nausea, or vomiting. A Gram stain reveals gram-negative rods. Which of the following is the most likely pathogen?

    (A) *Escherichia coli*

    (B) *Neisseria gonorrhoeae*

    (C) *Shigella dysenteriae*

    (D) *Streptococcus pneumoniae*

    (E) *Treponema pallidum*

32. Gram stain of the sputum from a patient with lobar pneumonia involving the left lower lobe demonstrates gram-positive, encapsulated, lancet-shaped diplococci. Which of the following is the most probable causative organism?

    (A) *Haemophilus influenzae*

    (B) *Neisseria gonorrhoeae*

    (C) *Pneumocystis carinii*

    (D) *Staphylococcus aureus*

    (E) *Streptococcus pneumoniae*

33. A 12-year-old girl has a temperature of 102.5 F and a sore throat. Two days later, she develops a diffuse erythematous rash and is taken to her pediatrician. On physical examination, there is circumoral pallor, and an erythematous rash with areas of desquamation is noted. The myocardial damage that can follow this infection is produced in a manner similar to the damage associated with which of the following disorders?

    (A) Atopic allergy

    (B) Contact dermatitis

    (C) Graft-versus-host disease

    (D) Graves disease

    (E) Idiopathic thrombocytopenic purpura

    (F) Myasthenia gravis

    (G) Rheumatoid arthritis

    (H) Serum sickness

    (I) Systemic lupus erythematosus

34. A 27-year-old IV drug user presents with difficulty swallowing. Examination of the oropharynx reveals white plaques along the tongue and the oral mucosa. Which of the following best describes the microscopic appearance of the microorganism responsible for this patient's illness?

    (A) Budding yeast and pseudohyphae

    (B) Encapsulated yeast

    (C) Mold with nonseptate hyphae

    (D) Mold with septate hyphae

35. A 40-year-old, otherwise healthy gardener presents with several subcutaneous nodules on his right hand, where he had cut himself on rose thorns. Physical examination reveals several erythematous fluctuant lesions. Which of the following organisms is most likely responsible for his condition?

    (A) *Aspergillus*

    (B) *Malassezia*

    (C) *Onchocerca*

    (D) *Rhizopus*

    (E) *Sporothrix*

36. An alcoholic is brought to the emergency department in respiratory distress. A chest x-ray film demonstrates lobar consolidation of the right lower lung. Which of the following organisms should be highest on the differential diagnosis?

    (A) *Klebsiella pneumoniae*

    (B) *Legionella* spp.

    (C) *Mycoplasma pneumoniae*

    (D) *Pneumocystis carinii*

    (E) *Staphylococcus aureus*

37. A diabetic patient has chronic sinusitis that has not responded to a 6-week course of antibiotics. The physician should suspect infection with which of the following organisms?

    (A) *Actinomyces*

    (B) *Aspergillus*

    (C) *Cryptococcus*

    (D) *Mucor*

    (E) *Pneumocystis*

38. A mother brings her 3-year-old boy into the emergency department because he has developed a harsh, "barking" cough with hoarseness. The virus responsible for this child's illness belongs to which of the following families?

    (A) Papovavirus

    (B) Paramyxovirus

    (C) Parvovirus

    (D) Picornavirus

    (E) Poxvirus

39. A 12-year-old boy with sickle cell disease develops sudden onset of fever and chills accompanied by intense pain and tenderness over the distal tibia. X-ray films and CT scan of the distal leg reveal swelling of the subcutaneous tissue and bone demineralization. A clinical diagnosis of acute osteomyelitis is made. Blood cultures and bone biopsy are arranged to confirm the diagnosis and isolate the offending agent. Which of the following infectious agents will most likely be identified?

    (A) Group B streptococci

    (B) *Hemophilus influenzae*

    (C) *Mycobacterium tuberculosis*

    (D) *Salmonella* spp.

    (E) *Staphylococcus aureus*

40. A 53-year-old woman with diarrhea and lower abdominal pain of 3 days' duration comes to her physician after various home remedies fail to relieve her symptoms. She denies any recent travel. There is blood and pus in her stool. Fecal cultures yield several flagellated, curved, oxidase-positive, gram-negative rods. Which of the following is the most likely pathogen?

    (A) *Campylobacter jejuni*

    (B) *Escherichia coli*

    (C) *Salmonella typhimurium*

    (D) *Shigella sonnei*

    (E) *Vibrio cholerae*

41. A 15-year-old high school student and several of her friends ate lunch at a local Chinese restaurant. They all were served the daily luncheon special, which consisted of sweet and sour pork with vegetables and fried rice. All of the girls developed nausea, vomiting, abdominal pain, and diarrhea within 4 hours of eating lunch. Which of the following is the most likely cause of these symptoms?

    (A) *Bacillus cereus*

    (B) *Clostridium botulinum*

    (C) *Clostridium perfringens*

    (D) EHEC (Enterohemorrhagic *Escherichia coli*)

    (E) *Staphylococcus aureus*

    (F) *Vibrio cholerae*

42. Three months after a needle-stick exposure to blood from a patient with hepatitis B, a nurse is evaluated for infection with the virus. Laboratory results reveal:

    | | |
    |---|---|
    | HBsAg | absent |
    | anti-HBs antibody | absent |
    | IgM anti-HBc | present |
    | IgG anti-HBc | absent |
    | HBeAg | absent |

    On the basis of these results, which of the following most accurately describes the nurse's hepatitis B status?

    (A) She had been effectively vaccinated against hepatitis B before the needle-stick exposure occurred

    (B) She has mounted an inappropriate antibody response to hepatitis B as a result of an immunocompromised state

    (C) She is a carrier of hepatitis B

    (D) She is actively infected with hepatitis B

    (E) She was not infected with hepatitis B

43. A 32-year-old physician who has spent the past several years in New Guinea presents with ulcerating granulomata of his genital skin. Microscopic evaluation of the papules with Wright-Giemsa stain reveals 1- to 2-μm, rounded structures contained within cystic areas of the cytoplasm of macrophages. Which of the following is the most likely pathogen?

    (A) *Calymmatobacterium donovani*

    (B) *Chlamydia trachomatis*

    (C) *Haemophilus ducreyi*

    (D) *Human papillomavirus*

    (E) *Neisseria gonorrhoeae*

    (F) *Treponema pallidum*

44. A 4-year-old girl is brought to the physician because of an enlarged spleen. Laboratory studies show an increased reticulocyte count, increased indirect bilirubin level, increased lactate dehydrogenase, and decreased haptoglobin level. A peripheral blood smear shows small red blood cells that have lost their central pallor. The red blood cells are abnormally vulnerable to swelling induced by hypotonic media. The Coombs test is negative. When told of the findings, the girl's mother reports that she has the same disorder. Infection with which of the following viruses is particularly dangerous for these patients?

    (A) Adenovirus

    (B) Cytomegalovirus

    (C) Herpes simplex virus

    (D) Measles virus

    (E) Parvovirus

45. A previously healthy 11-year-old girl develops a gastrointestinal infection with cramping and watery stools. After several days, she begins to pass blood per rectum and is hospitalized for dehydration. In the hospital, she has decreasing urine output with rising blood urea nitrogen (BUN). Total blood count reveals anemia and thrombocytopenia, and the peripheral smear is remarkable for fragmented red cells (schistocytes). Infection with which of the following bacterial genera is most likely responsible for this syndrome?

    (A) *Campylobacter*

    (B) *Clostridium*

    (C) *Salmonella*

    (D) *Shigella*

    (E) *Vibrio*

46. An 18-year-old college student presents to the student health center complaining of a sore throat and fever. He describes feeling tired for the past few days and reports a loss of appetite. On examination, he has pharyngitis with cervical lymphadenopathy. Blood tests reveal lymphocytosis and the presence of heterophile antibodies. Which of the following best describes the virus responsible for his illness?

    (A) Double-stranded, enveloped DNA virus

    (B) Double-stranded, nonenveloped DNA virus

    (C) Single-stranded, enveloped RNA virus

    (D) Single-stranded, nonenveloped DNA virus

    (E) Single-stranded, nonenveloped RNA virus

47. A 35-year-old, sexually active man presents to his internist with a painless penile vesicle. Physical examination reveals inguinal lymphadenopathy. The infecting organism is definitively diagnosed and is known to exist in distinct extracellular and intracellular forms. Which of the following is the most likely pathogen?

    (A) *Calymmatobacterium granulomatis*

    (B) *Chlamydia trachomatis*

    (C) *Haemophilus ducreyi*

    (D) *Neisseria gonorrhoeae*

    (E) *Treponema pallidum*

48. A 47-year-old grocer complains of diarrhea and painful arthritis. Physical examination is remarkable for lymphadenopathy and weight loss. Biopsy of his small bowel reveals PAS-positive macrophages within the lamina propria. Electron microscopic examination of the macrophages reveals small, rod-shaped structures. Which of the following is the most likely pathogen?

    (A) *Clostridium difficile*

    (B) *Enterotoxigenic Escherichia coli*

    (C) *Isospora belli*

    (D) *Salmonella* sp.

    (E) *Tropheryma whippelii*

49. A 38-year-old AIDS patient presents to the clinic complaining of nausea, occasional vomiting, and "bumps" on his groin. On physical exam, the bumps are nontender, pedunculated, reddish-purple nodules in the inguinal and perirectal areas. His liver is palpable 8 cm below the right costal margin. Routine laboratory tests are remarkable only for slightly elevated aminotransferases and alkaline phosphatase levels. He has two pet cats and denies any foreign travel. Which of the following agents is the most likely cause of this patient's infection?

    (A) *Bartonella henselae*

    (B) Human papillomavirus

    (C) Molluscum contagiosum

    (D) *Rickettsia prowazekii*

    (E) *Treponema pallidum*

50. A microbiologic laboratory studying the acquisition of drug resistance in gram-negative bacilli isolates a clone of bacteria with genetic resistance to chloramphenicol, tetracycline, sulfonamides, and streptomycin. The DNA from these bacteria is isolated and processed for nucleotide sequencing. The small segment of DNA containing the drug-resistance genes is found to contain three pairs of indirect repeats. What else is most likely to be found inside this linear segment of DNA?

    (A) A temperate phage

    (B) OriT

    (C) The tra operon

    (D) Three genes for transposase enzymes

    (E) Three pairs of direct repeats

**KAPLAN** MEDICAL

# Microbiology/Immunology Test Two: **Answers and Explanations**

## ANSWER KEY

| | | | | |
|---|---|---|---|---|
| 1. | B | | 26. | C |
| 2. | C | | 27. | A |
| 3. | D | | 28. | J |
| 4. | B | | 29. | C |
| 5. | C | | 30. | A |
| 6. | E | | 31. | A |
| 7. | E | | 32. | E |
| 8. | E | | 33. | E |
| 9. | D | | 34. | A |
| 10. | B | | 35. | E |
| 11. | B | | 36. | A |
| 12. | A | | 37. | D |
| 13. | C | | 38. | B |
| 14. | A | | 39. | D |
| 15. | A | | 40. | A |
| 16. | D | | 41. | A |
| 17. | A | | 42. | D |
| 18. | D | | 43. | A |
| 19. | A | | 44. | E |
| 20. | E | | 45. | D |
| 21. | D | | 46. | A |
| 22. | C | | 47. | B |
| 23. | A | | 48. | E |
| 24. | E | | 49. | A |
| 25. | E | | 50. | D |

1.  **The correct answer is B.** Reiter syndrome is a serious sequela that may follow enteric infections due to *Shigella*, *Salmonella*, *Yersinia*, or *Campylobacter* or sexually transmitted diseases caused by *Chlamydia* or *Ureaplasma*. Up to 80% of cases occur in HLA-B27 positive individuals. Male predominance is characteristic in cases following sexually transmitted infections. The role of infection is not clear, and infectious organisms have not been cultured from affected joints.

    *Borrelia burgdorferi* (**choice A**) is the causative agent of Lyme disease, a tick-borne infection that manifests in three stages and involves the skin (erythema chronicum migrans), joints, heart, and meninges.

    Enterotoxigenic *Escherichia coli* (**choice C**) causes a self-limited enteric infection that manifests with watery diarrhea.

    Infection by group A β-hemolytic streptococci (**choice D**), usually a pharyngitis, may result in rheumatic heart disease characterized by carditis, migratory polyarthritis, erythema marginatum, subcutaneous nodules, and Sydenham chorea.

    *Trichomonas vaginalis* (**choice E**) causes a vaginitis associated with malodorous yellow-green discharge. The infection remains localized, and there are no systemic manifestations.

2.  **The correct answer is C.** Carcinomas of the bladder and renal pelvis are usually transitional cell (**choices D and E**) carcinomas. However, *Schistosoma haematobium* infection (in which schistosomes lay eggs in the veins near the bladder, thereby inducing a marked inflammatory response) is associated with squamous metaplasia and squamous cell carcinoma of the bladder. Some authors have suggested that medications used to kill the worms may contribute to the etiology.

    Adenocarcinomas of the renal pelvis and bladder (**choices A and B**) are rare.

3.  **The correct answer is D.** This patient most likely has cytomegalovirus (CMV) retinitis. The best drug treatment for this infection is ganciclovir.

    Acyclovir (**choice A**) is not effective in CMV infections. It is used more for HSV type 1 and 2 infections.

    Amantadine (**choice B**) is used either therapeutically or prophylactically for the influenza A virus.

    Flucytosine (**choice C**) is an antifungal agent.

    Zidovudine (**choice E**) is a first-line drug for the treatment of AIDS. The drug by itself is ineffective against CMV retinitis.

4.  **The correct answer is B.** This patient has tuberculosis. The principal host defense in mycobacterial infections is cell-mediated immunity, which causes formation of granulomas. Unfortunately, in tuberculosis and many other infectious diseases characterized by granuloma formation, the organisms may persist intracellularly in the granulomas for years, and are a source of reactivation disease.

    Although antibody-mediated phagocytosis (**choice A**) is a major host defense against many bacteria, it is not the principal defense against mycobacteria.

    IgA-mediated hypersensitivity (**choice C**) does not exist. The only role of IgA is to prevent adherence of pathogens to mucosal surfaces.

    IgE-mediated hypersensitivity (**choice D**) is not involved in the body's defense against mycobacteria. It is important in allergic reactions.

    Neutrophil ingestion of bacteria (**choice E**) is a major host defense against bacteria but is not the principle defense against mycobacteria.

5.  **The correct answer is C.** This girl has streptococcal pharyngitis. The infecting organism is group A beta-hemolytic streptococcus (*Streptococcus pyogenes*); its growth is inhibited by the placement of a bacitracin disk on the throat culture plate. (Beta-hemolysis occurs as the result of the bacterial hemolysin streptolysin S.) This is a gram-positive bacterium and therefore possesses a very thick peptidoglycan layer that would protect it from lysis by detergents. (Note that gram-positives also contain teichoic acid.) In contrast, gram-negatives have a thin peptidoglycan layer.

    Keratin-like proteins in the spore coat (**choice A**) and calcium ion chelators (dipicolinic acid; **choice E**) are found in spores formed by species of *Bacillus* and *Clostridium*. These protect the spores from the elements: dehydration, heat, chemicals, radiation, etc.

    Lipopolysaccharide in the outer membrane (**choice B**) and a periplasmic space (**choice D**) are found in gram-negative organisms. The lipopolysaccharide is an endotoxin, and the periplasmic space contains beta-lactamases in some species.

6.  **The correct answer is E.** This is a straightforward question in which the introductory clinical details are really irrelevant. Ciprofloxacin and norfloxacin belong to a category of antibiotics called the fluoroquinolones. They are bactericidal and work by inhibiting topoisomerase II (DNA gyrase). They are effective against gram-negative rods and are the only oral agents effective against *Pseudomonas*. Ciprofloxacin is effective for treating urinary tract infections, gonorrhea, diarrheal diseases, and soft tissue infections. It is also used to treat *Pseudomonas* infections in cystic fibrosis.

Inhibition of dihydrofolate reductase (**choice A**) is the mechanism of action of trimethoprim, which is typically used in combination with sulfonamides (trimethoprim-sulfamethoxazole). Sulfonamides inhibit an earlier step in folate synthesis (dihydropteroate synthase), so the combination with trimethoprim is an effective "one-two" punch. Trimethoprim-sulfa is used in the treatment of *Shigella*, *Salmonella*, recurrent urinary tract infections, and *Pneumocystis carinii* pneumonia.

Inhibition of DNA-dependent RNA polymerase (**choice B**) is the mechanism of action of rifampin. Rifampin is used (along with other drugs) in the treatment of tuberculosis. You should also remember that rifampin can be used to treat individuals exposed to the meningococcus or *Haemophilus influenzae* type B.

Inhibition of the 30S ribosomal subunit (**choice C**) is the mechanism of action of two important classes of antibiotics—the tetracyclines (tetracycline, doxycycline, demeclocycline) and the aminoglycosides (gentamicin, tobramycin, streptomycin, etc.). The tetracyclines inhibit the attachment of the aminoacyl-tRNA to the ribosome, whereas the aminoglycosides inhibit the formation of the initiation complex.

Inhibition of the 50S ribosomal subunit (**choice D**) is the mechanism of action of the macrolides (e.g., erythromycin), the lincosamides (e.g., lincomycin, clindamycin), and chloramphenicol. Chloramphenicol inhibits the 50S peptidyl transferase, whereas erythromycin blocks translocation.

7. **The correct answer is E.** The symptoms described are characteristic of endemic or murine typhus, caused by *Rickettsia typhi*. The vector is the rat flea, and the reservoirs are the rat and the rat flea. Unlike other rickettsial infections, *R. typhi* is frequently acquired in cities in the developing world with inadequate rodent control.

*Bartonella henselae* (**choice A**) causes cat scratch disease and bacillary angiomatosis. Its reservoir is the domestic cat. The vector for the cat population is the cat flea, but most human infection is acquired through cat scratches or cat bites.

*Borrelia recurrentis* (**choice B**) is a spirochete that causes louse-borne, relapsing fever. Humans are the only reservoir.

*Coxiella burnetii* (**choice C**) is the cause of Q fever. It is acquired by inhalation, and its reservoirs are sheep, goat, and cattle.

*Ehrlichia chaffeensis* (**choice D**) is a cause of human ehrlichiosis, which is characterized by leukopenia, thrombocytopenia, and anemia. It is transmitted by ticks, and deer are the reservoir.

8. **The correct answer is E.** The disease described is trachoma, which is caused by serovars A, B, and C of *Chlamydia trachomatis*. *C. trachomatis* causes a conjunctival and corneal infection that is spread in developing countries by eye-seeking flies. The lesions begin with formation of lymphoid follicles in the conjunctiva. With disease progression, there is tissue necrosis, granulation tissue deposition, and scar formation, leading to lacrimal duct obstruction and distortion of the eyelids. With the loss of an adequate tear system, the cornea becomes vulnerable to dehydration and opacification. Also, the vigorous inflammatory response can directly involve the cornea, with resulting opacity. In developed countries, chlamydial eye infections are often transmitted venereally, rather than by flies, and may cause conjunctivitis in neonates and in sexually active young adults. Humans are the only reservoir for *C. trachomatis*. *Chlamydia* are obligate intracellular parasites that have morphologically distinct infectious and reproductive forms. The infectious form is called the elementary body; the intracellular form is the reticulate body. *Chlamydia* are also distinctive in that they require host ATP and have a cell wall that lacks muramic acid. *C. trachomatis* also causes lymphogranuloma venereum (serovars L1, L2, and L3), inclusion conjunctivitis in infants (serovars D–K), and a variety of relatively nonspecific inflammations of the male and female genital tract (serovars D–K).

*Bartonella henselae* (**choice A**) causes cat scratch disease and bacillary angiomatosis.

The test described in **choice B** is the Weil-Felix test, which is used to identify rickettsia, not chlamydia.

**Choices C and D** are incorrect because humans are the only known reservoir for *C. trachomatis*.

9. **The correct answer is D.** The patient described probably has systemic lupus erythematosus (SLE), which often presents with fatigue, malaise, fever, gastrointestinal symptoms, arthralgias, and myalgias. Hematologic abnormalities include anemia, leukopenia, lymphocytopenia, and thrombocytopenia. A circulating anticoagulant may prolong the activated partial thromboplastin time (APTT). Cutaneous manifestations include a malar rash and a generalized maculopapular eruption, both of which are photosensitive. Antibodies to the Smith antigen (core proteins of small ribonucleoproteins found in the nucleus) are present in only 20 to 30% of patients with SLE, but are quite specific for the disease, occurring only rarely in other autoimmune diseases.

Anti-centromere antibody (**choice A**) is specific for the CREST (Calcinosis, Raynaud syndrome, Esophageal dysfunction, Sclerodactyly, and Telangiectasia) variant of progressive systemic sclerosis (scleroderma).

Rheumatoid factor is actually an autoantibody directed against the Fc portion of the IgG molecule (**choice B**). It is found in more than two-thirds of patients with rheumatoid arthritis.

Around 95% of patients with SLE develop antinuclear antibodies (ANA; **choice C**), so this test is quite sensitive but not very specific for SLE. ANA occur in patients with other inflammatory disorders, autoimmune diseases, and viral diseases, as well as in a number of normal individuals. Antibodies to double-stranded DNA are more specific for SLE but are not included as an answer choice.

Anti-SS-A antigen (**choice E**) refers to antibodies to certain ribonucleoproteins, which are fairly specific for Sjögren syndrome.

10. **The correct answer is B.** Hand-foot-and-mouth disease is characterized by the appearance of ulcers in the mouth and a maculopapular or vesicular rash on the hands and feet. It is most frequently caused by coxsackievirus type A16, although other coxsackieviruses have occasionally been implicated. The disease usually affects young children. Systemic features and lymphadenopathy are absent, and recovery is uneventful.

Coronavirus (**choice A**) is a cause of the common cold.

Herpes simplex virus type 1 (**choice C**) causes a variety of diseases, including gingivostomatitis, pharyngotonsillitis, herpes labialis, genital herpes, keratoconjunctivitis, and encephalitis. It may cause painful ulcers of the oral region, but it is unlikely to have caused the maculopapular rash described here.

Parainfluenza virus (**choice D**) is responsible for croup. Croup, or acute laryngotracheobronchitis, is an acute febrile illness with stridor, hoarseness, and cough.

Rhinovirus (**choice E**) is a member of Picornaviridae. It is the most common cause of the common cold.

11. **The correct answer is B.** Viral meningitis is relatively common, accounting for 10,000 cases of meningitis per year in the U.S. The vast majority of cases occur in individuals younger than 30 years. Usually, the symptoms are relatively mild, and death is uncommon. Enteroviruses, arboviruses, and type 2 herpes simplex virus are the most common causes of viral meningitis. Also, up to 10% of HIV patients develop an acute meningitis, typically at the time of seroconversion.

Adenovirus (**choice A**) infection is associated with upper respiratory tract infections (URIs), sinusitis, ocular disease, enteric infections, and bladder infections. It does not typically cause aseptic meningitis.

Human papillomaviruses (**choice C**) are associated with warts on the skin and genital areas.

Poxviruses (**choice D**) include the causative agents of smallpox, cowpox, and molluscum contagiosum. These agents do not typically cause meningitis.

Reoviruses (**choice E**) cause URIs, hepatitis, gastroenteritis, and encephalitis, but not meningitis.

12. **The correct answer is A.** In the $F^+$ to $F^-$ conjugal cross, a single strand of the entire plasmid is transferred from the donor ($F^+$) to the recipient ($F^-$). The second strand of DNA is replaced in both donor and recipient, so that at the end of the process, all parties to the cross should have identical, double-stranded versions of the complete plasmid. Because the entire fertility factor is transferred (including the tra operon), all recipients become $F^+$, and would acquire the $Thr^+$ allele.

All clones would be $F^+$ but would require threonine in their growth medium (**choice B**) is not correct because it implies that the tra operon would be transferred without the $Thr$ allele. Because the entire plasmid is always transferred in the $F^+$ to $F^-$ cross, it is not possible to get one without the other.

Half of the clones would be $F^-$ and would grow on threonine-free medium (**choice C**) is not correct because it implies that in half of the cases at least, the $Thr$ allele was transferred without the tra operon. The entire plasmid is always transferred in this type of cross.

Half of the clones would be $F^+$ and would grow on threonine-free medium (**choice D**) is not correct because it implies that the transfer is only complete and successful in one half of the cases. The question stem stipulates that conditions have been optimized for conjugation and not for binary fission, so it is likely that conjugation will proceed to completion in all cases, and no new $F^-$ cells will be generated during the process of binary fission.

Half of the clones would be $F^+$ but would require threonine in their growth medium (**choice E**) is not correct because it implies that in half of the cases, the tra operon would be transferred without the $Thr$ allele. In this cross, it is assumed that the entire plasmid is always transferred.

13. **The correct answer is C.** The drug of choice for otitis media in children is amoxicillin. In refractory cases, often due to bacterial resistance, switching to a different drug class is often effective. You must look for another medication that is effective against common organisms responsible for pediatric otitis media, such as *Streptococcus pneumoniae* (a gram-positive diplococcus) and *Haemophilus influenzae* (a gram-negative

rod). A second-generation cephalosporin, such as cefaclor, should cover both and is the best choice. Consequently, it is commonly used in cases of amoxicillin-resistant otitis media. None of the other choices cover the proper spectrum of organisms.

Amphotericin B (**choice A**) is an antifungal polyene. It works by binding to ergosterol in the fungal cell membrane, creating an artificial pore. It is used to treat systemic mycoses such as those caused by *Aspergillus*, *Blastomyces*, *Candida*, *Coccidioides*, *Cryptococcus*, and *Histoplasma*.

Bacitracin (**choice B**) is a topical agent used to fight infection with gram-positive organisms. It interferes with cell wall synthesis.

Erythromycin (**choice D**) is a macrolide antibiotic that binds to the 23S rRNA portion of the 50S subunit of ribosomes, inhibiting release of uncharged tRNA and stopping protein synthesis. Though effective against *S. pneumoniae,* it is not particularly active against *H. influenzae.* Note that erythromycin may be used in amoxicillin-resistant otitis media, but only when administered with a sulfonamide such as sulfisoxazole.

Sulfamethoxazole (**choice E**) is a sulfonamide. It is bacteriostatic and works by inhibiting folic acid synthesis. It resembles p-aminobenzoic acid (PABA) structurally. When combined with trimethoprim (a dihydrofolate reductase inhibitor) it exerts a bactericidal effect and serves as the drug combination of choice for complicated urinary tract infections.

14. **The correct answer is A.** This boy probably has DiGeorge syndrome, as evidenced by his tetany (muscle spasms) due to hypocalcemia and his history of recurrent infections and neonatal seizures. The syndrome occurs because of an embryonic failure in the development of the third and fourth pharyngeal pouches. Patients have both hypoplastic parathyroids (producing hypocalcemia) and thymuses (producing T-cell deficiency and recurrent infections). Since cell-mediated immunity (which depends on T cells) is important in defense against infections caused by intracellular pathogens (such as viruses), patients with this condition are particularly susceptible to viral infections, such as chickenpox (varicella). They also have trouble with fungal pathogens (e.g., *Candida*) and mycobacteria.

Other clues to the diagnosis of DiGeorge syndrome include congenital cardiac defects, esophageal atresia, bifid uvula, short philtrum, hypertelorism, antimongoloid palpebral slant, mandibular hypoplasia, and low-set ears.

Diphtheria (**choice B**) is caused by *Corynebacterium diphtheriae,* which produces disease by the elaboration of a very potent exotoxin. Therefore, humoral immunity (antitoxin), which is not usually compromised in DiGeorge patients, is essential for defense against the organism. (Note that the *C. diphtheriae* exotoxin acts by causing the ADP-ribosylation of elongation factor-2 of eukaryotic cells, thereby inhibiting protein synthesis). The disease can be avoided by immunization with diphtheria toxoid.

Gas gangrene (**choice C**) is caused by *Clostridium perfringens,* which produces a potent alpha toxin that injures cell membranes. Therefore, humoral immunity would again play a predominant role in defense against this organism. Note that the disease occurs in wounds and would not be expected in an uninjured 4-year-old boy.

Gonorrhea (**choice D**) is caused by *Neisseria gonorrhoeae* and would not be expected in a 4-year-old boy unless there was evidence of sexual abuse. Virulence factors of this organism include pili, cell wall endotoxin and outer membrane, and IgA protease. Antibody responses, neutrophils, and complement are of prime importance in defense against gonococcal infections.

Tetanus (**choice E**) is caused by *Clostridium tetani* and serves as a tricky distracter, as you might have quickly associated the patient's muscle spasms with this answer choice. (This is why it is important to read the question stem carefully before prematurely jumping to the responses.) *C. tetani*, which gains entry through deep wounds, produces tetanus toxin (exotoxin) and can be prevented by immunization with tetanus toxoid.

15. **The correct answer is A.** This patient has *Pneumocystis carinii* pneumonia (PCP), which is caused by an agent now believed to be a fungus rather than a true bacterium. PCP is seen in immunocompromised patients, particularly those with AIDS, cancer, and, in children, prematurity or malnourishment. It can be the AIDS-defining illness.

Congestive heart failure (**choice B**) predisposes the patient to pulmonary edema.

Pulmonary embolus (**choice C**) can cause pulmonary infarction or sudden death.

Rheumatoid arthritis (**choice D**), particularly in miners, can cause formation of lung nodules similar to subcutaneous rheumatoid nodules.

Systemic lupus erythematosus (**choice E**) can cause pleuritis but is not associated with a significantly increased incidence of pneumonia.

16. **The correct answer is D.** Humans become infected with *Toxoplasma gondii* by ingesting cysts in contaminated food or through contact with cat feces. The veterinarian in question was therefore particularly at risk of

infection. *T. gondii* is especially hazardous in pregnant women because the organism can be transmitted to the fetus through the placenta. (It is part of the ToRCHeS group of congenital infections—*Toxoplasma*, Rubella, CMV, Herpes/HIV, Syphilis). Since infected mothers are usually asymptomatic, cases often go unnoticed. Occasionally, patients present with cervical lymphadenopathy, as did the veterinarian, and require treatment to prevent complications in the fetus. Though newborns are also often asymptomatic, they are at risk for developing the classic triad of chorioretinitis (at birth or later in life), hydrocephalus, and cerebral calcifications. Note that *T. gondii* is also a common cause of CNS infections (e.g., encephalitis) in HIV-positive patients.

*Isospora belli* (**choice A**) is an intestinal protozoan that causes watery diarrhea, particularly in immunocompromised patients. Fecal-oral transmission of oocysts allows invasion of small intestinal mucosa, destroying the brush border.

*Leishmania donovani* (**choice B**) causes kala-azar (visceral leishmaniasis), which is characterized by fever, weakness, weight loss, splenomegaly, and skin hyperpigmentation. It is prevalent in regions of the Mediterranean, Middle East, Russia, and China. The vector is the sandfly.

*Plasmodium vivax* (**choice C**) causes malaria and is transmitted by the female *Anopheles* mosquito, which introduces sporozoites into the blood. These differentiate into merozoites that destroy erythrocytes. Splenomegaly ensues. Other species of this organism that cause malaria are *P. malariae*, *P. ovale* and *P. falciparum* (which causes a more severe form of the disease). Note that sickle cell trait confers resistance to *P. falciparum*.

*Trypanosoma cruzi* (**choice E**) causes Chagas disease, characterized by unilateral facial edema and nodules, fever, lymphadenopathy, and hepatosplenomegaly. It affects cardiac muscle most severely and is a major cause of cardiac disease worldwide. The reduviid ("kissing") bug is the vector that infects humans by defecating in the bite wound. It is most prevalent in Central and South America, with rare cases in the southern U.S.

17. **The correct answer is A.** This patient has systemic sclerosis, also called scleroderma. Antibodies to topoisomerase I (anti-Scl-70) occur in up to 70% of patients with diffuse systemic sclerosis, but only rarely in other disorders. Systemic sclerosis is characterized initially by excessive fibrosis and edema of the skin, especially the hands and fingers, producing sclerodactyly (characteristic changes in the fingers, which resemble claws).

Raynaud phenomenon is common. The diffuse type of systemic sclerosis generally spreads to include visceral organs, such as the esophagus (producing dysphagia), the lungs (producing pulmonary fibrosis), the heart (leading to heart failure or arrhythmia), and the kidneys (renal failure causes 50% of scleroderma deaths). Females are affected more than males (3:1 ratio). A more restricted variant of systemic sclerosis, with a somewhat more benign course, is CREST syndrome (Calcinosis, Raynaud syndrome, Esophageal dysmotility, Sclerodactyly, and Telangiectasia), characterized by the presence of anti-centromere antibodies (although 10% of CREST patients will have anti-topoisomerase antibody as well).

Anti-ds DNA (**choice B**) and anti-Sm (Smith antigen; **choice D**) are characteristic of systemic lupus erythematosus (SLE) but are not common in patients with systemic sclerosis.

Rheumatoid factor is an autoantibody directed against IgG (**choice C**). It is found in patients with rheumatoid arthritis.

Anti-SS-A (**choice E**) is typically seen in Sjögren syndrome (although it may also be seen in SLE).

18. **The correct answer is D.** All of the organisms listed are protozoa. There are two intestinal protozoa specifically associated with AIDS that can cause transient diarrhea in immunocompetent individuals but can cause debilitating, and potentially life-threatening, chronic diarrhea in AIDS patients. These organisms are *Isospora belli* (treated with trimethoprim-sulfamethoxazole or other folate antagonists) and *Cryptosporidium parvum* (no treatment presently available).

*Diphyllobothrium latum* (**choice A**) is the fish tapeworm and occasionally causes diarrhea, which is not specifically associated with AIDS.

*Entamoeba histolytica* (**choice B**) and *Giardia lamblia* (**choice C**) are both causes of diarrhea, but they are not specifically associated with AIDS.

Microsporidia (**choice E**) are protozoa that cause diarrhea, but produce spores rather than oocysts.

19. **The correct answer is A.** The patient has Burkitt lymphoma. This high-grade B-cell lymphoma occurs endemically in Africa (it is the most common neoplasm in children in an equatorial belt that includes Africa and New Guinea) and sporadically in the U.S. and Europe. The sporadic form is often in an abdominal site and occurs in young adults. The African form of Burkitt lymphoma has been strongly associated with antibodies directed against Epstein-Barr virus; the association is weaker in sporadic cases. A characteristic translocation,

t(8;14) (q24.l3;q32.33) has been described. Malaria infection is a cofactor.

Hepatitis B (**choice B**) is associated with hepatocellular carcinoma. t(9;22) is the Philadelphia chromosome, which is seen in some cases of chronic myelogenous leukemia (CML) and acute myelogenous leukemia (AML).

Herpesvirus (**choice C**) type 8 is associated with Kaposi sarcoma. CD5 is a marker seen in small lymphocytic and mantle cell lymphomas.

HIV (**choice D**) is linked to AIDS. Some patients also develop primary lymphomas (not usually Burkitt). CD4 is a marker for helper T cells and some T cell lymphomas.

Human papillomavirus (**choice E**) is linked with common warts, genital condylomata, and genital cancers. t(2;5) is linked to anaplastic large cell lymphoma.

20. **The correct answer is E.** The combination of vomiting, anorexia, high fever (above 100.4 F), and a bulging fontanel equals neonatal meningitis until proven otherwise. *Streptococcus agalactiae* (group B strep) and *Escherichia coli* (not an answer choice) are the most common causes in neonates up to 1 month of age. The next most reasonable response would have been *Listeria monocytogenes* (**choice B**), another, though less common, cause of neonatal meningitis.

Most cases of meningitis caused by *Haemophilus influenzae* (**choice A**) occur in children aged 6 months to 6 years; 90% of these cases result from the capsular type b strain. It has become much less prevalent now that the *H. influenzae* type b conjugate vaccine is routinely administered to infants.

*Neisseria meningitidis* (**choice C**) is the most common cause of *epidemic* meningitis. The two organisms most often associated with sporadic cases are *Haemophilus influenzae* and *Streptococcus pneumoniae* (the most common cause in adults older than 30).

*Staphylococcus aureus* (**choice D**) is not a common cause of meningitis, except in patients with CSF shunts. It is often responsible for abscesses, osteomyelitis, endocarditis, toxic shock syndrome, and food poisoning.

21. **The correct answer is D.** *Pasteurella multocida* is a gram-negative rod that is normal flora of the oral cavity of dogs and cats. It often causes a local abscess following introduction under the skin by an animal bite. Most cases occur in children who are injured while playing with a pet.

*Bartonella henselae* (**choice A**) is a very small, gram-negative bacterium that is closely related to the rickettsia, although it is able to grow on inert media. It is the cause of cat-scratch disease (a local, chronic lymphadenitis most commonly seen in children) and

bacillary angiomatosis (seen particularly in AIDS patients). In this latter patient population, the organism causes proliferation of blood and lymphatic vessels causing a characteristic "mulberry" lesion in the skin and subcutaneous tissues of the afflicted individual.

*Brucella canis* (**choice B**) is a gram-negative rod that is a zoonotic agent. Its normal host is the dog, but when it gains access to humans, it causes an undulating febrile disease with malaise, lymphadenopathy and hepatosplenomegaly. The normal route of exposure is via ingestion of the organism.

*Clostridium tetani* (**choice C**) is a gram-positive spore-forming anaerobic rod. It causes tetanus [a spastic paralysis caused by tetanospasmin, which blocks the release of the inhibitory neurotransmitters glycine and gamma-aminobutyric acid (GABA)]. There may be no lesion at the site of inoculation, and exudation would be extremely rare.

*Toxocara canis* (**choice E**), a common intestinal parasite of dogs, is a metazoan parasite that causes visceral larva migrans. Young children are most likely to be affected, as they are most likely to ingest soil contaminated with eggs of the parasite.

22. **The correct answer is C.** Rotavirus is the most common cause of gastroenteritis in children aged 3 months to 2 years. It is most prevalent in the winter. Rotavirus, one of the reoviruses, looks like a wheel (which ROTAtes) and possesses a double-shelled icosahedral capsid with no envelope. Its genome consists of 11 segments of double-stranded RNA.

A complex double-stranded DNA genome (**choice A**) is found in enteric adenoviruses, the third most common cause of gastroenteritis in infants and children. This organism possesses an icosahedral nucleocapsid.

A partially double-stranded circular DNA genome (**choice B**) is characteristic of hepatitis B. Its envelope contains surface antigen (HBsAg). Its capsid is icosahedral and contains the genome, along with a DNA polymerase, which has reverse transcriptase activity.

A single-stranded circular RNA genome (**choice D**) is characteristic of hepatitis D virus. Its envelope consists of HBsAg. The virus is defective and can replicate only in cells infected with hepatitis B.

A single-stranded RNA genome (**choice E**) is characteristic of several viruses that cause gastroenteritis in children, including astrovirus and Norwalk virus. Astrovirus is the second most common cause of viral gastroenteritis in young children. Three structural proteins form its capsid. Norwalk virus is the most common cause of gastroenteritis outbreaks in older children and adults. Its capsid consists of one structural protein.

23. **The correct answer is A.** Amphotericin B is the most appropriate drug listed for the treatment of cryptococcal meningitis. It is a polyene antibiotic that binds to ergosterol in the fungal cell membrane, creating an artificial pore. Flucytosine is often prescribed as an adjunct medication. Fluconazole is used long-term to prevent recurrence in AIDS patients.

Isoniazid (**choice B**) inhibits the biosynthesis of mycolic acids in the mycobacterial cell wall. It is the primary drug used against tuberculosis. It is used alone for TB prophylaxis and in combination with other antituberculars to treat patients with active disease.

Ketoconazole (**choice C**) is an orally administered imidazole antifungal medication. It inhibits 14-alpha-demethylase to block the synthesis of fungal cell membrane ergosterol. Note the difference in mechanism between the polyenes, which alter ergosterol structure, and the imidazoles, which block ergosterol synthesis. Ketoconazole is often used to treat coccidioidomycosis (prevalent in California), histoplasmosis (prevalent in the Midwest), blastomycosis (prevalent in the eastern U.S.), paracoccidioidomycosis (prevalent in Latin America), and mucocutaneous candidiasis.

Metronidazole (**choice D**) is an antiprotozoal drug useful in treating a variety of parasitic infections. It is the drug of choice for trichomoniasis and giardiasis and provides general anaerobic coverage. This makes it useful for treating postsurgical abdominal and pelvic *Bacteroides fragilis* infections or flare-ups of intestinal diverticulitis.

Nystatin (**choice E**) is an antifungal polyene that is usually used topically but can be taken orally for oral and esophageal candidiasis. Candidal infections of the skin, mucous membranes, and vagina usually respond well to this drug. It may also be used to prevent intestinal fungal overgrowth in patients on chemotherapy.

24. **The correct answer is E.** This simple mathematical problem asks if the student understands the life cycle of the malaria parasite, specifically *Plasmodium vivax*. To answer the question, the student needs to understand the terminology and sequence of steps that this agent of "benign tertian" malaria goes through in the human host. The infectious form inoculated by the vector mosquito is the sporozoite. It immediately seeks out a hepatocyte, penetrates it, and undergoes the process of schizogony (asexual fission). The question stem tells us that one sporozoite is injected and within 10 days, 100 daughter merozoites will be produced from each sporozoite. Thus, at 10 days, 100 exoerythrocytic merozoites will be released. These parasitic forms will now seek out erythrocytes, and at 2-day intervals (for *P. vivax* and *P. ovale*) will again undergo

schizogony; this time, the question tells us to produce 10 merozoites per erythrocyte. There is no repetition of schizogony in the liver, but the cycle is repetitive in the erythrocytes, so that each crop of merozoites will repenetrate erythrocytes and undergo schizogony at 2-day intervals until the immune response or drug treatment stop the cycle. Thus, every 2 days after leaving the liver, there will be ten times the number of merozoites released as were released in the last cycle. The number of merozoites at 22 days will be 100 (day 10) × 10 (day 12) × 10 (day 14) × 10 (day 16) × 10 (day 18) × 10 (day 20) × 10 (day 22), or $100 \times 10^6$ or $1 \times 10^8$. If this question were posed for *P. malariae*, the erythrocytic schizogonic cycles would occur at 3-day intervals, and if the question were posed for *P. falciparum*, it would not be answerable because asynchronous schizogony and multiple infections of individual erythrocytes can alter the speed of multiplication.

25. **The correct answer is E.** *Proteus mirabilis* is a gram-negative rod that is a member of the family Enterobacteriaceae. It is lactose-negative and contains urease, which splits urea, raising the pH of the urine to create a more hospitable environment for the bacterium. Patients with stones are at increased risk for *Proteus* because the organism is able to hide in the stones, and patients with *Proteus* are more likely to get stones because the increased urinary pH contributes to their formation.

*Candida albicans* (**choice A**) is a yeast that can cause urinary tract infections in patients with poorly controlled diabetes because glucose in the urine enhances its growth.

*Enterococcus faecalis* (**choice B**) is a gram-positive coccus that commonly causes urinary tract infections in elderly men with prostate problems.

*Escherichia coli* (**choice C**) is a lactose-positive, oxidase-negative, gram-negative rod that is the most common cause of community-acquired urinary tract infections.

*Klebsiella pneumoniae* (**choice D**) is a lactose-positive, oxidase-negative, gram-negative rod. It can cause urinary tract infections in patients with poorly controlled diabetes because glucose in the urine enhances growth of this microorganism.

*Pseudomonas aeruginosa* (**choice F**) is a gram-negative rod. It can easily be distinguished from the family Enterobacteriaceae because it is oxidase-negative. It is an opportunistic pathogen that has an increased chance of causing urinary tract infections in patients who have catheters or are on antibiotics.

*Staphylococcus saprophyticus* (**choice G**) is a catalase-positive, coagulase-negative, gram-positive coccus that causes urinary tract infections in young, sexually active women.

26. **The correct answer is C.** This patient has disseminated gonococcal infection. Gonococcal arthritis and tenosynovitis typically involve both the upper and lower extremities equally. Vesicular skin lesions are characteristic of disseminated gonococcal disease. Females are at particular risk of gonococcemia during menstruation, since sloughing of the endometrium allows access to the blood supply, necrotic tissue enhances the growth of *Neisseria gonorrhoeae,* and there is an alteration of the pH. Patients who have a C6-C8 deficiency have both an increased risk of gonococcemia and a tendency to have multiple episodes. These patients are also at risk for bacteremia from *Neisseria meningitidis.*

C1 esterase inhibitor deficiency (**choice A**) can occur as an autosomal dominant disorder or may be acquired. Patients have angioedema without urticaria. The syndrome is also associated with recurrent attacks of colic and episodes of laryngeal edema.

Ciliary dysfunction (**choice B**) is a marker of Kartagener syndrome (immotile cilia syndrome). The syndrome includes infertility, bronchiectasis, sinusitis, and situs inversus. It is an autosomal recessive disorder caused by abnormalities in the dynein arm of the cilia.

Endothelial adhesion molecule deficiency (**choice D**), or beta-2 integrin deficiency, is characterized by failure of neutrophils to express CD18 integrins on their surface. Patients have impaired phagocyte adherence, aggregation, chemotaxis, and phagocytosis of C3b-coated particles. Clinically, there is delayed separation of the umbilical cord, sustained agranulocytosis, recurrent infections of skin and mucosa, gingivitis, and periodontal disease.

Eosinophil deficiency (**choice E**) or eosinopenia occurs with stressors such as acute bacterial infection and following administration of glucocorticoids. There is no known adverse effect of eosinopenia.

27. **The correct answer is A.** The clinical history suggests infant botulism. The clue here is that the mother feeds the infant honey. *Clostridium botulinum* (a common honey contaminant) was ingested and produced toxin in the infant. The toxin, which blocks the release of acetylcholine from nerve terminals, is responsible for the flacid paralysis. Acetylcholine is the neurotransmitter at the neuromuscular junction, and inhibition of release can lead to muscle weakness, failure to thrive, and, in more serious cases, respiratory impairment.

Glycine and GABA (**choice B**) release is inhibited by a toxin produced by *Clostridium tetani.* This leads to the muscular spasms of tetanus.

ADP-ribosylation of an elongation factor (**choice C**) is the mechanism of action of diphtheria and *Pseudomonas* exotoxins.

Alpha toxin from *Clostridium perfringens* is a lecithinase (**choice D**) responsible for the development of gas gangrene.

Guanylate cyclase (**choice E**) is stimulated by the heat-stable toxin produced by *Escherichia coli.*

28. **The correct answer is J.** The patient has cerebral toxoplasmosis. Toxoplasmosis is a major cause of neurologic symptoms in HIV-infected and other immunosuppressed patients. Domestic cats are the primary host for *Toxoplasma gondii* (a sporozoan) and shed oocysts in their feces. Uncooked meats are another source of *Toxoplasma* infection. Symptoms in humans arise from the ingestion of these cysts, leading to invasion of the gut wall and subsequent systemic dissemination. Parasites that migrate to the brain cause multiple necrotic lesions, particularly in the cortex and deep gray nuclei. Patients present with fever, headache, and focal neurologic symptoms. Ring-enhancing lesions are characteristic.

Coxsackievirus (**choice A**) can cause a variety of diseases, including herpangina, hand-foot-and-mouth disease, pleurodynia, myocarditis, and pericarditis. CNS complications include aseptic meningitis, mild paresis, and transient paralysis.

*Cryptococcus neoformans* (**choice B**) is an oval, budding yeast with a wide polysaccharide capsule. Infection results from the inhalation of the organism, which can then disseminate to the CNS (particularly in immunocompromised patients). CNS infection leads to a chronic meningitis characterized by high protein levels in the CSF. *C. neoformans* can be visualized in the CSF with an India ink preparation.

Cytomegalovirus (**choice C**) is prevalent in immunocompromised patients and causes chorioretinitis, esophagitis, colitis, interstitial pneumonitis, and meningoencephalitis. In infants infected *in utero,* it also causes chorioretinitis, hepatosplenomegaly, deafness, periventricular calcifications, and hemorrhages. It is not a likely cause of ring-enhancing lesions.

*Diphyllobothrium latum* (**choice D**), the fish tapeworm, is contracted through the ingestion of raw or inadequately cooked fish. Infection can cause abdominal discomfort, diarrhea, and in some cases a vitamin $B_{12}$ deficiency (the tapeworm absorbs all of the available vitamin $B_{12}$).

Herpes simplex virus (**choice E**) causes several forms of disease, including gingivostomatitis, herpes labialis, keratoconjunctivitis, and genital herpes. CNS complications include aseptic meningitis and, rarely, encephalitis. HSV encephalitis typically results in large necrotizing lesions of the inferomedial temporal lobes and the orbital gyri of the frontal lobes. It is usually heralded by sudden onset of headache, fever, and mental status changes. It is not a usual cause of ring-enhancing lesions.

*Mycobacterium leprae* (**choice F**) causes leprosy and preferentially infects the skin and superficial nerves (because it prefers cooler temperatures).

*Pasteurella multocida* (**choice G**) is a gram-negative rod that is part of the normal oral flora of domestic dogs and cats. It causes a rapid onset cellulitis at the site of an animal bite.

*Pneumocystis carinii* (**choice H**) is a fungus that causes pneumonia, particularly in immunocompromised patients.

*Taenia solium* (**choice I**) is the pork tapeworm that can cause cysticercosis. Cysticercosis results from the ingestion of tapeworm eggs in fecally contaminated food or water. The eggs hatch in the intestine, burrow through the gut wall, and disseminate throughout the body. The parasite frequently ends up in the eyes or the brain, where it encysts and produces a focal space-occupying mass until it is calcified and killed.

29.  **The correct answer is C.** The single finding of high autoantibody titers to histones, without any other autoantibodies, is characteristic of drug-induced lupus. The most commonly implicated drugs are procainamide, hydralazine (given for hypertension), and isoniazid. Patients typically have milder disease than in systemic lupus erythematosus (SLE), and tend to have arthritis, pleuro-pericardial involvement, and, less commonly, rash. CNS and renal disease are not usually observed.

CREST syndrome (**choice A**) is a milder variant of scleroderma characterized by calcinosis, Raynaud phenomenon, esophageal dysmotility, sclerodactyly and telangiectasia. Anti-centromere antibodies are diagnostic.

The diffuse form of scleroderma (**choice B**), also known as systemic sclerosis, causes fibrosis of the skin and internal viscera. This disorder is characterized by anti-SCI-70 and often low titers of many other autoantibodies.

Sjögren syndrome (**choice D**) is characterized by dry eyes and dry mouth. Sjögren syndrome in isolation is characteristically positive for anti-SS-A and anti-SS-B. If it accompanies rheumatoid arthritis, anti-RNP will be positive as well.

SLE (**choice E**) is a multisystem disorder that is distinguished from drug-induced lupus by the presence of a wide variety of autoantibodies, including anti-double-stranded DNA (anti-dsDNA).

30.  **The correct answer is A.** All the agents listed can infect the eyeball. The agent specifically associated with contact lens use is *Acanthamoeba*, which can infect lens solution. This amoeba is dangerous because it causes an intractable ulcerative keratitis that may progress to uveitis. If the lesion is suspected, the clinical laboratory should be notified, and specific directions for collecting samples for culture obtained. The parasites may be difficult to see in histologic sections or corneal scrapings.

Cytomegalovirus (**choice B**) and herpes (**choice C**) infections are most often seen in immunocompromised patients, particularly AIDS patients.

Circulating larvae of the helminth *Toxocara* (**choice D**) can lodge in the eye (particularly in the vitreous or retina); *Toxocara* infections are seen more commonly in children and would cause granulomatous, not ulcerative, change.

Toxoplasmosis (**choice E**) of the eye is most often congenital, but it can be acquired. It produces retinal scarring, not corneal ulceration.

31.  **The correct answer is A.** This patient has the symptoms of a urinary tract infection (UTI). *Escherichia coli* is the leading cause of community-acquired UTIs. The proximity of the urinary tract to the anus facilitates colonization of the tract by fecal flora.

Other gram-negative rods causing UTIs include *Enterobacter cloacae*, *Klebsiella pneumoniae*, *Serratia marcescens*, *Proteus mirabilis*, and *Pseudomonas aeruginosa*.

None of the other choices listed cause UTIs.

32.  **The correct answer is E.** This is the classic microscopic description of the pneumococcus *Streptococcus pneumoniae*, which is a common cause of lobar pneumonia. Most strains are still very sensitive to penicillins, although some drug-resistant strains have been isolated.

*Haemophilus influenzae* (**choice A**) is a gram-negative bacillus. Nontypeable strains may cause pneumonia in elderly patients with chronic respiratory disease.

*Neisseria gonorrhoeae* (**choice B**) is a gram-negative diplococcus that is not typically associated with pneumonia.

*Pneumocystis carinii* (**choice C**) is a small, hat-shaped fungus that is a common cause of pneumonia in HIV-positive patients.

*Staphylococcus aureus* (**choice D**) occurs as grape-like clusters of large, gram-positive cocci. It may cause pneumonia after surgery or after a viral respiratory infection, such as influenza, and is associated with empyema formation.

33. **The correct answer is E.** This is a case of rheumatic fever, which is an immunologically mediated sequela to *Streptococcus pyogenes* pharyngitis. It is a type II cytotoxic hypersensitivity, involving antibodies that bind to cardiac tissue, activate complement, and thereby cause cell destruction. It is therefore most similar to idiopathic thrombocytopenic purpura, which is also a form of type II cytotoxic hypersensitivity, in this case mediated by antibodies against platelets producing complement fixation and causing the clotting dyscrasia.

Atopic allergy (**choice A**) is a form of type I hypersensitivity, mediated by IgE antibodies, basophils, and mast cells.

Contact dermatitis (**choice B**) is a form of type IV hypersensitivity mediated by T cells and macrophages.

Graft-versus-host disease (**choice C**) is a form of type IV hypersensitivity mediated by T cells and macrophages.

Graves disease (**choice D**) is a form of type II hypersensitivity, but it is *not* cytotoxic in its action. Instead, antibodies to the TSH receptors on thyroid cells cause overstimulation of the gland and its eventual exhaustion.

Myasthenia gravis (**choice F**) is a form of type II hypersensitivity, but *not* of the cytotoxic variety. In this case, antibodies to the acetylcholine receptors on neurons diminish neurotransmission.

Rheumatoid arthritis (**choice G**) is a form of type III hypersensitivity, caused by immune complex deposition in joints and subsequent activation of complement.

Serum sickness (**choice H**) is a form of type III hypersensitivity, caused by immune complex deposition.

Systemic lupus erythematosus (**choice I**) is a form of type III hypersensitivity, caused by immune complex deposition.

34. **The correct answer is A.** This patient has *Candida* esophagitis. Any time a patient presents with dysphagia or odontophagia, along with white plaques in the oropharynx (thrush), you can assume that the *Candida* is affecting the esophagus as well. The fact that the patient is an IV drug user makes an opportunistic infection such as *Candida* more likely. *Candida* appears as budding yeast with pseudohyphae *in vivo*.

The other answer choices represent the morphology of other important opportunistic fungi:

*Cryptococcus* is an encapsulated yeast (**choice B**). You should think about *Cryptococcus neoformans* when you're presented with an immunocompromised patient with neurologic symptoms. The classic clue is the presence of encapsulated organisms observable in an India ink preparation.

*Mucor* and *Rhizopus* are molds with nonseptate hyphae (**choice C**). You should think about *Mucor* when you are presented with a diabetic (especially in ketoacidosis) or a leukemic patient with a severe sinus infection.

*Aspergillus* is a mold with septate hyphae (**choice D**). In immunocompromised patients, aspergillosis can present with acute pneumonia, often with cavitation (aspergillomas = fungus balls in the lungs).

35. **The correct answer is E.** Whenever you see a question about a gardener who works with roses, think "*Sporothrix schenckii.*" This organism is responsible for sporotrichosis, "rose gardener disease." The organism enters through skin breaks in the fingers or hands, causing a chancre, papule, or subcutaneous nodule with erythema and fluctuance. Ulcerating lesions appear along lymphatic channels, but the lymph nodes are not commonly infected. Potassium iodide is the treatment of choice for the subcutaneous manifestations.

*Aspergillus* (**choice A**) causes pulmonary aspergillosis—a systemic mycotic infection. There is an allergic type that is caused by a hypersensitivity reaction to the organism and an infectious type that occurs more commonly in the immunocompromised. Hemoptysis is a common symptom.

*Malassezia* (**choice B**), specifically *M. furfur*, causes tinea versicolor, a superficial mycotic infection.

*Onchocerca* (**choice C**), specifically *O. volvulus*, causes river blindness. This organism is a helminth that is transmitted by blackflies in Africa, Central America, and South America.

*Rhizopus* (**choice D**) causes rhinocerebral infections in diabetics with ketoacidosis.

36. **The correct answer is A.** Lobar pneumonia, in which an entire lobe of the lung becomes rapidly affected with pneumonia, is actually a relatively uncommon pattern for pneumonia. Common causative organisms include *Streptococcus pneumoniae* (pneumococcus), *Haemophilus influenzae*, and *Klebsiella pneumoniae*. *K. pneumoniae* is specifically associated with alcohol abuse, diabetes mellitus, and nosocomial infections.

*Legionella* spp. (**choice B**) most commonly causes a patchy atypical pneumonia not specifically associated with alcoholism. Instead, *Legionella* infection is associated with inspiration of aerosolized contaminated water.

*Mycoplasma pneumoniae* (**choice C**) causes atypical pneumonia (extensive patchy infiltrates) rather than lobar pneumonia. It is the most common cause of pneumonia in young adults.

*Pneumocystis carinii* (**choice D**) causes atypical pneumonia with diffuse interstitial and alveolar infiltrates, typically in patients immunosuppressed by AIDS, cytotoxic drug therapy, or cancer.

*Staphylococcus aureus* (**choice E**) produces a necrotizing, abscessing pneumonia. Staphylococcal pneumonia may complicate influenza during epidemics, or it may be a nosocomial infection. It is associated with empyema formation.

37. **The correct answer is D.** There is a specific association between diabetes (particularly in brittle diabetics who may have episodes of ketoacidosis) and chronic sinusitis due to saprophytic Zygomycetes, including *Mucor* and *Rhizopus*. These fungi can spread rapidly from the sinuses to the nearby skull bones and brain, potentially causing massive tissue destruction and death. The term "rhinocerebral mucormycosis" is used in these cases. Less commonly, other sites may be involved (lung, gastrointestinal tract), depending on the port of entry. The physician should suspect mucormycosis in any patient with chronic sinusitis who appears unusually ill and does not respond to antibiotic therapy. Unfortunately, most cases are diagnosed at autopsy.

*Actinomyces* (**choice A**) are part of the normal flora of the mouth. Actinomycosis also occurs in humans and may affect the cervicofacial region (typically following dental procedures or maxillofacial injuries), lungs, abdomen (typically following surgery, trauma, or intestinal penetration), or pelvis (related to IUD use). There is no specific association with diabetes mellitus.

*Aspergillus* (**choice B**) can be present in the sinuses, and does have a somewhat increased incidence in diabetics, but is not the organism about which the physician should be most concerned.

*Cryptococcus* (**choice C**) is found in pigeon feces and is usually introduced into the body via the respiratory tract. It can disseminate to the meninges and other sites in immunocompromised patients (often AIDS patients). It would not be of particular concern in this patient with sinusitis.

*Pneumocystis carinii* (**choice E**) causes pneumonia in severely immunosuppressed patients, e.g., AIDS patients.

38. **The correct answer is B.** This question is difficult for two reasons. First, it asks for the viral family instead of the virus itself. Second, it includes distracters that all look alike. You probably realized that the child in question has croup (laryngotracheobronchitis); the classic clue here is the "barking cough." You might have remembered that the virus responsible for croup is the parainfluenza virus. The toughest part was remembering that parainfluenza

virus (along with measles virus, mumps virus, and respiratory syncytial virus) belongs to the paramyxovirus family. These viruses all have negative-strand RNA and an enveloped helical nucleocapsid.

The papovaviruses (**choice A**) are DNA viruses with a naked icosahedral nucleocapsid. This family includes the human papilloma viruses, which cause warts and are associated with penile, laryngeal, and especially, cervical cancer; the BK virus, which can affect immunosuppressed patients; the JC virus, which is associated with progressive multifocal leukoencephalopathy; and the simian SV40 virus.

The parvoviruses (**choice C**) are small, single-stranded DNA viruses. Only one (B19) causes diseases in humans: erythema infectiosum in children (characteristic "slapped cheek" rash), aplastic crises in patients with hemolytic diseases, and hydrops fetalis or stillbirth in anemic fetuses.

The picornaviruses (**choice D**) are positive single-stranded RNA viruses with a naked icosahedral nucleocapsid. This family includes the polioviruses, echoviruses, coxsackieviruses, enterovirus 72 (HepA virus), and rhinoviruses (common cold).

The poxviruses (**choice E**) are double-stranded DNA viruses. This family includes the viruses responsible for smallpox and molluscum contagiosum.

39. **The correct answer is D.** Pyogenic osteomyelitis may result from hematogenous dissemination or local spread from a contiguous infectious focus. Patients with sickle cell disease are prone to osteomyelitis, and *Salmonella* spp. are the most common etiologic agents in this group. Bone pain, fever, and x-ray evidence of early bone demineralization and soft tissue swelling are the presenting clinical picture.

*Hemophilus influenzae* (**choice B**) and group B streptococci (**choice A**) are the most common causes of osteomyelitis occurring in infants.

Osteomyelitis caused by *Mycobacterium tuberculosis* (**choice C**) most commonly affects vertebral bones and develops in 3% of cases of disseminated tuberculosis. A chronic destructive infection of the lumbar vertebrae that tracks down along the iliopsoas muscle into the soft tissue of the inguinal fossa is referred to as Pott disease.

*Staphylococcus aureus* (**choice E**) is the major cause of osteomyelitis in all patients other than those who have sickle-cell disease.

40. **The correct choice is A.** *Campylobacter* is a motile, curved, oxidase-positive, gram-negative rod with polar flagella. The illness typically begins 1 to 7 days following ingestion of the organism. The presentation is usually

lower abdominal pain and diarrhea with blood and pus. The illness is self-limited after 3 to 5 days and can last up to 2 weeks. The organisms grow optimally at 42 C under microaerophilic conditions.

*Escherichia coli* (**choice B**) is a flagellated gram-negative, oxidative-negative organism. It is not a common cause of bloody diarrhea in this age group.

*Salmonella* (**choice C**) and *Shigella* (**choice D**) are incorrect because they are oxidase-negative.

*Vibrio cholerae* (**choice E**) has many physical features in common with *C. jejuni*. However, *V. cholerae* is not enteroinvasive and does not produce bloody diarrhea, but "rice water" stools.

41. **The correct answer is A.** *Bacillus cereus* produces a self-limited diarrhea due to ingestion of the preformed enterotoxin in contaminated fried rice and seafood. The incubation period is typically around 4 hours. The degree of vomiting is greater than the diarrhea. *B. cereus* is also associated with keratitis, producing a corneal ring abscess.

*Clostridium botulinum* (**choice B**) produces a neurotoxin that blocks the release of acetylcholine, resulting in a symmetric descending paralysis that may lead to respiratory complications causing death. Symptoms include blurred vision, photophobia, dysphagia, nausea, vomiting, and dysphonia. Most cases are associated with the ingestion of contaminated home-canned food.

*Clostridium perfringens* (**choice C**) produces a severe diarrhea with abdominal pain and cramping (sometimes called "church picnic" diarrhea). The incubation period is 8 to 24 hours after ingesting contaminated meat, meat products, or poultry. The meats have usually been cooked, allowed to cool, and then warmed, which causes germination of the clostridial spores.

EHEC—Enterohemorrhagic *Escherichia coli* (**choice D**), produces a bloody, noninvasive diarrhea due to the ingestion of verotoxin found in undercooked hamburger at fast food restaurants. The 0157:H7 serotype typically produces this syndrome. Some patients develop a life-threatening complication called hemolytic-uremic syndrome.

*Staphylococcus aureus* (**choice E**) produces a self-limited food poisoning syndrome with nausea, vomiting, and abdominal pain followed by diarrhea beginning 1 to 6 hours after ingestion of the enterotoxin. The organism is found in foods such as potato salad, custard, milk shakes, and mayonnaise.

*Vibrio cholerae* (**choice F**) typically produces a watery, nonbloody diarrhea with flecks of mucus (rice-water stools). Abdominal pain is not a feature. Massive fluid loss and electrolyte imbalance are complications. In the U.S., cases of cholera (El Tor 01 strain) are associated with the Gulf coast and ingestion of poorly cooked or poorly stored crabs, shrimp, or oysters. A strain of *V. cholerae* called non-01 is also found along the Gulf coast. Patients who ingest contaminated shellfish experience fever, copious watery diarrhea, and abdominal cramps within 48 hours after eating.

42. **The correct answer is D.** The nurse's elevated IgM anti-HBc indicates that she was infected with hepatitis B. Formerly, HBsAg (surface antigen) and anti-HBsAg (antibody to surface antigen) were used exclusively to determine this. Typically, HBsAg is positive for up to 6 months, and anti-HBsAg is positive for years after that. Unfortunately, this simple scheme has the disadvantage that many patients have a 2-week to 4-month "window" period, when the surface antigen (HBsAg) and the antibody (anti-HBs) are not detectable. Presumably, for a relatively brief period, HBsAg production exactly matches antibody production, and the two coprecipitate such that neither free species is present in adequate concentration to be detectable. This problem can be circumvented either by serial measurements of HBsAg and anti-HBs, or by concurrent measurement of other antigens and antibodies, including HBeAg, anti-HBe, and anti-HBc (HBcAg is not reliable). During the window period, IgM anti-HBc may be the only marker of recent HBV infection, as it is in this nurse.

If the nurse had been effectively vaccinated for hepatitis B (**choice A**), she would have had an elevated anti-HBs antibody level and no HBsAg present in the serum. Anti-HBc antibody would have been absent as well.

The antibody response to hepatitis B infection was appropriate in this person, which argues against immunocompromise (**choice B**).

Carriers (**choice C**) have elevated HBsAg and may have persistently elevated HBeAg (in approximately 10% of cases). IgG anti-HBc (not IgM) predominates in these chronic patients.

Had she not been infected with hepatitis B at all (**choice E**), IgM anti-HBc would be absent.

43. **The correct answer is A.** This patient presents with the classic findings of granuloma inguinale (Donovanosis). The clue that he had traveled to New Guinea clinches the diagnosis (granuloma inguinale is common in India and New Guinea and rare in the U.S.). This is a chronic, sexually transmitted disease (STD) that presents with ulcerating granulomata of the genital skin and mucous membranes. On biopsy, there is granulation tissue and microabscesses with macrophages containing diagnostic Donovan bodies (small, rounded coccobacilli within cystic areas of the cytoplasm seen with Wright-Giemsa

stain). This disease is caused by the bacterium *Calymmatobacterium donovani*.

*Chlamydia trachomatis* (**choice B**) causes lymphogranuloma venereum, an STD that is rare in the U.S. but common in the tropics. It can present with genital or anorectal lesions or regional lymphadenopathy. Cytoplasmic inclusion bodies would be seen in epithelial cells.

*Haemophilus ducreyi* (**choice C**) causes chancroid, an STD that presents with a painful chancre and regional lymphadenopathy. Remember that "ducreyi" makes you "cry" (because it's painful).

Human papillomavirus (**choice D**) comes in various strains, is associated with common warts as well as condylomata acuminata, and is a risk factor for cervical cancer in infected women and penile cancer in infected men.

*Neisseria gonorrhoeae* (**choice E**) causes gonorrhea. There may be purulent inflammation or abscesses.

*Treponema pallidum* (**choice F**) causes syphilis. Patients usually present with cutaneous manifestations followed by widespread dissemination. It occurs in three stages: primary syphilis is associated with a painless chancre; secondary syphilis is associated with condylomata lata; and tertiary syphilis involves the brain (neurosyphilis) and the aorta (aneurysm) with the development of gummas.

44. **The correct answer is E.** Parvovirus, especially type B19, is notorious for infecting bone marrow and causing an abrupt failure of erythropoiesis. This leads to the disappearance of all erythroblasts from the marrow. The marrow usually recovers in 10 to 12 days, and patients without anemia usually never realize that they had the infection. Unfortunately, patients with severe anemia of many different etiologies (e.g., hereditary spherocytosis, as these patients have, leukemia, post-chemotherapy, sickle cell anemia, thalassemia, and hemolytic anemia) may develop an "aplastic crisis," which requires multiple transfusions to maintain appropriate numbers of erythrocytes in the blood. Patients with hemolytic anemias are particularly vulnerable, since the lifetime of erythrocytes in peripheral blood in these patients may be as short as 10 days.

Adenovirus (**choice A**) causes upper and lower respiratory tract infections, conjunctivitis, and diarrhea.

Cytomegalovirus (**choice B**) is a herpesvirus associated with hepatitis, pneumonitis, congenital malformations from *in utero* infections, and retinitis and ophthalmitis in patients with HIV.

Herpes simplex viruses (**choice C**) cause cold sores and genital herpes. In rare cases, encephalitis may be produced by infection with these agents.

Measles virus (**choice D**) causes measles (rubeola).

45. **The correct answer is D.** This patient has hemolytic-uremic syndrome (HUS), a complication of the Shiga toxin or Shiga-like toxin (exotoxins released by *Shigella* species and the enterohemorrhagic *Escherichia coli*). In children, HUS usually develops after a gastrointestinal or flu-like illness and is characterized by bleeding, oliguria, hematuria, and microangiopathic hemolytic anemia. Presumably the Shiga toxin is toxic to the microvasculature, producing microthrombi that consume platelets and RBCs, and may fragment the red cell membrane.

The incorrect choices are all bacteria that may produce an enterocolitis but do not elicit HUS.

A long-term consequence of *Campylobacter* (**choice A**) infection is a reactive arthritis or full-blown Reiter syndrome.

Clostridial enterocolitis is produced by *Clostridium difficile* (**choice B**), a normal inhabitant of the gut that produces pseudomembranous colitis when other gut flora are suppressed by treatment with antibiotics.

In the U.S., *Salmonella* infections (**choice C**) are almost all nontyphoid inflammatory diarrhea, producing a simple enterocolitis that may proceed to sepsis in some cases. Typhoid fever (produced by *Salmonella typhi* and *Salmonella paratyphi*) causes a protracted illness that progresses over several weeks and includes rash and very high fevers, but not HUS.

*Vibrio* (**choice E**) infections produce copious amounts of watery diarrhea. The major risk of cholera and other *Vibrio* enteritides is shock due to hypovolemia or electrolyte loss.

46. **The correct answer is A.** In this case, the patient has all the hallmarks of mononucleosis (the heterophile antibodies should have confirmed your suspicion from the history and physical). Mononucleosis is caused by the Epstein-Barr virus, which, in turn, belongs to the herpesvirus family. The herpesviruses are enveloped viruses with double-stranded DNA. Remember that, in addition to Epstein-Barr virus, the herpesvirus family also includes herpes simplex (1 and 2), varicella-zoster (chickenpox, shingles), and cytomegalovirus (infection in immunocompromised patients). Cytomegalovirus also causes infectious mononucleosis, but the heterophile test is negative in these patients.

There are two families of viruses that are nonenveloped with double-stranded DNA (**choice B**): papovaviruses and adenoviruses.

There are many families of viruses that are enveloped with single-stranded RNA (**choice C**): arenaviruses, bunyaviruses, coronaviruses, filoviruses, flaviviruses, paramyxoviruses, orthomyxoviruses, retroviruses, rhabdoviruses, and togaviruses.

Parvoviruses are the only family of DNA virus with single-stranded DNA. They do not have an envelope (**choice D**).

There are two families of RNA virus that are single-stranded without an envelope (**choice E**): caliciviruses and picornaviruses.

47. **The correct answer is B.** This patient has lymphogranuloma venereum caused by *Chlamydia trachomatis* (type L1, L2, or L3). *Chlamydia* exhibit distinct infectious and reproductive forms. The extracellular infectious form is known as the elementary body (EB), which cannot reproduce. It attaches to the host cell and enters through endocytosis. Once inside the cell, the EB is transformed into the reticulate body (RB) within the endosome. The RB is capable of binary fission and divides within the endosome; fusion with other endosomes occurs to form a single large inclusion. Eventually, the RBs undergo DNA condensation and disulfide bond bridgings of the major outer membrane protein, forming EBs. The EBs are then released. Note that *C. trachomatis* is responsible for several sexually or perinatally transmitted diseases, including ocular trachoma (types A, B, and C), neonatal conjunctivitis, nongonococcal urethritis, cervicitis, and pelvic inflammatory disease (types D-K).

*Calymmatobacterium granulomatis* (**choice A**) is a gram-negative rod that causes superficially ulcerated genital or inguinal papules that coalesce to form substantial lesions. The appearance of Donovan bodies in histiocytes is diagnostic of this infection.

*Haemophilus ducreyi* (**choice C**) is a gram-negative rod that causes a soft, painful penile chancre, unlike that of a chlamydial or syphilitic lesion. This infection is common in the tropics.

*Neisseria gonorrhoeae* (**choice D**) is a gram-negative diplococcus responsible for gonorrhea. Patients typically present with purulent penile discharge, not genital lesions.

*Treponema pallidum* (**choice E**) is the spirochete responsible for syphilis. It may cause a firm, painless ulcer as a manifestation of primary syphilis, but the organism does not exist in distinct extracellular and intracellular forms as does *Chlamydia*. Secondary syphilis is associated with the appearance of condylomata lata—flat, gray, wart-like lesions.

48. **The correct answer is E.** For many years, Whipple disease was suspected of having a bacterial etiology because bacterial forms could be seen on electron microscopy. However, the identity of the causative agent remained elusive. It has recently been found to be a bacterium, which is now named *Tropheryma whippelii*.

*Clostridium difficile* (**choice A**) causes pseudomembranous colitis, generally after antibiotic administration.

Enterotoxigenic *Escherichia coli* (**choice B**) is associated with tropical sprue and traveler's diarrhea.

*Isospora belli* (**choice C**) is a cause of diarrhea in AIDS patients.

*Salmonella* sp. (**choice D**) can cause diarrheal illness after ingestion of contaminated poultry or beef.

49. **The correct answer is A.** Bacillary angiomatosis is a disease that occurs primarily in AIDS patients and is indicative of a defect in cell-mediated immunity. It is caused by either *Bartonella henselae* or *Bartonella quintana*. The domestic cat is the reservoir for these organisms, which are usually transmitted to humans via a cat scratch or bite. Patients with this illness usually have multiple skin lesions and extracutaneous manifestations involving liver and bone. Diagnosis is usually based on characteristic histopathologic findings, including plump "epithelioid" endothelial cells and mitotic figures. A macrolide, such as erythromycin or azithromycin, is the drug of choice for the infection.

Human papillomavirus (**choice B**) causes warts. It can present as sessile warts or as condylomata acuminata, which are fleshy soft growths that coalesce into large masses. When cellular immunity is depressed, as in AIDS, the condylomata acuminata proliferate.

Molluscum contagiosum (**choice C**) is caused by a poxvirus that is spread by close person-to-person contact. Infection produces a firm nodule that often becomes umbilicated and may resolve by discharging its contents. In AIDS, the lesions do not resolve, but enlarge and spread.

*Rickettsia prowazekii* (**choice D**) is the cause of epidemic typhus. It is spread by the human body louse *Pediculus humanus*. Its reservoirs are humans and flying squirrels.

*Treponema pallidum* (**choice E**) is the spirochete that causes syphilis. The primary lesion of syphilis is a chancre (a painless, indurated ulcer).

50. **The correct answer is D.** A small segment of DNA containing drug-resistance genes and three pairs of indirect repeats is a description of a group of three transposons. Transposons, or "jumping genes," are segments of DNA capable of movement from one location to another inside a cell. When they become accumulated in one location, particularly if that location is inside a fertility factor plasmid, then they can be transferred to new bacteria by conjugation. This is how multiple drug resistance plasmids are formed. Transposons are flanked by indirect repeats, which are sequences that are complementary and antiparallel to one another. Inside the indirect repeats, they carry the coding for the enzymes that mediate the actual movement from place to place, transposase genes, and other genetic coding (such as the drug-resistance genes described here).

A temperate phage (**choice A**) is a bacterial virus that incorporates its genome into the chromosome of the bacterium during its life cycle (lysogeny). There is no reason to expect that viral DNA would be found within a transposon.

OriT (**choice B**) is the genetic locus at which a break in the double-stranded DNA of either plasmid (fertility factor) or episome (Hfr chromosome) is made to begin transfer of DNA across a conjugal bridge. Transposons are not involved in the process of conjugation, although they can be transferred passively across a conjugal bridge if they become inserted in a fertility factor.

The tra operon (**choice C**) is the set of genes found in a fertility factor and that mediates the actual mechanism of conjugation. They encode sex pili, the enzymes of DNA metabolism, and those that mediate formation of the conjugal bridge. Because transposons move by site-specific recombination, it is not possible that the tra operon could be found inside the margins of a transposon.

Three pairs of direct repeats (**choice E**) could not be found inside the segment of DNA that includes three transposons. Direct repeats are formed by repair of the staggered breaks made in the recipient DNA when a transposon lands. Thus, with three transposons landing in a small area of DNA, two sets of direct repeats could be inside the margins, but the third set would have to be outside the outermost set of indirect repeats.

# Pathology and Pathophysiology: **Test One**

1. A 75-year-old man with a 5-year history of stable angina pectoris is brought to the emergency department with severe chest pain. EKG reveals profound ST segment elevations, and the CK-MB level is elevated. On stabilization, the patient is admitted to the coronary care unit for further management. Several days later, the patient again complains of chest pain. Physical examination is significant for fever, loud pericardial friction rub, mild pulmonary rales, and 1+ pitting edema of the lower extremities. Which of the following is the most likely diagnosis?

   (A) Caseous pericarditis

   (B) Fibrinous pericarditis

   (C) Hemorrhagic pericarditis

   (D) Serous pericarditis

   (E) Suppurative pericarditis

2. A 46-year-old woman presents to her physician complaining of weakness and fatigue. On physical examination, her physician notices a 10-lb weight gain since her last visit 6 months ago. Her blood pressure is 160/100 mm Hg. Blood tests reveal serum $Na^+$ 155 mEq/L, $K^+$ 2.8 mEq/L, and decreased serum renin. Which of the following is the most likely diagnosis?

   (A) Cushing syndrome

   (B) Diabetes mellitus

   (C) Pheochromocytoma

   (D) Primary aldosteronism

   (E) Secondary aldosteronism

3. A 24-year-old medical student comes to the student health center because of a "skin problem." She has no other complaints at this time. A physical examination is performed, and the physician gives the most likely diagnosis, explaining that her dermatologic condition is likely caused by hypersensitivity to an antigen that is taken up by Langerhans cells. These antigen-presenting cells process antigens and present them to naive CD4-positive T cells. Antigen re-exposure leads to recruitment of helper T cells and release of cytokines that mediate the inflammatory response. Which of the following dermatologic conditions is mediated by this type of hypersensitivity reaction?

   (A) Acne vulgaris

   (B) Bullous pemphigoid

   (C) Contact dermatitis

   (D) Dermatitis herpetiformis

   (E) Discoid lupus erythematosus

   (F) Urticaria

   (G) Pemphigus vulgaris

4. A 41-year-old obese woman with a history of biliary colic presents with right upper quadrant discomfort and pain in her right shoulder after eating a fatty meal. Physical examination is significant for marked right upper quadrant tenderness during inspiration. Which of the following structures is most likely involved in producing her shoulder pain?

   (A) Expiratory motor neuron

   (B) Inspiratory motor neuron

   (C) Intercostal nerve

   (D) Phrenic nerve

   (E) Vagus nerve

5. On a routine physical examination for medical insurance, a midsystolic ejection murmur is detected in the pulmonic area of a 35-year-old female executive. The cardiac examination also reveals a prominent right ventricular cardiac impulse and wide and fixed splitting of the second heart sound. An EKG shows right axis deviation, and a chest x-ray film shows enlargement of the right ventricle and atrium. Which of the following is the most likely diagnosis?

   (A) Aortic stenosis

   (B) Atrial septal defect

   (C) Mitral regurgitation

   (D) Mitral stenosis

   (E) Pulmonary valve stenosis

6. A 5-year-old boy, hospitalized for cellulitis, exhibits global denudation of the skin resulting from splitting of the epidermis at the stratum granulosum. Which of the following is the most likely diagnosis?

   (A) Impetigo

   (B) Melasma

   (C) Scalded skin syndrome

   (D) Tinea corporis

   (E) Vitiligo

7. A 6-month-old child has an eye surgically enucleated because it contains a retinoblastoma. To which of the following structures should the pathologist pay particular attention when evaluating the specimen?

   (A) Anterior chamber

   (B) Cornea

   (C) Lens

   (D) Optic nerve

   (E) Vitreous

8. A 14-year-old boy is brought to the physician because his mother noticed that his face looked puffy. The boy has no complaints, other than a recent upper respiratory infection that has resolved. No significant medical history is evident except for hay fever during the spring and summer. On examination, the boy is normotensive, has significant periorbital swelling, and 1+ pitting edema of both extremities. Urine dipstick reveals 3+ proteinuria and no blood. No casts are seen on microscopic examination. 24-hour urine reveals 3.7 g/day protein. Serum albumin is 2.4 g/dL, and LDL cholesterol is 290 mg/dL. A renal biopsy would reveal which of the following on light microscopic examination?

   (A) Diffuse mesangial proliferation

   (B) Multiple spikes in the glomerular basement membranes

   (C) Normal histologic appearance of glomeruli

   (D) Segmental sclerosis and hyalinization of various glomeruli

9. Conjoined twins are born attached at the chest. Examination of the placenta would likely reveal which of the following arrangements of the fetal membranes?

   (A) Diamnionic, dichorionic

   (B) Diamnionic, fused dichorionic

   (C) Diamnionic, monochorionic

   (D) Monoamnionic, dichorionic

   (E) Monoamnionic, monochorionic

10. A 36-year-old man with ulcerative colitis develops pruritus and fatigue. Alkaline phosphatase is elevated. The biliary tree appears beaded on barium radiograph. Which of the following is the most likely diagnosis?

   (A) Acute cholecystitis

   (B) Cholesterolosis

   (C) Chronic cholelithiasis

   (D) Gallstone ileus

   (E) Sclerosing cholangitis

11. A 14-year-old boy presents with a 1-month history of knee pain and a 6-pound weight loss. He is pale and afebrile. An x-ray film reveals a densely sclerotic lesion in the distal femur extending from the growth plate into the diaphysis. The periosteum is lifted, forming an angle with the cortex. The surrounding soft tissue resembles a "sunburst" on the radiograph. Which of the following is the most likely diagnosis?

    (A) Nonossifying fibroma

    (B) Osteochondroma

    (C) Osteomyelitis

    (D) Osteosarcoma

    (E) Paget disease

12. A gastroenterologist performs a colonoscopy on a patient with a family history of gastric and colon cancer and discovers multiple polyps. Biopsy of one lesion reveals a benign hamartoma. On physical examination the patient is noted to have dark pigmentation of the buccal mucosa and lips. What is the most likely diagnosis?

    (A) Adenomatous polyposis coli

    (B) Gardner syndrome

    (C) Peutz-Jeghers (PJ) syndrome

    (D) Turcot syndrome

13. A 36-year-old gravid woman notes vaginal bleeding. Ultrasound reveals small grape-like cystic structures without evidence of a developing embryo. A diagnosis of complete hydatidiform mole is made at the hospital. Further analysis is most likely to reveal that

    (A) the genotype of the mole is 46,XX and is completely paternal in origin

    (B) the genotype of the mole is triploid

    (C) human chorionic gonadotropin (hCG) levels are markedly decreased

    (D) serum levels of alpha fetoprotein are elevated

    (E) two or more sperm fertilized the ovum

14. A 22-year-old man with fatigue, recurrent fever, and enlarged cervical lymph nodes has numerous atypical lymphocytes in his peripheral blood smear. A biopsy from the patient's enlarged node shows expansion of lymphoid follicles with preservation of the underlying architecture. Numerous atypical lymphocytes are present in the paracortical areas. Which of the following is the most likely diagnosis?

    (A) AIDS

    (B) Burkitt lymphoma

    (C) Hodgkin disease

    (D) Mononucleosis

    (E) Non-Hodgkin lymphoma

15. A 70-year-old man experiences continuous lower abdominal discomfort with alternating constipation and diarrhea. His symptoms seem to improve on a high-fiber diet. If exploratory surgery were performed, which of the following would the surgeon most likely see?

    (A) An inflamed and fibrosed appendix

    (B) Multiple diverticula of the rectosigmoid colon

    (C) Normal small and large intestine

    (D) Thick, rubbery small and large intestinal walls

    (E) A trabeculated, dilated bladder

**KAPLAN** MEDICAL

16. A 45-year-old man is diagnosed with primary hypoaldosteronism. Which of the following laboratory results is most consistent with this diagnosis?

| | Serum sodium | Serum potassium | Serum bicarbonate | Urine sodium | Urine potassium |
|---|---|---|---|---|---|
| (A) | ↓ | ↑ | ↓ | ↑ | ↓ |
| (B) | ↓ | ↑ | ↑ | ↑ | ↓ |
| (C) | ↓ | ↓ | ↓ | ↑ | ↑ |
| (D) | ↑ | ↓ | ↑ | ↓ | ↑ |
| (E) | ↑ | ↑ | ↑ | ↓ | ↓ |

17. A 29-year-old woman with a history of pelvic inflammatory disease presents to the emergency department with severe left lower quadrant crampy pain and spotting, and amenorrhea for the past two cycles. Physical examination reveals a left adnexal mass with tenderness to palpation. The beta-human chorionic gonadotropin (hCG) level is elevated. Further studies would most likely reveal an implantation at which of the following locations in the fallopian tube?

(A) Ampulla

(B) Fimbriae

(C) Infundibulum

(D) Isthmus

(E) Uterine segment

18. A 13-year-old boy presents to the emergency department with a deep skin abrasion on his knee. He states that it has not stopped bleeding since it happened during recess approximately 20 to 30 minutes ago. Physical examination reveals a well-developed, well-nourished adolescent. There are multiple purpura over his legs and arms, and a few scattered petechiae on his chest and gums. His bleeding time = 22 minutes, platelets = 300,000/mm³, and hemoglobin = 11g/dL. A trial of cryoprecipitate transfusion does not improve his bleeding time, but a normal platelet transfusion does. Which of the following is the correct diagnosis?

(A) Bernard-Soulier syndrome

(B) Henoch-Schönlein purpura

(C) Idiopathic thrombocytopenic purpura

(D) Thrombotic thrombocytopenic purpura

(E) Von Willebrand disease

19. A patient with respiratory failure secondary to poliomyelitis is placed on a respirator accidentally set at too high a rate. Which of the following changes in arterial blood gas studies would you expect to see?

| | $P_{O_2}$ | $P_{CO_2}$ | pH |
|---|---|---|---|
| (A) | Markedly decreased | Slightly decreased | Increased |
| (B) | Markedly increased | Markedly increased | Decreased |
| (C) | Markedly increased | Slightly decreased | Decreased |
| (D) | Normal or slightly increased | Markedly decreased | Increased |
| (E) | Normal or slightly increased | Slightly decreased | Decreased |

20. A 27-year-old man presents with recurrent episodes of intensely pruritic vesicles symmetrically distributed on his trunk. On electron microscopy, granular deposition of IgA and complement is noted at the dermoepidermal junction. Which of the following underlying conditions predisposes patients to the described skin disorder?

(A) Celiac sprue

(B) Lactase deficiency

(C) Tropical sprue

(D) Ulcerative colitis

(E) Whipple disease

21. Which of the following histologic changes in the kidney would be caused by proteinuria?

    (A) Antibody deposition in the glomeruli

    (B) Complement deposition in the glomeruli

    (C) Hyaline droplets in the renal tubular epithelium

    (D) Increased mesangial cells in the glomeruli

    (E) Neutrophils in the glomeruli

22. Biopsy of a skin lesion shows marked intercellular edema that splays apart adjacent cells, leaving only thin dark lines between the cells. What is this process called?

    (A) Acantholysis

    (B) Acanthosis

    (C) Hyperkeratosis

    (D) Parakeratosis

    (E) Spongiosis

23. A 25-year-old, previously healthy man notices that he now develops painful muscle cramps after strenuous exercise. After shoveling 2 feet of snow off his driveway, his urine turns red, and he consults a physician. Which of the following genetic conditions does the patient most likely have?

    (A) Gaucher disease

    (B) McArdle syndrome

    (C) Niemann-Pick disease

    (D) Tay-Sachs disease

    (E) von Gierke disease

24. A 40-year-old alcoholic woman presents with intense pruritus and fatigue. Her medical history is significant for hypothyroidism. Physical examination reveals a slightly enlarged liver and xanthomas. Laboratory studies show a cholesterol of 538 mg/dL and an alkaline phosphatase of 571 IU/L. Which of the following serum values would most likely be elevated?

    (A) Alpha-fetoprotein

    (B) Antimitochondrial antibody

    (C) HBs antigen

    (D) Prothrombin time

    (E) Serum transaminases

25. A 56-year-old man presents with higher-than-normal language output and frequent paraphasic errors. Neurologic testing reveals that his comprehension of auditory and visual language is severely disturbed. He also exhibits an inability to repeat language. This patient has which of the following types of aphasia?

    (A) Broca (expressive)

    (B) Conduction

    (C) Global

    (D) Mixed transcortical

    (E) Transcortical motor

    (F) Transcortical sensory

    (G) Wernicke (receptive)

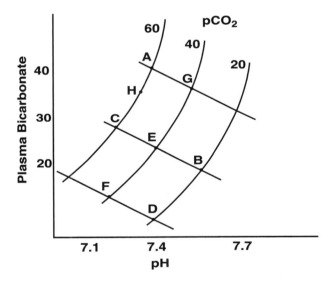

26. A 31-year-old stockbroker drives to a high-altitude mountain resort to do some rock-climbing. Later that day, he experiences headache, fatigue, dizziness, and nausea. Which point on the graph above best corresponds to the relationship between plasma bicarbonate, pH, and $P_{CO_2}$ in this patient?

    (A) A

    (B) B

    (C) C

    (D) D

    (E) E

    (F) F

    (G) G

    (H) H

27. A 45-year-old woman presents with recent onset of blood-tinged discharge from the right nipple. The nipple appears slightly retracted, and a ill-defined subareolar nodule can be appreciated on palpation. Mammographic examination reveals linear shadows attributable to calcification. An excisional biopsy is performed. Microscopically, the lesion consists of markedly dilated ducts that contain inspissated secretion and are surrounded by fibrosis and chronic inflammation. Focal calcium deposition is present. Which of the following is the most likely diagnosis?

    (A) Abscess

    (B) Adenocarcinoma

    (C) Fat necrosis

    (D) Fibrocystic changes

    (E) Foreign body reaction

    (F) Mammary duct ectasia

    (G) Mondor disease

28. A 53-year-old woman comes to the physician because of fatigue. She reports that she has been weak and tired for the past few months and has lately been feeling palpitations. She has no chronic medical conditions, does not take any medication or smoke cigarettes, and does not use drugs or alcohol. Laboratory studies show a normochromic anemia with no reticulocytes. The red blood cell morphology is normal. Platelets and myeloid cells are unaffected. Bone marrow biopsy is normocellular and is significant for a lack of erythroid precursors, but all other elements are normal. As part of the management of her condition she should be evaluated for which of the following?

    (A) Gastric adenocarcinoma

    (B) Pancreatic adenocarcinoma

    (C) Papillary thyroid cancer

    (D) Seminoma

    (E) Thymoma

29. During a routine pre-employment examination, a 37-year-old man is found to have a 4-cm mass on his left lung. A chest x-ray taken 3 years ago is normal. The patient does not smoke cigarettes, nor does anyone with whom he comes into daily contact. He works as manager of a supermarket and has no chronic medical conditions. Both of his parents are alive and well. He undergoes surgery, and pathologic examination of the lesion reveals that it is a primary lung cancer. Which of the following is the most likely type of cancer in this patient?

    (A) Bronchioloalveolar carcinoma

    (B) Bronchogenic adenocarcinoma

    (C) Large cell anaplastic carcinoma

    (D) Small cell (oat cell) carcinoma

    (E) Squamous cell carcinoma

30. The 10-year-old daughter of a United Nations ambassador in Turkey develops a severe sore throat, which resolves after a few days. Ten days later, the mother notices dark stains on the child's underwear and takes her to the pediatrician. A urine sample appears smoky, and red cell casts are noted in the urinary sediment. If a renal biopsy were obtained from this child it would probably show

    (A) dense deposits

    (B) fusion of podocyte foot processes

    (C) linear deposition of IgG

    (D) mesangial IgA deposits

    (E) subepithelial humps

31. A 37-year-old woman presents to her physician complaining of difficulty reading and fatigue. She reports having had a "pins and needles" feeling in her left arm several months ago that resolved without treatment. On examination, visual field deficits and mild hyperreflexia are noted. MRI confirms the suspected diagnosis. Which of the following is the underlying mechanism of this patient's disease?

    (A) Antibodies to acetylcholine receptors

    (B) Axonal degeneration

    (C) Demyelination of the peripheral nerves

    (D) Loss of oligodendrocytes

    (E) Loss of Schwann cells

32. A blood sample from a patient with polycythemia vera is sent for complete blood count. Which of the following blood components is most likely to be reported within normal limits?

    (A) Lymphocytes

    (B) Neutrophils

    (C) Platelets

    (D) Red blood cells

    (E) White blood cells

33. A 60-year-old man suddenly becomes completely blind in one eye, and angiography demonstrates occlusion of the central retinal artery. Which of the following is the most likely cause of the occlusion?

    (A) Atheroma or embolism

    (B) Cranial (temporal) arteritis

    (C) Hypertension

    (D) Polycythemia vera

    (E) Tumor

34. A 55-year-old man with a history of recurrent calcium-containing renal stones presents to the emergency department with excruciating flank pain and blood in the urine. This patient is likely to have which of the following underlying disorders?

    (A) Anemia of chronic disease

    (B) Chronic *Proteus* infection

    (C) Factor VIII deficiency

    (D) Hyperaldosteronism

    (E) Hyperparathyroidism

35. A 26-year-old woman accidentally inhales a peanut while laughing hysterically at a comedy club. Her friends bring her to a nearby emergency department, where it is revealed that the peanut lodged in her right mainstem bronchus. Which of the following is true about the blood flowing through the area of lung distal to the peanut?

    (A) The amount of dissolved oxygen is greater than normal

    (B) The oxygen dissociation curve is left-shifted

    (C) The $P_{CO_2}$ is lower than normal

    (D) The pH is lower than normal

    (E) The $P_{O_2}$ approaches that of arterial blood

36. A 40-year-old man who recently immigrated from Japan presents to his physician with abdominal discomfort characterized by sensations of fullness and mild pain after eating. He was previously diagnosed with a gastric ulcer, which has been refractory to traditional treatment. Biopsy of the lesion reveals gastric carcinoma. The cancer is most likely located in which of the following regions of the stomach?

    (A) Antropyloric region

    (B) Apex of the cardia

    (C) Greater curvature of the body

    (D) Lesser curvature of the body

    (E) Within 6 cm of the gastroesophageal junction

37. A 61-year-old woman has severe chest pain and shortness of breath. She has smoked a pack of cigarettes a day for the past 30 years and has a history of poorly controlled hypertension. An electrocardiogram shows ST segment elevations greater than 1 mm in two contiguous leads, and new Q waves. Laboratory studies show elevated levels of creatine kinase-MB and troponin I. The earliest pathologic evidence that this event has occurred consists of

    (A) infiltration of the myocardium with leukocytes

    (B) intercellular edema with "wavy change" of affected myocytes

    (C) necrosis with preservation of cell outlines

    (D) proliferation of fibroblasts

    (E) a softened, yellow plaque on the endocardial surface

38. A 65-year-old woman with an 8-year history of type 2 diabetes dies in the hospital. She had no other significant medical history. Which of the following was the most likely cause of death?

    (A) Diabetic ketoacidosis

    (B) Infection

    (C) Myocardial infarction

    (D) Renal failure

    (E) Stroke

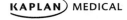

39. A 21-year-old woman attempts suicide by taking an overdose of barbiturates. On arrival in the emergency department, her blood pressure is 95/65 mm Hg, and her pulse is 105/min. The physician in the intensive care unit orders arterial blood gases. Which of the following values would you expect in this patient?

    (A) $P_{O_2} = 45$, $P_{CO_2} = 45$, pH = 7.45

    (B) $P_{O_2} = 55$, $P_{CO_2} = 70$, pH = 7.50

    (C) $P_{O_2} = 65$, $P_{CO_2} = 35$, pH = 7.45

    (D) $P_{O_2} = 75$, $P_{CO_2} = 60$, pH = 7.30

    (E) $P_{O_2} = 98$, $P_{CO_2} = 60$, pH = 7.20

40. An accident in a dry cleaning facility exposes an employee to massive amounts of carbon tetrachloride, both on the skin and by inhalation. Severe damage to which of the following organs is most likely to occur?

    (A) Heart

    (B) Intestine

    (C) Kidney

    (D) Liver

    (E) Stomach

41. A 65-year-old man complains of weakness, weight loss, and bone pain. He reports having progressive difficulty seeing. Physical examination is significant for hepatosplenomegaly and lymphadenopathy. Serum protein electrophoresis reveals an M-protein spike, with an elevated serum IgM level. Bone marrow aspiration shows intensely eosinophilic plasma cells. Urine contains Bence-Jones proteins. Which of the following is the most likely diagnosis?

    (A) Heavy chain disease

    (B) Monoclonal gammopathy of undetermined significance

    (C) Multiple myeloma

    (D) Plasmacytoma

    (E) Waldenström macroglobulinemia

42. A patient has a lymphoproliferative disorder containing mature B cells that mark weakly with kappa light chain on the plasma membrane, strongly with CD5, strongly with CD23, and weakly with CD22. Which of the following is the most likely diagnosis?

    (A) Chronic lymphocytic leukemia

    (B) Hairy cell leukemia

    (C) Non-Hodgkin lymphoma

    (D) Prolymphocytic leukemia

    (E) Sézary syndrome

43. The EKG of a 60-year-old man reveals QRS intervals of 0.14 seconds with distinctly abnormal configurations. Physical exam is significant for paradoxical splitting of the second heart sound. Which of the following conduction defects is likely in this patient?

    (A) Complete AV block

    (B) First-degree AV block

    (C) Mobitz Type I AV block

    (D) Mobitz Type II AV block

    (E) Wolff-Parkinson-White syndrome

44. A 56-year-old man presents with complaints of gnawing pain in the mid-epigastrium, with occasional radiation to the back. He also notes a 15-pound weight loss over the past 3 months. The clinician suspects pancreatic carcinoma. Which of the following tumor markers would aid in confirming this diagnosis?

    (A) Alpha-fetoprotein (AFP)

    (B) CA-125

    (C) Carcinoembryonic antigen (CEA)

    (D) Human chorionic gonadotropin (hCG)

    (E) Prostate-specific antigen (PSA)

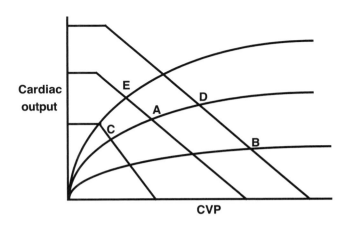

45. A 19-year-old man is brought into the emergency department with a gunshot wound to his leg. He is pale and tachypneic, his blood pressure is 90/65 mm Hg, and his pulse is weak and rapid at 130/min. This man's condition corresponds to which point (A–E) on the above graph?

    (A) A
    (B) B
    (C) C
    (D) D
    (E) E

46. A 25-year-old drug abuser with history of gonorrhea presents with fever and shortness of breath. Pulse oximetry reveals hypoxia. A chest x-ray film is significant for bilateral interstitial infiltrates. Which of the following findings is consistent with the most likely diagnosis?

    (A) Acid-fast organisms in sputum
    (B) Appearance of Curschmann spirals in mucus plugs
    (C) Elevated serum cold agglutinins
    (D) Positive methenamine-silver stain of lung tissue
    (E) Presence of Charcot-Leyden crystals in sputum

47. A 46-year-old woman who is clearly jaundiced is seen in clinic. Laboratory tests reveal conjugated hyper-bilirubinemia. Urine bilirubin levels are significantly above normal, while urine urobilinogen levels are significantly below normal. Which of the following mechanisms is the most likely cause of her jaundice?

    (A) Blockage of the common bile duct
    (B) Deficiency of glucuronyl transferase
    (C) Hemolytic anemia
    (D) Hepatocellular damage

48. A 35-year-old woman complains of vomiting dark, greenish material approximately 1 hour after eating. She is scheduled for a barium meal to evaluate the upper portion of the gastrointestinal tract. She denies pain and is anicteric. Which of the following is the most likely cause of this woman's condition?

    (A) Annular pancreas
    (B) Esophageal atresia
    (C) Gallstones
    (D) Meckel's diverticulum
    (E) Pyloric stenosis

49. A 73-year-old man is concerned about aging. He says that his skin is beginning to sag and his body "just doesn't work like it used to." He has no other complaints and leads a healthy lifestyle. Physical examination is consistent with a healthy man his age. Routine laboratory studies are within normal limits. On his way out of the physician's office, he sees a flyer asking for healthy, elderly volunteers. He enrolls in the study and undergoes a liver biopsy to evaluate the aging process. In this biopsy, which of the following substances will indicate aging at a cellular level?

    (A) Beta-carotene
    (B) Bilirubin
    (C) Hemosiderin
    (D) Lipofuscin
    (E) Melanin

50. A 57-year-old man presents with painless swelling in his neck. Physical examination is remarkable for splenomegaly. Biopsy of the neck mass reveals a neoplasm containing small, cleaved cells that recapitulate the normal follicular architecture of lymph nodes. Which of the following mechanisms is most likely involved in the development of this patient's neoplasm?

    (A) Amplification of L-*myc*
    (B) Homozygous loss of *p53*
    (C) Over-expression of *bcl-2*
    (D) Point mutation in *ras* decreasing its GTPase activity
    (E) Reciprocal translocation between chromosome 9 and 22

# Pathology and Pathophysiology Test One:
# Answers and Explanations

## ANSWER KEY

| | | | |
|---|---|---|---|
| 1. | B | 26. | B |
| 2. | D | 27. | F |
| 3. | C | 28. | E |
| 4. | D | 29. | B |
| 5. | B | 30. | E |
| 6. | C | 31. | D |
| 7. | D | 32. | A |
| 8. | C | 33. | A |
| 9. | E | 34. | E |
| 10. | E | 35. | D |
| 11. | D | 36. | A |
| 12. | C | 37. | B |
| 13. | A | 38. | C |
| 14. | D | 39. | D |
| 15. | B | 40. | D |
| 16. | A | 41. | E |
| 17. | A | 42. | A |
| 18. | A | 43. | D |
| 19. | D | 44. | C |
| 20. | A | 45. | C |
| 21. | C | 46. | D |
| 22. | E | 47. | A |
| 23. | B | 48. | A |
| 24. | B | 49. | D |
| 25. | G | 50. | C |

1. **The correct answer is B.** Pericarditis is inflammation of the pericardium. Fibrinous pericarditis is the most frequent form of pericarditis associated with myocardial infarction. Clinically, it may present as a loud pericardial friction rub with chest pain, fever, and, occasionally, symptoms of congestive heart failure (CHF).

   Caseous pericarditis (**choice A**) is usually caused by tuberculosis.

   Hemorrhagic pericarditis (**choice C**) is usually associated with tuberculosis or a malignant neoplasm.

   Serous pericarditis (**choice D**) is usually caused by an immunologic reaction, tumor, uremia, or viral infection; it can also be idiopathic.

   Suppurative pericarditis (**choice E**) may be caused by bacterial, fungal, or parasitic infections, and can clinically present with systemic signs of infection (fever, malaise) and a soft friction rub.

2. **The correct answer is D.** Primary aldosteronism (Conn syndrome) is a condition of hyperaldosteronism originating in the adrenal gland. The causes include an aldosterone-secreting adrenocortical adenoma, hyperplasia of the zona glomerulosa, and, very rarely, an adrenal carcinoma. It is characterized by hypertension secondary to sodium retention, hypokalemia, and a decreased serum renin due to a negative feedback of increased blood pressure on renin secretion.

   Cushing syndrome (**choice A**) is the result of increased glucocorticoid production, particularly cortisol. Physical signs typically include "moon facies," truncal obesity, "buffalo hump," and purple abdominal striae.

   Diabetes mellitus (**choice B**) is a condition of inadequate insulin production that presents with hyperglycemia and ketoacidosis.

   Pheochromocytoma (**choice C**) is a rare tumor of chromaffin cells occurring most commonly in the adrenal medulla. The tumor secretes epinephrine and norepinephrine, resulting in secondary hypertension.

   Secondary aldosteronism (**choice E**) results from activation of the renin-angiotensin system caused by renal ischemia, edema, and renal tumors. In contrast to primary aldosteronism, secondary aldosteronism is associated with increased serum renin.

3. **The correct answer is C.** Contact dermatitis is a form of *eczematous dermatitis*, characterized clinically by itchy vesicular eruption and histologically by epidermal spongiosis and chronic dermal inflammation. Contact dermatitis is initiated by hypersensitivity to an antigen that is taken up by Langerhans cells. These antigen-presenting cells process antigens and present them to naïve CD4 positive (helper) T lymphocytes. Antigen re-expo-

sure leads to recruitment of helper T cells and release of cytokines that mediate the inflammatory response.

The pathogenesis of acne vulgaris (**choice A**) is related to endocrine, familial, and environmental factors. Bacterial lipases from *Propionibacterium acnes* may play a role.

Bullous pemphigoid (**choice B**) and pemphigus vulgaris (**choice G**) are mediated by different types of autoantibodies that react with components of desmosomes or hemidesmosomes, disrupting intercellular junctions and resulting in bulla formation. Thus, the immune mechanism of these conditions can be regarded as type II hypersensitivity reactions.

Dermatitis herpetiformis (**choice D**) is a blistering disease that develops in individuals allergic to gliadin, a gluten component. IgA and IgG antibodies react with gliadin and deposit in the tips of dermal papillae, leading to inflammation and bulla formation. Type III hypersensitivity therefore appears to be the prevalent immunologic mechanism.

Discoid lupus erythematosus (**choice E**) is the localized cutaneous form of systemic lupus erythematosus. Skin lesions are associated with immune complex deposition along the dermal-epidermal junction. This is a form of type III hypersensitivity reaction.

Urticaria (**choice F**) is mediated by IgE-triggered degranulation of mast cells, which may follow exposure to a number of antigens, e.g., food, drugs, and pollen. This is a classic example of a type I hypersensitivity reaction.

4. **The correct answer is D.** This patient likely has cholelithiasis, with possible acute cholecystitis. The typical patient is "fat, female, fertile, and older than 40." The right upper quadrant tenderness on inspiration is called Murphy's sign and is characteristic of biliary inflammation. In this patient, inflammation of the gallbladder might produce irritation of the central diaphragmatic pleura, which is innervated by the phrenic nerve. The dermatome of the nerve root of the phrenic nerve (C3-C5) includes the right shoulder.

The expiratory motor neurons (**choice A**) are located in the lower medulla. They operate only during forced expiration to initiate contraction in expiratory muscles via alpha motor fibers.

The inspiratory motor neurons (**choice B**) are located in the upper part of the medulla and send impulses via alpha motor fibers to the muscles of inspiration. They play no role in Murphy's sign.

The intercostal nerves (**choice C**) innervate the costal and peripheral portions of the diaphragmatic pleura.

The vagus nerve (**choice E**) mediates the Hering-Breuer (stretch-inflation) reflex of breathing.

5. **The correct answer is B.** The classic findings in atrial septal defect are a prominent right ventricular cardiac impulse, a systolic ejection murmur heard in the pulmonic area and along the left sternal border, and fixed splitting of the second heart sound. These findings are due to an abnormal left to right shunt through the defect, creating a volume overload on the right side. The increase in volume on the right side creates the flow murmur, the dilatation of the right-sided chambers, and the delayed closure of the pulmonic valve, all of which are present in this case.

Aortic stenosis (**choice A**) is also associated with a systolic ejection murmur. The murmur is usually loudest at the right sternal border and radiates upward to the jugular notch. This condition is associated with left ventricular hypertrophy.

Mitral regurgitation (**choice C**) would present with a systolic murmur as well. However, left atrial enlargement would be seen before right ventricular enlargement.

Mitral stenosis (**choice D**) would present with an "opening snap" and a diastolic murmur.

Pulmonary valve stenosis (**choice E**) causes an increase in right ventricular pressure resulting in right ventricular hypertrophy and pulmonary artery dilatation. A crescendo-decrescendo murmur may be heard if the stenosis is severe. Right atrial enlargement would not be present.

6. **The correct answer is C.** Scalded skin syndrome is a pediatric condition caused by an exfoliative toxin produced by *Staphylococcus aureus* (which is a common cause of cellulitis). The toxin splits the epidermis at the level of the stratum granulosum, causing global denudation of the skin. Scalded skin syndrome is not associated with suntanning or sunburn.

Impetigo (**choice A**) is a superficial skin infection, usually caused by group A beta-hemolytic streptococci or staphylococci. Classic clues are eroded pustules covered by honey-colored crusts. Impetigo may lead to poststreptococcal glomerulonephritis, a sign of which is red cell casts in the urine.

Melasma (**choice B**) consists of irregular patches of hyperpigmentation on the face. It most commonly appears during pregnancy and may not completely regress.

Tinea corporis (**choice D**) is a fungal infection. It is also known as "ringworm" because it presents as an expanding round lesion with an erythematous circinate border.

Vitiligo (**choice E**) is characterized by irregular patchy depigmentation of the skin that exhibits melanocyte deficiency microscopically. It is possibly autoimmune in origin and may be related to stress. It is not associated with sun exposure and is a chronic condition.

7. **The correct answer is D.** Retinoblastomas are aggressive, malignant neoplasms derived from embryonic neuronal cells. Fortunately, they are rare. These tumors present in early childhood, often within the first 3 months of life. Retinoblastomas are very dangerous both because they can metastasize widely via a hematogenous route and because they show a marked propensity to invade the optic nerve and tract into the brain, where they quickly become inoperable. The pathologist should pay particular attention to the cut end of the optic nerve to make sure that the entire retinoblastoma was removed.

8. **The correct answer is C.** The most common cause of nephrotic syndrome in children is minimal change disease (lipoid nephrosis). The nephrotic syndrome is characterized by hypoalbuminemia, proteinuria >3.5 g/day, hyperlipidemia, and edema. The glomeruli of patients with this condition appear completely normal by light microscopy, thus the name "minimal change disease." Electron microscopy may reveal loss of epithelial foot processes.

Mesangial proliferation (**choice A**) is seen more often in glomerulonephritis.

Basement membrane spikes (**choice B**) are seen in membranous glomerulonephropathy.

Focal segmental glomerulosclerosis is associated with focal and segmental sclerotic lesions and hyalinization of various glomeruli (**choice D**). It is the most common glomerulonephropathy in AIDS.

9. **The correct answer is E.** This question may seem a bit challenging, but you have all the information you need to answer it. The type of fetal membranes produced in identical twin pregnancies depends on the timing of the twinning process. The chorion forms before the amnion, so the possible combinations for all twin pregnancies are monoamnionic and monochorionic, diamnionic and monochorionic, and diamnionic and dichorionic (with the chorions either separate or fused). The first two possibilities are seen only in identical twins, the last one can be seen in both identical and fraternal twins. Exactly what happens depends on the precise point at which twinning occurs.

Very early separation (at the two-cell stage) produces completely separate membranes with duplication of both the amnion and chorion (**choice A**).

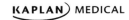

Slightly later separation results in two amnions and fused chorions (**choice B**).

Separation at a later stage, when the inner cell mass is present, produces twins with one chorion and two amnions (**choice C**). Very late separation results in one chorion and one amnion. Conjoined (Siamese) twins result from a very late twinning event, so the placenta will be monoamnionic and monochorionic.

Monoamnionic and dichorionic placentas (**choice D**) are not usually seen, as the chorion forms before the amnion.

10. **The correct answer is E.** Young men with ulcerative colitis are at increased risk for developing primary sclerosing cholangitis (PSC), a chronic cholestatic condition that leads to fibrosis of the bile ducts. A classic clue to the diagnosis is a beaded appearance of the biliary tree on barium radiograph.

Patients with acute cholecystitis (**choice A**) present with acute onset of right upper quadrant pain, fever, tenderness, and leukocytosis.

Cholesterolosis (strawberry gallbladder; **choice B**) refers to lipid foci deposited in the gallbladder wall. It is asymptomatic and unrelated to cholelithiasis.

Cholelithiasis (gallstones; **choice C**) is commonly asymptomatic but can cause biliary colic and may progress to acute cholecystitis.

Gallstone ileus (**choice D**), due to obstruction of the small bowel by gallstones, is associated with air in the biliary tree on abdominal radiograph.

11. **The correct answer is D.** This patient has osteosarcoma, a malignant bone tumor that produces osteoid and bone. Prognosis is poor. X-ray reveals bone destruction, soft tissue with "sunburst" appearance, and Codman's triangle (periosteal elevation that forms an angle with the cortex of the bone)—all classic clues to the diagnosis. Other hints were the patient's weight loss and pallor, which should have raised your suspicion that a malignancy existed. Choice D is the only malignant process among the answer choices. This tumor usually occurs in the second or third decades of life. At the same time, it is the most common bone tumor in the elderly and is often associated with Paget disease (**choice E**). A classic histologic finding for osteosarcoma is the presence of anaplastic cells with osteoid (a pink amorphous material that is variably mineralized).

Nonossifying fibroma (**choice A**), also known as fibrous cortical defect, is a common developmental abnormality seen in the bones of the lower extremities of children. This is a non-neoplastic lesion of bone cortex that is composed of fibrous connective tissue and usually resolves spontaneously. X-ray reveals irregular, well-demarcated radiolucent defects in the bony cortex with an intact subperiosteal shell of bone. In the metaphysis, there are whorls of connective tissue. These fibromas do not cross the epiphyses of bone, which distinguishes them from giant cell tumors of bone.

Osteochondromas (**choice B**) are hereditary multiple exostoses (bony metaphyseal projections capped with cartilage) that may be asymptomatic or may produce deformity and compromise the blood supply of bone. Five percent of them progress to sarcomas. If a patient presents with exostoses, sebaceous cysts, dermoid tumors, and colonic polyps, the likely diagnosis is Gardner syndrome.

Osteomyelitis (**choice C**) usually produces fever, localized pain, erythema, and swelling. The patient in question is afebrile, which decreases the likelihood of this diagnosis. Though x-ray films may show periosteal elevation, more specific findings would be expected in a patient with this condition, such as sequestrum (necrotic bone fragment), involucrum (new bone that surrounds the area of inflammation), and Brodie's abscess (localized abscess formation in the bone).

Paget disease (**choice E**), also known as osteitis deformans, is due to excessive bone resorption with replacement by soft, poorly mineralized matrix (osteoid) in a disorganized array. It generally affects the skull, pelvis, femur, and vertebrae. Skull involvement might produce deafness by impinging on the cranial nerves. Malignant transformation to osteosarcoma is seen in 1% of cases. X-ray reveals enlarged, radiolucent bones. Lab tests reveal extremely elevated alkaline phosphatase. If you see a patient who is older than 40 and has bone fracture, hearing loss, and increased alkaline phosphatase, suspect Paget disease. Note that this disease rarely occurs in the young and could have been ruled out as a possible answer by virtue of the patient's age.

12. **The correct answer is C.** All the choices are familial polyposes. The classic clue for Peutz-Jeghers (PJ) syndrome is the melanin pigmentation of the buccal mucosa and lips (the palms and soles may also be darkened). PJ presents with polyps of the entire gastrointestinal tract (thus the appearance of colonic lesions), but the small intestine is usually most severely affected. The polyps of PJ are hamartomas and are not premalignant, although there is an increased incidence of stomach, breast, and ovarian cancer associated with this disease.

Adenomatous polyposis coli (**choice A**) is also called familial multiple polyposis. Like PJ, it is inherited in an autosomal dominant fashion. Polyps typically begin in the rectosigmoid area and spread to the entire colon. Because almost all patients go on to develop cancer, colectomy is recommended once the diagnosis is made.

Gardner syndrome (**choice B**) refers to colonic polyps in the setting of other neoplasms (e.g., bone, skin) and desmoid tumors. Risk of colon cancer is close to 100%.

Turcot syndrome (**choice D**) is characterized by colonic polyps associated with brain tumors such as gliomas and medulloblastomas.

13. **The correct answer is A.** A complete hydatidiform mole is characterized by elevated human chorionic gonadotropin (hCG) and grape-like cystic structures filling the uterus with no detectable embryo on ultrasound. The genotype of a complete hydatidiform mole is purely paternal, caused by fertilization of an egg that has lost its chromosomes. Hydatidiform mole is associated with increasing maternal age and may be a precursor to choriocarcinoma.

Triploidy and even tetraploidy are characteristics of partial moles (**choice B**). Partial moles are thought to be due to fertilization of an egg with two different sperm, one with an X and one with a Y chromosome, typically leading to triploidy.

hCG levels are increased relative to normal values for dates, rather than decreased (**choice C**), in a molar pregnancy.

Alpha fetoprotein (AFP; **choice D**) is a marker for endodermal yolk sac tumors, embryonal tumors in men, and hepatocellular carcinoma. It is made by the fetus. In a complete hydatidiform mole, AFP is not detectable since there is no fetus.

Two or more sperm may fertilize an ovum, leading to a triploid fetus and partial mole (**choice E**).

14. **The correct answer is D.** Infectious mononucleosis is a benign infection caused by the Epstein-Barr virus (EBV), a herpesvirus. Although B lymphocytes are infected by the virus, the characteristic atypical cells are activated cytotoxic and suppressor T cells—thus the paracortical location (T cell zone) in the lymph node. Lymph nodes in viral infections show expansion of germinal centers without loss of normal architecture. All lymphomas, including Burkitt, Hodgkin, and non-Hodgkin lymphomas, destroy the normal architecture of the lymph node.

AIDS (**choice A**) is associated with a number of neoplastic and infectious processes that may alter the lymph node structure. The characteristic lymph node changes in AIDS are progressive transformation of the germinal centers, not paracortical hyperplasia.

Burkitt lymphoma (**choice B**) produces a sea of monotonous, mitotically active cells in a "starry sky" appearance.

Hodgkin lymphoma (**choice C**) also can show nodular or diffuse patterns but is characterized by the presence of Reed-Sternberg cells.

Other non-Hodgkin lymphomas (**choice E**) show either a nodular appearance or diffuse sheets of cells that replace the germinal centers.

15. **The correct answer is B.** This is a presentation of colonic diverticulosis, although only about 20% of affected individuals develop clinical symptoms. Patients are typically older than 40. The diverticula are small, flask-like outpouchings of the colonic mucosa and submucosa. They are often found at sites of focal weakness of the colonic wall, particularly adjacent to the taeniae coli, where the nerves and arterial vasa recta penetrate the inner circular muscle coat. High-fiber diets appear to improve the symptoms, but it is unclear whether such diets can impede disease progression. Note that irritable bowel syndrome may also present with alternating constipation and diarrhea, but is more common in younger females. No organic changes are evident in this disease.

An inflamed appendix (**choice A**) is more likely to be seen in a younger individual.

Crohn disease, which produces rubbery small and large intestinal walls (**choice D**), usually presents at a much younger age, with intermittent attacks of abdominal pain and relatively mild diarrhea.

A dilated bladder (**choice E**) would produce urinary rather than colonic symptoms.

16. **The correct answer is A.** Aldosterone is an adrenal hormone that maintains intravascular volume by promoting sodium and water reabsorption at the distal convoluted tubule. Hypoaldosteronism results in salt-wasting, thereby decreasing serum sodium and increasing urine sodium. Since water follows sodium, the patient may develop orthostatic hypotension or become frankly hypotensive. In response to the electrical gradient established by sodium reabsorption, aldosterone induces the passive secretion of potassium at the distal convoluted tubule, promoting potassium excretion. Hypoaldosteronism would, in contrast, increase serum potassium and decrease urine potassium. Aldosterone causes hydrogen ions to be actively secreted into the distal tubule. Therefore, in hypoaldosteronism, $H^+$ ions are retained, creating a metabolic acidosis (decreased serum bicarbonate).

A comment on strategy: A good way to approach this question is to break it down into parts. Begin by looking for answer choices in which the serum sodium values are decreased. This allows you to eliminate **choices D and E**. Next, look for increased urine sodium. This does not allow you to eliminate any more choices, so you must move on and look for increased serum potassium. **Choice C** can now be eliminated. As both of the remaining choices show decreased urinary potassium, decreased serum bicarbonate is the deciding factor, and the correct answer is **choice A**.

17. **The correct answer is A.** This patient has an ectopic (tubal) pregnancy. Patients with a history of pelvic inflammatory disease are more susceptible to this disorder. The ampulla is the most common site of fertilization within the fallopian tube, as well as the most common site for tubal pregnancy. It is the longest region of the tube and has thin walls.

The fimbriae (**choice B**) of the fallopian tubes are highly unlikely locations for tubal pregnancy. They are mucosal ridges located at the funnel-shaped end of the oviduct that are covered with ciliated cells. They beat toward the mouth of the tube, "brushing" the ovum released from the ovary into the fallopian tube.

The infundibulum (**choice C**) is the technical term for the "funnel-shaped end of the fallopian tube." It opens to the peritoneal cavity.

The isthmus (**choice D**) is the narrow, thick-walled segment of the fallopian tube nearest to the uterine wall.

The uterine (interstitial) segment (**choice E**) is the portion of the tube that traverses the uterine wall. Ectopic pregnancies occurring here are at particularly high risk for catastrophic rupture.

18. **The correct answer is A.** Bernard-Soulier syndrome is an autosomal recessive disease of platelet adhesion that causes prolonged bleeding times in the presence of normal platelet counts. These patients' platelets cannot bind to subendothelial collagen properly because of a deficiency or dysfunction of the glycoprotein Ib-IX complex. Clinically the patients have impaired hemostasis and recurrent severe mucosal hemorrhage. The only treatment for an acute episode is a transfusion of normal platelets. This patient has a slightly decreased hemoglobin because of blood loss.

Henoch-Schönlein purpura (**choice B**) is a self-limited autoimmune vasculitis that affects children and young adults, usually following an upper respiratory infection. Affected individuals develop purpuric rashes on the extensor surfaces of their arms, legs, and buttocks. They also have abdominal pain and hematuria from glomerulonephritis. Despite the tendency toward hemorrhage, the bleeding times and platelet count would be normal.

Idiopathic thrombocytopenic purpura (**choice C**) causes an increase in the bleeding time, but, as the name implies, platelet counts are decreased. There is bleeding from small vessels, especially of the skin, gastrointestinal tract, and genitourinary tract. Purpura and petechiae frequently develop. It is considered a self-limited autoimmune disorder, typically affecting children after a recent viral infection.

Thrombotic thrombocytopenic purpura (**choice D**), which is characterized by an increased bleeding time but a decreased platelet count, is a rare disorder of unknown etiology. It is thought to be initiated by endothelial injury, which releases certain procoagulant materials into the circulation, causing platelet aggregation. It causes purpura, fever, renal failure, microangiopathic hemolytic anemia, and microthrombi, generally in young women. In this disorder, platelet transfusion is actually contraindicated, as it can precipitate thrombosis.

Von Willebrand disease (**choice E**) causes increased bleeding times with normal platelet counts. It is the most common inherited bleeding disorder, caused by a defect in von Willebrand factor, which aids the binding of platelets to collagen. Even though the platelets themselves are normal, binding is impaired, thus a platelet transfusion would not correct the problem. Cryoprecipitate, a plasma fraction rich in von Willebrand factor, would help in the case of von Willebrand disease but would not help with Bernard-Soulier syndrome.

19. **The correct answer is D.** This situation is analogous to the voluntary hyperventilation that can occur during anxiety. $CO_2$ is "blown off," potentially leading to a markedly decreased $P_{CO_2}$ with resulting increase in pH (dissolved $CO_2$ combines with water to form carbonic acid, which lowers pH). In an individual with normal lungs, the hemoglobin becomes nearly fully saturated (97.5%) during the normal passage of blood through the alveolar capillaries. So, hyperventilation does not usually change $P_{O_2}$ significantly.

20. **The correct answer is A.** Patients with celiac sprue (nontropical sprue or gluten-sensitive enteropathy) are prone to the development of dermatitis herpetiformis, the dermatologic diagnosis in this patient. This gastrointestinal malabsorption syndrome is caused by an allergic, immunologic, or toxic reaction to the gliadin component of gluten and has a genetic predisposition. There is reversal of symptoms of celiac sprue with a gluten-free diet.

Hint: Even if you were unaware of the association between celiac sprue and dermatitis herpetiformis, the mention of IgA and complement as an element in the skin pathology should have increased your suspicion that the associated condition was immunologically related.

Lactase deficiency (**choice B**) is the most common disaccharidase deficiency (lactase is absent from the brush border of the small intestine). It results in milk intolerance, with symptoms of bloating, diarrhea, and cramping following ingestion of dairy products.

Tropical sprue (**choice C**) is a disorder of malabsorption of unknown etiology that may be caused by enterotoxigenic *Escherichia coli*. There is a high incidence in the tropics, where it occasionally occurs in epidemics. Treatment is with tetracycline and folic acid.

Ulcerative colitis (**choice D**) is associated with a dermatologic condition called pyoderma gangrenosum. This disorder is characterized by blue-red ulcerations that surround purulent necrotic bases.

Whipple disease (**choice E**) is a systemic disorder characterized by clumps of periodic acid-Schiff (PAS)-positive macrophages (full of and surrounded by small bacilli) in the lamina propria of intestines and in mesenteric lymph nodes. It also leads to malabsorption and responds to tetracycline.

21. **The correct answer is C.** In cases of proteinuria, hyaline (dark-staining) droplets can be found in the epithelium of the proximal convoluted tubule. These droplets are protein-containing, pinocytotic vesicles that have fused with lysosomes (to produce phagolysosomes). This change is a sensitive histologic indicator of proteinuria.

Glomerular changes (**choices A, B, D, and E**) can cause proteinuria, but are not usually produced by it.

22. **The correct answer is E.** Spongiosis is the name used for intercellular edema of the epidermis. Fluid accumulates between the cells, pulling them apart. However, the intercellular connections (desmosomes) remain largely intact. This produces a distinctive microscopic appearance in which each cell is surrounded by a broad white band with tiny dark cross-stripes, somewhat reminiscent of a closed zipper.

Acantholysis (**choice A**) is the process of cell separation seen in some blistering diseases. The intercellular connections are broken in acantholysis, producing "rounded-up" cells that are dissociated from each other.

Acanthosis (**choice B**) is a marked thickening of the epidermis due to an increase in the number and size of the epithelial cells.

Hyperkeratosis (**choice C**) is an increase in the thickness of the superficial keratin layer of the epidermis.

The term parakeratosis (**choice D**) is used when nuclei are present in the normally anuclear superficial keratin layer.

23. **The correct answer is B.** This is a typical clinical history for patients with the glycogen storage disease (glycogenosis) known as McArdle syndrome (type V glycogenosis). These patients are deficient in muscle phosphorylase and accumulate glycogen in skeletal muscle tissue without accumulating glycogen in the liver. Their muscles are typically weak, owing to impaired energy production, although they may never have specifically noticed this (on careful questioning, they may instead say they never liked exercise). Obvious clinical onset is typically in the 20s, and measurement of very low serum lactate in these patients during exercise is helpful in establishing the diagnosis. Myoglobinuria (with reddish urine) may occur. The heart is typically not particularly affected, and longevity is normal. A similar presentation can be seen in muscle phosphofructokinase deficiency (type VII glycogen storage disease) and in mild forms of the generalized glycogenosis known as Pompe disease (type II glycogenosis).

Gaucher disease (**choice A**) is a lysosomal disorder of cerebroside metabolism that typically involves the reticuloendothelial system; the brain is not affected.

Niemann-Pick disease (**choice C**) is a lysosomal disorder of sphingomyelin metabolism that typically involves the CNS and the reticuloendothelial system.

Tay-Sachs disease (**choice D**) is another lysosomal storage disease with defective ganglioside degradation. It principally affects the brain.

von Gierke disease (**choice E**) is a hepatorenal form of glycogen storage disease that is not compatible with normal longevity.

24. **The correct answer is B.** Primary biliary cirrhosis is an autoimmune disease associated with elevated antimitochondrial antibodies. Note that Hashimoto thyroiditis, an autoimmune disease that is the most common cause of hypothyroidism, is also associated with increased levels of this antibody.

Elevated alpha-fetoprotein (**choice A**) is associated with hepatocellular carcinoma.

HBs antigen (**choice C**) is usually elevated in active hepatitis B (unless the patient is tested during the window period).

Elevated prothrombin time (**choice D**) and increased serum transaminases (**choice E**) are indicative of liver failure. These values are usually normal in primary biliary cirrhosis.

25. **The correct answer is G.** The question stem describes Wernicke, or receptive, aphasia. It is caused by a lesion in Wernicke's area, which is located in the posterior part of the superior temporal gyrus of the language-dominant hemisphere.

    Broca (expressive) aphasia (**choice A**) is a disorder primarily of language output. Speech is slow and effortful, phrase length is short, and the patient tends to use only common nouns, verbs, and, occasionally, adjectives. Comprehension is relatively intact. Repetition is generally disturbed comparable to the amount of spontaneous output. It is produced by a lesion of Broca's area, which is in the posterior part of the inferior frontal gyrus of the language-dominant hemisphere.

    Conduction aphasia (**choice B**) is produced by a lesion in the arcuate fasciculus, which is in the posterior inferior part of the parietal lobe of the language-dominant hemisphere. This effectively disconnects Broca's area from Wernicke's area, resulting in the inability to repeat.

    Global aphasia (**choice C**) occurs with the destruction of Broca's area, Wernicke's area, and the arcuate fasciculus, resulting in a combination of both Broca and Wernicke aphasias.

    Mixed transcortical aphasia (**choice D**) results from damage to much of both Broca's and Wernicke's areas, but leaves the arcuate fasciculus intact. The patient has little spontaneous language output or comprehension but is still able to repeat.

    Transcortical motor aphasia (**choice E**) is a variation of Broca aphasia in which repetition is preserved. The lesion is generally superior or anterior to Broca's area or may involve the supplementary motor area.

    Transcortical sensory aphasia (**choice F**) is similar to Wernicke aphasia, but the ability to repeat is preserved. The lesion is generally posterior or superior to Wernicke's area.

26. **The correct answer is B.** Acute mountain sickness is caused by hypoxemia and alkalosis due to exposure to high altitude. Hyperventilation occurs in response to the hypoxemia, which helps bring the oxygen saturation back toward normal, but "blows off" excessive amounts of $CO_2$, producing acute respiratory alkalosis.

    **Choice A** represents respiratory acidosis with renal compensation or metabolic alkalosis with respiratory compensation.

    **Choice C** represents uncompensated respiratory acidosis.

    **Choice D** represents either metabolic acidosis with respiratory compensation or respiratory alkalosis with renal compensation.

**Choice E** represents normal values.

**Choices F and G** represent metabolic acidosis.

**Choice H** represents partially compensated chronic respiratory acidosis.

27. **The correct answer is F.** Mammary duct ectasia may simulate cancer clinically. It is a disorder of premenopausal age that manifests often with nipple retraction or inversion and sometimes with nipple discharge. Characteristic histologic features include marked dilatation (ectasia) of large ducts with fibrosis and chronic inflammation. The pathogenesis is obscure but may be a reaction to stagnant colostrum.

    Abscesses (**choice A**) develop most often in the lactating breast and are associated with an exquisitely painful mass with systemic signs of infection. *Staphylococcus aureus* is the most common etiologic agent.

    The histologic features of the lesion exclude a diagnosis of adenocarcinoma (**choice B**), which is composed of atypical cells arranged in duct-like or glandular structures.

    Fat necrosis (**choice C**) refers to a focus of necrotic adipose tissue with secondary histiocytic infiltration. Physical findings may mimic cancer. It is often related to localized trauma.

    Fibrocystic changes (**choice D**) are among the most common breast changes and include varying combinations of cysts, fibrosis, apocrine metaplasia, calcification, chronic inflammation, and epithelial hyperplasia. The latter, if florid or associated with atypia, is associated with an increased risk of cancer transformation.

    A foreign body reaction (**choice E**) may develop to silicone used for mammoplasty and simulate a tumor. There is prominent infiltration of histiocytes and multinucleated giant cells.

    Mondor disease (**choice G**) is a rare condition consisting of thrombophlebitis developing in the breast and manifesting as a nodular cord in the thoracic wall. It is self-limited and possibly related to trauma, and often follows radical mastectomy.

28. **The correct answer is E.** In the rare pure red cell aplasia, the erythroid marrow elements are absent or nearly absent, while granulopoiesis and thrombopoiesis remain unaltered. This condition occurs in both primary and secondary forms, both of which are thought to be related to autoimmune destruction of erythroid precursors. There is a relatively weak general association between cancers and red cell aplasia, which is probably due to triggering of autoimmune disease by the cancers. In addition, be aware that there is a specific association between thymic tumors (thymoma) and autoimmune

hematologic diseases, specifically pure red cell aplasia. This association is strong enough that a patient with pure red cell aplasia should be specifically evaluated for thymoma.

The other answer choices are distracters with no specific association with red cell aplasia, although cancer in general can be a predisposing factor.

29. **The correct answer is B.** Bronchogenic adenocarcinoma is only weakly associated with smoking. This disorder is the most common lung cancer seen in nonsmokers and in women.

Bronchioloalveolar carcinoma (**choice A**) is a relatively uncommon form of carcinoma of the lung. It arises in the lung periphery and does not appear to be clearly related to smoking.

Large cell (anaplastic) carcinomas (**choice C**) are unusual and probably represent undifferentiated variants of squamous cell and bronchogenic adenocarcinomas.

Small cell (oat cell) carcinoma (**choice D**) is very strongly associated with smoking.

Squamous cell carcinoma (**choice E**) is very strongly associated with smoking.

30. **The correct answer is E.** The history suggests streptococcal pharyngitis, followed by poststreptococcal glomerulonephritis. Subepithelial humps composed of proteinaceous material can be seen projecting outward from the outer capillary wall to the urinary space by light or electron microscopy. Granular deposits of IgG and C3 can be seen by immunofluorescence microscopy.

Dense deposits (**choice A**) are characteristic of type II membranoproliferative glomerulonephritis.

Fusion of podocyte processes (**choice B**) is seen in minimal change disease.

Linear deposition of IgG (**choice C**) is seen in Goodpasture syndrome.

Mesangial IgA deposits (**choice D**) are characteristic of Berger disease.

31. **The correct answer is D.** This woman presents with the classic signs and symptoms of multiple sclerosis (MS). A key to the diagnosis is different neurologic signs that are separated by space and time. (Another classic clue might have been oligoclonal bands on electrophoresis of the CSF.) MS is a demyelinating disease of the CNS, characterized by loss of oligodendroglial cells, which are responsible for producing myelin in the CNS. Diagnosis can be confirmed by an MRI revealing sharply delineated regions of demyelination (plaques) throughout the CNS white matter (especially in periventricular areas).

Antibodies to acetylcholine receptors (**choice A**) have been implicated in the etiology of myasthenia gravis, not MS.

MS is generally characterized by axonal preservation, rather than degeneration (**choice B**).

Demyelination of peripheral nerves (**choice C**) occurs in a number of diseases (e.g., Guillain-Barré), but not in MS. Guillain-Barré is characterized by ascending muscle weakness, areflexia, and paralysis.

Oligodendrocytes are responsible for producing myelin in the CNS; Schwann cells (**choice E**) are responsible for myelination in the peripheral nervous system and are not affected in MS.

32. **The correct answer is A.** Polycythemia vera is an example of a myeloproliferative disorder, a neoplastic disease of multipotential myeloid stem cells with the capacity to differentiate into erythrocytes, megakaryocytes, or granulocytes. The only hematologic cell line that is not increased in polycythemia vera is the lymphocytic line, and the lymphocyte count is generally normal. The complications of polycythemia vera are generally due to increased blood viscosity and a tendency toward thrombosis. Without regular phlebotomy, death usually occurs within months of diagnosis.

Clonal expansion of granulocyte precursors leads to markedly increased neutrophil counts (**choice B**) and white blood cell counts (**choice E**).

Increased megakaryocyte production often produces platelet counts (**choice C**) above 500,000 cells/mL.

Dramatic increases in erythroid cell production (**choice D**) dominate the hematologic picture in polycythemia vera, and patients may have hematocrits as high as 60%.

33. **The correct answer is A.** The point of this question is that sometimes the obvious explanation is the correct one. Occlusion of the central retinal artery rapidly causes irreversible blindness with loss of the inner retinal layers. (The photoreceptor rod and cone cells are maintained by the pigment epithelium.) The site of occlusion is typically just posterior to the cribriform plate. A garden-variety atheroma or embolism is overwhelmingly the most common cause of central retinal artery occlusion.

Despite all of the teaching about the risk of blindness in temporal arteritis (**choice B**), this disorder causes only 10% of central retinal artery occlusions.

Hypertension (**choice C**) is more likely to cause bleeding than thrombosis.

Polycythemia vera (**choice D**) could (rarely) cause occlusion because of increased blood viscosity and a tendency for thrombosis.

Tumor (**choice E**) might also cause retinal artery thrombosis, but this would be far rarer than atheroma.

34. **The correct answer is E.** This patient is experiencing the very painful passage of a renal stone, which is often accompanied by hematuria. His history of recurrent urolithiasis with calcium-containing stones implies a disorder in the regulation of calcium concentration. Hyperparathyroidism is associated with increased parathormone (PTH) levels, which can produce hypercalcemia, hypercalciuria, and, ultimately, renal stones.

Anemia of chronic disease (**choice A**) does not produce calcium stones. It is an attractive distracter because the patient presents with a chronic condition and hematuria. Note that urinary blood loss is not usually significant enough to produce an anemic state.

Chronic *Proteus* infection (**choice B**) would produce struvite (magnesium-ammonium phosphate), not calcium stones. Staghorn calculi are also seen.

Factor VIII deficiency (**choice C**) occurs in hemophilia, a hereditary clotting disorder. It is not associated with calcium stones.

Hyperaldosteronism (**choice D**) results in potassium depletion, sodium retention, and hypertension. Primary hyperaldosteronism (Conn syndrome) is associated with adrenocortical adenomas in 90% of patients and is characterized by decreased renin. Secondary hyperaldosteronism results from excessive stimulation by angiotensin II, which is caused by excess renin production (plasma renin-angiotensin levels are high). Neither condition is associated with renal stones.

35. **The correct answer is D.** This woman sustained an obstruction of a major airway such that the area of the lung distal to the obstruction was perfused, but not ventilated. In this area of lung, there will be no gas exchange, and the V/Q ratio will approach zero. As a result, the $P_{O_2}$ and $P_{CO_2}$ of the pulmonary blood (and alveolar gas) approaches that of venous blood ($P_{O_2}$ = 40 mm Hg, $P_{CO_2}$ = 45 mm Hg). Therefore, the $P_{O_2}$ will be lower, and the $P_{CO_2}$ will be higher than normal. Because the $P_{CO_2}$ is high, pH will be low.

The amount of dissolved oxygen will be lower than normal, not greater (**choice A**). Dissolved oxygen is equal to 0.003 mL $O_2$/100 mL blood times $P_{O_2}$. Because the $P_{O_2}$ is low in this situation, so must be the dissolved oxygen.

$P_{CO_2}$ will be elevated and pH will be diminished in this lung area. Both of these factors cause the curve to shift to the right, not to the left (**choice B**).

$P_{CO_2}$ will be higher than normal, not lower (**choice C**).

$P_{O_2}$ is decreased and approaches that of venous blood, not arterial blood (**choice E**).

36. **The correct answer is A.** Gastric carcinomas involve the antropyloric region in 50 to 60% of cases. Note that gastric carcinoma is the most common malignancy in Japan and typically presents with early satiety and pain after eating large meals.

Gastric carcinoma occurs at the apex of the cardia (**choice B**) in 25% of cases. These patients generally present with dysphagia due to esophageal outlet obstruction.

The greater curvature of the body (**choice C**) is involved in only about 12% of cases of gastric carcinoma. However, when an ulcerating lesion does occur in this region, it is quite likely to be malignant.

The antropyloric region is involved more often than the lesser curvature of the body (**choice D**), where lesions typically present with symptoms of peptic ulcer, not early satiety.

Gastric carcinoma occurs much more commonly in the antropyloric region than near the gastroesophageal junction (**choice E**).

Although the lesser curvature of the antropyloric region is a favored site, any nonhealing ulcer at any site in the stomach should be biopsied, as it may be cancer.

37. **The correct answer is B.** The earliest microscopic signs of a myocardial infarct are intercellular edema and "wavy change" at the periphery of the affected area. The wavy change in the myocytes is thought to be due to the effects of nearby, intact myocyte contraction on the ischemic myocytes situated at the periphery of the lesion. Such changes can be observed as early as 1 hour after infarction.

Neutrophilic infiltration (**choice A**) is observed within about 12 hours of infarction.

Necrosis with preservation of cell outlines (**choice C**) is a definition of coagulative necrosis, the type that characterizes the myocardium. Coagulative necrosis appears within the first days after an infarct but is not evident during the first hour or so, when wavy change is apparent.

Proliferation of fibroblasts (**choice D**) is a component of scar formation, which occurs weeks after an infarct (if the patient survives).

A softened, yellow plaque (**choice E**) is generally visible about 1 week after infarction.

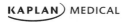

**38.** **The correct answer is C.** Myocardial infarction is the leading cause of death in diabetics. The advanced glycosylated products associated with long-standing diabetes mellitus accelerate the atherosclerotic process. Other risk factors for coronary artery disease (CAD) include hypertension, smoking, hypercholesterolemia, family history of CAD at a young age, male sex, or being a postmenopausal female.

Diabetic ketoacidosis (DKA; **choice A**) carries a high mortality rate for type 1 diabetics. However, this patient had type 2 diabetes, which is associated with hyperosmolar coma, not with DKA.

Although the remaining choices (**B, D, and E**) are all common causes of morbidity and mortality in diabetics, myocardial infarction is the most frequent cause.

**39.** **The correct answer is D.** Barbiturate overdose causes respiratory depression, resulting in carbon dioxide retention (producing increased $P_{CO_2}$ and decreased pH) and hypoxemia (decreased $P_{O_2}$). In other words, the patient has respiratory acidosis. You should look for low $P_{O_2}$, high $P_{CO_2}$, and acidotic pH. **Choices A, B, C, and E** do not fulfill these requirements. Note that **choice C** might be expected in a patient who is hyperventilating to the point of respiratory alkalosis: diminished $O_2$ (the usual drive for hyperventilation in nonpsychiatric hyperventilation), diminished $CO_2$, and mildly alkalotic pH.

**40.** **The correct answer is D.** The most important risk to this patient is liver damage by free radical species derived from carbon tetrachloride ($CCl_4$), notably $CCl_3$. These species are produced when the hepatic P-450 microsomal system attempts to degrade the $CCl_4$. They can cause severe, sometimes fatal, fatty liver damage by reacting with the polyenoic (multiple double bonds) acids present in the membrane phospholipids. The reaction is particularly harmful because peroxides are often formed as a byproduct. Peroxides can be autocatalytic, in that the peroxide radicals themselves form new free radicals capable of more damage to membranes and other cellular structures. Clinically, patients may have an extremely rapid (30 min to 2 hours) decline in hepatic function after the carbon tetrachloride exposure. Other organs are not affected to the same degree, because of the relatively lower concentration of the toxic metabolites there.

**41.** **The correct answer is E.** The challenge in answering this question arises from the difficulty in differentiating the very similar diseases that cause monoclonal gammopathy. The key to answering correctly is making sure not to use only one piece of information as the sole distinguishing factor. You must look at the whole picture—clinical presentation, physical exam, and laboratory findings—just as will be expected when you practice medicine in the future. This 65-year-old patient has Waldenström macroglobulinemia (WM), a disease resulting from neoplasms of lymphocytoid plasma cells that produce monoclonal IgM. Peak incidence is between ages 60 and 70. This patient's symptoms and signs are due to hypergammaglobulinemia and tumorous infiltration (weakness, weight loss, bone pain, hepatosplenomegaly, and lymphadenopathy). His visual disturbance is a symptom of blood hyperviscosity (this creates a resistance to blood flow that may create dysfunction in organs supplied by small arteries such as the retinal artery). The M-protein spike found on serum protein electrophoresis is consistent with WM but not specific for it since this result is also associated with the other answer choices. The intensely eosinophilic plasma cells discovered on bone marrow aspiration are known as "flame cells" and are classic for WM. Although Bence-Jones proteins in the urine are classically associated with multiple myeloma (MM; **choice C**), they are also found in about 10% of patients with WM. This highlights the importance of not jumping to the answers prematurely.

Heavy chain disease (**choice A**) occurs rarely, when a neoplastic clone of plasma cells or lymphocytes produces a monoclonal alpha, gamma, or M chain.

Patients with monoclonal gammopathy of undetermined significance (**choice B**) are generally asymptomatic. Incidence increases with age. Patients with this disorder have a predisposition for developing myeloma, lymphoma, amyloidosis, or WM. They should be followed with periodic evaluations for serum and urine immunoglobulins.

Patients with multiple myeloma (**choice C**) present with susceptibility to infection, proteinuria, bone pain, and hypercalcemia. Renal insufficiency commonly develops. Peak incidence is from age 50 to 60. Tumor-secreted osteoclast-activating factor (OAF) results in osteolytic lesions and "punched out" defects on x-ray films. Bone marrow aspiration would reveal plasma cells in various stages of maturation that may resemble lymphoid precursors with cytoplasmic inclusions (Russell bodies).

Plasmacytoma (**choice D**), or solitary myeloma, is a rare, isolated plasma cell neoplasm in bone or soft tissues. If the primary cancer is in bone, it is likely to disseminate; extraosseous tumors tend to remain localized.

**42.** **The correct answer is A.** The immunophenotype of chronic lymphocytic leukemia is distinctive among clonal B-cell disorders. There is usually strong expression of both CD5 and CD23, and weak expression of surface immunoglobulin (either kappa or lambda chain) and CD22.

In contrast, other disorders that contain mature B cells, such as hairy cell leukemia (**choice B**), non-Hodgkin lymphoma (**choice C**), including follicular and mantle cell lymphomas, and prolymphocytic leukemia (**choice D**), typically have strong expression of surface immunoglobulin and CD22. There is usually absent expression of CD5 (may be seen in prolymphocytic leukemia and some non-Hodgkin lymphomas) and CD23 (may be seen in some non-Hodgkin lymphomas).

Sézary syndrome (**choice E**) is a form of T-cell lymphoma/leukemia.

43. **The correct answer is D.** This patient has bundle branch block, as implied by the QRS interval greater than 0.12 seconds and by paradoxical splitting of the second heart sound. Mobitz II block is frequently associated with bundle branch block. Mobitz II block is characterized on EKG by a constant PR interval before failure of AV conduction occurs. The anatomic site of this type of block is usually below the AV node.

Complete AV block (**choice A**) represents the failure of any impulses to be conducted from the atria to the ventricles. The ventricles are depolarized by an AV nodal or ventricular escape rhythm. It is manifested by a slow ventricular rate, wide pulse pressure, a variable first heart sound, and prominent jugular venous pulsations.

First-degree AV block (**choice B**) represents a delay in conduction of the impulse from the atria to the ventricles, due most commonly to abnormalities in the AV node. It is reflected by a prolonged PR interval, usually exceeding 0.20 seconds.

Mobitz Type I AV block (Wenckebach; **choice C**) is usually due to a problem in the AV node and can result from a variety of cardiac or systemic disorders, including myocardial infarction.

Wolff-Parkinson-White syndrome (**choice E**) is also known as pre-excitation syndrome because conduction occurs by way of an auxiliary pathway between the atria and ventricles. Findings on EKG include a short PR interval and a delta wave (slurred QRS upstroke).

44. **The correct answer is C.** Tumor markers can be very helpful in narrowing the possible primary sources for metastatic lesions. Carcinoembryonic antigen (CEA) can be seen in any tumor derived from gut epithelium, notably colon cancer and pancreatic cancer. Tumor markers should not be used as the primary tool for cancer diagnosis, but they have considerable utility in the confirmation of the diagnosis, as well as for monitoring recurrence or response to therapy.

Alpha-fetoprotein (AFP; **choice A**) is seen in hepatocellular carcinoma, embryonal cell tumor of the testis, and malignant teratoma.

CA-125 (**choice B**) is produced by ovarian cancer.

The beta subunit of human chorionic gonadotropin (hCG; **choice D**) is seen in choriocarcinoma, hydatidiform mole, and germinoma.

Prostate-specific antigen (PSA; **choice E**) is seen in prostatic carcinoma.

You should also remember that serum elevations of many of these markers can also be seen in some benign conditions of similar tissues. hCG, for example, is elevated normally in pregnancy.

45. **The correct answer is C.** This is essentially a Frank-Starling curve that plots cardiac output against central venous pressure (CVP). This patient is in hemorrhagic shock due to trauma. Both cardiac output and CVP should be reduced.

**Point A** represents normality.

**Point B** represents diminished cardiac output despite elevated preload and implies intrinsic cardiac pathology (cardiogenic shock).

**Point D** represents a state in which cardiac output increases normally in response to increased preload.

**Point E** represents elevated cardiac output despite diminished preload and corresponds to septic shock.

46. **The correct answer is D.** This patient has two major risk factors for HIV: drug abuse and a prior sexually transmitted disease (STD), implying high-risk behavior. *Pneumocystis carinii* is the most common cause of pneumonia in HIV-positive patients and is diagnosed by demonstration of organisms via methenamine-silver stain or fluorescent antibody in lung tissue. Bilateral interstitial infiltrates are characteristic of this disease.

Acid-fast bacteria found in the sputum (**choice A**) is associated with tuberculosis (TB), which is also commonly found in HIV-positive patients. Primary TB is usually asymptomatic, whereas reactivation of the infection (secondary TB) is associated with chronic cough, hemoptysis, fever, weight loss, and night sweats. The presence of both a calcified peripheral lung nodule (Ghon complex) and a calcified perihilar lymph node is characteristic of this disease.

Curschmann spirals in mucus plugs (**choice B**), which are shed epithelia that have assumed a spiral configuration, and the presence of Charcot-Leyden crystals (**choice E**), which are eosinophils and membrane proteins forming a crystalloid collection, are characteristic of asthma.

Elevated serum cold agglutinins (IgMs; **choice C**) are found in 50% of patients with *Mycoplasma pneumoniae* infection, the most common cause of pneumonia in young adults. Clinical features include fever, malaise, and a dry hacking cough. Twenty percent of patients with adenovirus exhibit this finding as well.

47. **The correct answer is A.** Cholestasis due to obstruction of the common bile duct results in an increase in serum conjugated bilirubin, an increase in urine bilirubin, and a decrease in urine urobilinogen. This form of jaundice is caused by a deficit in bilirubin excretion, since the process of bilirubin conjugation is normal. Because the conjugated bilirubin cannot be excreted through the biliary tree, it refluxes back into the serum, resulting in increased serum and urine bilirubin levels. In addition, because very little (if any) of the bilirubin is excreted into the gastrointestinal tract, there is very little urobilinogen produced by the enteric flora, resulting in decreased urobilinogen levels.

A deficiency in glucuronyl transferase (**choice B**) would result in impaired bilirubin conjugation, leading to an unconjugated hyperbilirubinemia.

Increased erythrocyte destruction caused by hemolytic anemia (**choice C**) would release more free bilirubin into the bloodstream than the liver could immediately process, resulting in a predominantly unconjugated hyperbilirubinemia.

Hepatocellular damage (**choice D**) results in a mixed conjugated/unconjugated bilirubinemia, since the hepatic mechanisms for both bilirubin conjugation and excretion are disrupted.

48. **The correct answer is A.** An annular pancreas may exert pressure on the duodenum, causing the patient to vomit bile-stained material. This condition is the result of the ventral pancreatic bud's failure to migrate normally.

Esophageal atresia (**choice B**) is diagnosed shortly after birth. Milk cannot reach the stomach and is therefore quickly regurgitated in an undigested state.

The lodging of one or more gallstones (**choice C**) in the extrahepatic biliary apparatus may cause indigestion, severe pain, and jaundice.

Meckel's (ileal) diverticulum (**choice D**) is persistence of a portion of the embryonic vitelline duct (yolk stalk). It is usually asymptomatic but may cause bleeding or ulceration because of the presence of ectopic gastric tissue.

Pyloric stenosis (**choice E**) is a congenital thickening of the smooth muscle in the wall of the pyloric portion of the stomach. It is usually diagnosed in infants following episodes of projectile vomiting.

49. **The correct answer is D.** Lipofuscin is a brown pigment that accumulates with aging. It is believed to be produced from the peroxidation of lipids. Lipofuscin accumulation does not necessarily impair the ability of the cell to function and can be found in the hearts and livers of healthy elderly patients.

Beta-carotene (**choice A**) is a carotenoid ingested in the diet (found in yellow vegetables such as squash, pumpkins, and carrots) and converted to vitamin A. Excessive beta-carotene can cause a benign yellow-orange discoloration of the skin in a condition known as carotenemia.

Bilirubin (**choice B**) is a pigment derived from the metabolism of the heme group of hemoglobin. As hemoglobin is broken down, it first forms biliverdin, which is subsequently converted to bilirubin. Bilirubin can be conjugated (to glucuronic acid) or unconjugated. The conjugated form (also called the direct reacting portion) accumulates in biliary obstructions. The unconjugated form of bilirubin (indirect-reacting) accumulates in hemolytic processes.

Hemosiderin (**choice C**) is the storage form of iron and stains blue with Prussian blue. Hemosiderin accumulation from breakdown of red cells is seen in chronic passive congestion of the lung (inside hemosiderin-laden macrophages called "heart failure cells"). Hemosiderin deposition is also seen in hemochromatosis, a disorder characterized by abnormal iron storage. Hemochromatosis is seen in patients with increased iron uptake from the gastrointestinal tract and in patients receiving repeated blood transfusion therapy.

Melanin (**choice E**) is a brown-black pigment made by melanocytes in the skin. Melanin is also found in the iris, giving the eye its color. Neuromelanin is a type of melanin found in catecholamine neurons in the brain.

50. **The correct answer is C.** This patient has a non-Hodgkin lymphoma of the follicular type. *Bcl-2* is a very important gene that normally acts to prevent apoptosis, or programmed cell death. In approximately 85% of B-cell lymphomas (especially follicular and undifferentiated), this gene is over-expressed as a result of a translocation [t(14;18)(q32;q21)] that links *bcl-2* (at 18q21) to the Ig heavy chain gene (14q32). It is thought that the resultant over-expression of *bcl-2* causes other mutations, which then produce the frank lymphoma.

Amplification of L-*myc* (**choice A**) is associated with the development of small cell (oat cell) carcinoma of the lung.

Homozygous loss of *p53* (**choice B**) is associated with a number of different kinds of human neoplasms, including colon, breast, and lung cancer.

**KAPLAN** MEDICAL

Point mutation in *ras* (**choice D**) may alter its ability to bind GTPase activating proteins (GAPS), thereby preventing termination of the signal transduced by the *ras* protein. The net result is excessive activation of a mitogenic cellular pathway, as well as tumor formation. Approximately 30% of human tumors are associated with *ras* mutations.

Reciprocal translocation between chromosome 9 and chromosome 22 (**choice E**) forms the Philadelphia chromosome, which is associated with chronic myelocytic leukemia.

# Pathology and Pathophysiology: **Test Two**

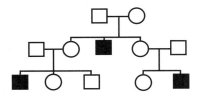

1. A teenage boy with a history of peripheral neuropathy and ocular abnormalities has multiple purplish nodules diffusely over his skin. Other family members have been similarly affected, as shown in the pedigree above. Laboratory tests reveal the young man has a deficiency of α-galactosidase A. Biopsy of the skin lesions would most likely reveal that they were

   (A) basal cell carcinomas

   (B) cavernous hemangiomas

   (C) cystic hygromas

   (D) neurofibromas

   (E) squamous cell carcinomas

2. A Guatemalan child with a history of meconium ileus is brought to a clinic because of a chronic cough. The mother notes a history of respiratory tract infections and bulky, foul-smelling stools. After assessment of the respiratory tract illness, the physician should also look for signs of

   (A) cystinuria

   (B) hypoglycemia

   (C) iron deficiency anemia

   (D) sphingomyelin accumulation

   (E) vitamin A deficiency

3. A 38-year-old man comes to the physician because of severe stiffness and pain in his hips, back, and knees. Physical examination shows bluish-gray discoloration of ear cartilage and sclerae and decreased joint mobility. A spinal x-ray reveals disk degeneration combined with dense calcification, particularly in the lumbar area. This patient most likely has a deficiency of which of the following enzymes?

   (A) Arylsulfatase A

   (B) Glucose-6-phosphatase

   (C) Hexosaminidase A

   (D) Homogentisic oxidase

   (E) Muscle phosphorylase

4. A neonate develops marked unconjugated hyperbilirubinemia. No hemolysis can be demonstrated, and other liver function tests are normal. No bilirubin is found in the urine. This infant's condition continues to deteriorate, and he dies at 2 weeks of age. To which of the following conditions did the infant most likely succumb?

   (A) Crigler-Najjar syndrome, Type I

   (B) Crigler-Najjar syndrome, Type II

   (C) Dubin-Johnson syndrome

   (D) Gilbert syndrome

   (E) Rotor syndrome

5. A 59-year-old man complains of headache and decreasing visual ability. History reveals that the patient has also "outgrown" his pants and shirts within the past year. The man exhibits a marked overbite. Which of the following is the best method to diagnose this patient?

   (A) Measuring growth hormone (GH) and insulin growth factor-1 (IGF-1) levels before and after administrating glucose

   (B) Measuring resting corticotropin (ACTH) levels

   (C) Measuring resting prolactin levels

   (D) Measuring the patient's height and comparing it with last year's value

   (E) Measuring the patient's shoe size and comparing it with last year's value

6. A 36-year-old alcoholic man is brought to the emergency department because he is jaundiced and exhibits inappropriate somnolence. Past medical history is significant for depression and seizures, both of which are well controlled with medications. Physical exam is significant for icterus, asterixis, and tachypnea. Slit lamp examination reveals greenish-golden crescents on the cornea. AST is 2489 IU/L, ALT is 4873 IU/L, bilirubin is 29 mg/dL, alkaline phosphatase is 112 IU/L, hematocrit is 29%, prothrombin time (PT) is 19.1 seconds, and serum ceruloplasmin is decreased. Which of the following is the most likely diagnosis?

   (A) Alcoholic hepatitis

   (B) Budd-Chiari syndrome

   (C) Drug-induced hepatitis

   (D) Hepatitis B

   (E) Wilson disease

7. A 9-year-old Mexican girl develops rapid, purposeless movements, an expanding erythematous rash, and subcutaneous nodules 3 weeks after recovery from a severe sore throat. A biopsy of the subcutaneous nodules would most likely reveal

   (A) caseous necrosis with epithelioid cells and Langhans giant cells

   (B) fibrinoid necrosis with lymphocytes, macrophages, and Anitschkow cells

   (C) focal collections of hemosiderin-laden macrophages

   (D) lymphoid nodules with a "starry-sky" appearance

   (E) Reed-Sternberg cells in a background of lymphocytes with occasional eosinophils

8. A 35-year-old IV drug abuser is brought to the hospital with high fever, chills, and hematuria. Physical examination reveals splenomegaly, erythematous, nontender lesions on the palms and soles, and hemorrhages in the nail beds. An echocardiogram is ordered. On which of the following heart valves would the appearance of vegetations be expected?

   (A) Aortic

   (B) Mitral

   (C) Pulmonic

   (D) Tricuspid

9. A 55-year-old man comes to the physician after being told at a health fair that he has type 2 diabetes mellitus. He is asymptomatic and, besides being a "big eater," he has no other bad habits. He does not smoke cigarettes, and he drinks only two or three glasses of wine a week. In 5 years he is most likely to exhibit which of the following?

   (A) Fatty liver

   (B) Intermittent claudication

   (C) Motor neuropathy

   (D) Retinopathy

   (E) 3+ proteinuria

10. A 20-year-old man presents with an enlarged right testicle that was undescended at birth but had self-corrected by age 1. Serum AFP is elevated. A testicular tumor is biopsied and reveals multiple mitoses, along with hemorrhage and necrosis. The surgeon decides to perform an orchiectomy because the tumor type is not particularly radiosensitive. Which of the following is the most likely diagnosis?

   (A) Embryonal carcinoma

   (B) Interstitial cell tumor

   (C) Seminoma

   (D) Sertoli cell tumor

11. A 28-year-old woman comes to the office because of fatigue. Lately she has been having difficulty making it through the day without taking a nap. She is generally healthy and takes no medications other than NSAIDs for menstrual cramps. Her last menstrual period was 3 weeks ago and was "very heavy," as usual. Physical examination shows tachycardia and tachypnea but is otherwise normal. Laboratory studies show decreased levels of iron and ferritin and an increased total iron-binding capacity. A peripheral blood smear shows hypochromic, microcytic erythrocytes. She was placed on oral ferrous sulfate and makes an appointment to return 1 month later. What will the peripheral blood smear look like at the scheduled return visit?

    (A) Almost all larger than normal erythrocytes

    (B) Almost all normal erythrocytes

    (C) Almost all small, but no longer hypochromic, erythrocytes

    (D) Almost all small hypochromic erythrocytes

    (E) A mix of small hypochromic and normal erythrocytes

12. A 35-year-old man presents to the physician with intensely pruritic skin lesions on his axillary folds, nipples, waistband, wrists, interdigital spaces of the hand, and genitalia. Linear burrows are apparent in affected areas. Which of the following is the most likely diagnosis?

    (A) Dermatitis herpetiformis

    (B) Lichen planus

    (C) Photosensitivity

    (D) Scabies

    (E) Seborrhea

13. A patient complains to her physician that she feels lightheaded and has even fainted during defecation. This is most probably an example of syncope due to which of the following mechanisms?

    (A) Anoxia

    (B) Hyperventilation

    (C) Hypovolemia

    (D) Sinus node disease

    (E) Valsalva mechanism

14. Radiographic studies of a 2-year-old child brought to an emergency department reveal a new fracture of the humerus and evidence of multiple old fractures in ribs and long bones of the extremities. A social worker wants to initiate prosecution of the parents for child abuse, but an alert emergency department physician notices that, despite the broken arm, the toddler shows minimal bruising. A very careful, directed, physical examination reveals that the toddler has "peculiar teeth," a blue tinge to the sclera, and unusually mobile joints. The physician suspects a disease that is characterized by an abnormality of which of the following biochemical functions?

    (A) Collagen type I synthesis

    (B) Collagen type II synthesis

    (C) Collagen type III synthesis

    (D) Collagen type IV synthesis

    (E) Collagen type V synthesis

15. A 35-year-old roofer presents to his primary care physician complaining of dyspnea and chronic dry cough. A chest x-ray film reveals pulmonary hyperinflation with "honeycombing" and calcified parietal pleural plaques. Which of the following is the most likely diagnosis?

    (A) Anthracosis

    (B) Asbestosis

    (C) Berylliosis

    (D) Byssinosis

    (E) Silicosis

16. A concerned mother brings her 6-year-old son to the pediatrician because he has developed a "puffy face." On examination, the child has a blood pressure of 90/60 mm Hg, marked periorbital edema, and pitting edema of both the hands and feet. Cardiac examination is unremarkable, and he has no splenomegaly or signs of liver disease. Laboratory values are notable for decreased serum albumin and increased total cholesterol. A urinalysis reveals 4+ proteinuria but no red blood cells, white blood cells, or casts. Which of the following is the most likely diagnosis?

    (A) Goodpasture syndrome

    (B) minimal change nephropathy

    (C) poststreptococcal glomerulonephritis

    (D) systemic lupus erythematosus

    (E) Wegener granulomatosis

17. A 50-year-old industrial chemist presents with painless hematuria. On further questioning he also describes urinary frequency and urgency. After additional testing, a diagnosis of bladder cancer is made. The patient's cancer is most likely which of the following types?

    (A) Adenocarcinoma

    (B) Papilloma

    (C) Sarcoma

    (D) Squamous cell carcinoma

    (E) Transitional cell carcinoma

18. A 42-year-old man previously diagnosed with kidney stones complains of gnawing, burning epigastric pain. On questioning, he also notes moderate to severe diarrhea. Measurement of the patient's basal gastric acid output reveals that it is markedly elevated. These symptoms are likely the result of which of the following neoplastic syndromes?

    (A) Familial polyposis coli

    (B) Multiple endocrine neoplasia type I (MEN I)

    (C) MEN IIA

    (D) MEN IIB

    (E) MEN III

19. A 40-year-old woman comes to the physician for a periodic health maintenance examination. She has no complaints at this time, but she is concerned about a story that she heard on the local news. The story was about the progeny of women who took diethylstilbestrol (DES) and their increased risk for disease, but she missed the end of the story and is not sure of the disease. This woman is particularly concerned because her mother took DES for the prevention of spontaneous abortion. This woman should be told that she has an increased risk for developing which of the following diseases?

    (A) Bladder cancer

    (B) Endometrial carcinoma

    (C) Ovarian carcinoma

    (D) Renal cell carcinoma

    (E) Vaginal clear cell adenocarcinoma

20. A 3-day-old, full-term male newborn has not passed meconium since birth. History reveals that the infant was born to a 24-year-old primigravid mother after an uneventful pregnancy. The delivery was by cesarean section due to fetomaternal disproportion. The baby weighed 3.2 kg at birth and had normal Apgar scores. He was started on formula feeding, which was tolerated without any incidence of vomiting. He passed urine shortly after birth, but passage of meconium has not been observed. On examination, he appears in no distress and feeds vigorously. There are no dysmorphic features, and the abdomen is not distended. Liver and spleen are not enlarged and the bowel sounds are present. Examination of the perineum reveals normal male genitalia and a normally placed anal atresia. Which of the following is the most likely cause for the newborn's constipation?

    (A) Anal atresia

    (B) Duodenal atresia

    (C) Hirschsprung disease

    (D) Meckel diverticulum

    (E) Pyloric stenosis

21. A 65-year-old man with a history of smoking and alcohol abuse complains of poor appetite and difficulty swallowing both solid and liquid foods over the course of the past 4 months. He has lost 20 lb and occasionally vomits blood. A mass is detected in his esophagus and is subsequently biopsied. What is the most likely histologic appearance of the biopsy?

    (A) Glandular epithelium associated with desmoplasia

    (B) Malignant tumor of mesenchymal origin

    (C) Squamous cell morphology

    (D) Tumor derived from all three germ layers

    (E) Tumor of epithelial origin demonstrating transitional cell morphology

22. A 7-year-old boy with chickenpox is given aspirin to reduce his fever. He develops severe vomiting, mental status changes, and seizures, and eventually falls into a coma. Which of the following would you expect to see on a biopsy specimen of his liver?

    (A) Diffuse fibrosis with areas of regeneration

    (B) Fatty change

    (C) Hemosiderin deposits

    (D) Hepatocyte necrosis

    (E) Mallory bodies

23. An 18-year-old Japanese woman presents to her physician with fever and conjunctivitis. Physical exam is significant for oral erythema and fissuring along with a generalized maculopapular rash and cervical lymphadenopathy. The patient's 3-year-old sister experienced the same symptoms 1 week ago. Which of the following is the most likely diagnosis?

    (A) Henoch-Schönlein purpura

    (B) Kawasaki disease

    (C) Polyarteritis nodosa

    (D) Rheumatic fever

    (E) Takayasu arteritis

24. A 24-year-old man presents to his physician with gynecomastia and testicular enlargement. Serum urine and human chorionic gonadotropin (hCG) levels are elevated. Biopsy of the testicular mass reveals a cytotrophoblastic and syncytiotrophoblastic structure. Which of the following is the most likely diagnosis?

    (A) Choriocarcinoma

    (B) Sertoli cell tumor

    (C) Teratoma

    (D) Yolk sac tumor

25. A 57-year-old woman is found unconscious on her kitchen floor after having suffered a myocardial infarction. She has pulmonary edema and distended jugular and peripheral veins. A midsystolic gallop is heard on chest auscultation. EKG shows prominent Q waves in leads II, III, and aVF. Which of the following is most consistent with the patient's condition?

| | Preload | Cardiac output | PAWP | CVP | Vascular resistance | Mixed venous |
|---|---|---|---|---|---|---|
| (A) | ↑ | ↓ | ↓ | ↑ | ↑ | ↓ |
| (B) | ↑ | ↑ | ↓ | ↓ | ↓ | ↑ |
| (C) | ↑ | ↓ | ↑ | ↑ | ↑ | ↓ |
| (D) | ↑ | ↑ | ↑ | ↑ | ↓ | ↓ |
| (E) | ↓ | ↓ | ↑ | ↓ | ↑ | ↓ |
| (F) | ↓ | ↑ | ↓ | ↑ | ↓ | ↑ |
| (G) | ↓ | ↓ | ↑ | ↓ | ↓ | ↓ |

26. A 68-year-old, well-developed, well-nourished black man presents to the emergency department complaining of shortness of breath. He denies chest pain. He has no significant past medical history and takes no medications. A chest x-ray film shows clear lung fields, mild cardiomegaly, and a widened thoracic aorta with linear calcifications. An MRI of the chest shows aortic dilatation in the thorax, extending proximally, with atrophy of the muscularis and wrinkling of the intimal surface. What is the most likely etiology of this condition?

    (A) Atherosclerosis
    (B) Hypertension
    (C) Marfan syndrome
    (D) Syphilis infection
    (E) Takayasu arteritis

27. A 32-year-old woman is diagnosed with breast cancer. Her mother had cervical cancer at age 35, her grandfather had colon cancer at age 36, and her brother was recently diagnosed with lung cancer. If genetic analysis is performed, what would be the likely genotype of this individual at the p53 tumor suppressor gene locus?

    (A) One deleted allele
    (B) Two deleted alleles
    (C) Two wild-type alleles
    (D) Three wild-type alleles
    (E) Fusion of one p53 allele with another gene

28. Bronchoalveolar lavage is performed in a patient with long-standing congestive heart failure exacerbated by periodic acute pulmonary edema. Which of the following findings would be consistent with this patient's history of cardiac failure?

    (A) Anthracotic macrophages
    (B) Charcot-Leyden crystals
    (C) Curschmann spirals
    (D) Fat-laden macrophages
    (E) Ferruginous bodies
    (F) Goblet cells
    (G) Iron-laden macrophages
    (H) Squamous pearls

29. A 23-year-old African American woman presents to the emergency department with severe abdominal pain and evidence of dehydration. Her past medical history is significant for numerous pulmonary infections and effusions of the knees. This patient's erythrocytes would be expected to exhibit

    (A) an absence of central pallor
    (B) deletion of all four alpha Hb genes
    (C) denaturation during deoxygenation
    (D) Heinz bodies on RBC staining

30. A young man presents to his physician's office for a physical examination. He is concerned because his father died of a heart attack in his late 40s. The physician finds that the patient has elevated serum cholesterol and LDL levels, but his VLDL and triglyceride levels are normal. Further investigation reveals an LDL receptor deficiency. This patient has which of the following types of hyperlipidemia?

    (A) I
    (B) IIa
    (C) IIb
    (D) III
    (E) IV
    (F) V

31. A brief occlusion of the right femoral artery produces transient ischemia in the forelimb of a laboratory animal. The cellular edema seen in reversibly injured cells in a muscle biopsy taken from the animal is most closely related to an increase in which of the following?

    (A) Intracellular $Ca^{2+}$
    (B) Intracellular $K^+$
    (C) Intracellular $Mg^{2+}$
    (D) Intracellular $Na^+$
    (E) $Na^+/K^+$ ATPase pump activity

32. A 28-year-old woman presents to the physician complaining of syncopal episodes that last a few minutes. She is not taking any medications and has no previous medical history. EEG and EKG studies are performed and are unremarkable. An echocardiogram shows a single ball-shaped mass dangling in the left atrium near the mitral valve. Which of the following is the most likely diagnosis?

    (A) Angiosarcoma

    (B) Mesothelioma

    (C) Myxoma

    (D) Rhabdomyoma

    (E) Rhabdomyosarcoma

33. Biopsy of the lung from a patient with chronic lung disease demonstrates a honeycomb appearance on gross inspection and fibrosis with inflammation of the alveolar walls on microscopic examination. The patient's blood gas studies are within normal limits. If spirometry were performed on this patient, which of the following would most likely be seen?

    (A) Decreased airway resistance

    (B) Decreased compliance

    (C) Increased functional residual capacity (FRC)

    (D) Increased lung volume

    (E) Increased tidal volume

34. An infant born at 33 weeks' gestation exhibits signs of respiratory distress at birth. Her mother had gestational diabetes. Which of the following would have indicated lung immaturity in the fetus prior to birth?

    (A) <0.5 L of amniotic fluid

    (B) Alpha-1 antitrypsin deficiency in amniotic fluid

    (C) Amniotic lecithin:sphingomyelin ratio less than 2:1

    (D) Elevated maternal $HbA_{1c}$

    (E) Elevated maternal serum alpha-fetoprotein (AFP)

35. A patient is observed to have an abnormal breathing pattern characterized by cyclical changes in tidal volume. The tidal volume first increases and then decreases to the point of apnea. What term best describes this breathing pattern?

    (A) Apneustic

    (B) Biot's

    (C) Cheyne-Stokes

    (D) Hysterical

    (E) Kussmaul

36. A cyanotic infant is discovered to have a ventricular septal defect, an overriding aorta, right ventricular hypertrophy, and complete pulmonic stenosis. Which of the following accompanying congenital anomalies permits survival in this patient?

    (A) Bicuspid aortic valve

    (B) Ostium secundum defect

    (C) Patent ductus arteriosus

    (D) Patent foramen ovale

    (E) Preductal coarctation of aorta

37. A 45-year-old man presents to the physician with muscle cramps, perioral numbness, and irritability over the past 3 to 4 months. Laboratory results reveal hypocalcemia, normal albumin level, mild hypomagnesemia, and hyperphosphatemia. Parathyroid hormone (PTH) level is decreased. Alkaline phosphatase level is normal. Which of the following is most likely causing this clinical scenario?

    (A) Bone metastases

    (B) Hashimoto thyroiditis

    (C) Hypervitaminosis D

    (D) Hypomagnesemia

    (E) Previous subtotal thyroidectomy

38. A patient with systemic lupus erythematosus (SLE) very much wants to become pregnant. What should her physician should tell her regarding pregnancy in lupus patients?

    (A) There is no increased risk to the baby

    (B) There is an increased risk of cardiovascular malformations

    (C) There is an increased risk of nervous system malformations

    (D) There is an increased risk of renal malformations

    (E) There is an increased risk of spontaneous abortions and prematurity

39. To make extra money, a healthy medical student participates in a hematology study. Because the study only involves having her blood drawn multiple times, she is not particularly concerned. A few weeks after her first blood test, the hematologist calls her into his office and asks if she is aware that she has a hematologic disorder. When she says she is not, he tells her that she should not be too concerned, inasmuch as there are usually no complications associated with this disorder, but that there is a risk of thrombosis. The student most likely has a deficiency of which of the following factors?

    (A) V

    (B) VIII

    (C) IX

    (D) X

    (E) XII

40. A 32-year-old woman with one child has tried unsuccessfully to conceive for the past 2 years. She tells her physician that she has had problems putting on weight and is often anxious and irritable. On physical examination, her thyroid is enlarged with no palpable nodules. Which of the following laboratory findings would be most suggestive of a diagnosis of secondary hyperthyroidism?

    (A) Decreased thyroxine-binding globulin (TBG)

    (B) Elevated triiodothyronine (T3)

    (C) Elevated thyroxine (T4)

    (D) Elevated thyroid-stimulating hormone (TSH)

    (E) Presence of serum thyroid-stimulating autoantibodies

41. A hospitalized man with hemoglobinuria and symptoms of anemia undergoes a complete hematologic evaluation. The reticulocyte count is elevated. The remaining laboratory results are pending. Which of the following diagnoses is most consistent with the information available thus far?

    (A) Chronic renal disease

    (B) Folate deficiency

    (C) G6PD deficiency

    (D) Iron deficiency

    (E) Pernicious anemia

42. A 62-year-old man presents with progressive, pruritic erythroderma, exfoliation, and lymphadenopathy. Peripheral smear reveals T cells with cerebriform nuclei. Which of the following is the most likely diagnosis?

    (A) Burkitt lymphoma

    (B) Histiocytic lymphoma

    (C) Lymphoblastic lymphoma

    (D) Lymphocytic lymphoma

    (E) Sézary syndrome

43. A 32-year-old man with a history of chronic drug abuse presents to his primary care physician complaining of uncontrollable shaking in his hands. He moves very slowly and walks with a stooped posture and shuffling gait. Physical examination reveals cogwheel rigidity, a pill-rolling tremor, and masked facies. His condition deteriorates, and he eventually dies. Structures similar to which of the following would be expected on autopsy?

    (A) Hirano bodies

    (B) Lewy bodies

    (C) Lipofuscin granules

    (D) Negri bodies

    (E) Neurofibrillary tangles

44. A 45-year-old woman complains of difficulty speaking, chewing, and swallowing. She experiences generalized weakness that increases with effort and as the day goes on. Symptoms are significantly improved after taking neostigmine. Autoantibodies responsible for causing the patient's condition are directed against which of the following?

    (A) Acetylcholine receptors

    (B) Double-stranded DNA

    (C) Dystrophin

    (D) Erythrocyte surface antigens

    (E) Myelin

45. A patient has severe arthritis involving the lower back. Before making a diagnosis of ankylosing spondylitis, the patient should be questioned about which of the following diseases?

    (A) Carcinoid syndrome

    (B) Celiac disease

    (C) Crohn disease

    (D) Peptic ulcer

    (E) Whipple disease

46. A 3-year-old child develops severe generalized edema following a viral infection. On the basis of clinical chemistry tests, a renal biopsy is performed, with normal light microscopic findings. Which of the following abnormal laboratory values might be expected in this individual?

    (A) Decreased alpha$_2$ globulin levels

    (B) Decreased fibrinogen

    (C) Increased serum calcium levels

    (D) Low serum albumin levels

    (E) Red blood cell casts in the urine

47. A patient with long-standing hypertension dies in a car accident. At autopsy, multiple, small, cavitary lesions are observed in the basal ganglia. This finding is most consistent with pathology of which of the following arteries?

    (A) Anterior cerebral

    (B) Lateral striate

    (C) Posterior cerebral

    (D) Superior cerebellar

    (E) Vertebral

48. The clinical pathology lab at the hospital receives a specimen from the pediatrics inpatient unit. Laboratory studies show a marked susceptibility of the red cells to lysis in hypotonic solutions. This finding is most useful for the diagnosis of which of the following disorders?

    (A) Alpha thalassemia minor

    (B) Beta thalassemia major

    (C) Hereditary spherocytosis

    (D) Sickle cell anemia

    (E) Sickle cell trait

49. A 75-year-old man with angina pectoris has recurrent episodes of atrial tachycardia (240/min). A rapid sequence of normal QRS waves is seen on EKG. The episodes are controllable by the patient's performance of vagal maneuvers. Which of the following is the most likely etiology of this arrhythmia?

    (A) Atrial re-eentry

    (B) Automatic atrial conduction

    (C) AV dissociation

    (D) AV nodal re-entry

    (E) Wandering atrial pacemaker

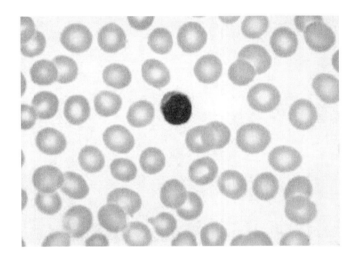

50. A 2-year-old girl has an infection. A complete blood count reveals increased numbers of the white blood cell type shown above. Which of the following diseases is most consistent with this laboratory result?

    (A) Bronchiolitis

    (B) Cellulitis

    (C) Diphtheria

    (D) Epiglottitis

    (E) Pertussis

# Pathology and Pathophysiology Test Two: **Answers and Explanations**

## ANSWER KEY

| | | | | |
|---|---|---|---|---|
| 1. | B | | 26. | D |
| 2. | E | | 27. | A |
| 3. | D | | 28. | G |
| 4. | A | | 29. | C |
| 5. | A | | 30. | B |
| 6. | E | | 31. | D |
| 7. | B | | 32. | C |
| 8. | D | | 33. | B |
| 9. | D | | 34. | C |
| 10. | A | | 35. | C |
| 11. | E | | 36. | C |
| 12. | D | | 37. | E |
| 13. | E | | 38. | E |
| 14. | A | | 39. | E |
| 15. | B | | 40. | D |
| 16. | B | | 41. | C |
| 17. | E | | 42. | E |
| 18. | B | | 43. | B |
| 19. | E | | 44. | A |
| 20. | C | | 45. | C |
| 21. | C | | 46. | D |
| 22. | B | | 47. | B |
| 23. | B | | 48. | C |
| 24. | A | | 49. | D |
| 25. | C | | 50. | A |

1. **The correct answer is B.** Fabry disease is a lysosomal storage disease with sex-linked genetics caused by deficiency of a-galactosidase, which leads to the accumulation of ceramide trihexoside in many tissues (reticuloendothelial, myocardial, ganglion, renal glomeruli and tubules, and connective tissue). Fabry disease is characterized by angiokeratoma corporis diffusum (cavernous hemangioma with epidermal keratosis), thickened blood vessels (with risk of myocardial infarction and stroke), and progressive renal failure and hypertension in adult life.

   Multiple basal cell carcinomas (**choice A**) are seen in familial basal cell nevus syndrome, which is not a lysosomal storage disease.

   Cystic hygromas (**choice C**) are seen in Turner syndrome and are associated with a "webbed" neck.

   Neurofibromas (**choice D**) are seen in neurofibromatosis.

   Multiple squamous cell carcinomas (**choice E**) are seen in skin badly damaged by the sun or radiation, in xeroderma pigmentosa, and in albinism.

2. **The correct answer is E.** This child probably has cystic fibrosis. In this disorder, an abnormality of chloride channels causes all exocrine secretions to be much thicker and more viscous than normal. Pancreatic secretion of digestive enzymes is often severely impaired, with consequent steatorrhea and deficiency of fat-soluble vitamins, including vitamin A.

   Cystinuria (**choice A**) is a relatively common disorder in which a defective transporter for dibasic amino acids (<u>c</u>ystine, <u>o</u>rnithine, <u>l</u>ysine, <u>a</u>rginine; *COLA*) leads to saturation of the urine with cystine, which is not very soluble in urine, and precipitates out to form stones.

   Hypoglycemia (**choice B**) is not a prominent feature in children with cystic fibrosis who are on a normal diet. <u>Hy</u>perglycemia may occur late in the course of the disease.

   Iron deficiency anemia (**choice C**) is not regularly found in children with cystic fibrosis.

   Sphingomyelin accumulation (**choice D**) is generally associated with deficiency of sphingomyelinase, as seen in Niemann-Pick disease.

3. **The correct answer is D.** The patient has alkaptonuria (ochronosis), a deficiency in the phenylalanine-tyrosine pathway that specifically blocks the metabolic degradation of homogentisic acid. The disease is hereditary (autosomal recessive) but does not typically become clinically evident until about the fourth decade of life, when the degenerative arthropathy becomes a problem.

Arylsulfatase A (**choice A**) is deficient in metachromatic leukodystrophy, one of the lysosomal storage diseases.

Glucose-6-phosphatase (**choice B**) is deficient in von Gierke disease, one of the glycogenoses.

Hexosaminidase A (**choice C**) is deficient in Tay-Sachs disease, one of the lysosomal storage diseases.

Muscle phosphorylase (**choice E**) is deficient in McArdle disease, one of the glycogenoses.

4. **The correct answer is A.** All the diseases listed are inherited disorders of bilirubin metabolism, and they are usually discussed together. Crigler-Najjar syndrome (**choices A and B**) and Gilbert syndrome (**choice D**) are both unconjugated hyperbilirubinemias, whereas Dubin-Johnson syndrome (**choice C**) and Rotor syndrome (**choice E**) are conjugated hyperbilirubinemias. Crigler-Najjar syndrome (particularly the type I variant) is rare and extremely serious (with the presentation given in the question stem), whereas Gilbert syndrome is completely benign. The type II variant of Crigler-Najjar is intermediate in severity between Gilbert and the Type I. Dubin-Johnson and Rotor syndromes are also relatively benign; Dubin-Johnson is distinguished from Rotor syndrome by the presence of a black pigment of unknown composition in the liver.

5. **The correct answer is A.** Acromegaly is most commonly caused by a pituitary adenoma. Acromegalic persons secrete excessively high levels of growth hormone (GH) and insulin growth factor-1 (IGF-1) from pituitary gland tissue. These hormones are not suppressed by glucose, as they would be in a normal person.

   Measuring resting corticotropin (ACTH) levels (**choice B**) may be indicated in a person with Cushing syndrome.

   Measuring resting prolactin levels (**choice C**) would be indicated in a person with a suspected prolactinoma.

   Measuring the height (**choice D**) of a 59-year-old patient would not be indicated. Acromegaly, or excess GH, in individuals who have already experienced closure of bone growth centers results in a broadening of the skeletal bones, not a lengthening. Lengthening of skeletal bones occurs in gigantism, before the closure of bone growth centers.

   Measuring a patient's shoe size and comparing it with last year's size (**choice E**), although indicative of a broadening of skeletal bones, is not a clinically used standard for the diagnosis of acromegaly.

6. **The correct answer is E.** Acute liver failure (implied by the abnormal liver function tests) in this young patient with depression strongly suggests Wilson disease (WD).

In conjunction with a low serum ceruloplasmin level, the presence of Kayser-Fleischer rings (greenish-golden crescents on the cornea) on slit lamp examination is diagnostic of WD.

Alcoholic hepatitis (**choice A**) very rarely causes elevation of transaminases in the range of 3000 to 4000, but it is classically associated with an AST twice the value of the ALT.

Budd-Chiari syndrome (**choice B**), or hepatic vein thrombosis, is a rare condition that presents with abdominal pain, large, tender liver, and ascites. Micropathology is similar to chronic passive congestion of the liver, with central hemorrhagic necrosis and rupture at Disse's spaces. The liver develops a "nutmeg" appearance, which is also seen in patients with severe heart failure.

Drug-induced hepatitis (**choice C**) may be caused by phenytoin, which the patient may have been taking for seizures. However, drug-induced hepatitis usually presents with fever, rash, joint pain, and eosinophilia, which are not evident in this patient. Other medications causing drug-induced hepatitis include isoniazid, methyldopa, and halothane.

Patients with hepatitis B (**choice D**) typically present with nausea, vomiting, malaise, diarrhea, and dark urine. Jaundice, tender hepatomegaly, and low-grade fever may be evident on physical exam. Serum transaminases are usually elevated, but serum ceruloplasmin would likely be normal. The detection of hepatitis antigens and antibodies in serum is diagnostic.

7.  **The correct answer is B.** The history of a recent severe sore throat in a young person is a classic clue suggesting rheumatic fever. The histologic description given is that of an Aschoff body, which classically occurs in the heart in rheumatic heart disease. Erythema marginatum (the expanding erythematous rash) and Sydenham chorea (rapid, purposeless movements) also accompany this disorder. The subcutaneous nodules characteristic of rheumatic fever are basically "giant" Aschoff bodies.

    Caseous necrosis with epithelioid cells and Langhans giant cells (**choice A**) are characteristic of the granulomas of tuberculosis.

    Hemosiderin-laden macrophages (**choice C**) may be found in chronic passive congestion of the liver.

    Burkitt lymphoma is characterized by dense collections of lymphoid cells with macrophages intermixed. The macrophages often have a clear space around them, giving the tissue a "starry sky" appearance (**choice D**).

    Reed-Sternberg cells (**choice E**) are characteristic of Hodgkin lymphoma. Occasional eosinophils are often admixed with the proliferating lymphocytes in this disorder.

8.  **The correct answer is D.** This patient's symptoms (fever, chills, hematuria) and signs [erythematous, nontender lesions (Janeway lesions) and nail-bed hemorrhages (splinter hemorrhages)] are most consistent with acute bacterial endocarditis (ABE). ABE in IV drug abusers most often affects the tricuspid valve and is usually caused by *Staphylococcus aureus*, although *Pseudomonas*, *Bacillus*, and *Candida albicans* can also be involved.

    The aortic (**choice A**), mitral (**choice B**), and pulmonic (**choice C**) valves are less commonly affected in this particular population.

9.  **The correct answer is D.** Diabetic retinopathy usually precedes the development of diabetic nephropathy and proteinuria (**choice E**).

    Fatty liver (**choice A**) occurs in alcohol abuse and toxic insults to the liver. It is not associated with diabetes.

    Intermittent claudication (**choice B**) and coronary artery disease, when solely associated with diabetes and no other risk factors (e.g., hypertension, smoking), usually occur later in the disease.

    Motor neuropathy (**choice C**) is rare in diabetes and usually occurs later in the disease (at about 10 years). It is usually manifested by foot or wrist drop (peroneal and radial nerve palsies, respectively).

10. **The correct answer is A.** Embryonal carcinomas occur most commonly in the 20 to 30 age group and are more aggressive than seminomas. These tumors present with testicular enlargement, and 30% have metastasized at the time of diagnosis. Serum AFP is usually elevated. They are less radiosensitive than seminomas.

    Interstitial (Leydig) cell tumors (**choice B**) can produce androgens, estrogens, or corticosteroids. In children, they often present with masculinization or feminization. In adults, they often present with gynecomastia. Microscopically, tumor cells resemble normal Leydig cells with round nuclei, eosinophilic cytoplasm, and lipid granules. Approximately half the tumors contain cigar-shaped crystalloids of Reinke.

    Seminomas (**choice C**) occur most commonly in the fourth decade of life. Microscopic exam reveals sheets of uniform polyhedral cells divided by fibrous septa of connective tissue; lymphocytes and multinucleated giant cells may also be present. These tumors are highly radiosensitive.

    Sertoli cell tumors (**choice D**) can produce small amounts of androgens or estrogens, but usually not enough to cause endocrinologic changes. They may present with testicular enlargement. Microscopic exam reveals uniform, tall, polyhedral cells with clear cytoplasm, growing in cords resembling spermatic tubules.

11. **The correct answer is E.** Erythrocytes have a life-span of about 110 days in the bloodstream. Since the circulating erythrocytes have no nucleus, produce no RNA, and make no protein, there is no way for the circulating erythrocytes to utilize the newly available iron. Thus the older cells, many of which will still remain in the bloodstream, will have an unchanged appearance after iron therapy. The erythrocytes newly released into the bloodstream had an adequate iron supply during their development and will consequently be normal. The result is that the peripheral blood smear shows a mixture of normal red cells and hypochromic, microcytic red cells.

12. **The correct answer is D.** This pattern of lesions is seen in scabies, a contagious skin disease characterized by intense itching. Scabies is caused by infestation with small, burrowing mites *(Sarcoptes scabiei).*

    Dermatitis herpetiformis (**choice A**) typically affects the scalp, shoulders, anterior surface of the knees, elbows, and the small of the back.

    Lichen planus (**choice B**) affects the mouth, anterior forearms, genitalia, the small of the back, and the posterior aspect of the leg below the knee.

    Photosensitivity (**choice C**) produces skin changes in the face and anterior neck except below the chin, the back of the neck, and the dorsum of the hands.

    Seborrheic rashes (**choice E**) affect the scalp, posterior surface of the head, neck, and shoulders, the perianal region, chin, groin, umbilicus, and sternum.

13. **The correct answer is E.** Syncope has a broad differential diagnosis, since fainting can be produced by a wide variety of mechanisms. All of the mechanisms listed in the answers can produce syncope, but only the Valsalva mechanism (in which high intra-abdominal pressures trigger a reflex fall in cardiac output) is specifically associated with defecation. This mechanism can also produce fainting during weight-lifting and with the use of wind instruments.

    Anoxic "seizures" (nonepileptic; **choice A**) are fainting spells that occur because a patient holds his/her breath while experiencing severe pain or intense emotion.

    Hyperventilation (**choice B**), typically related to anxiety, can also cause fainting.

    Patients who are hypovolemic (**choice C**) because of medical reasons (e.g., hemorrhage, acute sodium or water loss, burns, Addison disease) tend to be hypotensive and may faint.

    Patients with cardiac arrhythmias (**choice D**) are prone to fainting spells.

14. **The correct answer is A.** The child has the most common variant (type I) of osteogenesis imperfecta, which is an autosomal dominant genetic defect in the synthesis of type I collagen, due to decreased synthesis of the procollagen $alpha_1(1)$ amino acid chain. This defect (unlike that of the perinatal, lethal, type II form of osteogenesis imperfecta) is compatible with survival but does cause skeletal fragility, dentinogenesis imperfecta (abnormal teeth), blue sclera, joint laxity, and hearing impairment. Unfortunately, a number of children with this defect have been removed from their parents because of "abuse," only to have the broken bones continue in the new environment. Type I collagen is found in skin, bone, tendons, and most other organs.

    Type II collagen (**choice B**) is found in cartilage and vitreous humor.

    Type III collagen (**choice C**) is found in blood vessels, uterus, and skin.

    Type IV collagen (**choice D**) makes basement membranes.

    Type V collagen (**choice E**) is a minor component of interstitial tissues and blood vessels. There are also type VI-XI collagens, which are minor constituents of various tissues.

15. **The correct answer is B.** This question concerns a USMLE-favorite topic—pneumoconioses. Be sure to know the classic clues associated with each of the answer choices to this question. Asbestosis is a disease caused by a family of fibrous silicates commonly found in shipyards, insulation, and roofing industries. Many years after exposure, patients complain of dyspnea and chronic dry cough, along with recurrent respiratory infections (especially viral) and weight loss. A classic pathologic finding is lower lobe interstitial fibrosis with septal wall widening that is worse near the periphery of the lung. Chest x-ray film often reveals hyperinflation of the normal parenchyma leading to "honeycombing." Calcified parietal pleural plaques are also commonly present. Secondary bronchiectasis may complicate the picture.

    Anthracosis (**choice A**) is due to the inhalation of carbonaceous particles by city dwellers, cigarette smokers, and miners. Deposition of carbon dust can be seen as black pigment in lung parenchyma, pleura, and lymph nodes. When isolated, it is not associated with systemic disease.

    Berylliosis (**choice C**) is due to heavy exposure to airborne beryllium or its salts. Because of its high tensile strength and resistance to heat and fatigue, beryllium is used in the electronic, ceramic, aerospace, and nuclear energy industries. Disease due to beryllium probably represents a type IV hypersensitivity reaction, with noncaseating granuloma formation and eventual fibrosis. There is increased risk of bronchogenic carcinoma.

Byssinosis (**choice D**) is a type of hypersensitivity pneumonitis that can occur with exposure to cotton, linen, or hemp. It is associated with histamine-related bronchospasm.

Silicosis (**choice E**) occurs with prolonged exposure to silica dust (mining, glass production, sand blasting, farming, and road construction). This insidious disease can progress to respiratory failure and death and is associated with increased risk for tuberculosis. Classic x-ray findings include calcified lymph nodes that produce an "eggshell" pattern. The disease initially involves the upper lobes and perihilar region. Pleural involvement creates dense fibrous plaques and adhesions that may obliterate the pleural cavities. Uninvolved parenchyma tends to be hyperinflated and emphysematous.

16. **The correct answer is B.** This boy has nephrotic syndrome: edema, heavy proteinuria with a benign urinary sediment, hypoalbuminemia, and hypercholesterolemia. Of the choices listed, only minimal change nephropathy is a recognized cause of nephrotic syndrome. It is the most common cause of nephrotic syndrome in children.

None of the other choices are consistent with the clinical history; they are causes of nephritis, not nephrosis. Remember that nephritic patients present with hypertension, moderate proteinuria, hematuria, and an active urinary sediment with red blood cell casts.

17. **The correct answer is E.** In this item, the clinical information is really just "window dressing" for the actual question. All you are being asked is, "What is the most common type of cancer seen in the bladder?" The answer is that 90% of primary bladder cancers are transitional cell carcinomas, derived from bladder urothelium (a transitional cell epithelium). Let's take a moment to review the classic clues associated with bladder carcinoma: exposure to industrial chemicals, cigarette smoking, and infection with *Schistosoma haematobium* (predisposes to squamous cell type). Remember that a patient's occupation is usually stated for a reason.

All of the other answer choices are quite rare by comparison.

18. **The correct answer is B.** Pancreatic islet tumors, which may produce gastrin and secondarily Zollinger-Ellison syndrome, are a feature of multiple endocrine neoplasia type I (MEN I). Other features of MEN I are tumors of the parathyroid (the resulting hypercalcemia and hypercalciuria leads to kidney stones), adrenal *cortex*,

and pituitary gland. In general, the tumors in the MEN syndromes may be expressed at different times in a patient's life, and not all patients exhibit the full syndromes.

Endocrine tumors are not a feature of familial polyposis coli (**choice A**), which is instead characterized by colonic polyps and colon cancer.

MEN type IIA (**choice C**) features tumors of the adrenal *medulla* (pheochromocytoma), medullary carcinoma of the thyroid, and parathyroid hyperplasia or adenoma.

MEN type IIB (**choice D**) closely resembles type IIA but also includes mucosal neuromas, and less often includes parathyroid diseases.

MEN type III (**choice E**) is now considered to be the same as MEN type IIB.

19. **The correct answer is E.** Diethylstilbestrol, or DES, is an estrogen analog that was prescribed in the 1950s to 1970s for prevention of spontaneous abortion. The progeny of woman taking DES were often diagnosed with clear cell vaginal or cervical adenocarcinoma, which is rarely seen in unexposed women.

Bladder cancer (**choice A**) is often seen in individuals exposed to beta-naphthalene dyes or phenacetin.

Endometrial carcinoma (**choice B**) is seen in individuals on long-term estrogen therapy, but was not seen in the progeny of DES-treated women.

Ovarian carcinoma (**choice C**) is increased in nulliparous women and in those with a family history of the disorder.

Renal cell carcinoma (**choice D**) has been linked to such epidemiologic factors as smoking. The incidence is increased in patients with von Hippel-Lindau syndrome.

20. **The correct answer is C.** An infant who has not passed meconium for over 48 hours should be investigated for intestinal obstruction. Normal full-term infants will pass meconium by 36 hours, and most will do so within the first 24 hours. Hirschsprung disease is caused by absence of ganglion cells in the bowel wall, starting from the internal anal sphincter and extending proximally for a variable length of the bowel. It is the most common cause of lower intestinal obstruction in the newborn period and more commonly affects males. Diagnosis is based upon radiographic evidence and rectal suction biopsy, which demonstrates absence of ganglion cells.

Anal atresia (**choice A**) can also present similar to Hirschsprung disease in the newborn period but can be detected during the newborn examination when an ectopic or absence of anal opening can be detected.

Newborns with duodenal atresia (**choice B**) or pyloric stenosis (**choice E**) typically present with vomiting as the predominant symptom. Vomiting starts soon after birth in duodenal atresia, whereas patients with pyloric stenosis often present in the second or third week of life.

Meckel diverticulum (**choice D**), which occurs in 2 to 3% of all infants, can present with lower gastrointestinal tract bleeding or bowel obstruction due to intussusception. The symptoms, however, typically start in the first decade of life, and the disorder does not present at birth.

21. **The correct answer is C.** The most common esophageal cancer is squamous cell in origin (although the incidence of adenocarcinoma is rising). Recall that the esophageal mucosa consists of stratified, nonkeratinized, squamous epithelium. Smoking and alcohol increase the risk for the development of esophageal squamous cell carcinoma. Suspect cancer when there are signs like rapid weight loss in a short period of time and symptoms such as dysphagia, hematemesis, and anorexia.

Glandular epithelium (**choice A**) is associated with adenocarcinoma, which is often associated with Barrett's esophagus. This is not as common as squamous cell carcinoma, especially in smokers.

A mesenchymal tumor (**choice B**) is a sarcoma.

A teratoma can be derived from all three germ layers (**choice D**), e.g., a dermoid cyst in the ovary.

Transitional cell morphology (**choice E**) is found in the urinary system and not in the esophagus, unless a urinary tract tumor was metastatic to that location.

22. **The correct answer is B.** This is a two-step question. First, you need to make a diagnosis. In this case, the combination of viral illness plus aspirin followed by neurologic symptoms should have led you straight to the diagnosis of Reye syndrome. Next, what are the liver changes associated with this condition? The answer is that the liver will characteristically show microvesicular fatty changes. Note that the neurologic symptoms result from encephalopathy and that the brain will develop cerebral edema that may lead to herniation.

Diffuse fibrosis, with areas of regeneration (**choice A**), is characteristic of cirrhosis.

Hemosiderin deposits (**choice C**) would be seen in patients with hemochromatosis.

There is no hepatocyte necrosis (**choice D**) in Reye syndrome, although mitochondrial effects can be seen on electron microscopy.

Mallory bodies (**choice E**) can be seen in alcoholic hepatitis, Wilson disease, hepatocellular carcinoma, and primary biliary cirrhosis. They are not seen in Reye syndrome.

23. **The correct answer is B.** This patient presents with five of the six clinical criteria associated with Kawasaki disease: fever, conjunctivitis, oral involvement, rash, and cervical lymphadenopathy. Edema, erythema, or desquamation of the hands and feet is the sixth sign. (Fulfillment of at least five criteria is necessary to make the diagnosis.) The disease usually occurs in children younger than 4 years, but has been reported in patients up to 34 years of age. Multiple members of the same household might be affected. The syndrome was first described in Japan and is still more common there. The etiology is still unknown, but a viral or immunologic basis for the disease is suggested suspected. The disease involves inflammation and necrosis of the blood vessel wall and possible aneurysm formation. The most hazardous potential complication is the development of coronary aneurysm, thrombosis, or rupture.

Henoch-Schönlein purpura (**choice A**) is a hypersensitivity angiitis that occurs in children. It is characterized by nonthrombocytopenic purpura, skin lesions, joint involvement, colicky abdominal pain, and renal lesions. A classic clue to the diagnosis is the appearance of lesions on the extensor surfaces of the limbs and across the buttocks.

Polyarteritis nodosa (**choice C**) is a systemic necrotizing vasculitis. Though the disease is most common in young adults (which may have led you to choose this answer), patients present with low-grade fever, weakness, and weight loss. They may also have abdominal pain, hematuria, renal failure, hypertension, and leukocytosis.

Rheumatic fever (**choice D**) is a recurrent inflammatory disease that typically follows streptococcal pharyngitis. Onset is typically 1 to 3 weeks after infection. The major Jones criteria are migratory polyarthritis, erythema marginatum, Sydenham chorea, subcutaneous nodules, and carditis. The minor criteria are previous rheumatic fever, elevated temperature, arthralgias, prolonged PR interval, elevated erythrocyte sedimentation rate (ESR), leukocytosis, and elevated C-reactive protein. These are very testable concepts (not only on the USMLE but also during your pediatrics rotation), so memorize them.

Takayasu arteritis (**choice E**) is a granulomatous inflammation of medium-to-large arteries, often branches of the aortic arch. Although it commonly affects Asian women between the ages of 15 and 45 (which might have led you to choose this answer), its clinical presentation includes ocular disturbances, neurologic abnormalities, and weak pulses in the upper extremities. Weakness, fever, malaise, and arthralgias may also occur.

24. **The correct answer is A.** Choriocarcinomas are most common in men aged 15 to 25 years. These tumors are highly malignant and are associated with gynecomastia or testicular enlargement. Laboratory studies typically show elevated serum and urine human chorionic gonadotropin (hCG) levels.

Sertoli cell (**choice B**) tumors can produce small amounts of androgens or estrogens, but usually not enough to cause endocrinologic changes. They may present with testicular enlargement. Microscopic exam reveals uniform, tall, polyhedral cells with clear cytoplasm, growing in cords resembling spermatic tubules.

Teratomas (**choice C**) can occur at any age but are most common in infants and children. This type of tumor appears as a testicular mass. Microscopically, it may show differentiation into any of the three germ layers: endoderm, mesoderm, or ectoderm.

Yolk sac tumors (**choice D**) are most common in infants and children; they are rare in adults. They can also coincide with embryonal carcinomas. Serum AFP is elevated.

25. **The correct answer is C.** This case depicts the classic picture of cardiogenic shock, which typically occurs after ischemic myocardial injury, acute valve dysfunction associated with endocarditis, blunt chest trauma, acute myocarditis, or end-stage cardiomyopathy. Left ventricular function is compromised; therefore, *cardiac output* is diminished. *Preload* is increased because blood from the right side of the heart and pulmonary circulation is pumped into an already filled left ventricle (this explains the S3 and S4 sounds that presented as a midsystolic gallop). *Pulmonary artery wedge pressure*, measured with a Swan-Ganz catheter, reveals left atrial pressure as well as left ventricular end-diastolic pressure and is elevated in heart failure. Left ventricular failure causes increased left atrial pressure, which results in increased hydrostatic pressure in the pulmonary vasculature. Once hydrostatic pressure is higher than oncotic pressure, fluid from the circulation leaks into the alveolar spaces, causing pulmonary edema and dyspnea. Eventually, the right ventricle can no longer pump blood against the increased pulmonary pressure and fails. This causes a backup of blood, which results in increased *central venous pressure*. *Systemic vascular resistance* is increased in an attempt to compensate for the diminished cardiac output. *Mixed venous oxygen levels* are reduced because of increased tissue demand for oxygen.

26. **The correct answer is D.** Although rare now because of advances in treatment, syphilitic aortitis and aneurysm are still seen, especially in underserved populations. This complication generally occurs 10 to 40 years after initial infection. The vasa vasorum of the aorta undergoes obliterative endarteritis, leading to atrophy of the muscularis and elastic tissues of the aorta and dilatation. Linear calcifications are often seen in the ascending aorta by x-ray. The intimal wrinkling or "tree barking" is also a common feature. Syphilitic aneurysm can be associated with respiratory distress, cough, congestive heart failure, and, rarely, rupture.

Atherosclerosis (**choice A**) is the most common cause of aortic aneurysms. These are most often located in the abdominal aorta, distal to the renal arteries. Intimal wrinkling and linear calcifications are not seen.

Hypertension (**choice B**) is usually responsible for dissecting aneurysms located within 10 cm of the aortic valve. Patients present with sudden chest pain that is usually severe and tearing in nature. The chronic hypertension causes a cystic medial necrosis, allowing the separation of vessel layers.

Marfan syndrome, an autosomal dominant connective tissue disorder (**choice C**), is also associated with dissecting aneurysms, usually of the ascending aorta. The patients are often very tall with arachnodactyly and ligamentous laxity. Their life-span is generally shortened. This patient's description and age are not consistent with this diagnosis.

Takayasu arteritis (**choice E**) is a syndrome characterized by ocular disturbances and weak pulses in the arms. It occurs most frequently in young females. It is considered a giant cell arteritis and does not cause aneurysms.

27. **The correct answer is A.** Typically, cancers are precipitated by a number of "hits" or mutation/deletion events that endow the transformed cell with a survival and/or growth advantage such that it is no longer restricted by the normal cellular checks and balances. The mutation events commonly include *1*) loss of function of both copies of a tumor suppressor gene; *2*) mutation of a proto-oncogene; or *3*) fusion of a proto-oncogene with a strong promoter/enhancer. p53 is a tumor suppressor gene that, when mutated or deleted, seems to play a role in many different types of cancers. If an individual inherits a mutated allele of a tumor suppressor, the chance of acquiring a second mutation in the other allele is extremely high. This second mutation "knocks-out" the normal tumor suppressor function, giving the cell a growth/survival advantage that can lead to the cancer phenotype. Members of families

that are strongly predisposed to many different types of cancer may have an inherited mutant allele of p53, referred to as Li-Fraumeni syndrome. Note that although the cells of the tumor may have lost both copies of the tumor suppressor gene, analysis of the blood sample would reveal only the one mutant or deleted allele in other cells.

In a normal blood sample, one would not find deletions in both alleles (**choice B**) of p53. Loss of both copies of p53 is not compatible with normal cellular function.

Normally, being diploid, individuals have two wild-type copies of each allele (**choice C**).

Amplification of certain proto-oncogenes (e.g., *neu* in breast cancers or N-*myc* in neuroblastomas) is associated with a poor prognosis, but an extra copy of a tumor suppressor gene (**choice D**) would probably not contribute to the early development of cancer.

Some cancers are precipitated by the fusion of a proto-oncogene with a second gene or with a new promoter/enhancer region, leading to the unregulated overexpression of the proto-oncogene (e.g., the Philadelphia chromosome in chronic myelogenous leukemia [CML]). In contrast to **choice E**, mutations in tumor suppressor genes that produce cancer are generally "loss of function" mutations resulting from deletions, frameshift mutations, or nonsense mutations.

28. **The correct answer is G.** Many different types of structures and cells, normal and pathologic, can be found in bronchial and alveolar cavities. These can be observed in bronchial washings obtained by bronchoalveolar lavage—a procedure in which buffered saline is injected into a peripheral bronchus and then reaspirated. Hemosiderin-laden macrophages, or *heart failure cells*, indicate prior episodes of pulmonary edema or intra-alveolar hemorrhage of any cause (e.g., Goodpasture syndrome).

Anthracotic macrophages (**choice A**) contain black cytoplasmic carbon particles, phagocytosed from polluted air or cigarette smoke.

Charcot-Leyden crystals (**choice B**) are rhomboid structures derived from enzymes present within eosinophils. They are commonly found in patients with allergic conditions (asthma).

Curschmann spirals (**choice C**) are corkscrew-shaped casts resulting from mucus plugs present in smaller bronchi and commonly found in association with chronic obstructive disease.

Fat-laden macrophages (**choice D**) have been observed in cases of lipid pneumonia.

Ferruginous bodies (**choice E**) are needle-shaped structures surrounded by an iron-protein coat. Ferruginous bodies are also known as *asbestos bodies*, since asbestos is the most common (although not the sole) source of these structures.

Goblet cells (**choice F**) constitute a normal finding in bronchial washings and result from exfoliation of mucus-secreting cells of the bronchial epithelium.

Squamous pearls (**choice H**) are concentrically arranged layers of keratinized squamous cells dislodged from the bronchial epithelium by the procedure itself.

29. **The correct answer is C.** Whenever the Step 1 exam specifies a patient's ethnic background, there is a good chance that it provides an important clue to the question. The patient described is an African American woman with symptoms and history suggestive of sickle cell anemia. The woman is experiencing the most frequent type of vaso-occlusive crisis seen in patients with this disease (infarctive). Crises may be precipitated by dehydration or infection. Hb electrophoresis is used to diagnose the illness, which is caused by an amino acid substitution of valine for glutamate in position 6 of the beta Hb chain. The resulting abnormal hemoglobin (HbS) tends to polymerize during low oxygen states, causing the red blood cells to assume a sickle shape.

Absence of central pallor (**choice A**) may be observed in patients with hereditary spherocytosis (usually autosomal dominant) resulting from abnormal red cell membrane proteins (e.g., spectrin, ankyrin). Spherocytes will exhibit increased osmotic fragility because they have decreased surface area per unit volume.

Deletion of all four alpha genes (**choice B**) occurs in the most severe form of alpha thalassemia and is incompatible with life. It can result in hydrops fetalis and intrauterine death.

Heinz bodies (**choice D**) are clumps of Hb-degradation products seen when RBCs are stained with methylene blue. They are found in the peripheral blood smears of people with G6PD deficiency, especially common in males of Mediterranean or West African descent. Hemolysis occurs in response to oxidant stress that may be caused by drugs (e.g., antimalarials, sulfonamides, or nitrofurantoin) or the ingestion of fava beans.

30. **The correct answer is B.** There are many clues in the question that should have guided you to this choice. The laboratory findings are classic for type IIa hyperlipidemia. These patients have LDL receptor deficiencies and are at a great risk of advanced coronary atherosclerosis. Since it is autosomal dominant, the patient's father could have been affected as well.

Type I hyperlipidemia (**choice A**), or familial hyperchylomicronemia, is caused by a lipoprotein lipase deficiency. These patients have high serum triglycerides and normal cholesterol. They do not have a substantially higher risk of atherosclerosis.

Type IIb hyperlipidemia (**choice C**), or familial combined hyperlipidemia, presents as elevated serum LDL, VLDL, cholesterol, and triglycerides. These patients have an increased incidence of atherosclerosis.

Type III hyperlipidemia (**choice D**), or familial dysbetalipoproteinemia, presents as increased serum cholesterol and triglycerides. The mode of inheritance is not understood, but apoprotein E is affected and the risk of atherosclerosis is great.

Type IV hyperlipidemia (**choice E**), or familial hypertriglyceridemia, presents as increased triglycerides with normal cholesterol and LDL. The disease may be sporadic and is possibly associated with an increased risk for atherosclerosis.

Type V hyperlipidemia (**choice F**), or mixed hypertriglyceridemia, is not common. Cholesterol is slightly increased, and triglycerides are greatly increased. There is deficient apoprotein CII. The risk of atherosclerosis is not clear.

31. **The correct answer is D.** The cellular edema observed during reversible cell injury is usually due to decreased ATP levels. In the presence of lower ATP levels, there is less activity of the $Na^+/K^+$ ATPase on the plasmalemma. This, in turn, leads to a shift of $Na^+$ into the cell and $K^+$ out of it. The pump does not normally transport the same amount of $Na^+$ out of and $K^+$ into the cell, so when the pump fails there is a net flow of solute in the form of $Na^+$ into the cell. When this solute adds to the higher intracellular osmotic pressure relative to the extracellular osmotic pressure (due to all of the proteins and small molecules trapped in the cell), water flows into the cell to "dilute" its constituents.

$Ca^{2+}$ (**choice A**) and $Mg^{2+}$ (**choice C**) do not play a direct role in cellular edema.

Both the $Na^+/K^+$ ATPase activity (**choice E**) and intracellular $K^+$ (**choice B**) are usually decreased during cellular edema.

32. **The correct answer is C.** The vignette illustrates a typical presentation for a tumor of the heart. Primary cardiac tumors are rare and usually require a intensive work up to pinpoint the diagnosis. Seventy-five percent of primary cardiac tumors are benign; among these, myxoma is the most common. The tumors are usually single, and the most common location is the left atrium. They may cause syncopal episodes or even shock and death due to obstruction by a "ball valve" mechanism.

Angiosarcoma (**choice A**) is a malignant tumor of vascular origin that can occur as a primary cardiac tumor. It is the most common malignant primary cardiac tumor, but it is still very rare. Angiosarcoma usually affects the right side of the heart.

Mesothelioma (**choice B**) is a benign tumor of mesothelial origin that can rarely present as a primary cardiac tumor. It is usually a small intramyocardial tumor that presents with disturbances of the conduction system of the heart.

Rhabdomyoma (**choice D**) is a benign tumor of muscle origin. It can occur as a primary cardiac tumor, typically in infants and children, in whom it may be associated with tuberous sclerosis. It usually occurs in the ventricles.

Rhabdomyosarcoma (**choice E**) is a malignant neoplasm that can also occur as a rare primary cardiac tumor. It is of muscle origin and usually affects the right heart.

33. **The correct answer is B.** This patient has pulmonary fibrosis, which markedly decreases the compliance of the lung, thereby producing a small lung that is difficult to inflate (restrictive lung disease).

The airway resistance (**choice A**) would not be expected to change.

The functional residual capacity (FRC; **choice C**) would be expected to decrease, rather than increase.

The lung volume (**choice D**) is generally smaller than normal in patients with this disorder.

The tidal volume (**choice E**) would be expected to decrease, rather than increase.

34. **The correct answer is C.** Neonatal respiratory distress syndrome (hyaline membrane disease) occurs in premature infants as the result of a deficiency in pulmonary surfactant (composed primarily of dipalmitoyl lecithin). This is due to inadequate lecithin synthesis by immature type II pneumocytes. It can be diagnosed before birth by analyzing the amniotic fluid: a lecithin:sphingomyelin ratio greater than 2:1 and the presence of phosphatidylglycerol implies lung maturity. The syndrome is the most common cause of death in premature neonates. Risk factors include birth before the 37th week of gestation, birth by cesarean section, and maternal diabetes.

Less than 0.5 L of amniotic fluid (**choice A**) is the definition of oligohydramnios, which can be associated with renal agenesis. (Failure of the fetal kidneys to produce urine will result in a low amniotic fluid volume.)

Alpha-1 antitrypsin deficiency in amniotic fluid (**choice B**) is not associated with lung immaturity.

However, deficiency of this enzyme is associated with both emphysema and liver failure in adults.

Elevated maternal $HbA_{1c}$ (**choice D**) would indicate poor glycemic control in the mother and a potentially increased risk for fetal abnormalities, but it does not serve as direct evidence of lung immaturity.

Elevated maternal serum alpha-fetoprotein (AFP; **choice E**) would be expected in fetal neural tube defects. A low maternal AFP is associated with fetal Down syndrome.

35. **The correct answer is C.** Cheyne-Stokes breathing is characterized by the pattern described in the question stem, and is considered an ominous prognostic sign when observed in a seriously ill patient. This form of respiratory dysfunction suggests that central respiratory mechanisms are no longer functioning adequately.

Apneustic breathing (**choice A**) is seen after head trauma and is characterized by inspiratory breath-holding that lasts many seconds, followed by brief exhalations.

Biot's breathing (**choice B**) is seen in some patients with CNS disease (e.g., meningitis). It consists of periods of normal breathing interrupted suddenly by periods of apnea.

Hysterical breathing (**choice D**) may produce hyperventilation, i.e., rapid, intense breathing that causes the $Paco_2$ to decrease.

Kussmaul breathing (**choice E**) occurs in diabetic coma and consists of continuous, rapid, deep breathing.

36. **The correct answer is C.** The ductus arteriosus connects the aorta with the pulmonary artery. If it remains patent after birth, it allows oxygenated blood to flow from the aorta to the pulmonary artery. In this patient, who has tetralogy of Fallot with complete right ventricular outflow obstruction, this anastomosis is a crucial source of blood to the pulmonary vasculature.

A bicuspid aortic valve (**choice A**) may be asymptomatic but can lead to infective endocarditis, left ventricular overload, and sudden death. It is a common cause of aortic stenosis. It would not benefit a patient with tetralogy of Fallot in any way.

Ostium secundum defect (**choice B**) is the most common form of atrial septal defect (ASD). ASD is an acyanotic congenital heart disease that would not improve cardiovascular function in a patient with tetralogy of Fallot.

A patent foramen ovale (**choice D**) is a slit-like remnant of communication between the left and right atria in the fetus. It is usually not of clinical significance.

A preductal coarctation of the aorta (**choice E**) involves narrowing of the aorta proximal to the opening of the ductus arteriosus. This would prevent adequate blood flow through a possible life-preserving patent ductus arteriosus and would result in the patient's death.

37. **The correct answer is E.** This patient is experiencing symptoms of hypocalcemia secondary to diminished parathyroid hormone (PTH) secretion. This must always be considered in a patient who undergoes total or subtotal thyroidectomy, because the parathyroids are nestled in the tissue surrounding the thyroid gland. Surgical attempts to leave portions of the parathyroids intact are sometimes unsuccessful. Other causes of decreased PTH include neck irradiation, autoimmune phenomena (polyglandular autoimmune syndromes), dysembryogenesis (as in DiGeorge syndrome), and heavy metal damage (Wilson disease, hemosiderosis, hemochromatosis).

Bone metastases (**choice A**) would cause hypercalcemia, as a result of osteolysis.

Hashimoto thyroiditis (**choice B**) is the most common cause of hypothyroidism and results in decreased thyroid hormone and elevated thyroid-stimulating hormone (TSH) levels. Serum calcium and PTH should be normal.

Hypervitaminosis D (**choice C**) would cause hypercalcemia.

Hypomagnesemia (**choice D**) may cause a functional hypoparathyroidism, because magnesium is needed for PTH activity in tissue. In such a case, however, actual PTH levels would not be decreased. Severe hypomagnesemia (levels below 0.4 mmol/L [1 mg/dl] blocks release of PTH, but mild hypomagnesemia can actually enhance PTH release.

38. **The correct answer is E.** Systemic lupus erythematosus (SLE) predominantly affects younger women, and so the question of lupus and pregnancy may arise frequently in clinical practice. Patients with SLE have an increased incidence of spontaneous abortion, fetal death *in utero*, and prematurity. The mother may experience an exacerbation in the activity of her disease in the third trimester or peripartum period, and it may be difficult to distinguish between active SLE and preeclampsia. Therapy of pregnant patients with SLE is problematic, and the generalist should consult the literature or a specialist when such a patient is encountered.

Congenital malformations (**choices B, C, and D**) are not a complication of pregnancies in patients with SLE.

39. **The correct answer is E.** Factor XII is unusual among coagulation factors in that its deficiency is associated

with thrombosis rather than hemorrhage. The mechanism appears to be a deficient activation of fibrinolysis, and both thrombophlebitis and myocardial infarction have occurred in severely affected patients. The condition is inherited in an autosomal recessive manner. Many patients with mild-to-moderate factor XII deficiency are never detected; others are identified when a routine preoperative clotting screen demonstrates a greatly prolonged partial thromboplastin time.

Deficiency of each of the other factors (**choices A, B, C, and D**) is associated with hemorrhage.

40. **The correct answer is D.** Secondary hyperthyroidism presents in a similar clinical fashion to primary hyperthyroidism. However, secondary hyperthyroidism is the result of a pituitary hyperfunction resulting in an excess production of thyroid-stimulating hormone (TSH) and a secondary elevation of thyroid hormones T4 and T3. Some of the symptoms of hyperthyroidism include nervousness, anxiety, heat intolerance, increased sweating, tachycardia, amenorrhea, and infertility.

Decreased thyroxine-binding globulin (TBG; **choice A**) is not by itself diagnostic.

Elevated T3 (**choice B**) and T4 (**choice C**) are found in both secondary and primary hyperthyroidism.

The presence of serum thyroid-stimulating autoantibodies (**choice E**) is diagnostic of Graves disease, a cause of primary hyperthyroidism.

41. **The correct answer is C.** Hemoglobinuria means that there is hemoglobin in the urine and suggests hemolysis in a patient with symptoms of anemia. The patient's reticulocytosis further supports this suspicion. Reticulocytosis refers to an increase in the number of circulating reticulocytes. Reticulocytes are immature red blood cells that typically constitute approximately 1% of circulating red blood cells. The reticulocyte count is used to differentiate between anemias due to decreased erythropoiesis (low reticulocyte count since marrow can't produce reticulocytes) and anemias secondary to blood loss or peripheral red blood cell destruction (hemolysis; reticulocyte count elevates as marrow tries to compensate).

Of the choices listed, only G6PD deficiency leads to hemolysis. (In the absence of G6PD, there is a deficiency of NADPH and, therefore, a deficiency of reduced glutathione. This causes oxidative stress on the erythrocyte that leads to hemolysis.) Other causes of hemolytic anemia include hereditary spherocytosis, sickle cell disease, thalassemias, autoimmune hemolytic anemia, red blood cell trauma, and paroxysmal nocturnal hemoglobinuria.

All the distracters would lead to anemia secondary to decreased erythropoiesis and would therefore be associated with low reticulocyte counts.

Chronic renal disease (**choice A**) results in decreased production of the hormone erythropoietin, leading to decreased reticulocyte (and therefore erythrocyte) production.

Folate deficiency (**choice B**) results in decreased red blood cell production and a megaloblastic anemia characterized by macrocytic red blood cells and hypersegmented neutrophils.

Iron deficiency (**choice D**) results in a microcytic, hypochromic anemia. An elevated reticulocyte count after administration of ferrous sulfate would indicate improvement of the anemia with therapy.

Pernicious anemia (**choice E**) refers to vitamin $B_{12}$ malabsorption secondary to antibodies against intrinsic factor or intrinsic factor receptors. $B_{12}$ deficiency leads to megaloblastic anemia.

42. **The correct answer is E.** Sézary syndrome is a rare chronic disease associated with progressive, pruritic erythroderma, exfoliation, and lymphadenopathy. It is related to the cutaneous T-cell lymphoma mycosis fungoides, and may be a leukemic variant of this condition.

Burkitt lymphoma (**choice A**) is endemic in Africa and sporadic in the U.S. It usually affects children or young adults. In Africa, it often arises in the mandible or maxilla. In the U.S., it often arises in the abdomen. It is related to EBV infection, which may act as a mitogen, initiating a sustained polyclonal activation of B cells. This eventually leads to a neoplastic proliferation of a single B-cell clone after a chromosomal translocation occurs. Microscopic examination reveals a uniform sea of moderately large cells with round nuclei, multiple nucleoli, moderately basophilic cytoplasm with lipid-containing vacuoles, frequent mitoses, and many macrophages with ingested debris ("starry sky pattern").

Histiocytic lymphoma (**choice B**) is one of the most common non-Hodgkin lymphomas. It is usually diffuse but may be nodular. The diffuse form typically presents with nodal involvement (usually on one side of the diaphragm), extranodal involvement (gastrointestinal tract, skin, brain, bone), or, rarely, liver and spleen involvement. Microscopic examination shows large tumor cells with vesicular nuclei and prominent nucleoli. The cells may be pleomorphic.

Lymphoblastic lymphoma (**choice C**) is a diffuse lymphoma that is most common in adolescents and young adults, but there is a bimodal age distribution with a second peak in the 70s. The male:female ratio is 2.5:1.

The disease is often associated with a mediastinal mass (thymoma), suggesting thymic origin for the neoplastic cells. These cells often express T-cell markers and resemble the lymphoblasts of ALL. They have uniform size, scant cytoplasm, delicate chromatin, and absent nucleoli. The nuclear membrane may be loculated or convoluted. There are frequent mitoses.

Lymphocytic lymphoma (**choice D**) occurs in two forms: well differentiated (WDLL) and poorly differentiated (PDLL). WDLL usually affects older patients, who present with generalized lymphadenopathy and mild hepatosplenomegaly. Microscopic examination reveals small round lymphocytes with scant cytoplasm, dark nuclei, and rare mitoses. PDLL patients are usually middle-aged or older. Most present with lymphadenopathy and with infiltration of bone marrow, liver, and spleen at the time of diagnosis. Microscopic examination reveals atypical lymphocytes, often larger than in WDLL. Nuclei are irregular, angular, and indented, and have coarse chromatin. Mitoses are rare.

43. **The correct answer is B.** This patient has irreversible parkinsonism induced by a contaminant of illicit drugs—methylphenyltetrahydropyridine (MPTP), a meperidine analog. The parkinsonism is caused by the drug's destruction of dopaminergic neurons in the substantia nigra. The clinical signs and symptoms described in the question are classically associated with parkinsonism. Lewy bodies are neuronal inclusions that are characteristic of Parkinson disease. The latest research suggests that structures resembling immature Lewy bodies appear in MPTP-induced parkinsonism.

Hirano bodies (**choice A**) are intraneuronal, eosinophilic rod-like inclusions in the hippocampus that are associated with Alzheimer disease. They may occur in normal elderly brains as well.

Lipofuscin granules (**choice C**) are pigmented cytoplasmic inclusions that commonly accumulate with aging. They are believed to be residual bodies derived from lysosomes.

Negri bodies (**choice D**) are intracytoplasmic inclusions that are pathognomonic for rabies. They are found in the pyramidal cells of the hippocampus, the brainstem, and the Purkinje cells of the cerebellum.

Neurofibrillary tangles (**choice E**) consist of intracytoplasmic degenerated neurofilaments and are seen in patients with Alzheimer disease. Amyloid plaques are also commonly seen in these patients.

44. **The correct answer is A.** The patient has myasthenia gravis (MG), which typically produces weakness worsening over the course of the day. It often affects the eye muscles and can produce diplopia. Neostigmine, an acetylcholinesterase inhibitor, would temporarily improve the patient's condition, which is associated with antibodies against nicotinic acetylcholine receptors present on skeletal muscle.

Antibodies to double-stranded DNA (**choice B**), as well as anti-Smith antibodies, are found specifically in systemic lupus erythematosus. Peripheral nuclear staining is observed on immunofluorescence.

Antibodies to dystrophin (**choice C**) do not produce recognized pathology. Abnormal or absent dystrophin, resulting from mutations in the X chromosome, is associated with Becker and Duchenne muscular dystrophy, respectively. Pelvic girdle weakness and ataxia are classic symptoms.

Antibodies to erythrocyte surface antigens (**choice D**) can be found in warm antibody autoimmune hemolytic anemia. Patients with this condition would have a positive direct Coombs test.

Antibodies to myelin (**choice E**) may play a role in multiple sclerosis, which is presumed to be of autoimmune etiology. This demyelinating disease is characterized by the spontaneous appearance and remission of symptoms such as hyperreflexia, weakness, spasticity, dysarthria, tremor, ataxia, and visual disturbances. Neostigmine would not produce any improvement.

45. **The correct answer is C.** Ten to twenty percent of patients with Crohn disease and ulcerative colitis develop an arthritis that resembles ankylosing spondylitis. Similar arthropathies are seen in psoriasis or Reiter syndrome (arthritis, urethritis, conjunctivitis, and rash following chlamydial infection), as well as related syndromes seen following *Shigella, Salmonella,* or *Yersinia* enterocolitis. The other answers are distracters.

46. **The correct answer is D.** This child has minimal change disease, which is the major cause (more than 90% of cases) of nephrotic syndrome in children aged 2 to 6 years. The most prominent clinical chemistry finding in these patients is massive proteinuria. The urinary protein in minimal change disease, in contrast to other causes of nephrotic syndrome, is often composed predominantly of albumin. Many other clinical chemistry changes may also be seen, including decreased serum albumin levels, hyperlipidemia, increased serum levels of alpha$_2$- and beta-globulins, decreased IgG, and increased fibrinogen. Minimal change disease characteristically shows normal or near normal appearance of the glomeruli by light microscopy and extensive fusion of foot processes of the glomerular podocytes by electron microscopy. A point not always recognized by beginners is that the podocyte alterations may represent a reaction to, rather than a cause of, the proteinuria (e.g., an

attempt to "seal the holes" in the glomerulus), since varying degrees of foot process fusion (together with more specific features) may sometimes be seen in other glomerular diseases associated with the nephrotic syndrome.

Alpha$_2$-globulin levels (**choice A**) are increased, rather than decreased, in minimal change disease.

Fibrinogen levels are increased, rather than decreased (**choice B**).

Serum calcium levels (**choice C**) are typically decreased in the nephrotic syndrome, possibly because of renal loss of vitamin D binding protein.

Red blood cell casts in the urine (**choice E**) are indicative of glomerulonephritis, rather than the nephrotic syndrome.

47. **The correct answer is B.** The lateral striate arteries are penetrating branches of the middle cerebral artery that supply the caudate, putamen, globus pallidus, and internal capsule. Lacunar infarcts, small cavitary lesions that commonly occur in the distribution of the lateral striate and lenticulostriate arteries, are relatively common in the context of long-standing hypertension. The basal ganglia and thalamus are favorite sites for lacunar infarcts.

The anterior cerebral artery (**choice A**) supplies the medial surface of the cerebral hemispheres extending from the frontal pole to the parieto-occipital sulcus. It therefore supplies the leg and foot area of the motor and sensory cortices.

The posterior cerebral artery (**choice C**) supplies the occipital lobe, which contains the visual cortex. Occlusion of this vessel results in contralateral hemianopia with macular sparing. This vessel also supplies the inferior surface of the temporal lobe (which contains the hippocampal formation) and the thalamus, and provides the major blood supply to the midbrain.

The superior cerebellar artery (**choice D**) supplies the superior cerebellar peduncle, the superior surface of the cerebellum, and the deep cerebellar nuclei. It also supplies the dorsolateral tegmentum of the rostral pons.

The vertebral artery (**choice E**), a branch of the subclavian artery, gives rise to the posterior inferior cerebellar artery (PICA) and the anterior spinal artery. PICA supplies the dorsolateral quadrant of the medulla and the inferior surface of the cerebellum. The anterior spinal artery supplies the anterior two thirds of the spinal cord.

48. **The correct answer is C.** Hereditary spherocytosis is due to an intrinsic abnormality in the membrane support structure of the red cell. A distinctive feature of this disorder is marked susceptibility of the red cells to lysis in hypotonic solutions. This feature is the basis of the osmotic fragility test, which is quite specific for spherocytosis.

Neither thalassemias (**choices A and B**) nor sickle cell disease (**choices D and E**) are characterized by a positive osmotic fragility test.

49. **The correct answer is D.** This patient has paroxysmal supraventricular tachycardia (PSVT), which is a regular, rapid (150-250/min) arrhythmia originating in the atria or AV node. AV nodal re-entry is the most common cause of this arrhythmia (about 70% of patients). In this condition, the AV node is pathologically divided into two functional pathways. The electrical impulse usually proceeds anterograde down the slow pathway and retrograde up the fast pathway. The P waves are recorded nearly simultaneously with the QRS complexes (which occur in rapid sequence) and are therefore obscured on EKG. This arrhythmia is commonly seen in older patients, about half of whom have underlying heart disease. Re-entry PSVTs can be reverted to normal sinus rhythm by interrupting the re-entry pathway. For example, the performance of vagal maneuvers often improves the condition by increasing AV nodal refractoriness.

Atrial re-entry (**choice A**) causes about 10% of all PSVTs. The re-entrant pathway is in the atria. The P wave is recorded before the QRS complex. This arrhythmia is frequently associated with organic heart disease.

Automatic atrial conduction (**choice B**) results in about 5% of PSVTs. Often, these are not paroxysmal, last days to years, and are resistant to treatment. The P wave has an abnormal configuration.

AV dissociation (**choice C**) is caused by accelerated junctional rhythms, in which a normally latent pacemaker in the AV nodal area depolarizes at a regular, accelerated rate of 60 to 150/min. When the rate of the accelerated pacemaker approaches the rate of the SA node, the ectopic impulses are often conducted to the ventricles only, while the atria remain under the control of the SA node, producing AV dissociation.

Wandering atrial pacemaker (**choice E**) is a usually benign arrhythmia. The dominant pacemaker "wanders" from one atrial focus to another and in and out of the SA node.

Test-taking strategy: If you are unsure of an answer to a question, have tried to reason through the problem to no avail, and believe you must randomly guess, choose the "most common" item from among the given answer choices. Remember, the USMLE tends to test common concepts, so the odds should be in your favor.

50. **The correct answer is A.** The figure shown depicts a lymphocyte. Lymphocytosis is commonly associated with viral infections; therefore, you should have looked for a viral disease in the answer choices. Bronchiolitis in a 2-year-old is most likely caused by respiratory syncytial virus. The rest of the diseases listed have bacterial etiologies.

Cellulitis (**choice B**) is a bacterial infection usually attributed to *Staphylococcus* or *Streptococcus*.

Diphtheria (**choice C**) is due to *Corynebacterium diphtheriae*.

Epiglottitis (choice D) in a 2-year-old is most likely due to *Haemophilus influenzae*.

Pertussis (choice E) is caused by *Bordetella pertussis*.

# Pathology and Pathophysiology: **Test Three**

1. A patient presents to his physician because of a chronic cough. He notes occasional streaks of blood in his sputum. A chest x-ray film reveals multi-nodular, cavitating lesions in the apical posterior segments of both lungs, with evident satellite lesions. The condition described is likely to occur in the apices of the lungs, rather than in the base, because the apices

   (A) are better perfused
   (B) are more acidic
   (C) contain more alveolar macrophages
   (D) have a higher $P_{O_2}$
   (E) ventilate better

2. A 50-year-old man presents to his physician with diarrhea, flushing, and wheezing. Physical examination is significant for a grade II/VI diastolic murmur located at the right sternal border at the fourth intercostal space. Which of the following substances is most likely to be elevated in this patient's urine?

   (A) 5-Hydroxyindoleacetic acid (5-HIAA)
   (B) Homovanillic acid (HVA)
   (C) Phenylalanine
   (D) Selegiline
   (E) Vanillylmandelic acid (VMA)

3. Many patients with cirrhosis, particularly alcoholic cirrhosis, develop gynecomastia, testicular atrophy, and impotence. Which of the following is thought to be the underlying mechanism producing these changes?

   (A) Both decreased testosterone secretion and decreased extraction of androstenedione
   (B) Decreased hepatic extraction of androstenedione
   (C) Increased estrogen secretion by Leydig cells
   (D) Increased estrogen secretion by Sertoli cells
   (E) Testosterone deficiency alone

4. A 29-year-old woman comes to her physician's office complaining of headaches, fatigue, and weakness over the past several months. Physical examination is significant for pallor, tachycardia, dizziness on standing up, and koilonychia (spooning of the nails).

   Laboratory studies show:

   | | |
   |---|---|
   | Hemoglobin | 10.2 g/dL |
   | Hematocrit | 30.8% |
   | Serum iron | 24 mg/dL |
   | Serum ferritin | 30 ng/mL |
   | Total iron binding capacity | 713 mg/dL |

   A peripheral blood smear would likely show which of the following?

   (A) Macrocytosis with hypersegmented neutrophils
   (B) Microcytosis with basophilic stippling
   (C) Microcytosis with hypochromia
   (D) Numerous schistocytes

5. A 27-year-old African American man visits his primary care physician because of recent onset of "yellowness in the whites of his eyes." His recent history is significant for a "chest cold," for which he is taking trimethoprim-sulfamethoxazole; he is also taking fluoxetine for depression. On examination, the sclera are icteric and the mucosa beneath the tongue appears yellow. No hepatosplenomegaly is present.

Laboratory studies are as follows:

| | |
|---|---|
| Hemoglobin | 11.1 g/dL |
| Hematocrit | 34% |
| Total bilirubin | 6.2 mg/dL |
| Conjugated (direct) bilirubin | 0.8 mg/dL |
| Alkaline phosphatase | 77 U/L |
| AST (SGOT) | 24 U/L |
| ALT (SGPT) | 22 U/L |

The most likely cause of this patient's jaundice is which of the following?

(A) Acute infectious hepatitis

(B) Cholestatic liver disease

(C) Drug reaction from fluoxetine

(D) Drug reaction from trimethoprim-sulfamethoxazole

6. Autopsy investigations on a 70-year-old man with a history of peripheral vascular disease reveal an atherosclerotic plaque in the left anterior descending coronary artery, which results in 80% luminal stenosis. This atheroma is covered by a smooth endothelial lining without evidence of thrombosis, ulceration, or hemorrhage. The remaining coronary vessels are relatively spared. Which of the following clinical syndromes would most likely have resulted from this pathologic lesion?

(A) Chest pain awakening the patient in the early morning

(B) Chest pain occurring with progressive frequency and severity

(C) Chest pain precipitated by exercise and consistently relieved by rest

(D) Progressive development of congestive heart failure without chest pain

(E) Prolonged (more than 30 minutes) chest pain accompanied by shock

7. A 31-year-old woman comes to the physician for a periodic health maintenance examination. She has no complaints at this time. She has a normal menstrual period every 28 days. She had an appendectomy at the age of 18 and has had no other surgeries. She takes no medications and is allergic to sulfa. She lives with her husband and works as a computer programmer. Physical examination, including breast and pelvic examinations, is normal. She is planning on becoming pregnant in the next few months. The physician should advise her to begin taking folate supplements to reduce the risk of which of the following fetal abnormalities?

(A) Arnold-Chiari malformations

(B) Germinal matrix hemorrhage

(C) Holoprosencephaly

(D) Neural tube defects

(E) Syringomyelia

8.  A patient develops an acute febrile illness with shivers, nonproductive cough, and pleuritic chest pain. Five days later, he presents to the emergency department after abruptly having "coughed up" nearly a cup of blood-stained sputum. Which of the following is most likely to be seen on a chest x-ray film?

    (A) Blunting of diaphragmatic costal angles

    (B) A cavity with a fluid level

    (C) Complete opacification of one lobe with no additional findings

    (D) Patchy consolidation centered on bronchi

    (E) Prominent bronchi that can be followed far out into the lung fields

9.  A 30-year-old woman has chronic, silver-white, scaly patches with an erythematous border on the skin of her knees and elbows. Which of the following is the most likely etiology of this condition?

    (A) Autoimmune disease

    (B) Bacterial disease

    (C) Fungal disease

    (D) Granulomatous disease

    (E) Large vessel vasculitis

10. An infant born with a congenital infection has excessive growth of new bone on the anterior surface of the tibia with anterior bowing of the bone. This finding is due to which of the following processes?

    (A) Neoplastic cortical bone deposition

    (B) Neoplastic medullary bone deposition

    (C) Neoplastic periosteal bone deposition

    (D) Reactive medullary bone deposition

    (E) Reactive periosteal bone deposition

11. A 22-year-old man is evaluated for mitral regurgitation due to mitral valve prolapse. Examination reveals a tall, slender young man with long extremities and long tapering fingers. Pupillary dilation followed by slit-lamp examination reveals bilateral dislocation of the lenses of the eyes. This patient is potentially at increased risk for development of which of the following?

    (A) Aortic dissection

    (B) Lisch nodules

    (C) Noncaseating granulomata

    (D) Progressive dementia

    (E) Rapidly progressive renal failure

12. A 6-cm length of rectosigmoid colon containing a 2-cm diameter sessile polyp is surgically removed. On sectioning, the lesion shows finger-like papillae with cores of scant lamina propria. The surfaces of the papillae are covered by dysplastic columnar epithelium with considerable nuclear pleomorphism. No glandular structures are seen in the base of the lesion or in the adjacent muscle tissue. The margins of the specimen are free of dysplastic epithelium. What further therapy does this person most likely require?

    (A) Adjunct chemotherapy

    (B) Complete colectomy

    (C) Radiation therapy

    (D) Resection of regional lymph nodes

    (E) No further therapy is required

13. A 65-year-old man presents with a productive cough and difficulty breathing. His sputum culture is positive for encapsulated gram-positive cocci, which are often seen in pairs. The patient's dyspnea is primarily due to which of the following mechanisms?

    (A) Inadequate perfusion

    (B) Inadequate ventilation

    (C) Increased airway resistance

    (D) Increased lung compliance

    (E) Poor oxygen diffusion

14. A previously healthy 20-year-old woman presents to the emergency department with fever, jaundice, and confusion. Her examination is notable for a temperature of 102.0 F, scleral icterus, scattered petechiae on her palate and extremities, and disorientation on mental status examination. Laboratory studies reveal a platelet count of 20,000/mm³, a hemoglobin of 8 g/dL, an elevated indirect bilirubin level, and a creatinine of 5 mg/dL. Her prothrombin time (PT) and partial thromboplastin time (PTT) are both normal. Her peripheral blood smear reveals decreased platelets and numerous fragmented red blood cells. Which of the following is the most likely diagnosis in this patient?

(A) Autoimmune hemolytic anemia

(B) Disseminated intravascular coagulation (DIC)

(C) Idiopathic thrombocytopenic purpura (ITP)

(D) Thrombotic thrombocytopenic purpura (TTP)

(E) Von Willebrand disease

15. A 52-year-old man is brought into the emergency department by his wife because he has been complaining of a severe headache. Physical examination reveals ptosis of the right eyelid with the right eye facing down and out. There is a fixed and dilated right pupil with an inability to accommodate. Subarachnoid blood appears on non contrast CT scan. Magnetic resonance angiography (MRA) would be expected to reveal an aneurysm of which of the following arteries?

(A) Anterior cerebral

(B) Anterior choroidal

(C) Anterior communicating

(D) Middle cerebral

(E) Ophthalmic

(F) Posterior communicating

(G) Posterior inferior cerebellar

16. During a routine pediatric examination, a 12-year-old boy is noted to be in growth arrest. The child is obese and has multiple small bruises on his arms and legs. The patient has difficulty rising from a crouching position. Measurements of blood pressure demonstrate hypertension when compared with age-based standards. This patient most likely has which of the following disorders?

(A) Diabetes mellitus

(B) Graves disease

(C) Hypothyroidism

(D) Parathyroid adenoma

(E) Pituitary microadenoma

17. A 15-year-old white boy presents with a hemarthrosis of the right knee joint and a recent history of protracted bleeding from cuts or scrapes. He has no family history of bleeding disorders. The patient also notes a long history of chronic abdominal discomfort and diarrhea, which has been worse for the past 6 months, occasionally accompanied by fever. Physical examination reveals a patient at the fifth percentile for both height and weight; an actively bleeding rectal fissure is also noted. Both prothrombin time (PT) and the partial thromboplastin time (PTT) are prolonged. Laboratory evaluation of the blood is likely to reveal low levels of which of the following?

(A) Factor VIII

(B) Factor IX

(C) Factors II, VII, IX, and X

(D) Factors II, V, VII, IX, and X

(E) von Willebrand factor

18. A 63-year-old woman presents to her physician complaining of right facial numbness and weakness. Six months earlier she presented with moderate diplopia. Neurologic examination reveals a decrease of all sensation over the right face. There is decreased strength and bulk of the right masseter and temporalis muscles, decreased abduction of the right eye, and weakness of all facial muscles on the right. What would testing of the corneal reflex most likely reveal?

    (A) A consensual reflex but no direct reflex of the left eye

    (B) A consensual reflex but no direct reflex of the right eye

    (C) A direct reflex and a consensual reflex of the left eye

    (D) A direct reflex and a consensual reflex of the right eye

    (E) No direct reflex and no consensual reflex of the left eye

    (F) No direct reflex and no consensual reflex of the right eye

19. A 30-year-old patient presents to a physician because his morning urine had a dark red-brown color. He describes having had several months of increasing weakness and dyspnea on exertion, several episodes of cramping abdominal pain, and a recent cold. Physical examination reveals pallor and mild jaundice. A urine sample appears yellow and clear. Which of the following additional tests is most likely to yield an abnormal result?

    (A) Urine complete cell count

    (B) Urine free hemoglobin

    (C) Urine free myoglobin

    (D) Urine hemosiderin

    (E) Urine red cell count

20. Primary immunodeficiencies can be investigated by injecting tetanus toxoid into the medial aspect of the thigh, followed by ipsilateral inguinal node biopsy 7 days later. If this test is performed on an immunocompetent individual, which of the following would be the predominant change observed in the biopsied lymph node?

    (A) Follicular hyperplasia

    (B) Necrotizing lymphadenitis

    (C) Paracortical lymphoid hyperplasia

    (D) Sinus histiocytosis

    (E) Stellate abscesses

    (F) Suppurative lymphadenitis

21. A 16-year-old boy sustains multiple fractures over the course of an intramural basketball season and is referred to a radiologist. X-ray examination of the boy's upper extremities reveals diffusely sclerotic bones with enlarged, flask-shaped radial and ulnar metaphyses. The boy's father had a similar condition as a child, but he lived in a rural area and was not further evaluated. The boy's condition is most likely due to which of the following?

    (A) Deficiency of vitamin D

    (B) Deficient osteoblastic activity

    (C) Deficient osteoclastic activity

    (D) Deficient synthesis of type I collagen

    (E) Primary hyperparathyroidism

22. A 32-year-old woman with insomnia undergoes an electroencephalogram (EEG) in a sleep disorder clinic. At 3:00 AM, the EEG technician notes that the woman is exhibiting vertex waves, sleep spindles, and K complexes. Which stage of sleep is she in at this time?

    (A) REM

    (B) Stage 1

    (C) Stage 2

    (D) Stage 3

    (E) Stage 4

23. A 65-year-old man comes to the emergency department because of chest pain and shortness of breath. An electrocardiogram shows ST elevations and new Q waves. Despite appropriate care, the patient dies. The family agrees to an autopsy, which shows extensive atherosclerotic disease. The finding of which of the following features in an atherosclerotic plaque indicates that it has become a complicated lesion?

    (A) Cholesterol crystals

    (B) Chronic inflammatory cells

    (C) Intimal smooth muscle

    (D) Lines of Zahn

    (E) Necrotic cell debris

24. A 40-year-old woman with polycythemia vera develops progressive severe ascites and tender hepatomegaly over a period of several months. Liver function tests are near normal. Which of the following tests would be most likely to establish the probable diagnosis?

    (A) Endoscopic retrograde cholangiopancreatography

    (B) Hepatic venography

    (C) Serum alpha-fetoprotein

    (D) Serum ceruloplasmin studies

    (E) Serum iron studies

25. A 4-year-old girl is brought to her pediatrician for a checkup. The child's skin is slightly jaundiced, and she has mild splenomegaly. Her hemoglobin and hematocrit are reduced. Her mean corpuscular volume is 90 $\mu m^3$, and her reticulocyte count is 7%. A Coombs test is performed and is negative. A hemoglobin electrophoresis shows an abnormal component, constituting less than 25% of the total. A blood smear shows inclusion bodies within the RBCs. Which of the following is the most likely diagnosis?

    (A) Beta thalassemia

    (B) Heinz body anemia

    (C) Hereditary spherocytosis

    (D) Pernicious anemia

    (E) Sickle cell anemia

26. A high school basketball player passes out in the middle of a game. He is rushed to the emergency department, where he regains consciousness. He claims that just before he fainted, he had difficulty breathing and experienced palpitations. On physical examination, he has a bifid apical impulse and a coarse systolic murmur at the left sternal border. The echocardiogram reveals ventricular hypertrophy with asymmetric septal thickening. Which of the following would increase the intensity of his heart murmur?

    (A) Elevating his legs

    (B) Increasing sympathetic tone

    (C) Performing the Valsalva maneuver

    (D) Squatting

27. An MRI reveals a cerebellomedullary malformation in which the vermis of the cerebellum and the medulla are elongated and flattened and protrude through the foramen magnum into the vertebral canal. Which of the following is the most likely diagnosis?

    (A) Arnold Chiari malformation

    (B) Dandy-Walker syndrome

    (C) Holoprosencephaly

    (D) Lissencephaly

    (E) Polymicrogyria

    (F) Schizencephaly

28. Two weeks after starting a course of methicillin, a pneumonia patient develops fever, hematuria, proteinuria, skin rash, and eosinophilia. Which of the following is the most likely diagnosis?

    (A) Acute interstitial nephritis

    (B) Acute renal tubular necrosis

    (C) Crescentic glomerulonephritis

    (D) Minimal change disease

    (E) Pyelonephritis

29. A woman is brought into the emergency department following an automobile accident in which her chest was hit by the steering wheel. Her blood pressure is 120/90 mm Hg. When she inhales, her systolic blood pressure drops to 100 mm Hg. This finding defines which of the following terms?

    (A) Pulsus alternans

    (B) Pulsus bisferiens

    (C) Pulsus paradoxus

    (D) Pulsus parvus

    (E) Pulsus tardus

30. A 13-year-old girl complaining of visual deficits is diagnosed with a brain tumor. The mass is detectable on x-ray by the presence of opaque calcifications. MRI reveals destruction of more than 75% of the anterior pituitary gland. Which of the following clinical manifestations would be most likely in this patient?

    (A) Amenorrhea and galactorrhea

    (B) Bilateral exophthalmos and palpitations

    (C) Coarse facial features and enlarged hands and feet

    (D) Polydipsia, polyuria, and low urine osmolality

    (E) Weight gain, sluggishness, and depression

31. A 47-year-old alcoholic presents with fever and a tender, enlarged liver. His AST is 150 U/L, and his SGPT ALT is 70 U/L. His prothrombin time is 25 seconds, and his partial thromboplastin time is 30 seconds. This patient has a deficiency of which of the following clotting factors?

    (A) II

    (B) V

    (C) VII

    (D) VIII

    (E) IX

    (F) X

    (G) XII

32. A 23-year-old construction worker presents to the emergency department after falling down on his outstretched right hand. An x-ray film reveals a fracture of one of the wrist bones. The physician is concerned about the risk for avascular necrosis. Which of the following bones was fractured?

    (A) Capitate

    (B) Lunate

    (C) Pisiform

    (D) Scaphoid

    (E) Trapezoid

33. A 50-year-old woman presents with complaints of difficulty rising from a chair and combing her hair. Physical examination is remarkable for erythema and edema of cheeks, eyelids, and the backs of her hands. The lesions have a distinctive mauve color, and mauve papules are noted on the knuckles. Approximately 30% of patients with this disorder also may have

    (A) abnormal circulating lymphocytes with cerebriform nuclei

    (B) bacillary bodies in macrophages in the lamina propria of the intestine

    (C) flattening and blunting of villi in the jejunum

    (D) a mutation in a skeletal muscle protein

    (E) an underlying malignancy

34. A patient presents to a dermatologist because of skin changes. The skin is hyperpigmented and thickened and feels velvety. Multiple skin tags are present. The changes are worst in the axillae, groin, and anogenital area, but are very widespread. This patient should be specifically evaluated for which of the following diseases?

    (A) Hepatic cirrhosis

    (B) Lung cancer

    (C) Polycystic renal disease

    (D) Systemic lupus erythematosus

    (E) Ulcerative colitis

35. A 48-year-old woman presents to the physician with lower back pain. She states that she has had the pain for about 2 weeks and that it has become steadily more severe. An x-ray film shows a lytic bone lesion in her lumbar spine. Review of systems reveals the recent onset of mild headaches, nausea, and weakness. Her CBC shows a normocytic anemia, and her erythrocyte sedimentation rate is elevated. Urinalysis shows heavy proteinuria, and a serum protein electrophoresis shows a monoclonal peak of IgG. Which of the following is responsible for this patient's spinal lesion?

    (A) Bence-Jones proteins

    (B) Lymphoplasmacytoid proliferation

    (C) Osteoblast activating factor

    (D) Osteoclast activating factor

    (E) Primary amyloidosis (AL)

36. Biopsy of a 4-mm rough, tan, and slightly raised skin lesion on the face of a 65-year-old man demonstrates atypical basal cells with eosinophilic cytoplasm but persistent intercellular bridges. The stratum corneum is thickened, and parakeratosis is present; the remainder of the epidermis is thinned. Which of the following features would also probably be seen in the dermis?

    (A) Benign nevus cells

    (B) Blue-gray elastic fibers

    (C) Large numbers of spindle-shaped fibroblasts

    (D) Malignant nevus cells

    (E) Touton giant cells

37. During a bitterly cold winter, an elderly couple is found dead in their apartment. All their windows are closed, and their leaky old furnace is on full. Which of the following is the primary mechanism by which the toxin involved led to the death of this couple?

    (A) Decreasing intracellular calcium

    (B) Inhibition of cytochrome oxidase

    (C) Inhibition of $Na^+/K^+$ ATPase

    (D) Irreversible binding to hemoglobin

    (E) Stimulation of cellular apoptosis

38. A 25-year-old-man presents with weight loss, abdominal pain, and bloody diarrhea. Sigmoidoscopy/colonoscopy reveals mucosal erythema and ulceration extending in a continuous fashion proximally from the rectum. Which of the following pathologic findings would also be characteristic of this patient's illness?

    (A) Bowel wall thickening

    (B) Cobblestone appearance of mucosa

    (C) Fistulas

    (D) Pseudopolyps

    (E) Transmural lesions

39. A 61-year-old woman comes to the office because of an enlarging breast mass. She noticed the lesion about 10 months ago and has been "following it" on her own ever since. She decided to seek medical advice because she thinks that it might be cancer. Examination reveals a firm, fixed, 3-cm mass in the right upper outer quadrant. A biopsy of the mass reveals loss of cell differentiation and lack of tissue organization. Which of the following terms best corresponds to this finding?

    (A) Anaplasia

    (B) Desmoplasia

    (C) Dysplasia

    (D) Hyperplasia

    (E) Metaplasia

40. A 1-month-old infant is in the clinic for routine well child care. He was born at full term with a birth weight of 8 lb, 2 oz, and the perinatal period was uncomplicated. He has been breastfed since birth, and there have been no feeding problems. His current weight is 9 lb, and the length and head circumference are at the 50th percentile. The baby is alert and appears well. Physical examination shows a loud holosystolic murmur in the left parasternal region with an associated systolic thrill. The first and second heart sounds are normal. There is no gallop or diastolic murmur. The peripheral pulses are well palpable, and the blood pressure is normal in all four extremities. There is no peripheral edema or cyanosis. The remainder of the examination is unremarkable. A chest x-ray reveals cardiomegaly with increased pulmonary vascular markings. An echocardiogram is most likely to reveal which of the following findings?

    (A) Atrial septal defect

    (B) Patent ductus arteriosus

    (C) Patent foramen ovale

    (D) Pulmonic stenosis

    (E) Ventricular septal defect

41. A 62-year-old indigent woman with a long history of uncontrolled hypertension presents to the emergency department with headache, vomiting, and patchy loss of vision. Her blood pressure is 210/155 mm Hg, and her blood chemistry reveals marked azotemia. Which of the following would most likely be associated with her condition?

    (A) Berry aneurysm

    (B) Granulomatous arteritis

    (C) Hyperplastic arteriolitis

    (D) Phlebosclerosis

    (E) Thromboangiitis obliterans

42. A 40-year-old female diabetic has glycosuria. This finding may be attributed to inadequate glucose reabsorption at which of the following sites?

    (A) Collecting duct

    (B) Distal convoluted tubule

    (C) Glomerulus

    (D) Loop of Henle

    (E) Proximal convoluted tubule

43. A woman delivers a stillborn boy at 31 weeks' gestation. Examination of the boy shows severe generalized edema and ascites with hepatosplenomegaly. Laboratory studies show that this boy had thalassemia. Which of the following is the most likely genotype?

    | | **Beta-Chain Genes** | **Alpha-Chain Genes** |
    |---|---|---|
    | (A) | Four abnormal | Two normal |
    | (B) | Two abnormal | Four normal |
    | (C) | Two normal | Four abnormal |
    | (D) | Two normal | Two normal |

44. A 3-year-old patient with short stature has hepatosplenomegaly, skeletal abnormalities, mental retardation, and corneal clouding. Electron microscopy of lysosomes reveals laminated structures. Which of the following substances would accumulate in this patient?

    (A) Galactocerebroside

    (B) Glucocerebroside

    (C) $GM_2$ ganglioside

    (D) Heparan sulfate

    (E) Sphingomyelin

    (F) Sulfatide

45. During the summer after her second year of medical school, a student is volunteering at the Centers for Disease Control and Prevention. As part of her project, the student is trying to determine which forms of cancers can theoretically be prevented by a vaccine targeted against an oncogenic virus. Which of the following diseases might be prevented by such a vaccine?

    (A) Acute lymphocytic leukemia

    (B) Acute myelogenous leukemia

    (C) Adult T-cell leukemia

    (D) Chronic myelogenous leukemia

    (E) Hairy cell leukemia

    (F) Hodgkin lymphoma

    (G) Multiple myeloma

    (H) Mycosis fungoides

46. A patient develops a pea-sized, translucent nodule on the wrist, which when excised shows cystic degeneration of connective tissue without a true cell lining. Which of the following is the most likely diagnosis?

    (A) Ganglion cyst

    (B) Gout

    (C) Pseudogout

    (D) Synovial cyst

    (E) Villonodular synovitis

47. A thin, 32-year-old Jewish man develops left hip pain and fever. A diagnosis of septic arthritis is established and he undergoes surgical drainage of the left hip joint. On the third day after surgery, it is noted that the fluid draining from the joint has become green and frothy, looking suspiciously like enteric contents. He is given charcoal granules by mouth, and the granules are clearly visible in the hip drainage 6 hours later. In response to directed questions, he gives a history of occasional episodes of colicky abdominal pain going back at least 10 years, sometimes accompanied by diarrhea. He never had blood in his stools before. Which of the following is the most likely diagnosis?

    (A) Appendiceal abscess

    (B) Chronic ulcerative colitis

    (C) Crohn disease

    (D) Sigmoid diverticulitis

    (E) Surgical damage to nearby intestinal loops

48. A 35-year-old, obese, former football player complains of joint stiffness of the knees and distal interphalangeal joints of the fingers. Physical examination reveals decreased range of motion of the affected joints, crepitus, and bony swelling. X-ray films display narrowing of the affected joint spaces. Which of the following is the most likely etiology of this patient's disorder?

    (A) Accumulation of calcium pyrophosphate in joint fluid

    (B) Antibodies against the $F_c$ fragment of IgG

    (C) Chondrocyte injury and abnormal collagen activity

    (D) Hematogenous seeding of joints during bacteremia

    (E) Inborn error of purine metabolism

49. A 15-year-old boy who very recently immigrated to the U.S. presents to the physician with fever, headache, and stiff neck. Examination is remarkable for asymmetric weakness and hyporeflexia. He has a poor immunization history, and poliomyelitis is diagnosed. What is the primary mechanism by which poliovirus causes paralytic disease?

    (A) Demyelination of lower motor neuron axons

    (B) Demyelination of upper motor neuron axons

    (C) Destruction of cell bodies of lower motor neurons

    (D) Destruction of muscle cells

    (E) Destruction of synapses between the axon and the muscle

50. A severely ill patient in shock develops acute renal failure with oliguria and azotemia. The urine osmolality approaches that of the glomerular ultrafiltrate (specific gravity 1.010). A renal biopsy would most likely show which of the following?

    (A) Acute pyelonephritis

    (B) Acute tubular necrosis

    (C) Chronic pyelonephritis

    (D) Crescentic glomerulonephritis

    (E) Renal cell carcinoma

# Pathology and Pathophysiology Test Three:
# Answers and Explanations

## ANSWER KEY

| | | | | |
|---|---|---|---|---|
| 1. | D | | 26. | C |
| 2. | A | | 27. | A |
| 3. | A | | 28. | A |
| 4. | C | | 29. | C |
| 5. | D | | 30. | E |
| 6. | C | | 31. | C |
| 7. | D | | 32. | D |
| 8. | B | | 33. | E |
| 9. | A | | 34. | B |
| 10. | E | | 35. | D |
| 11. | A | | 36. | B |
| 12. | E | | 37. | D |
| 13. | E | | 38. | D |
| 14. | D | | 39. | A |
| 15. | F | | 40. | E |
| 16. | E | | 41. | C |
| 17. | C | | 42. | E |
| 18. | F | | 43. | C |
| 19. | D | | 44. | D |
| 20. | A | | 45. | C |
| 21. | C | | 46. | A |
| 22. | C | | 47. | C |
| 23. | D | | 48. | C |
| 24. | B | | 49. | C |
| 25. | B | | 50. | B |

1. **The correct answer is D.** The presentation is typical for reactivation pulmonary tuberculosis. The patient may also note fever, malaise, and weight loss. The high $P_{O_2}$ found in the upper portion of the lungs provides a favorable environment for growth of *Mycobacterium tuberculosis*, leading to reactivation tuberculosis. (In contrast, primary tuberculosis tends to occur in the lower and middle lobes, where small infectious particles are most likely to lodge after being inhaled.)

   Ventilation increases from the top to the bottom of the lung, so **choice E** is wrong. Perfusion increases even more rapidly than ventilation, so **choice A** is also wrong. As a result, the ventilation-perfusion ratio decreases from the top to the bottom of the lung. The higher ratio at the apex of the lung results in a relatively elevated $P_{O_2}$ at that location.

   The apex of the lung has a higher pH than the base, so **choice B** is wrong. Because the ventilation-perfusion ratio is higher at the apex, $P_{CO_2}$ would be lower, thus increasing the pH.

   Regional differences in the density of alveolar macrophages (**choice C**) are not known to cause the described predisposition.

2. **The correct answer is A.** 5-Hydroxyindoleacetic acid (5-HIAA) is a metabolite of serotonin, a major secretory product of carcinoid tumors. The signs and symptoms of carcinoid syndrome include diarrhea, flushing, and wheezing. The cardiac abnormalities are commonly concentrated in the right heart because carcinoid secretory products are degraded or detoxified in the lung.

   Homovanillic acid (HVA; **choice B**) is a breakdown product of dopamine through the monoamine oxidase (MAO) or catechol-*o*-methyltransferase (COMT) metabolism pathways.

   Phenylalanine (**choice C**) is an essential amino acid that is used to synthesize tyrosine, the precursor of the catecholamines (dopamine, norepinephrine, and epinephrine).

   Selegiline (**choice D**) is a MAO-B inhibitor that inhibits the degradation of dopamine. It is used in the treatment of Parkinson disease.

   Vanillylmandelic acid (VMA; **choice E**) is a metabolite of epinephrine that is elevated in the urine of individuals with pheochromocytoma.

3. **The correct answer is A.** The secondary sexual changes seen in alcoholic cirrhosis appear to be due to both decreased testicular secretion of testosterone and decreased hepatic extraction of the androgen androstenedione. Thus, androstenedione is available for extrasplanchnic aromatization (occurring mostly in peripheral adipose tissue) to form compounds with estrogenic activity.

   **Choices B and E** do not fully explain the secondary sexual changes.

   Although tumors of Leydig and/or Sertoli cells may excrete both androgens and estrogens, the normal Leydig (**choice C**) and Sertoli cells (**choice D**) do not usually secrete estrogens.

4. **The correct answer is C.** This is a classic description of iron deficiency anemia (up to 20% of adult women are iron deficient!). Iron deficiency anemia is very common in menstruating women and is associated with the signs and symptoms described (fatigue, weakness, pallor). It can also be associated with epithelial changes, such as brittle nails and atrophic tongue. The typical laboratory values are those presented, along with a decreased reticulocyte count. On peripheral blood smear, the RBCs are small (microcytic) and pale (hypochromic, due to low hemoglobin levels from inadequate iron stores).

   Vitamin $B_{12}$/folate deficiency would produce macrocytosis with hypersegmented neutrophils (**choice A**).

   Lead poisoning would produce microcytosis with basophilic stippling (**choice B**).

   Schistocytes (**choice D**) are RBC fragments seen when the cells are destroyed by shearing forces in the vascular system, such as those present in prosthetic heart valves and microangiopathic hemolytic anemias.

5. **The correct answer is D.** This man has glucose-6-phosphate dehydrogenase (G6PD) deficiency (as do 10% of African American males). G6PD serves to protect the RBC from oxidative damage by maintaining high intracellular levels of NADPH. People of Mediterranean descent can also have G6PD deficiency, but to a much greater degree. Therefore, hemolytic episodes in this population are more severe (and can be fatal) as compared with those of the African American type, which are usually mild and self-limited. Common oxidative stressors that initiate hemolysis are drug reactions (especially sulfa drugs), febrile illnesses, and fava bean ingestion.

   Acute infectious hepatitis (**choice A**) would more likely present with abdominal pain, hepatomegaly, and high elevations of AST and ALT (often into the 1000s).

   Cholestatic liver disease (**choice B**) more often presents with elevation of alkaline phosphatase, along with mild AST and ALT elevations. This patient has elevated unconjugated bilirubin levels, as in hemolytic disorders. Both hepatocellular (hepatitis) and cholestatic liver disease cause more conjugated (as opposed to unconjugated) hyperbilirubinemia.

The most common side effects of fluoxetine (a selective serotonin reuptake inhibitor; **choice C**) are anxiety, agitation, and insomnia.

6. **The correct answer is C.** The atherosclerotic lesion described here is referred to as *fixed coronary obstruction*, which becomes clinically manifest with chest pain when increased myocardial demand cannot be compensated by vasodilatation. This usually occurs when the obstruction is more than 75% the cross-sectional area of the lumen, unless there are additional predisposing factors. Fixed coronary artery obstruction manifests with *stable angina*, i.e., chest pain triggered by exercise or emotional strain and promptly relieved by rest.

Chest pain that awakens a patient in the early morning (**choice A**) is characteristic of *Prinzmetal angina*, which is due to coronary artery vasospasm and is not often associated with atherosclerotic lesions.

Chest pain occurring with progressive frequency and severity (**choice B**) refers to *unstable angina*, in which chest pain manifests with relatively unpredictable patterns. Pain becomes increasingly frequent and less responsive to rest or medication. This form is related to plaque rupture, hemorrhage, ulceration, and superimposed thrombosis.

Progressive development of congestive heart failure without chest pain (**choice D**) defines chronic ischemic heart disease, which is usually due to involvement of all three coronary branches and associated with diffuse loss of myofibers and fibrosis throughout the ventricles.

Prolonged (more than 30 minutes) chest pain accompanied by shock (**choice E**) is most likely due to myocardial infarction. This is usually caused by occlusive thrombosis complicating acute plaque changes, such as ulceration or rupture.

7. **The correct answer is D.** Neural tube defects result from failure of the primitive neural tube to close, which may affect either end of the neuraxis and lead to anomalies involving both the neural tissue and overlying skin and bone. Anencephaly and encephalocele may develop at the cranial end, whereas various forms of spina bifida, myelomeningocele, and meningocele occur at the caudal end. Folate deficiency has been linked to neural tube defects. Elevated alpha-fetoprotein in the maternal blood allows antenatal diagnosis.

Arnold-Chiari malformations (**choice A**), which affect the craniospinal junction, have two forms. Type 1 is frequent but usually asymptomatic and consists of downward displacement of the cerebellar tonsils. Type 2 is much more complex and manifests with early signs and symptoms of hydrocephalus.

Germinal matrix hemorrhage (**choice B**) is one cause of perinatal brain injury and consists of hemorrhage within the germinal matrix, the periventricular layer of neuronal and glial precursors. This injury affects premature infants and may lead to significant neurologic impairment or death.

Holoprosencephaly (**choice C**) is a severe malformation in which lack of separation between hemispheres leads to a single central ventricle. It is usually associated with trisomy 13.

Syringomyelia (**choice E**) refers to the formation of an ependymal-lined cavity within the spinal cord, parallel to and connected with the central canal. It is associated with Arnold-Chiari type 1, traumas, or spinal tumors and leads to progressive neurologic deficits.

8. **The correct answer is B.** This is a classic presentation of a pulmonary abscess. Chronic courses with less severe symptoms (with intermittent improvement following short courses of antibiotics) are also sometimes seen, particularly if the diagnosis was not suspected. A chest x-ray film typically shows pneumonic opacification in which a cavity, often with a fluid level, is visible. Pulmonic abscesses can be caused by anaerobes (most common, particularly if aspiration initiated the abscess), gram-negative aerobic bacilli, and staphylococci. Therapy is based on the organisms isolated and should be continued for at least 4 to 6 weeks. In cases that fail to resolve, the possibility of coexisting carcinoma should be considered.

**Choice A** is the x-ray appearance of pleural effusion.

**Choice C** is the x-ray appearance of lobar pneumonia.

**Choice D** is the x-ray appearance of bronchopneumonia.

**Choice E** is the x-ray appearance of bronchiectasis.

9. **The correct answer is A.** The patient has psoriasis. This chronic disease, which affects 1 to 2% of people in the U.S., typically involves the elbows, knees, scalp, intergluteal cleft, penis, and lumbosacral area. Well established lesions show extensive parakeratotic scales overlying a thinned or absent stratum granulosum. The mitotic rate in the underlying epidermis is increased, and mitotic figures can be seen well above the basal cell layer. Collections of neutrophils (Munro abscesses) can be seen within the parakeratotic stratum corneum. The pathogenesis of psoriasis is not well understood, but evidence has been accumulating that autoimmunity may play a role. The theory is that exogenous or endogenous damage to the stratum corneum of the skin exposes antigens against which complement-fixing autoantibodies are directed. Activation of the complement cascade draws neutrophils to the site, further damaging the

**KAPLAN** MEDICAL

stratum corneum and perpetuating the process. The damage also triggers release of proliferative factors for epidermal cells, leading to increased epithelial turnover, hyperplasia, and scale formation (an alternative theory is that the underlying process begins with an enhanced ability of the endothelial cells of the superficial dermal microvessels to recruit neutrophils).

Bacterial (**choice B**) or fungal (**choice C**) diseases may trigger psoriasis but are not the primary etiologies.

Psoriasis is not associated with granuloma formation (**choice D**), but rather with the formation of microabscesses (Munro abscesses—see above) in the stratum corneum.

Large vessel vasculitis (**choice E**) does not seem to play a role in the pathogenesis of psoriasis.

10. **The correct answer is E.** The infant has congenital syphilis. The tibial deformity develops when spirochetes localize in the periosteum, where they produce an active inflammation with many plasma cells. This then causes a massive, reactive, periosteal deposition of bone on the medial and anterior surfaces of the tibia ("saber shin"). "Saddle nose" deformity, another feature of congenital syphilis, is due to inflammatory destruction of the nasal and palatal bones. Gummas, in which a central necrotic focus is surrounded by layers of granulomatous and nonspecific chronic inflammation, can also be found in and near the saber shin and saddle nose.

The bone changes are not neoplastic (**choices A, B, and C**), and involvement of the medulla (**choice B and D**) and cortical layer of the bone is less marked than are the periosteal changes.

11. **The correct answer is A.** This young man is displaying features of Marfan syndrome, a genetic (often autosomal dominant) disease of connective tissues that affects the skeleton (tall stature, long fingers and toes, hyperextensible joints), eyes (often subluxation of the lenses bilaterally), and the cardiovascular system (cystic medial necrosis predisposing to aortic dissection, or aortic valve incompetence). Marfan syndrome is due to mutations in the fibrillin gene, leading to defects in the structure of elastic tissue.

Lisch nodules (**choice B**) are pigmented nodules found on the iris of the eye. They are associated with type I neurofibromatosis.

Noncaseating granulomata (**choice C**) can be seen in a variety of disorders, including sarcoidosis and berylliosis.

Progressive dementia (**choice D**) is a feature of a number of disorders, including Alzheimer disease, Huntington disease, and Pick disease.

Rapidly progressive renal failure (**choice E**) is not a feature of Marfan disease. It occurs in a number of other disorders, such as Goodpasture disease.

12. **The correct answer is E.** The patient has a villous adenoma, which has been adequately treated by complete resection. If dysplastic epithelium had been found at the surgical resection margins, re-excision to remove the dysplastic epithelium would be required, since villous adenomas are considered to be a premalignant condition.

Adjunct chemotherapy (**choice A**) or radiation therapy (**choice C**) are not indicated since villous adenoma is a premalignant condition rather than an actual malignancy.

Complete colectomy (**choice B**) is typically performed for inflammatory bowel disease rather than for carcinoma of the colon, and would certainly not be indicated for the treatment of villous adenoma.

The presence of clearly invasive glands would have indicated that the patient had a true adenocarcinoma, and examination of regional lymph nodes (**choice D**) would be required to evaluate the extent of the disease.

13. **The correct answer is E.** The patient has pneumococcal pneumonia. In many bacterial pneumonias, alveoli in large areas of the lungs fill with viscous fluid containing proteinaceous debris and many neutrophils. This filling limits the rate at which oxygen can diffuse into the capillary bed and, in many filled alveoli, may even completely block oxygen diffusion into the bloodstream.

Inadequate ventilation (**choice B**) is not initially as important as poor diffusion.

Changes in perfusion (**choice A**), airway resistance (**choice C**), and lung compliance (**choice D**) usually play lesser roles, although a perfusion/ventilation mismatch may also develop as blood is shunted through poorly ventilated lung tissue.

14. **The correct answer is D.** This woman is exhibiting the classic pentad of thrombotic thrombocytopenic purpura (TTP)—fever, encephalopathy, renal dysfunction, thrombocytopenia, and microangiopathic hemolytic anemia.

Autoimmune hemolytic anemia (**choice A**) can cause anemia and an elevated indirect bilirubin, but generally produces only mild symptoms, is not associated with thrombocytopenia, and does not cause fragmentation of red blood cells on the peripheral smear.

Disseminated intravascular coagulation (DIC; **choice B**) can cause thrombocytopenia and microangiopathic hemolytic anemia, but is also associated with prolongation of both the prothrombin time (PT) and activated partial thromboplastin time (PTT).

Idiopathic thrombocytopenic purpura (ITP; **choice C**) causes thrombocytopenia with minimal symptoms along with normal hemoglobin and PT/PTT. The peripheral smear in ITP reveals only a decreased number of platelets.

Von Willebrand disease (**choice E**) is an inherited coagulopathy that causes abnormal bleeding. The PTT is typically prolonged.

15.  **The correct answer is F.** Aneurysm of the posterior communicating artery is the second most common aneurysm of the circle of Willis (anterior communicating artery is most common) and can result in third cranial nerve palsy (paralysis). The oculomotor nerve (CN III) innervates the levator palpebrae muscle. CN III paralysis would therefore result in ptosis (drooping of the upper eyelid). CN III also innervates all of the extraocular muscles, except for the superior oblique (CN IV) and the lateral rectus muscles (CN VI). Thus, CN III palsy would result in unopposed action of the superior oblique and lateral rectus muscles, causing the affected eye to look down and out. CN III also supplies parasympathetic innervation to the sphincter muscle of the iris (which constricts the pupil) and to the ciliary muscle. Interruption of this pathway leads to a dilated and fixed pupil and to paralysis of accommodation.

The symptoms described probably resulted from subarachnoid hemorrhage (SAH), in this case, due to rupture of a posterior communicating artery aneurysm. A classic clue to the diagnosis is a patient presenting with "the worst headache of his or her life." When you are presented with a case of sudden severe headache, SAH should rank highly on your differential diagnosis list.

The anterior cerebral artery (**choice A**) supplies the medial surface of the cerebral hemisphere, from the frontal pole to the parieto-occipital sulcus. Occlusion may produce hypesthesia and paresis of the contralateral lower extremity.

The anterior choroidal artery (**choice B**) arises from the internal carotid artery and is not part of the circle of Willis. It perfuses the lateral ventricular choroid plexus, the hippocampus, parts of the globus pallidus, and the posterior limb of the internal capsule.

The anterior communicating artery (**choice C**) connects the two anterior cerebral arteries. It is the most common site of aneurysm in the circle of Willis and may cause aphasia, abulia (impaired initiative), and hemiparesis.

The middle cerebral artery (**choice D**) supplies the lateral convexity of the cerebral hemisphere, including Broca's and Wernicke's speech areas and the face and arm areas of the motor and sensory cortices. It also gives rise to the lateral striate arteries, which supply the internal capsule, caudate, putamen, and globus pallidus. The middle cerebral artery is the most common site of stroke.

The ophthalmic artery (**choice E**) enters the orbit with the optic nerve (CN II) and gives rise to the central artery of the retina. Occlusion results in blindness.

The posterior inferior cerebellar artery (**choice G**) supplies the dorsolateral medulla and the inferior surface of the cerebellar vermis. Occlusion may result in Wallenberg syndrome: cerebellar ataxia, hypotonia, loss of pain and temperature sensation of the ipsilateral face, absence of corneal reflex ipsilaterally, contralateral loss of pain and temperature sensation in the limbs and trunk, nystagmus, ipsilateral Horner syndrome, dysphagia, and dysphonia.

16.  **The correct answer is E.** The child has features of Cushing syndrome, which can be caused by excess corticotropin (ACTH), due to pituitary adenoma or ectopic ACTH production, or can occur independently of ACTH production, due to adrenal adenoma, adrenal carcinoma, alcohol, or exogenous steroids. The presentation of Cushing syndrome, as classically stressed to medical students, includes truncal obesity, moon facies, and "buffalo hump." However, these features cannot always be clearly distinguished from ordinary obesity, particularly in unusual populations such as children. It is consequently of great help to be aware of other features that may suggest the diagnosis. Children with Cushing syndrome almost inevitably have growth arrest, which may, as in this patient, be the initial diagnostic clue that more than simple obesity is present. Some children also show precocious puberty, secondary to androgen excess. Features present in both children and adults that are particularly helpful in discriminating Cushing syndrome from obesity include easy bruising and a mild proximal myopathy that can be demonstrated by asking the patient to rise from a crouching position. Hypertension is another prominent feature, which tends to be more common in patients with Cushing syndrome than in those who are obese. A predisposition to infections can be another helpful clue. Other features that can be present (usually in adult cases) include psychiatric abnormalities, most commonly depression and lethargy; osteoporotic vertebral collapse leading to lost height, seen in long-standing Cushing syndrome; red-purple striae of the abdomen or thighs; plethorics appearance secondary to skin thinning; and, sometimes, skin pigmentation in ectopic

ACTH syndrome and with some pituitary tumors. Once Cushing syndrome is suspected, it can be investigated with a variety of endocrine techniques, including urinary free cortisol, dexamethasone suppression tests, and plasma ACTH, and can be treated surgically if an adrenal or pituitary tumor is found.

17. **The correct answer is C.** Low levels of factors II, VII, IX, and X are seen in vitamin K deficiency, leading to prolonged prothrombin time (PT) and partial thromboplastin time (PTT). Vitamin K deficiency is occasionally severe enough in obstructive jaundice, pancreatic disease, or small bowel disease to cause a bleeding diathesis. This patient has evidence of small bowel disease and a history suggestive of Crohn disease (chronic abdominal discomfort, diarrhea and fever). Crohn disease, which is also characterized by rectal fissures, growth retardation, and malabsorption, causes malabsorption of fat-soluble vitamins (A,D,E,K) by several mechanisms. It most often involves the terminal ileum, which is responsible for the recycling of bile acids necessary for the transport and proper absorption of lipids. Small intestinal Crohn disease itself can cause malabsorption by reducing the surface area available for absorption of nutrients. Finally, the disease can cause the development of fistulae, which can lead to exclusion of loops of bowel, also reducing available absorptive surface area.

Factor VIII deficiency (**choice A**) is the cause of hemophilia A. This answer is incorrect because hemophilia A is characterized by an elevated PTT but a normal PT, since only factor VIII is involved. Although hemophilia A can cause gastrointestinal hemorrhage and pain, a 6-month crisis with abdominal discomfort as the only symptom would be extremely rare. Also, hemophilia would likely be characterized by black tarry stools rather than diarrhea. Hemophilia A is inherited as an X-linked recessive; thus, affected individuals are usually male, whereas carriers are female.

Low levels of factor IX (**choice B**) is the cause of Christmas disease. Like hemophilia A, factor IX deficiency is characterized by prolonged APTT and normal PT. Specific coagulation factor assays distinguish these two diseases, as they are otherwise identical in both presentation and inheritance.

Low levels of factors II, V, VII, IX, and X (**choice D**) could be characteristic of liver disease, but in such a case both PT and APTT would be elevated. Note that in liver disease, all other factors (except for Factor VIII) would also be low.

Low levels of von Willebrand factor (**choice E**) cause a prolonged or normal APTT, a normal PT, and a pro-

longed bleeding time. Von Willebrand disease is inherited in an autosomal dominant pattern with incomplete penetrance.

18. **The correct answer is F.** This woman has lesions of the right trigeminal (CN V; right facial numbness, decreased bulk of the right masseter and temporalis muscles), right abducens (CN VI; diplopia, decreased abduction of the right eye), and right facial (CN VII; weakness of all facial muscles on the right) nerves. A corneal reflex is elicited by touching a cotton wisp to the eye, resulting in bilateral blinking. The afferent limb of this reflex is carried by CN V (V1), and the efferent limb is mediated by CN VII. Touching the cotton to this patient's right eye would not produce blinking in either eye. The right eye would not blink because of CN V and CN VII lesions, and the left eye would not blink because of a lesion of CN V. Touching cotton to the left eye would result in blinking of the left eye, but not the right (lesion of right CN VII).

19. **The correct answer is D.** The patient has paroxysmal nocturnal hemoglobinuria (PNH), which can cause a striking hemoglobinuria with red-brown to black urine and an elevated urine hemosiderin level. The condition usually presents between 20 and 40 years of age. The hemoglobinuria is intermittent, but a regular, rhythmic nocturnal pattern is actually observed in only a minority of patients. PNH is an acquired disease, and, surprisingly, may be related to erythroleukemia. (The erythrocytes that lyse in PNH appear to be derived from a clone arising from somatic mutation.) Factors that may trigger lysis include infection (even with the common cold), menstruation, surgical procedures, exposure to cold, vaccines, and possibly "stress." These patients are prone to venous thrombosis (thought to result from inappropriate platelet activation), which may be the cause of the abdominal pain that is frequently experienced. Thrombosis and thromboembolism are the most frequent immediate cause of death in PNH patients, with the intrahepatic veins being a favorite site for thrombosis (producing Budd-Chiari syndrome). Other complications include pigment gallstones (secondary to chronic hemolysis) and granulocytopenia, leading to frequent infections.

Urine complete cell counts (**choice A**) are generally uninformative.

In practice, urine hemosiderin levels are a more reliable indicator of the condition than urine free hemoglobin (**choice B**), which is typically present only during episodes of frank hemolysis. Because the patient's urine sample was yellow, it is unlikely that he is experiencing hemolysis at the present time; however, in all likelihood, the urine would still contain hemosiderin.

Myoglobin (**choice C**) would not be expected to be present in the urine in PNH.

Urine red cell counts (**choice E**) are generally uninformative.

20. **The correct answer is A.** The antigenic challenge in this case would result in activation of B-lymphocytes and production of antigen-specific immunoglobulins. The B-dependent areas of lymph nodes would consequently become hyperplastic. These are the germinal centers of lymphoid follicles, where maturation of B-cells takes place. Thus, a picture characterized by enlargement of germinal centers develops. This is called follicular hyperplasia.

Necrotizing lymphadenitis (**choice B**) is seen in a few specific infections (namely tularemia, bubonic plague, anthrax, and typhoid fever) and in Kikuchi lymphadenitis, a rare noninfectious form.

Paracortical lymphoid hyperplasia (**choice C**) refers to hyperplasia of the interfollicular zones, which are predominantly populated by T-cells. This change is seen in response to phenytoin, viral infections, and antiviral vaccinations.

Sinus histiocytosis (**choice D**) is characterized by enlarged lymphatic sinuses filled with reactive histiocytes. This nonspecific change is seen frequently in nodes draining sites with chronic infections or a neoplasia.

Stellate abscesses (**choice E**) occur in nodes involved by cat-scratch disease, tularemia, and lymphogranuloma venereum.

Suppurative lymphadenitis (**choice F**) develops in response to acute infection by pyogenic organisms, most frequently *Staphylococcus aureus.*

21. **The correct answer is C.** The patient described is exhibiting signs of osteopetrosis, characterized by abnormally brittle bones with increased density throughout the body. In this condition, the ends of long bones also show a characteristic widening (Erlenmeyer flask deformity) on x-ray films. Deficient osteoclast activity underlies this rare hereditary disorder. In the autosomal dominant form, which this boy (and his father) presumably has, the defect is fairly mild, characterized by multiple fractures and anemia (due to filling of the medullary cavities of bone with immature bone). The autosomal recessive form is much more severe, with only a few afflicted children surviving into infancy.

Deficiency of vitamin D (**choice A**) causes rickets in children and osteomalacia in adults. Both are characterized by inadequate mineralization of an exuberant cartilage matrix.

Deficient osteoblastic activity (**choice B**) would produce decreased bone density, not increased density, as in this patient.

Deficient synthesis of type I collagen (**choice D**) underlies some forms of osteogenesis imperfecta. This disorder is characterized by multiple fractures; however, these fractures are related to the production of smaller amounts of abnormal bone, rather than too much bone, as in osteopetrosis.

Hyperparathyroidism (**choice E**) produces characteristic bone demineralization, in contrast to the diffuse, symmetric, skeletal sclerosis seen in osteopetrosis.

22. **The correct answer is C.** Stage 2 sleep is characterized by low-amplitude, mixed-frequency EEG activity with more theta waves than Stage 1. In addition, vertex waves (sharply contoured potentials at the vertex), sleep spindles (short bursts of 12-16 Hz activity), and K complexes (high-amplitude waves with superimposed sleep spindles) occur intermittently. Muscle tone is slightly reduced, and eye movements are absent.

REM sleep (**choice A**) is characterized by low-amplitude, mixed-frequency activity. Ponto-geniculo-occipital (PGO) spikes, which are transient, larger amplitude potentials, occur over the occipital areas. There are also episodic bursts of rapid eye movements (REMs), and skeletal muscle tone is decreased.

Stage 1 sleep (**choice B**), or drowsiness, is characterized by a transition from alpha rhythms (relaxed wakefulness) to theta rhythms. Electromyographic (EMG) activity is decreased, compared with relaxed wakefulness, and there are slow, roving eye movements.

Stages 3 (**choice D**) and 4 (**choice E**) are also known as slow-wave sleep. They are characterized by high-amplitude slow waves, especially delta waves. Eye movements are absent, and EMG activity is decreased compared with relaxed wakefulness.

23. **The correct answer is D.** Complicated lesions indicate advanced atherosclerotic disease. They arise in atherosclerotic plaques and render them more susceptible to sudden occlusion and acute infarction of the supplied tissues. Commonly, the plaque ulcerates or ruptures, and the exposed surfaces, being highly thrombogenic, precipitate thrombus formation. Thrombi are typified by the lines of Zahn, alternating layers of platelets and fibrin (the pale lines), and layers of blood (the dark lines). Beyond thrombus formation, other features of a complicated plaque include hemorrhage into the lesion itself, and microembolism by cholesterol crystals or calcified debris. Furthermore, the weakened media underlying the plaque may develop an aneurys-

**KAPLAN) MEDICAL**

mal dilatation. In general, the clinical significance of atherosclerosis is related to the consequences of complicated lesions.

The incorrect options all include features of atheromatous plaques but do not indicate complicated lesions:

Beneath the endothelium of a plaque there is a fibrous cap composed of smooth muscle (**choice C**), chronic inflammatory cells (**choice B**), and lipid laden macrophages (foam cells), as well as extracellular material.

The core of the lesion, which lies between the intima and the media, is composed of necrotic cellular debris (**choice E**), with cholesterol crystals (**choice A**), calcium, and more foam cells.

24. **The correct answer is B.** The clinical presentation is most consistent with Budd-Chiari syndrome (hepatic vein obstruction), which may occur as a complication of thrombogenic and myeloproliferative disorders including polycythemia vera. The presentation illustrated is the most common; alternative presentations include fulminant liver failure and cases in which intractable abdominal pain is the most prominent initial finding. Hepatic venography is the best technique of those listed to demonstrate the occlusion of the hepatic venous system.

Endoscopic retrograde cholangiopancreatography (**choice A**) is most useful in demonstrating lesions of the biliary tree.

Serum alpha-fetoprotein (**choice C**) is a marker for hepatocellular carcinoma.

Ceruloplasmin (**choice D**) levels are decreased in Wilson disease.

Serum iron studies (**choice E**) are useful when considering hemochromatosis as a cause of cirrhosis.

25. **The correct answer is B.** Heinz body anemia is an autosomal dominant disease that causes an abnormal hemoglobin variant. The mutant hemoglobin precipitates within the RBC, forming an inclusion, or Heinz body. The RBC is then either phagocytosed or removed by the spleen. Patients present with hemolytic anemia, jaundice, splenomegaly, and dark colored urine. The MCV is normal, and electrophoresis usually reveals the abnormal component as a small percentage of the total. The reticulocyte count is increased as the body tries to make new blood to compensate. If the Coombs test were positive, this would indicate that the problem was extracorpuscular.

Beta thalassemia (**choice A**), an inherited defect in or absence of the beta chain of hemoglobin, causes a microcytic, rather than a normocytic, anemia. It results in red cells containing excess alpha globin chains that

form insoluble aggregates, leading to hemolysis. The presenting symptoms are anemia, jaundice, splenomegaly, hepatomegaly, and certain developmental abnormalities, depending on the subtype of the disease.

Hereditary spherocytosis (**choice C**) can cause a normocytic anemia with an increased reticulocyte count, but the hemoglobin electrophoresis would be normal in these patients. Jaundice and splenomegaly are often present. The disease is caused by an autosomal dominant defect in the erythrocyte membrane spectrin molecule that makes the cell less pliable and more easily destroyed.

Pernicious anemia (**choice D**) causes a megaloblastic anemia, ruled out in this patient by the normal MCV. It presents in children younger than 10 years (juvenile form) or in adults in the 6th decade. It is caused by lack of intrinsic factor from the gastric mucosa, causing a lack of vitamin $B_{12}$ uptake in the terminal ileum. Patients present with pallor, slight jaundice, tachycardia, a smooth red tongue, diarrhea, and possibly CNS symptoms.

Sickle cell anemia (**choice E**) causes a microcytic, rather than normocytic, anemia. It is a hereditary disorder characterized by a substitution of valine for glutamic acid in the beta hemoglobin chain. With hypoxemia, the red cell changes to a sickle shape. Patients present with pain, jaundice, splenomegaly, and anemia.

26. **The correct answer is C.** This patient has hypertrophic cardiomyopathy (idiopathic hypertrophic subaortic stenosis)—the most common cause of sudden cardiac death in young patients. It usually causes problems during exertion. Clues to the diagnosis include dyspnea, palpitations, bifid apical impulse, coarse systolic murmur at the left sternal border, and ventricular hypertrophy with asymmetric septal thickening on echocardiogram. Left ventricular outflow obstruction typically plays an important role in the pathophysiology of this condition. Maneuvers that decrease preload, such as the Valsalva maneuver, will accentuate the heart murmur because they result in less ventricular filling, contributing to greater outflow obstruction.

Elevating his legs (**choice A**), increasing sympathetic tone (**choice B**), and squatting (**choice D**) would all increase venous return and therefore diminish the murmur.

27. **The correct answer is A.** The findings in this patient indicate the presence of an Arnold Chiari malformation. There are also variable defects of the hindbrain and skeletal structure. Hydrocephalus and myelomeningocele are often present.

In Dandy-Walker syndrome (**choice B**), the cerebellar vermis is hypoplastic or aplastic, and the posterior fossa is instead filled with a large cyst produced by expansion of the roofless (lacking the cerebellar vermis) fourth ventricle.

Holoprosencephaly (**choice C**) is a failure of the prosencephalon to cleave, also leading to a defect of midline facial development. The most severe form results in cyclopia. In the form that results from trisomy 13 (Patau syndrome) there are bilateral cleft lip and palate, low-set ears, microcephaly, ocular anomalies, hypotelorism, mental retardation, convulsions, deafness, and ventricular septal defects.

Lissencephaly (**choice D**) is agyria, which means "smooth brain." The cerebral hemispheres are devoid of gyri or sulci.

Polymicrogyria (**choice E**) describes a brain in which the gyri are too small and too numerous.

Schizencephaly (**choice F**) is characterized by symmetric clefts that extend from the cortical surface to the underlying ventricle. The cleft is generally hypoplastic.

28. **The correct answer is A.** This is a typical presentation for drug-induced acute interstitial nephritis, which usually resolves when the offending drug is removed. Half of the cases progress to acute renal failure. Additional offending drugs include other penicillin derivatives, sulfonamides, and some diuretics.

Acute renal tubular necrosis (**choice B**) has been associated with exposure to aminoglycosides, amphotericin, and methoxyflurane.

Crescentic glomerulonephritis (**choice C**) is not typically associated with methicillin exposure, but rather with immunologic mechanisms or unknown causes.

Minimal change disease (**choice D**), or lipoid nephrosis, is an important cause of the nephrotic syndrome in children and is sometimes associated with a recent respiratory infection or a vaccination.

Pyelonephritis (**choice E**) is a tubulointerstitial kidney disease caused by bacterial infection, with elements of obstruction or vesicoureteral reflux in many cases.

29. **The correct answer is C.** Pulsus paradoxus is defined as a fall in systolic blood pressure >10 mm Hg on inspiration. It can be associated with cardiac tamponade and chronic obstructive pulmonary disease (COPD).

Pulsus alternans (**choice A**) is a repeated variation in the amplitude of the pulse pressure. It can be associated with profound left ventricular dysfunction.

Pulsus bisferiens (**choice B**) is a double pulsation occurring during systole. It can be associated with aortic regurgitation and hypertrophic cardiomyopathy.

Pulsus parvus (**choice D**) is a weak pulse upstroke caused by diminished stroke volume. It can be associated with hypovolemia, aortic stenosis, mitral stenosis, and left ventricular failure.

Pulsus tardus (**choice E**) is a delayed pulse upstroke. It can be associated with aortic stenosis.

30. **The correct answer is E.** This patient has panhypopituitarism induced by her brain mass This condition is associated with decreased serum levels of thyroid-stimulating hormone (TSH), adrenocorticotropic hormone (ACTH), follicle-stimulating hormone (FSH), luteinizing hormone (LH), prolactin, and growth hormone. The x-ray findings (opaque calcifications) and patient description suggest a craniopharyngioma, the most common pituitary tumor in children. Note that nonsecreting-chromophobe adenomas may also present with hypopituitarism. Weight gain, sluggishness, and depression are all signs of hypothyroidism, resulting from the decreased TSH levels caused by anterior pituitary hypofunction.

Amenorrhea and galactorrhea (**choice A**) are associated with hyperpituitarism, which is most often associated with a pituitary adenoma that secretes prolactin, growth hormone, or ACTH.

Bilateral exophthalmos and palpitations (**choice B**) are symptoms of Graves disease. This condition is associated with a decrease in TSH, which occurs in response to elevated thyroid hormone levels; it is not a result of anterior pituitary hypofunction.

Coarse facial features and enlarged hands and feet (**choice C**) are signs of acromegaly, which may result from increased growth hormone levels associated with hyperpituitarism.

Polydipsia, polyuria, and low urine osmolality (**choice D**) are symptoms of diabetes insipidus. Central diabetes insipidus is associated with disorders of the posterior pituitary or the hypothalamus (decreased antidiuretic hormone [ADH]). Remember that nephrogenic diabetes insipidus stems from renal unresponsiveness to ADH, not from diminished levels of the hormone.

31. **The correct answer is C.** This vignette had some clinical information that was irrelevant in terms of answering the question. This is a common USMLE question format—providing a clinical context for a straightforward basic science question. It is important that you don't spend too much time analyzing data (for example the liver function tests in this case) before you've read the

actual question. This is especially true on the even longer vignettes you may occasionally see on the test. You'll also note that this question has more than five answer choices. The USMLE has been including an increasing number of such items, making it more difficult to guess correctly.

To answer this question, you need to know that the prothrombin time (PT) measures the extrinsic pathway, that the partial thromboplastin time (PTT) measures the intrinsic pathway, and which of the factors listed is unique to the extrinsic system (so that a deficiency would elevate the PT without affecting the PTT). The only factor listed that is unique to the extrinsic pathway is factor VII. The reason that the PT is elevated in patients with liver damage (alcoholic hepatitis in this patient) is that all the coagulation factors (with the exception of factor VIII) are synthesized solely by the liver. The reason the PT is elevated before the PTT is affected is that factor VII has the shortest circulating half-life of any of the coagulation factors. You should be aware that in severe liver damage, the PTT eventually will also rise as the patient develops a deficiency in all the coagulation factors (except VIII).

Factors II (**choice A**), V (**choice B**), and X (**choice F**) are part of the final common pathway and are not unique to either the intrinsic or extrinsic systems. Deficiencies in any of these factors would elevate both the PT and the PTT.

Factors VIII (**choice D**), IX (**choice E**), and XII (**choice G**) are exclusive to the intrinsic pathway. Patients with deficiencies in any of these factors (e.g., hemophilia) will have elevated PTTs with normal PTs.

Here are some useful mnemonics:

To remember that PT measures the extrinsic pathway: PET

To remember that PTT measures the intrinsic pathway: PITT

To remember the factors in the final common pathway: $1 \times 2 \times 5 = 10$ (factors I, II, V, and X)

32. **The correct answer is D.** Suspect fracture of the scaphoid (navicular) bone in any young adult who has "fallen on an outstretched hand" (classic clue). The physician was concerned about the risk of avascular necrosis because, in some people, the blood supply of the bone is located distally, and a fracture will deprive the proximal region of the bone of its arterial nourishment. Osteoarthritis is a common complication of scaphoid fractures that do not heal properly.

The lunate bone (**choice B**) is commonly dislocated in patients who have fallen on an outstretched hand. Median

nerve injury is a frequently associated occurrence.

The capitate (**choice A**), pisiform (**choice C**), and trapezoid (**choice E**) bones of the wrist are less commonly associated with falls on an outstretched hand.

33. **The correct answer is E.** This is a typical presentation of dermatomyositis. Approximately 30% of middle-aged patients who present with this condition have an underlying malignancy. A wide variety of cancers, particularly adenocarcinomas, can cause dermatomyositis. The mauve papules are known as Gottron's sign and, together with the eyelid involvement, are helpful in distinguishing the rash of dermatomyositis from that of systemic lupus erythematosus.

Abnormal lymphocytes with cerebriform nuclei (**choice A**) circulate in Sézary syndrome, which is a leukemic variant of mycosis fungoides, a cutaneous T-cell lymphoma.

Bacillary bodies in macrophages within the intestinal lamina propria (**choice B**) are characteristic of Whipple disease.

Flattening and blunting of villi in the jejunum (**choice C**) are characteristic of celiac sprue, or gluten-sensitive enteropathy.

Duchenne-type muscular dystrophy is caused by a mutation in a skeletal muscle protein (**choice D**), dystrophin.

34. **The correct answer is B.** The condition described is acanthosis nigricans. Mild forms are common and may be associated with obesity and endocrine abnormalities. More extensive forms, such as in this patient, may be associated with malignant disease: usually an adenocarcinoma (often lung), less commonly a lymphoma. The pattern is important to recognize because the eruption may precede other symptoms of the malignancy by several years.

35. **The correct answer is D.** The disease described above is multiple myeloma, a plasma cell neoplasm in which the neoplastic plasma cells elaborate a single, or monoclonal, type of immunoglobulin. In this case, and most commonly, IgG is produced. Patients with this disease are usually older than 40 and may have normocytic anemia. They often complain of skeletal pain from lytic bone lesions and may report headaches and nausea caused by hyperviscosity of the blood due to the excessive amounts of immunoglobulins. The lytic bone lesions are caused by the production of osteoclast activating factor by the neoplastic plasma cells. This can also lead to hypercalcemia.

Bence Jones proteins (**choice A**) are immunoglobulin light chains. They are often overproduced in multiple myeloma and are filtered in the urine. They are not usually detected in serum unless there is renal impairment, but they can be detected in the urine by electrophoresis and immunofixation. They do not cause bony lytic lesions.

Lymphoplasmacytoid proliferation (**choice B**), describes a normal type of B lymphocyte that is morphologically between a lymphocyte and a plasma cell. Lymphoplasmacytoid lymphocytes produce IgM; in Waldenstrom macroglobulinemia, they undergo neoplastic proliferation and produce IgM peaks. Bone lesions are not seen in this disease.

Osteoblast activating factor (**choice C**) would not produce osteolytic lesions and is not seen in multiple myeloma. There is a rare osteoblastic variant of multiple myeloma with dense bony osteosclerosis rather than lytic lesions, but osteoblast activating factor has not been shown to be involved.

Primary amyloidosis (AL; **choice E**), is a primary light-chain type of amyloidosis associated with multiple myeloma. The insoluble proteinaceous deposits occur in the tongue, heart, kidney, and skin. This does not cause bony lytic lesions.

36.  **The correct answer is B.** The lesion described is an actinic keratosis. This common premalignant lesion is caused by solar damage, which also characteristically damages the elastic fibers (changing their color in stained tissue to blue-gray) of the superficial dermis.

Benign nevocellular nevus cells (**choice A**) are found in common moles (nevocellular nevi).

Large numbers of spindle-shaped fibroblasts (**choice C**) are found in dermatofibromas.

Malignant nevus cells (**choice D**) are found in melanoma.

Touton giant cells (**choice E**) are found in xanthomas.

37.  **The correct answer is D.** This couple died of carbon monoxide poisoning. Carbon monoxide has approximately 240 times the affinity for hemoglobin than does oxygen. In a sense, the hemoglobin-CO dissociation curve is shifted very far to the left compared with the hemoglobin-$O_2$ dissociation curve. This means that the binding of hemoglobin to carbon monoxide is virtually irreversible. (The carbon monoxide that cigarette smokers inhale is cleared only when senescent red cells are phagocytized in the spleen and the hemoglobin is degraded.) In addition, the carbon monoxide shifts the hemoglobin-$O_2$ dissociation curve to the left, making the unloading of $O_2$ to the tissues very difficult. When too much hemoglobin is tied up with carbon monoxide, the person dies. The carbon monoxide-hemoglobin complex has a bright red color; a distinctive feature of

carbon monoxide poisoning that can be helpful either at autopsy or in living patients is that this color makes the skin and organs also appear bright cherry red.

Generally, intracellular calcium levels increase, rather than decrease (**choice A**), with cellular injury or death.

Cytochrome oxidase is inhibited by cyanide (**choice B**).

Ouabain is an example of a poison that inhibits the $Na^+/K^+$ ATPase (**choice C**).

Apoptosis (programmed cell death) is stimulated (**choice E**) by certain genes (e.g., *p53, ced 3,4*), glucocorticoids, and aging.

38.  **The correct answer is D.** This is a question that tests your ability to distinguish between ulcerative colitis (UC) and Crohn disease. First, you need to figure out which one this patient has. The key clues here are the bloody diarrhea (much more common in UC), the rectal involvement, and, especially, the continuous nature of the mucosal damage. Once you've figured out that the patient has UC, you need to identify the answer choice that is characteristic of UC. The correct answer is pseudopolyps, which are inflammatory polyps found in ulcerative colitis and not Crohn disease.

All the other choices are features of Crohn disease. Especially diagnostic is the transmural nature of the inflammation, which can lead to the development of fissures and fistulas. Remember also that although Crohn disease can involve any part of the gastrointestinal tract, it typically does not involve the rectum and is usually found in the terminal ileum and/or colon. In contrast to UC, the lesions are discontinuous (skip lesions).

39.  **The correct answer is A.** Anaplasia is a loss of cell differentiation and tissue organization. It is associated with malignancy and is an ominous prognostic sign.

Desmoplasia (**choice B**) is excessive fibrous tissue formation in tumor stroma.

Dysplasia (**choice C**) is abnormal atypical cellular proliferation.

Hyperplasia (**choice D**) is an increase in the number of cells.

Metaplasia (**choice E**) is a reversible change of one cell type to another, usually in response to irritation.

40.  **The correct answer is E.** The differential diagnosis of an acyanotic congenital cardiac defect includes several lesions that cause either a left-to-right shunt or cardiac outflow obstruction. Ventricular septal defects (VSDs) are the most common congenital cardiac defects and are frequently detected incidentally in otherwise healthy infants through the presence of a loud murmur. The murmur of a VSD is loud, holosystolic,

and often associated with a thrill. The presence of a gallop or diastolic murmur indicates that the defect is large.

Atrial septal defects (ASDs) (**choice A**) are also incidentally discovered in healthy children. The classic findings are related to a systolic flow murmur and a widely split and fixed second heart sound.

Patent ductus arteriosus (PDA) is more commonly seen in premature babies (**choice B**), although occasional cases occur in full-term infants. The physical findings include a continuous murmur and hyperdynamic peripheral pulses. Pulmonary vascularity is increased.

Children with an isolated patent foramen ovale (**choice C**) are asymptomatic and have no physical findings. These defects are detected by an echocardiogram.

Pulmonic stenosis (**choice D**) causes a loud ejection systolic murmur at the upper left sternal border. The pulmonary vascularity is not increased with pulmonic stenosis.

41.  **The correct answer is C.** This patient has developed malignant hypertension, a syndrome of end-organ damage associated with long-standing hypertension, usually occurring with blood pressures greater than 200/140 mm Hg. Severe elevations of blood pressure are frequently associated with hyperplastic arteriolitis (truly an arteriolosclerosis), typified by concentric, laminated smooth muscle proliferation narrowing the arteriolar lumen (onion skinning). Necrotizing arteriolitis, characterized by fibrinoid degeneration and acute inflammation in the arteriolar wall, may also be seen.

Berry aneurysms (**choice A**) arise at points of weakness in the arterial media, especially branch points in the circle of Willis. Although hypertension may play a role in atherosclerosis and the development of dissecting aortic aneurysms, berry aneurysms are believed to be congenital.

Granulomatous arteritis (**choice B**) is typical of several large and medium vessel diseases, especially giant cell arteritis, Takayasu arteritis, and Wegener granulomatosis. It is identified histologically with mural inflammation with clusters of macrophages, often containing multinucleated giant cells. The arteriolar inflammation in malignant hypertension involves neutrophils, not granulomata.

Phlebosclerosis (**choice D**) is the characteristic change in varicose veins, in which dilated and tortuous veins show elastic degeneration and calcifications in the venous media.

Thromboangiitis obliterans (**choice E**), also known as Buerger disease, is a disease of cigarette smokers. It is characterized by segmental vascular occlusion with luminal thrombus formation and microabscesses within small to medium-sized arteries and veins in the extremities.

42.  **The correct answer is E.** The proximal convoluted tubule is the site of reabsorption (via $Na^+$/glucose cotransporters) of nearly 100% of the glucose filtered at the glomerulus. In diabetes mellitus, sugar spills into the urine when the proximal convoluted tubule's capacity for reabsorption is exceeded.

The collecting duct (**choice A**) is the site of reabsorption of water (and urea) when antidiuretic hormone (ADH) is present.

The distal convoluted tubule (**choice B**) is one of the sites of sodium reabsorption.

The glomerulus (**choice C**) is the site of filtration of the plasma entering via the afferent arteriole.

In the initial part of the loop of Henle (**choice D**), water moves out into the hypertonic interstitium. In the ascending limb, sodium and chloride are reabsorbed, but water cannot follow, so the filtrate becomes more hypotonic.

43.  **The correct answer is C.** Hydrops fetalis is a form of alpha-thalassemia, which results from deletion of the four genes responsible for alpha-chain synthesis. Deletion of one gene produces a silent carrier. Deletion of two genes causes alpha-thalassemia trait (with a mild hypochromic anemia; **choice D**). Deletion of three genes results in HbH disease (with hemolysis), and deletion of four genes leads to the condition known as hydrops fetalis and death *in utero*. Beta-thalassemia is due to a genetic abnormality at a single site that results in defects in mRNA processing. Since a person receives genetic material from both parents, the patient can have zero, one, or two abnormal genes at this site, but not four (**choice A**). Homozygotes for beta-thalassemia (**choice B**) have beta-thalassemia major. Heterozygotes have beta-thalassemia minor.

44.  **The correct answer is D.** This patient has a mucopolysaccharidosis, which exists in several different forms. In Hurler syndrome and Sanfilippo syndrome, lysosomes contain characteristic laminated structures on electron microscopy. In Hurler syndrome, a defect in α-L-iduronidase causes accumulation of heparan and dermatan sulfate. In Sanfilippo syndrome, heparan sulfate accumulates.

Accumulation of galactocerebroside (**choice A**) occurs in Krabbe disease, which is due to galactocerebrosidase deficiency.

Accumulation of glucocerebroside (**choice B**) occurs in Gaucher disease, which is due to defects in β-glucocerebrosidase. The reticuloendothelial cells and CNS are affected.

Accumulation of $GM_2$ ganglioside (**choice C**) occurs in Tay-Sachs disease because of hexosaminidase A deficiency. The swollen ganglion cells of the retina contribute to a classic sign of Tay-Sachs—the macular cherry-red spot.

Accumulation of sphingomyelin (**choice E**) in a variety of organs occurs in Niemann-Pick disease, which is due to a defect in sphingomyelinase.

Accumulation of sulfatide (**choice F**) occurs in metachromatic leukodystrophy, caused by arylsulfatase A deficiency.

45. **The correct answer is C.** The only disease listed that has been established as related to an oncogenic virus is adult T-cell leukemia. This disease is endemic in Japan. It is caused by the human T-cell leukemia virus known as HTLV-1.

For the USMLE, you should also be aware of the other neoplastic diseases thought to be caused by viruses: Burkitt lymphoma (Epstein-Barr virus), hepatocellular carcinoma (hepatitis B virus), cervical/penile/anal carcinoma (human papillomavirus), and Kaposi sarcoma. Note: Kaposi sarcoma is associated with HIV but is now thought to be caused by a specific Kaposi sarcoma-associated herpesvirus—HHV 8 (human herpesvirus type 8).

46. **The correct answer is A.** Ganglion cysts are common, benign degenerations of connective tissue that are almost always located near a joint capsule or tendon sheath, often in the wrist. Ganglion cysts characteristically lack a true lining, which distinguishes them morphologically from synovial cysts.

Gout (**choice B**) and pseudogout (**choice C**) produce crystal deposition rather than fluid-filled cavities.

A synovial cyst (**choice D**) is due to herniation of synovium through a joint capsule and is characteristically lined by synovium.

Villonodular synovitis (**choice E**) is a benign, synovial proliferation that produces a shaggy mass in the synovium.

47. **The correct answer is C.** Fistulas between the gastrointestinal tract and the hip joints are very rare, but clearly this man has developed one. Crohn disease is notorious for its propensity to develop fistulas. These are typically within the abdomen, but they can form at rather unexpected locations, like this one. His age, ethnicity, and prior history are highly suggestive for this diagnosis.

An appendiceal abscess (**choice A**) could eventually point into the groin, following the psoas muscle. Such migration of pus would occur on the right side rather than the left, however, and it would produce a groin mass rather than a septic hip. There would not be a history extending for 10 years.

Chronic ulcerative colitis (**choice B**) rarely fistulizes and often has bloody diarrhea.

Sigmoid diverticulitis (**choice D**) can fistulize, but usually it does so into the urinary bladder. It is preferentially a disease of older people. It has been described in young, obese men of Mexican American decent. This patient does not fit the profile.

It would be quite a surgical tour de force to get into the bowel by way of the hip joint (**choice E**), but even if we assume that such complication could occur, we must remember that in this case the hip joint had become infected before an operation was performed.

48. **The correct answer is C.** This patient has osteoarthritis, a degenerative joint disease that is very common in the elderly and in those with a history of "wear and tear" or overuse of the joints (as found in football players). Chondrocyte injury occurs along with abnormal collagen activity. Predisposing factors include obesity, previous joint injury, and synovial disease. Clinically, patients have joint stiffness, decreased range of motion, effusions, crepitus, and bony swelling. The most commonly affected joints include the vertebrae, hips, knees, and distal interphalangeal (DIP) joints of the fingers. (Note that Heberden's nodes [terminal phalanx] and Bouchard's nodes [proximal phalanx] are characteristic of this disease.) Symptoms of nerve compression may occur secondary to compression by osteophytes and bone spur development. A classic finding on x-ray is joint space narrowing. Joint fluid shows few cells and normal mucin.

Accumulation of calcium pyrophosphate in joint fluid (**choice A**) is associated with pseudogout (which is also known as calcium pyrophosphate dihydrate (CPPD) crystal deposition disease).

Antibodies against the $F_c$ fragment of IgG (**choice B**) are associated with rheumatoid arthritis (RA).

Hematogenous seeding of joints during bacteremia (**choice D**) is the etiology of suppurative arthritis (septic).

An inborn error of purine metabolism (**choice E**) results in the development of gout.

Be careful not to confuse your crystals! Remember:

Gout = negatively birefringent urate crystals

*P*seudogout = *p*ositively birefringent calcium pyrophosphate crystals

Don't confuse your nodules either!

Gout = tophi

Osteoarthritis = Heberden's and Bouchard's nodes

Rheumatoid arthritis = subcutaneous nodules on extensor surfaces

49. **The correct answer is C.** The poliovirus kills alpha motor neurons present in the ventral horns of the spinal cord. These lower motor neurons are the cells whose axons form the motor nerves that innervate the muscles of the body.

Guillain-Barré syndrome is an acute, inflammatory, demyelinating disease of peripheral nerves, including the axons of lower motor neurons (**choice A**).

Multiple sclerosis can cause demyelination of upper motor neurons (**choice B**).

Trauma, including extremely strenuous exercise, is an example of a process that can directly damage muscle (**choice D**).

Selective destruction of synapses between the muscle and the lower motor neurons (**choice E**) is not directly involved in the pathology of poliomyelitis.

50. **The correct answer is B.** This is the typical clinical scenario in which acute tubular necrosis develops secondary to shock, and further destabilizes an already desperately ill patient. Acute tubular necrosis can also occur following exposure to nephrotoxins or as a manifestation of acute rejection in a transplanted kidney. The prognosis depends on the patient's overall health. In patients who recover, the initial oliguric phase (lasting 1-2 weeks) is followed by a diuretic phase (weeks to months) before eventual restoration of tubular function.

Acute pyelonephritis (**choice A**) is not typically a cause of renal failure with loss of concentrating ability.

Chronic pyelonephritis (**choice C**) actually refers to chronic interstitial nephritis, which usually does not produce loss of concentrating ability (except in rare cases in which the reaction is so severe that acute tubular necrosis ensues).

Crescentic glomerulonephritis (**choice D**) is associated with rapidly progressive renal failure, characterized by hypertension, hematuria, proteinuria, and an active urinary sediment.

Renal cell carcinoma (**choice E**) is not a typical cause of renal failure with loss of concentrating ability. Hematuria is the most common presenting symptom.

# Pathology and Pathophysiology: **Test Four**

1. Following an upper respiratory infection, a 5-year-old develops large purpuric lesions on the buttocks and extensor surfaces of the arms and legs. The patient also has abdominal pain, vomiting, and arthralgias. Dipstick analysis of the urine shows microscopic hematuria. Renal biopsy would probably show which of the following distinctive features?

   (A) IgA in the mesangial region

   (B) Marked interstitial nephritis

   (C) Subepithelial electron-dense deposits

   (D) Tumor

   (E) Vasculitis

2. A 29-year-old man presents with hemoptysis and hematuria. Renal biopsy shows inflammation of the glomeruli. An x-ray film shows focal pulmonary infiltrates. Which of the following is likely to be found with an immunofluorescence study of the glomeruli and alveoli?

   (A) Electron-dense humps on the epithelial side of basement membrane

   (B) Linear IgG deposits on alveolar and glomerular basement membranes

   (C) Mesangial deposition of IgA

   (D) Spike and dome IgG deposits on the glomerular basement membrane

3. A farmer develops acute attacks of fever, dyspnea, cough, and leukocytosis whenever he works around wet, harvested hay. Lung biopsy would be most likely to show which of the following?

   (A) Alveoli filled with dense, amorphous, proteinaceous material

   (B) Ferruginous bodies

   (C) Interstitial pneumonitis with eosinophils, and interstitial fibrosis

   (D) Interstitial pneumonitis with lymphocytes, plasma cells, and macrophages, and interstitial fibrosis

   (E) Linear immune deposition along the alveolar basement membrane

4. A 57-year-old man who has lived in New York City his entire life comes to the emergency department because of chest pain and shortness of breath. He is diagnosed with a massive pulmonary embolism and dies before receiving treatment. An autopsy confirms the diagnosis and also reveals a soft, yellow, greasy, grossly enlarged liver. Histologic evaluation of the liver shows lipid accumulation within the hepatocytes, compressing and displacing the nucleus to the periphery of the hepatocyte. Which of the following is the most likely cause of these hepatic findings?

   (A) Alcohol abuse

   (B) Carbon tetrachloride exposure

   (C) Diabetes mellitus

   (D) Malnutrition

   (E) Obesity

**KAPLAN) MEDICAL**

5.  A 25-year-old man presents to his physician after finding a lump in the left side of his neck. He also states that he has recently lost 10 pounds and sometimes awakens dripping in sweat. Biopsy of a cervical node reveals Reed-Sternberg cells. The remainder of his workup reveals nodal involvement limited to the neck and axilla. How should his disease be staged?

    (A) IA

    (B) IB

    (C) IIA

    (D) IIB

    (E) IIIA

    (F) IIIB

    (G) IVA

    (H) IVB

6.  A 60-year-old man complains of difficulty arising from a chair and initiating new movements. On examination, the physician notices a resting hand tremor and cogwheel rigidity. Which of the following amino acids is the precursor for the neurotransmitter that is deficient in the brain of this patient?

    (A) Glutamate

    (B) Glycine

    (C) Histidine

    (D) Tryptophan

    (E) Tyrosine

7.  A patient with a history of easy bruising is diagnosed with Bernard-Soulier syndrome. Which of the following would you expect to find in this patient?

    (A) Decreased circulating von Willebrand factor (vWF)

    (B) Prolonged bleeding time

    (C) Prolonged partial thromboplastin time (PTT)

    (D) Prolonged prothrombin time (PT)

    (E) Thrombocytopenia

8.  A normal ovum is fertilized by two separate sperm. All genetic material is retained. Which of the following terms best describes the product of this conception?

    (A) Complete hydatidiform mole

    (B) Normal infant

    (C) Partial hydatidiform mole

    (D) Placenta accreta

    (E) Placenta previa

9.  A neurologic examination of a 47-year-old woman reveals a normal corneal reflex in her right eye, but no consensual corneal reflex in her left eye. Which of the following additional findings might be expected?

    (A) Absence of pupillary light reflex of the left eye

    (B) Hyperacusis of the left ear

    (C) Inability to abduct the right eye

    (D) Loss of pain and temperature of the left face

    (E) Loss of taste from the anterior two thirds of the right tongue

    (F) Ptosis of the left eye

10. A 25-year-old woman presents with a 12-month history of palpitations, intermittent diarrhea, anxiety, and a 1-month history of "bulging of both eyes." What is the most likely cause of her symptoms?

    (A) Graves disease

    (B) Hashimoto thyroiditis

    (C) Multinodular toxic goiter

    (D) Papillary carcinoma

    (E) Subacute thyroiditis

11. A 17-year-old girl complains of fatigue. She has difficulty making it through the entire school day. She recently began to feel her heart beating in her chest. Examination shows pale mucosal membranes. A peripheral blood smear shows hypochromic, microcytic red blood cells. Which of the following is the most likely diagnosis?

    (A) Folate deficiency

    (B) Hereditary spherocytosis

    (C) Iron deficiency anemia

    (D) Sickle cell anemia

    (E) Vitamin $B_{12}$ deficiency

12. A 67-year-old woman with advanced metastatic breast cancer comes to the clinic for a followup visit. Her chief complaint at this time is weight loss and a reduced appetite. She is very concerned because she believes that this is making her very weak and she is therefore not able to "do much during these final days." Which of the following is thought to be a major contributor to her chief complaint?

    (A) Clathrin

    (B) Histamine

    (C) Interferon

    (D) Interleukin-2

    (E) Tumor necrosis factor (TNF)

13. A 47-year-old alcoholic presents with acute upper left abdominal pain with tenderness on palpation. The pain is referred to his back. Laboratory results reveal a low serum calcium level. His hypocalcemia probably reflects which of the following?

    (A) Caseous necrosis

    (B) Coagulative necrosis

    (C) Enzymatic fat necrosis

    (D) Gangrenous necrosis

    (E) Liquefactive necrosis

14. A 70-year-old woman presents to her physician prior to beginning chemotherapy for newly diagnosed small cell lung carcinoma. Her examination is notable for obesity, blood pressure of 180/110 mm Hg, facial hair, abdominal striae, and an acneiform rash on her chest and back. Laboratory values are normal except for a serum glucose of 250 mg/dL. Her chest x-ray film shows a right perihilar mass and severe diffuse osteoporosis. Which of the following most likely accounts for her physical examination, laboratory, and x-ray findings?

    (A) Adrenal gland destruction by metastases

    (B) Anterior pituitary gland disruption by metastases

    (C) Ectopic production of corticotropin (ACTH)

    (D) Ectopic production of gastrin

    (E) Ectopic production of parathyroid hormone (PTH)

15. A 35-year-old woman presents to her physician with paresthesias of the left shoulder and arm. She has also noticed a hard, bony structure on the left side of her neck above the clavicle. Which of the following diagnoses best accounts for her symptoms?

    (A) Horner syndrome

    (B) Osteopetrosis

    (C) Pancoast tumor

    (D) Shoulder dislocation

    (E) Thoracic outlet obstruction

16. A young girl develops dilation of the lateral ventricles as a consequence of a massive astrocytoma involving the cerebellum and compressing the fourth ventricle. Which of the following is the most likely diagnosis?

    (A) Arnold Chiari malformation

    (B) Communicating hydrocephalus

    (C) Dandy-Walker syndrome

    (D) Noncommunicating hydrocephalus

    (E) Syringomyelia

17. A 60-year-old alcoholic with a 50 pack-year history of smoking presents with hoarseness and dysphagia. Physical examination reveals cervical lymphadenopathy. Laryngoscopy reveals an ulcerated nodule on the laryngeal surface. Which of the following is the most likely diagnosis?

    (A) Adenocarcinoma

    (B) Anaplastic carcinoma

    (C) Malignant papilloma

    (D) Squamous cell carcinoma

    (E) Transitional cell carcinoma

18. A patient presents to the emergency department in the middle of the night with acute abdominal pain. Which of the following descriptions of the patient's pain would be consistent with a diagnosis of diverticulitis?

    (A) Burning substernal pain after meals

    (B) Severe, diffuse ache in the periumbilical region

    (C) Steady ache in the left lower quadrant with referral to the back

    (D) Steady, boring epigastric pain with referral to the back

    (E) Sudden, severe pain in the lower quadrant with referral to the flank

19. A 60-year-old alcoholic who appears malnourished presents to his physician complaining of shortness of breath and gasping for air on awakening. Cardiac exam reveals an S3 heart sound, a diastolic murmur, and jugular venous distention. Pulmonary rales and peripheral edema are evident. An echocardiogram would be expected to reveal which of the following?

    (A) A carotid pulse tracing with spike and dome configuration

    (B) Bilateral atrial enlargement and ventricular thickening

    (C) Depressed left ventricular function with pericardial effusion

    (D) Left and right ventricular dilatation with poor contraction throughout

    (E) Left ventricular hypertrophy with asymmetric septal hypertrophy

**KAPLAN)** MEDICAL

20. A 67-year-old man presents with decreased sensation and tingling in his fingers and toes. He appears fatigued and malnourished. Physical examination is remarkable for hyperactive deep tendon reflexes, spasticity, and the presence of Romberg sign. Blood tests reveal a hematocrit of 22% and a hemoglobin level of 6 mg/dL. What other hematologic values would be expected in this patient?

|  | MCV | Reticulocyte Count | WBC Count | Folate Level | Target Cells | Hypersegmented Neutrophils |
|---|---|---|---|---|---|---|
| (A) | 65 | Increased | Low | Normal | None | None |
| (B) | 85 | Normal/Low | Normal | Low | None | Present |
| (C) | 110 | Normal/Low | Low | Normal | None | Present |
| (D) | 115 | Increased | Normal | Normal | None | Present |
| (E) | 120 | Increased | Normal | Normal | Present | None |

21. A 64-year-old man presents with increased language output, most of which is incomprehensible. Neurologic testing reveals that he cannot comprehend verbal or written language. What is the location of his lesion?

    (A) Basal ganglia
    (B) Diencephalon
    (C) Frontal lobe
    (D) Occipital lobe
    (E) Parietal lobe
    (F) Temporal lobe

22. A 34-year-old woman who has had no prenatal care comes to the emergency department at 39 weeks' gestation because of contractions and a loss of fluid. She delivers an apparently healthy girl 4 hours later. The medical student in the room cuts the umbilical cord and places the placenta in a container. While examining the neonate, the pediatricians become concerned because of uncontrolled bleeding from the umbilical stump. This finding suggests a deficiency of which of the following coagulation factors?

    (A) Factor VIII
    (B) Factor IX
    (C) Factor XII
    (D) Factor XIII
    (E) Von Willebrand's factor

23. Which of the following Starling force changes is the primary cause of the edema seen in patients with nephrotic syndrome?

    (A) Decreased capillary hydrostatic pressure ($P_c$)
    (B) Decreased capillary oncotic pressure ($\pi_c$)
    (C) Decreased interstitial hydrostatic pressure ($P_i$)
    (D) Decreased interstitial oncotic pressure ($\pi_i$)
    (E) Increased capillary hydrostatic pressure ($P_c$)
    (F) Increased capillary oncotic pressure ($\pi_c$)
    (G) Increased interstitial hydrostatic pressure ($P_i$)
    (H) Increased interstitial oncotic pressure ($\pi_i$)

24. A 68-year-old woman who recently had a cholecystectomy develops a temperature of 103.0 F and has persistent drainage from her biliary catheter. She is given cephalothin and gentamicin for 10 days. Her serum creatinine level increases to 7.6 mg/dL. Her urine output is 1.3 L/day and has not diminished over the past few days. There is no history of hypotension, and her vital signs are normal. Renal ultrasonography shows no evidence of obstruction. The most likely etiology of the patient's condition is which of the following?

    (A) Acute glomerulonephritis
    (B) Acute renal failure secondary to cephalothin
    (C) Gentamicin nephrotoxicity
    (D) Renal artery occlusion
    (E) Sepsis

25. A 52-year-old woman complains of sudden visual abnormalities. She has a 30 pack-year history of smoking, as well as hypertension, and hypercholesterolemia. A head CT shows a lesion in the right occipital lobe, and an angiogram reveals an embolic stroke of the right posterior cerebral artery. Which of the following types of visual deficits is she most likely experiencing?

    (A) Bitemporal hemianopia

    (B) Central scotoma

    (C) Left homonymous hemianopia

    (D) Left superior quadrantanopia

    (E) Right homonymous hemianopia

    (F) Right superior quadrantanopia

    (G) Total left eye blindness

    (H) Total right eye blindness

26. A 46-year-old woman has bone pain. Radiographic evaluation reveals a bone mass in the femur. Histologic evaluation of a bone biopsy taken from the mass reveals the accumulation of osteoclasts, reactive multinucleated giant cells, and hemosiderin deposits in areas of microfracture. Which of the following is the most likely diagnosis?

    (A) Cushing syndrome

    (B) Graves disease

    (C) Hyperparathyroidism

    (D) Hypoparathyroidism

    (E) Hypothyroidism

27. A neonate is admitted to the neonatal intensive care unit because of respiratory distress. His mother did not receive any prenatal care. Despite treatment, at 2 weeks of age the boy dies of respiratory distress syndrome. The mother grants permission for an autopsy. Histologic evaluation of his lungs will most likely reveal which of the following findings?

    (A) Alveoli filled with neutrophils

    (B) Dense fibrosis of the alveolar walls

    (C) Enlarged air spaces

    (D) Hyaline membranes and collapsed alveoli

    (E) Normal lung histology for age

28. An abdominal x-ray performed on a 54-year-old man demonstrates a large, irregular, calcified mass with multiple broad projections filling one renal pelvis. Which of the following laboratory findings might be expected in this patient?

    (A) Decreased urine pH

    (B) Hypercalcemia

    (C) Hyperuricemia

    (D) Increased ammonia concentration in the urine

    (E) Increased cystine concentration in the urine

29. A 37-year-old woman comes to the emergency department because of a severe headache and a stiff neck. The headache came on suddenly when she was getting ready to go to work, and the nuchal rigidity began soon after. A lumbar puncture reveals grossly bloody cerebrospinal fluid with an elevated opening pressure, high protein, and low glucose. Which of the following is the most likely diagnosis?

    (A) Amyloid angiopathy

    (B) Hypertensive vascular changes

    (C) Rupture of a berry aneurysm

    (D) Tear of bridging veins

    (E) Tear of middle meningeal artery

30. A premature infant develops progressive difficulty breathing over the first few days of life. Deficient surfactant synthesis by which of the following cell types may have contributed to the infant's respiratory problems?

    (A) Alveolar capillary endothelial cells

    (B) Bronchial mucous cells

    (C) Bronchial respiratory epithelium

    (D) Type I pneumocytes

    (E) Type II pneumocytes

31. A chronic alcoholic presents with confusion, impaired balance, and nystagmus. Administration of thiamine leads to rapid symptomatic improvement. Which of the following neuropathologic changes accounts for this presentation?

    (A) Axonal degeneration of posterior and lateral columns of spinal cord

    (B) Demyelination affecting the central region of basis pontis

    (C) Demyelination involving corpus callosum and anterior commissure

    (D) Hemorrhagic necrosis of mammillary bodies and periaqueductal gray matter

    (E) Loss of neocortical neurons, Purkinje cells, and hippocampal pyramidal neurons

32. An HIV-positive, 38-year-old woman is suspected of having a B-cell lymphoma. Which of the following pathologic findings would be most likely in this patient?

    (A) Evidence of infection with human T-cell leukemia virus-1

    (B) Greatly elevated levels of serum IgG

    (C) Greatly elevated levels of serum IgM

    (D) Positive Epstein-Barr virus (EBV) titer

    (E) Presence of Bence-Jones proteins in a urine sample

    (F) Presence of Reed-Sternberg cells in a lymph node biopsy

    (G) Translocation between chromosomes 9 and 22 in white blood cells

33. A 59-year-old retired construction worker comes to the physician for a periodic health maintenance examination. He has no complaints at this time. He is generally healthy, exercises regularly, does not smoke cigarettes, and drinks a few bottles of beer a week. He has a history of asbestos exposure. Physical examination is unremarkable. Which of the following malignancies is most likely to occur in this patient?

    (A) Bladder carcinoma

    (B) Bronchogenic carcinoma

    (C) Lymphoma

    (D) Malignant mesothelioma

    (E) Scrotal carcinoma

34. A 76-year-old man presents to his physician complaining of an inability to empty his bladder for the past 3 days and a continual leakage of urine for the past 2 days. A cystometrogram reveals that his bladder has an abnormally large capacity, and an MRI reveals a lesion limited to the sacral spinal cord. Which of the following is the most likely diagnosis?

    (A) Automatic neurogenic bladder

    (B) Autonomous neurogenic bladder

    (C) Motor neurogenic bladder

    (D) Sensory neurogenic bladder

    (E) Uninhibited neurogenic bladder

35. A 70-year-old woman undergoes a bilateral hip replacement for osteoarthritis. Which of the following pathologic changes will the removed femoral heads most likely demonstrate?

    (A) Marked synovial proliferation with pannus formation

    (B) Multiple small fractures in the cartilage

    (C) Multiple white flecks in the synovium

    (D) No visible change

    (E) Pus covering the articular surface

36. A 60-year-old man who is being evaluated for abdominal pain and a 30-lb weight loss undergoes endoscopy, which demonstrates a broad region of the gastric wall in which the rugae are flattened. Biopsy of this area shows infiltration by numerous polygonal tumor cells with small, dark, round, or ovoid nuclei pushed to the margin of the cell by large, clear, cytoplasmic structures. These cells might be expected to have which of the following properties?

    (A) Keratohyalin granules observed by electron microscopy

    (B) Melanosomes and premelanosomes by electron microscopy

    (C) Positive staining for gastrin by light microscopy

    (D) Positive staining for leukocyte common antigen by light microscopy

    (E) Positive staining for mucin by light microscopy

37. A 30-year-old woman is diagnosed with cervical intraep-ithelial neoplasia (CIN) associated with a previous viral infection. Which of the following viral products is (are) implicated in producing this type of dysplasia?

    (A) EBNA proteins

    (B) E1A and E1B proteins

    (C) E6 and E7 proteins

    (D) Large tumor antigen

38. A tall man with gynecomastia and testicular atrophy has a testicular biopsy that shows sparse, completely hyalinized seminiferous tubules with a complete absence of germ cells and only rare Sertoli cells. Leydig cells are present in large clumps between the hyalinized tubules. Which of the following genetic disorders should be suspected?

    (A) Testicular feminization syndrome

    (B) Trisomy 18

    (C) Trisomy 21

    (D) 45,XO

    (E) 47,XXY

39. A male infant begins to have persistent, projectile, non-bilious vomiting at age 2 to 3 weeks. Which of the fol-lowing conditions is likely responsible for these symp-toms?

    (A) Caroli disease

    (B) Cystic fibrosis

    (C) Diaphragmatic hernia

    (D) Gastric ulcer

    (E) Pyloric stenosis

40. A patient with severe iron-deficiency anemia refractory to oral ferrous sulfate therapy is given multiple blood transfusions in preparation for surgery. She develops hemosiderosis. Which of the following microscopic findings would be expected?

    (A) Hepatocytes damaged by intracellular iron accu-mulation

    (B) Intense lysosomal staining with methylene blue

    (C) Storage of excess copper in hepatocytes

    (D) Yellow-brown granules in cell cytoplasm

41. Over a span of years, an individual develops thickening of the fascia of one palm, which eventually causes a flex-ion contracture of the hand, most markedly involving the fourth and fifth fingers. The patient most probably has which of the following conditions?

    (A) Desmoid

    (B) Dupuytren contracture

    (C) Neurofibroma

    (D) Peyronie disease

    (E) Plantar fibromatosis

42. A 25-year-old woman is discovered on physical exam to have a midsystolic click and a high-pitched heart mur-mur. Which of the following additional cardiovascular findings is she most likely to exhibit?

    (A) Atrial fibrillation

    (B) Decreased peripheral pulse pressure

    (C) Premature ventricular contractions

    (D) Slowed carotid upstroke

    (E) Wide pulse pressure

43. A patient presents with hypertension, hypernatremia, hypokalemia, low renin levels, and metabolic alkalosis. Which of the following is the most likely diagnosis?

    (A) Bartter syndrome

    (B) Conn syndrome

    (C) Empty sella syndrome

    (D) Kimmelstiel-Wilson syndrome

    (E) Sheehan syndrome

    (F) Waterhouse-Friderichsen syndrome

44. A child with cystic fibrosis presents with signs of a bleeding diathesis. Deficiency in which of the following factors is the most likely cause of this child's coagulo-pathy?

    (A) Factor V

    (B) Factor VIII

    (C) Factor XII

    (D) Protein C

    (E) Prothrombin

45. A 64-year-old man with atherosclerosis suffers an embolic stroke that leaves him with a left leg paresis. Physical examination reveals a Babinski sign on the left and diminished sensation over his left leg. Blockade of which of the following vessels is responsible for his symptoms?

    (A) Left anterior cerebral artery

    (B) Left middle cerebral artery

    (C) Left posterior cerebral artery

    (D) Right anterior cerebral artery

    (E) Right middle cerebral artery

    (F) Right posterior cerebral artery

46. A 42-year-old man develops acute renal failure. Laboratory studies also reveal hypocalcemia. What is the most likely mechanism underlying this electrolyte disturbance?

    (A) Hyperphosphatemia

    (B) Hyponatremia

    (C) Increased sensitivity to 1,25-dihydroxyvitamin D

    (D) Increased sensitivity to parathyroid hormone (PTH)

    (E) Metabolic alkalosis

47. A patient with lung cancer has one lung removed. When he is at rest, his pulmonary artery pressure is within normal limits. However, when he tries to exercise, the pulmonary artery pressure rises rapidly. Which of the following best explains this finding?

    (A) The airway resistance of the lung is limiting during exercise

    (B) The compliance of the lung limits blood flow

    (C) Pulmonary vessels constrict during exercise

    (D) Recruitment of additional pulmonary vessels is not adequate during exercise

    (E) The volume of the single lung is inadequate during exercise

48. A 4-year-old child with chronic tonsillitis presents with a swollen cervical lymph node. Biopsy of the node would most likely reveal which of the following?

    (A) Acute nonspecific lymphadenitis

    (B) Follicular hyperplasia form of chronic nonspecific lymphadenitis

    (C) Hodgkin lymphoma

    (D) Paracortical lymphoid hyperplasia form of chronic nonspecific lymphadenitis

    (E) Sinus histiocytosis form of chronic nonspecific lymphadenitis

49. A 30-year-old woman complains of breast tenderness that becomes worse during the premenstrual period. Multiple small masses are appreciable on palpation. Cytologic examination of a fine needle aspirate reveals no malignant cells. A subsequent biopsy shows multifocal cyst formation, areas of fibrosis, calcification, and apocrine metaplasia. This condition is associated with an increased risk of cancer if

    (A) apocrine metaplasia is marked

    (B) calcification is prominent

    (C) cysts are larger than 0.5 cm

    (D) epithelial hyperplasia is florid

    (E) fibrosis is predominant

50. A 70-year-old woman dies 3 days after admission to the ICU. The clinical picture is characterized by fever, purulent sputum, and pulmonary infiltrates on chest radiograph. An autopsy shows patchy areas of consolidation in both lungs, with neutrophilic exudate filling bronchi and bronchioles on microscopic examination. Gram staining reveals colonies of small gram-negative bacilli. Which of the following is the most likely diagnosis?

    (A) Anaerobic pneumonia

    (B) Community-acquired pneumonia

    (C) Hospital-acquired pneumonia

    (D) Lipid pneumonia

    (E) Primary atypical pneumonia

# Pathology and Pathophysiology Test Four:
# Answers and Explanations

## ANSWER KEY

| | | | |
|---|---|---|---|
| 1. | A | 26. | C |
| 2. | B | 27. | D |
| 3. | D | 28. | D |
| 4. | A | 29. | C |
| 5. | D | 30. | E |
| 6. | E | 31. | D |
| 7. | B | 32. | D |
| 8. | C | 33. | B |
| 9. | B | 34. | B |
| 10. | A | 35. | B |
| 11. | C | 36. | E |
| 12. | E | 37. | C |
| 13. | C | 38. | E |
| 14. | C | 39. | E |
| 15. | E | 40. | D |
| 16. | D | 41. | B |
| 17. | D | 42. | C |
| 18. | C | 43. | B |
| 19. | D | 44. | E |
| 20. | C | 45. | D |
| 21. | F | 46. | A |
| 22. | D | 47. | D |
| 23. | B | 48. | B |
| 24. | C | 49. | D |
| 25. | C | 50. | C |

1. **The correct answer is A.** The presentation in the question stem is classic for Henoch-Schönlein purpura. The distinctive renal biopsy finding is deposition of IgA (together with IgG and complement) in the mesangium of the glomeruli. IgA can also be present in small dermal vessels within the characteristic skin lesions, which consist of subepidermal hemorrhages with necrotizing vasculitis. Vasculitis (**choice E**) can also be present in gastrointestinal organs (hence the abdominal symptoms) but is not present in the kidney. The condition typically occurs in young children, between the ages of 3 and 8 years, but it can occur in adults. Adults are more likely to develop severe renal disease with crescentic glomerulonephritis. The clinical course is variable; patients who have more extensive renal damage and proteinuria are more likely to progress to eventual renal failure. Some patients have recurrent hematuria for years.

Subepithelial electron dense "humps" (**choice C**) are a feature of post-streptococcal glomerulonephritis, which can also follow an upper respiratory infection but differs from Henoch-Schönlein purpura by the absence of vasculitis and purpura.

Interstitial nephritis (**choice B**) and tumor (**choice D**) are distracters that are unrelated to Henoch-Schönlein purpura.

2. **The correct answer is B.** This is a classic case of Goodpasture syndrome, which is autoimmune in origin and characterized by hemorrhagic pneumonitis leading to hemoptysis and glomerulonephritis progressing to renal failure. Most cases involve the presence of anti-basement membrane antibodies. It occurs mostly in young men. Under immunofluorescence, there are linear deposits of IgG on alveolar and glomerular basement membranes.

Electron-dense humps (**choice A**) are found with electron microscopy, not immunofluorescence. These humps are found in poststreptococcal glomerulonephritis; immunofluorescence in this case would show C3, IgM, and IgG granular deposits.

Mesangial deposition of IgA (**choice C**) occurs in Berger disease or IgA nephropathy.

Spike and dome IgG deposits (**choice D**) are found in membranous nephropathy, a cause of the nephrotic syndrome.

3. **The correct answer is D.** Hypersensitivity pneumonitis constitutes a spectrum of interstitial lung disorders that occur in response to a variety of environmental (often occupational) antigens. Farmer's lung, which this patient has, is one example of a hypersensitivity pneu-

monitis and is related to antigens found in the spores of thermophilic actinomycetes, which grow in warm, moist hay. Other examples of hypersensitivity pneumonitis include pigeon breeder's lung (bird excreta), humidifier lung (thermophilic bacteria), and mushroom picker's lung. Although one might expect to see eosinophils, the interstitial pneumonitis is instead composed of lymphocytes, plasma cells, and macrophages. Long-standing cases additionally show permanent disease features that may include interstitial fibrosis, obliterative bronchiolitis, and granuloma formation.

Alveoli filled with dense, amorphous, proteinaceous material (**choice A**) are a feature of pulmonary alveolar proteinosis.

Ferruginous bodies (**choice B**) are a feature of asbestosis.

Interstitial pneumonitis with eosinophils and interstitial fibrosis (**choice C**) is a feature of Loeffler syndrome.

Linear deposition of antibody and complement along the alveolar basement membrane (**choice E**) is a feature of Goodpasture syndrome.

4. **The correct answer is A.** All the conditions listed can cause steatosis (fatty change) of the liver. In industrialized nations, however, the most common cause is alcohol abuse. The steatosis may take the form of either microsteatosis (multiple, very small, lipid vacuoles) or macrosteatosis (a single, large, coalesced lipid vacuole in each cell); the two forms may also coexist. The triglyceride accumulation underlying the changes is related to alcohol-induced damage to mitochondrial and microsomal functions that normally degrade triglycerides.

5. **The correct answer is D.** This patient has Hodgkin disease (Reed-Sternberg cells were the classic clue), affecting more than one lymph node region but limited to one side of the diaphragm. This corresponds to Stage II (Stage I is only one node region; Stage III is both sides of diaphragm; Stage IV means disseminated disease to nonlymphoid organs). The A/B designation depends on the presence of constitutional symptoms such as weight loss, fever, chills, or night sweats. A = no constitutional symptoms, and B = presence of constitutional symptoms. Therefore, this patient has Stage IIB disease.

6. **The correct answer is E.** This question requires three steps of logic. First, figure out the diagnosis (a classic case of Parkinson disease), then remember which neurotransmitter is involved in the disease (dopamine), and, finally, recall which amino acid serves as the precursor for that neurotransmitter (tyrosine). The hydroxylation of tyrosine by tyrosine hydroxylase results in DOPA, which is then decarboxylated to

dopamine. Note that norepinephrine and epinephrine are also tyrosine derivatives, as are the melanins and the thyroid hormones thyroxine and triiodothyronine.

Glutamate (**choice A**) can be converted to the inhibitory neurotransmitter GABA by the action of glutamate decarboxylase.

Glycine (**choice B**) is involved in the synthesis of both creatine (along with arginine and S-adenosylmethionine) and heme (along with succinyl-CoA).

Histidine (**choice C**) can be decarboxylated to histamine, an important inflammatory mediator.

Tryptophan (**choice D**) can be converted to serotonin by a hydroxylation reaction (tryptophan hydroxylase) followed by a decarboxylation reaction.

7. **The correct answer is B.** Bernard-Soulier syndrome is caused by a deficiency in the platelet membrane glycoprotein GPIb. GPIb serves as the platelet receptor for von Willebrand factor (vWF), which, in turn, is required for normal platelet adhesion to exposed collagen. A defect in platelet adhesion will result in a prolonged bleeding time. Remember that the bleeding time is a measure of platelet plug formation; it is not related to the functioning of the coagulation cascade.

Although vWF will not be able to bind to platelets in patients with Bernard-Soulier, the amount of vWF will not be affected (**choice A**).

As noted above, platelet adhesion defects do not affect the functioning of the coagulation cascade; thus, patients with Bernard-Soulier will have a normal PTT (**choice C**) and PT (**choice D**).

Bernard-Soulier represents a qualitative, not a quantitative, platelet defect. These patients do not have thrombocytopenia (**choice E**).

8. **The correct answer is C.** Hydatidiform moles can be considered an aberrant form of pregnancy. The moles are found in the uterus and are characterized by dilated chorionic villi and production of human chorionic gonadotropin (hCG). Moles are subclassified into partial moles (which contain a triploid genome derived from the egg and two sperm) and complete moles (which contain a diploid genome derived completely from one duplicated or two separate sperm with loss of maternal genetic material; **choice A**). The two types can be distinguished grossly (partial moles have fewer enlarged villi) and microscopically (partial moles often have blood vessels containing fetal erythrocytes). Treatment is by removal of the mole with followup of serum hCG levels.

Fertilization of an egg by two sperm is not generally associated with placental abnormalities (**choices D and E**).

9. **The correct answer is B.** The first trick to this question is to determine where the lesion is. The corneal reflex is tested by touching a cotton wisp to the eye. A normal response would be blinking of the ipsilateral eye as well as the contralateral eye (consensual reflex). The afferent limb of the corneal reflex is contained within the ophthalmic division of the ipsilateral ophthalmic nerve (V1), the efferent limb is by both (right and left) facial nerves (VII). This woman had a normal corneal reflex in her right eye, indicating a normal right V1 and right VII. However, she lacked a consensual reflex, indicating an abnormal left VIIth nerve. The next trick to this question is to determine what other signs a lesion in the left VIIth nerve could produce. A lesion in the left VIIth would also produce hyperacusis (increased sensitivity to sound) in the left ear because of paralysis of the stapedius muscle, which ordinarily dampens sound transmission through the middle ear.

Absence of a pupillary light reflex of the left eye (**choice A**) could be caused either by a lesion of the left optic nerve (CN II; afferent limb) or by a lesion of the left oculomotor nerve (CN III; efferent limb).

Inability to abduct the right eye (**choice C**) could be caused by a lesion of the right abducens nerve (CN VI), which innervates the lateral rectus muscle.

Loss of pain and temperature of the left face (**choice D**) could be caused by a lesion of the spinal nucleus of V. This nucleus is located in the medulla and receives pain and temperature information from the face via the trigeminal nerve (CN V).

Loss of taste from the anterior two thirds of the right tongue (**choice E**) could result from a lesion of the *right* CN VII.

Ptosis of the left eye (**choice F**) could result from a lesion of the left oculomotor nerve (CN III) because of denervation of the levator palpebrae muscle. A lesion of the left VII would result in the inability to close the left eye.

10. **The correct answer is A.** Graves disease is the most common cause of hyperthyroidism in a young female and is the only one that causes exophthalmos ("bulging of both eyes"). Graves disease is an autoimmune disorder in which a thyroid-stimulating IgG immunoglobulin (TSI) binds to the thyroid-stimulating hormone (TSH) receptors, causing increased release of thyroid hormone. The exophthalmos is caused by lymphocytic infiltration of the extraocular muscles.

Hashimoto thyroiditis (**choice B**) results in hypothyroidism and is associated with a diffusely enlarged thyroid gland and antimicrosomal antibodies against the thyroid parenchyma.

Multinodular toxic goiter (**choice C**) causes hyperthyroidism but does not result in exophthalmos.

Papillary carcinoma (**choice D**) will only very rarely present as a hypersecreting nodule. Most cases will be nonsecreting, cold nodules. There is no exophthalmos. This is the most common thyroid cancer and has the best prognosis of all thyroid cancers.

Subacute thyroiditis (**choice E**) is an uncommon form of thyroiditis that lasts approximately 8 months and is self-limited. Early on, with destruction of thyroid tissue, there may be release of thyroid hormone and symptoms of hyperthyroidism, but exophthalmos is generally absent.

11. **The correct answer is C.** Conditions that produce microcytic anemia include iron deficiency, thalassemia minor, anemia of chronic disease, and the anemia produced by erythrocyte fragmentation.

Folate deficiency (**choice A**) and vitamin $B_{12}$ deficiency (**choice E**) usually produce a macrocytic anemia.

Hereditary spherocytosis (**choice B**) and sickle cell anemia (**choice D**) usually produce an anemia with cells of normal volume.

12. **The correct answer is E.** Weight loss of more than 5% of body weight is considered a very adverse prognostic feature in cancer since it usually indicates the presence of widespread disease. (Uncommonly, a relatively small primary lesion that has not yet metastasized can cause cachexia.) Both tumor necrosis factor (TNF) and interleukin 1-beta have been implicated in the production of cachexia with weight loss, loss of appetite, and alteration in taste. Large tumor burdens may additionally alter protein and energy balance, often with negative nitrogen balance. Therapy, in whatever form (surgery, radiation, chemotherapy), may also contribute to cachexia late in the course secondary to effects on the digestive system.

Clathrin (**choice A**) is a protein that helps to form pinocytotic vesicles.

Histamine (**choice B**) is released by mast cells and basophils and contributes to allergic responses.

Interferon (**choice C**) is important in the body's response to viral infection.

Interleukin 1-beta, not 2 (**choice D**), is produced by activated monocytes and macrophages and has been implicated in cachexia. Interleukin 2 is released by helper T cells and augments B-cell growth as well as antibody production.

13. **The correct answer is C.** The patient most likely has acute pancreatitis, which is commonly caused by either alcoholism or impaction of a small gallstone in the common bile duct. Acute pancreatitis causes the release of many digestive enzyme precursors, which are then converted to the active form in the damaged tissues. These enzymes degrade the adipose tissue around the pancreatic lobules, producing enzymatic fat necrosis. As part of this process, many free fatty acids are produced that can bind as soaps with extracellular calcium in chemical equilibrium with serum calcium. This will often cause a significant decrease in serum calcium levels.

Caseous necrosis (**choice A**) is seen in granulomata produced by infection with *Mycobacterium tuberculosis*.

Coagulative necrosis (**choice B**) preserves the outlines of cells in affected tissue. This common type of necrosis is seen in the heart following an infarct.

Gangrenous necrosis (**choice D**) is massive necrosis associated with loss of vascular supply and is generally accompanied by bacterial infection.

Liquefactive necrosis (**choice E**) results in liquefaction of tissues due to the release of lysosomal enzymes. Cellular outlines are not preserved. This type of necrosis characterizes bacterial infections and CNS infarcts.

14. **The correct answer is C.** This woman has all the classic findings of Cushing syndrome: obesity, hypertension, hirsutism, acne, striae, glucose intolerance, and osteoporosis. Cushing syndrome may be caused by excess production of cortisol due to bilateral adrenal hyperplasia or an adrenal neoplasm; by excess production of corticotropin (ACTH) by a pituitary adenoma; or by ectopic production of ACTH by a tumor, most commonly a small cell lung carcinoma (major clue in the question stem!).

Destruction of the adrenal glands bilaterally (**choice A**) or of the anterior pituitary by metastases (**choice B**) would cause a deficiency of cortisol and ACTH, respectively, and would lead to a syndrome of cortisol deficiency with orthostatic hypotension, malaise, nausea, and weight loss.

Ectopic production of gastrin (**choice D**), as seen in Zollinger-Ellison syndrome, causes severe refractory peptic ulcer disease.

Ectopic production of parathyroid hormone (PTH; **choice E**), which can be seen in squamous cell lung carcinoma, would result in hypercalcemia.

15. **The correct answer is E.** The patient has a left cervical rib. This anatomic variant, which is typically bilateral but can occur on only one side, is due to formation of an extra rib at the C7 level. Cervical ribs, while often asymptomatic, can cause thoracic outlet obstruction. This results in pain due to distortion of blood vessels;

pain or paresthesias related to brachial plexus impingement (notably sensory disturbances in the distribution of the ulnar nerve); and palpable abnormalities in the greater supraclavicular fossa.

Horner syndrome (ptosis, anhidrosis, and miosis; **choice A**) occurs with Pancoast tumors (**choice C**) at the apex of the lung, as well as with certain brainstem or spinal cord lesions.

Osteopetrosis (**choice B**) is a hereditary disease characterized by increased density and thickening of bone cortex with narrowing of medullary cavities. Bones are brittle and fracture easily.

Shoulder dislocation (**choice D**) does not present with a supraclavicular bony structure.

16. **The correct answer is D.** Noncommunicating hydrocephalus is caused by a block in cerebrospinal fluid (CSF) circulation in the ventricles or in the foramina of Luschka and Magendie, by which the fourth ventricle communicates with the subarachnoid space. Tumor compression of the fourth ventricle is a good example of acquired noncommunicating hydrocephalus.

Arnold Chiari malformation (**choice A**) is a congenital form of noncommunicating hydrocephalus in which an elongated medulla oblongata blocks passage of CSF through the subarachnoid space at the level of the foramen magnum.

In communicating hydrocephalus (**choice B**), the block occurs outside the brain proper. The arachnoid villi (which resorb CSF in the subarachnoid space) are often dysfunctional.

Dandy-Walker syndrome (**choice C**) is a congenital, noncommunicating hydrocephalus in which a failure of development of the cerebellar vermis leads to obstruction of the foramina of Luschka and Magendie.

Syringomyelia (**choice E**) is a cystic dilatation of the spinal cord (usually cervical) that may extend into the brainstem.

17. **The correct answer is D.** Malignant tumors of the larynx are relatively uncommon, except for those arising from surface epithelium. Most occur on the vocal cords, although they can occur anywhere. 95% of laryngeal cancers are squamous cell carcinomas, which can cause hoarseness, difficulty swallowing, pain, hemoptysis, and, eventually, respiratory compromise (by obstructing the airway). Ulceration can lead to superinfection. Complications arise because of direct extension, metastases, and infection. Risk factors include smoking, alcohol abuse, and chronic irritation (as might occur in singers).

Adenocarcinomas (**choice A**), anaplastic carcinomas (**choice B**), and transitional cell carcinomas (**choice E**) usually occur in the nasopharynx.

A papilloma (**choice C**) is usually a soft, friable nodule on the true vocal cords. It frequently ulcerates and bleeds with manipulation. It appears as multiple finger-like projections composed of fibrous tissue covered with squamous epithelium. It rarely undergoes malignant transformation.

18. **The correct answer is C.** Diverticulitis commonly produces a steady, aching pain, localized to the left lower quadrant of the abdomen, with referral to the back in some cases. In addition, a mass (due to inflammation) may be appreciated on abdominal examination, and the patient may be febrile with an increased white count. Remember, if a patient presents with symptoms and signs similar to appendicitis, but the complaints concern the left rather than the right side of the abdomen, think of diverticulitis as a likely diagnosis. Also, take note that diverticul<u>osis</u>, not diverticul<u>itis</u>, is the most common cause of massive lower gastrointestinal bleeding in adults.

Burning substernal pain after meals (**choice A**) is suggestive of reflux esophagitis. The pain may be referred to the left arm.

A severe, diffuse ache in the periumbilical region (**choice B**) is suggestive of bowel infarction, although it must be distinguished from the early pain of appendicitis. The pain of bowel infarction is often aching and severe, whereas appendicitis can (but doesn't always) produce crampy pain.

Steady, boring epigastric pain with referral to the back (**choice D**) and little relation to meals may indicate pancreatitis. Nausea and vomiting frequently accompany the pain.

Sudden, severe, left lower quadrant pain that the patient describes as "tearing" or "ripping," with referral to the flank (**choice E**), may indicate a distal dissecting aortic aneurysm. The pain may also be periumbilical.

19. **The correct answer is D.** Dilated cardiomyopathy can be caused by ethanol abuse. Malnourishment often accompanies severe alcoholism and implies thiamine deficiency, which can lead to heart disease (wet beriberi). Suspect this diagnosis in any alcoholic presenting with symptoms and signs of congestive heart failure. In this patient, an echocardiogram would be expected to reveal bilateral ventricular dilatation with impaired contraction throughout both chambers.

**KAPLAN) MEDICAL**

A carotid pulse tracing with spike and dome configuration (**choice A**) and left ventricular hypertrophy with asymmetric septal hypertrophy (**choice E**) are both associated with hypertrophic cardiomyopathy, also known as idiopathic hypertrophic subaortic stenosis.

Bilateral atrial enlargement and ventricular thickening (**choice B**) is associated with restrictive cardiomyopathy. Common causes of this condition are amyloidosis (in the elderly) and sarcoidosis (in the young).

Depressed left ventricular function with pericardial effusion (**choice C**) would be consistent with myocarditis accompanied by pericarditis.

20. **The correct answer is C.** This patient's low hematocrit and hemoglobin indicate that he has an anemia. It useful to divide anemias into three categories: low mean corpuscular volume (MCV), normal MCV, and high MCV (these are referred to as micro-, normo-, and macrocytic anemias). The only anemia associated with these neurologic symptoms is a megaloblastic anemia caused by a cobalamin (vitamin $B_{12}$) deficiency. This is a macrocytic anemia characterized by hypersegmented neutrophils, leukopenia, and a normal-to-low reticulocyte count. This makes sense, since $B_{12}$ is required for DNA synthesis. Without it, RBC precursors cannot divide as often and consequently produce larger RBCs in fewer numbers, hence the high MCV and normal-to-low reticulocyte count (compare with **choices A, D, and E**). Similarly, fewer WBCs can be made. The array of neurologic symptoms is characteristic of subacute combined degeneration, caused by demyelination of the dorsal and lateral columns of the spinal cord and peripheral sensory nerves.

Although folate deficiency (**choice B**) can also cause a megaloblastic anemia, it does not cause neurologic symptoms. Also, the MCV here was too low to qualify as megaloblastic anemia.

Target cells (**choice E**) are associated with impaired hemoglobin production, as in thalassemia, and are found in micro- to normocytic anemias, not in macrocytic anemia as in this distracter.

Remember that a good way to approach questions like these is to isolate one lab value, such as MCV, in order to eliminate incorrect distracters. This will greatly facilitate solving the problem and will save you precious time.

21. **The correct answer is F.** This patient has Wernicke aphasia, which is caused by a lesion of Wernicke's area, located in the posterior part of the superior temporal gyrus (area 22) of the language-dominant hemisphere.

Lesions of the basal ganglia (**choice A**) produce extrapyramidal motor symptoms.

Lesions of the diencephalon (**choice B**), which includes the thalamus, hypothalamus, subthalamus, and epithalamus, can lead to myriad sensory, endocrine, and motor defects, but would not selectively affect language.

Lesions of the frontal lobe (**choice C**) can produce spastic paralysis, Broca's aphasia (expressive, nonfluent aphasia), disorders of higher order thinking, and deviation of the eyes. (Mnemonic: Broca's aphasia is associated with broken speech).

Lesions of the occipital lobe (**choice D**) can produce visual disturbances.

Lesions of the parietal lobe (**choice E**) can produce a variety of higher cortical dysfunctions and a loss of sensation, but would not produce the type of language problem seen in this patient.

22. **The correct answer is D.** Hereditary factor XIII deficiency is an autosomal recessive condition that is unusual among the factor deficiencies in that the presentation is often at birth, when the umbilical stump bleeds excessively, sometimes leading to the neonate's death. Factor XIII is necessary to stabilize clot formation; in its absence, clots will rapidly lyse. Cutaneous and muscular hematomas are common in affected patients. Bleeding after surgery and trauma can occur, including bleeding into the CNS. Spontaneous abortion in affected women is common. A factor XIII concentrate is available for treatment.

23. **The correct answer is B.** This question illustrates an important strategy: knowing what you're looking for before you consider the answer choices. If you thought about the answer before considering the choices, this question was very straightforward and simple. If, on the other hand, you considered each answer choice in turn, you no doubt got pretty confused and wasted a lot of precious test time.

The first thing to remember is that nephrotic syndrome is defined as proteinuria (>3.5 g/day) with concurrent hypoalbuminemia and hyperlipidemia. The loss of protein in the urine results in a decreased oncotic pressure in the vascular space (decreased $\pi_c$). This decrease in capillary oncotic pressure promotes movement of fluid into the interstitium and the development of edema. This is also the cause of edema in patients with liver disease.

Decreased interstitial oncotic pressure ($\pi_i$; **choice D**) would actually promote the movement of fluid into the vasculature; it would not lead to edema. The same thing would occur with decreased capillary hydrostatic forces ($P_c$; **choice A**).

Although decreased interstitial hydrostatic pressure ($P_i$; **choice C**) would lead to edema, it is not the mechanism of action in nephrotic syndrome.

Although increased capillary hydrostatic pressure (**choice E**) does lead to edema, it is not the mechanism at work in nephrotic syndrome. It is, however, the mechanism of edema in the setting of both congestive heart failure (increased capillary hydrostatic pressure due to inefficient pumping of the heart, leading to pooling) and glomerulonephritis (increased intravascular volume due to inefficient excretion by the kidney).

Increased capillary oncotic pressure (**choice F**) would not lead to edema.

Increased interstitial hydrostatic pressure (**choice G**) would not lead to edema.

Increased interstitial oncotic pressure (**choice H**) would cause edema, but not in the setting of nephrotic syndrome. Instead, this is the mechanism of edema (typically localized) in the setting of burns and inflammation (increased capillary permeability allows protein to leak into the interstitium and increase oncotic pressure).

24.  **The correct answer is C.** A small percentage of patients (5 to 10%) develop a nonoliguric form of acute renal failure when treated with aminoglycosides such as gentamicin. Gentamicin can accumulate in the kidneys to produce a delayed form of acute renal failure with elevation of the serum creatinine level. The nonoliguric form of renal failure seen in this patient is the typical presentation for gentamicin nephrotoxicity.

Acute glomerulonephritis (**choice A**) is typically associated with hypertension and the appearance of an active urinary sediment containing casts and red blood cells.

Cephalothin (**choice B**) is a first-generation cephalosporin commonly used in the treatment of severe infection of the genitourinary tract, gastrointestinal tract, and respiratory tract, as well as skin infections. This antibiotic can produce an acute interstitial nephritis; however, the patient's presentation is consistent with gentamicin nephrotoxicity. Interstitial nephritis is associated with acute renal failure, fever, rash, and eosinophilia.

Renal artery occlusion (**choice D**) is commonly caused by thrombosis or embolism. The clinical features of acute renal artery occlusion are hematuria, flank pain, fever, nausea, elevated LDH, elevated AST, and acute renal failure.

Since the patient has normal vital signs and no history of hypotension, a diagnosis of sepsis (**choice E**) is unlikely.

25.  **The correct answer is C.** The posterior cerebral arteries supply the cortical surfaces of the occipital and medial temporal lobes. Damage to one occipital lobe (e.g., by trauma or by ischemia/infarction due to stroke) usually produces a contralateral homonymous hemianopia. Occlusion of the right posterior cerebral artery would therefore result in a left homonymous hemianopia—blindness in the left half of the visual field in both eyes. In addition, involvement of the medial temporal lobe might give rise to peduncular hallucinosis—visual illusions or elementary (unformed) hallucinations. Bilateral lesions would cause "cortical" blindness, which does not affect the pupillary reflexes.

Bitemporal hemianopia (**choice A**) is a loss of vision in the temporal quadrants of the visual field. (It is also termed heteronymous hemianopia). This occurs in lesions of the optic chiasm, which may occur with pituitary tumors.

Central scotoma (**choice B**) is a loss of vision in the center of the visual field, with preservation of the peripheral fields. It is associated with optic neuritis, a common complication of multiple sclerosis.

Superior quadrantanopia (**choices D and F**) is caused by lesions in the upper portion of the contralateral temporal lobe.

Right homonymous hemianopia (**choice E**) would result from left posterior cerebral artery occlusion.

Total blindness in one eye (**choices G and H**) occurs when its optic nerve is severed.

26.  **The correct answer is C.** This brief histologic description refers to *brown tumors*, which develop in association with hyperparathyroidism. These lesions result from repeated microfractures, with subsequent accumulation of hemosiderin-laden macrophages and reactive osteoclastic and fibroblastic proliferation. The brown color is due to hemosiderin deposition.

Cushing syndrome (**choice A**) is caused by excess of cortisol from endogenous or exogenous sources. Administration of glucocorticoids for therapeutic purposes is the most common form. Osteoporosis is the most significant effect of excess glucocorticoids.

Graves disease (**choice B**) is due to a hyperfunctioning thyroid, stimulated by autoantibodies to TSH-receptors. Excessive production of thyroid hormone results in a complex clinical picture, in which bone changes are not seen.

Hypoparathyroidism (**choice D**) is an uncommon disorder most often due to surgical removal of the parathyroids. The most characteristic manifestation is *tetany*, resulting from decreased calcemia and consequent neuromuscular hyperexcitability.

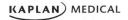

Hypothyroidism (**choice E**) is a disorder of diminished thyroid function, most commonly due to previous Hashimoto thyroiditis. If hypothyroidism is present *in utero*, infancy, or early childhood, short stature, mental retardation, and other abnormalities develop (*cretinism*).

27. **The correct answer is D.** Neonatal respiratory distress syndrome is a disease of immaturity. The immature lung is not able to produce sufficient surfactant to prevent collapse of many alveoli. Severe diffuse damage to alveoli causes precipitation of protein ("hyaline membranes") adjacent to many alveolar walls. In infants who survive, particularly if oxygen was used for therapy, the lungs eventually become heavily fibrotic (misnamed bronchopulmonary dysplasia).

    Abundant neutrophils (**choice A**) would not be seen unless the patient had also developed pneumonia.

    Fibrosis (**choice B**) is a late, not early, feature of respiratory distress syndrome.

    The air spaces are collapsed, not enlarged (**choice C**), in this condition.

    The histology in these patients is usually markedly abnormal (**not choice E**).

28. **The correct answer is D.** The patient has a stag-horn calculus. These very large calculi are almost always principally composed of magnesium ammonium phosphate (often with enough calcium to be radio-opaque) and form in the setting of infection by urea-splitting bacteria, such as *Proteus*.

    Increased urine ammonia concentrations are a byproduct of the bacterial metabolism of urea and tend to increase urine pH (compare with **choice A**).

    Hypercalciuria, with or without hypercalcemia (**choice B**), is a cause of calcium oxalate stones.

    Uric acid stones can be seen in patients with hyperuricemia (**choice C**) secondary to gout, or in conditions in which a very rapid cell turnover occurs (e.g., leukemias).

    Genetically determined defects in the renal transport of amino acids are associated with cystine stones (**choice E**).

29. **The correct answer is C.** The presence of blood in the spinal tap indicates bleeding within the subarachnoid space, and rupture of berry aneurysms represents the most frequent cause leading to this form of intracranial bleed. Berry aneurysms develop as outpouchings of the arterial wall in the circle of Willis and consist of intima and adventitia; the media is absent. Congenital weakness at branching points is thought to be the underlying pathogenetic mechanism, but hypertension plays a facilitating role in their development and rupture.

Amyloid angiopathy (**choice A**) usually leads to hemorrhages occurring in the neocortex in a "lobar" distribution. The amyloid depositing in the vessel walls is Aβ, the same type as the amyloid in senile plaques of Alzheimer disease. Blood is usually absent in a spinal tap.

Hypertensive vascular changes (**choice B**) affect intraparenchymal arterioles and small arteries. These changes constitute the predisposing condition for the development of hypertensive bleeding, which is intraparenchymal and often involves the basal ganglia, cerebellum, or pons. The subarachnoid space is free of blood, unless the bleeding extends into the subarachnoid space.

Tearing of bridging veins (**choice D**) is the most frequent mechanism of *subdural hemorrhage*, occurring most commonly in people with cerebral atrophy. In this setting, such veins become stretched and thus more vulnerable to trauma.

Tearing of the middle meningeal artery (**choice E**) is the most common cause of epidural hemorrhage, usually resulting from trauma and often associated with calvarial fracture. Blood collects rapidly between the dura and the overlying bone, leading to increased intracranial pressure and impending danger of cerebral herniation.

30. **The correct answer is E.** This child has neonatal respiratory distress syndrome (hyaline membrane disease), which is caused by the inability of the immature lungs to synthesize adequate amounts of surfactant. Surfactant, which reduces surface tension, helps keep alveoli dry, and aids in expansion of the lungs, is synthesized by type II pneumocytes.

    Alveolar capillary endothelial cells (**choice A**) are important in maintaining the capillary structure and permitting flow of gases into and out of the blood stream.

    Bronchial mucous cells (**choice B**) produce the usually thin (in healthy individuals) coat of mucus that lines the bronchi.

    The ciliated bronchial respiratory epithelium (**choice C**) is responsible for moving the dust-coated mucus layer out of the bronchi.

    Type I pneumocytes (**choice D**) are the squamous cells that line alveoli and permit easy gas exchange. These cells tend to be immature (and thick) in premature infants but do not produce surfactant.

31. **The correct answer is D.** The clinical picture of confusion, ataxia, and variable disturbances of eye movements (e.g., nystagmus and ophthalmoplegia) is due to *Wernicke encephalopathy*, which results from thiamine deficiency. Hemorrhage and necrosis in the abovementioned areas are the underlying pathologic changes. Alcoholics are particularly prone to this condition.

Axonal degeneration of posterior and lateral columns of spinal cord (**choice A**), or *subacute combined degeneration*, results from two different etiologies: vitamin $B_{12}$ deficiency and HIV myelopathy. Ataxia, numbness, and spastic paresis of the lower extremities are the clinical manifestations.

Demyelination affecting the central region of the basis pontis (**choice B**) is known as *central pontine myelinolysis*. This complication is most commonly encountered in severely malnourished and dehydrated alcoholics. Rapid correction of hyponatremia triggers this condition.

Demyelination involving the corpus callosum and anterior commissure (**choice C**), or *Marchiafava-Bignami disease*, is a rare disorder associated with chronic alcoholism. It is probably related to some dietary deficiency.

Loss of neurons in the neocortex, cerebellar Purkinje cells, and hippocampal pyramidal neurons (**choice E**) results from hypoxia or hypoglycemia-related necrosis. These neurons are the most vulnerable to hypoxic or hypoglycemic injury.

32.  **The correct answer is D.** Infectious mononucleosis is caused by the Epstein-Barr virus (EBV), although most EBV infections do not result in acute disease. In patients with the African form of Burkitt lymphoma, and in some AIDS patients with B-cell lymphomas, there is evidence of EBV infection. In these patients, leukemic cells contain multiple copies of the EBV genome. A translocation between the cellular proto-oncogene *myc* on chromosome 8 and immunoglobulin chains on chromosomes 2, 14, or 22 is a typical finding in these cells. Evidence of EBV infection is therefore relevant (but not required) for the diagnosis of B-cell lymphoma.

Infection with HTLV-1 (**choice A**) is, as the name suggests, associated with adult T-cell leukemia. HTLV-1 is a retrovirus that activates proto-oncogenes when it inserts its genome upstream of these genes.

Severely elevated levels of IgG (**choice B**) represent a form of macroglobulinemia. This is not typical of either chronic myelogenous leukemia (CML) or B-cell lymphomas. Patients with multiple myeloma may have elevated levels of a monoclonal IgG.

Severely elevated levels of IgM (**choice C**) are found in patients with Waldenström macroglobulinemia. Levels of IgM are high enough to cause hyperviscosity syndrome and to interfere with blood clotting. Waldenström macroglobulinemia can eventually lead to an aggressive B-cell lymphoma.

Bence-Jones proteins (**choice E**) are immunoglobulin light chains that have "spilled" into the urine. This is seen primarily in patients with multiple myeloma or its advanced stages, known as plasma cell leukemia. These cells overproduce antibodies and their building blocks, such as light chains, which are then excreted in the urine.

The diagnostic marker of Hodgkin disease is the presence of Reed-Sternberg cells (**choice F**) in lymph node biopsies. Reed-Sternberg cells are multinucleated, often with mirror-image nuclei, and contain giant nucleoli.

More than 95% of patients with CML have a translocation between chromosomes 9 and 22 in their leukemic cells (**choice G**). The "new" chromosome that is generated by this event is referred to as the Philadelphia chromosome. Different translocations are responsible for other hematologic malignancies. For example, Burkitt lymphoma often shows a translocation between chromosomes 8 and 14.

33.  **The correct answer is B.** A little knowledge, such as the "knee-jerk" association between asbestos exposure and malignant mesothelioma (**choice D**), can get you into trouble on this type of USMLE question. Malignant mesothelioma is a very rare tumor that is much more common in individuals with a history of asbestos exposure. However, bronchogenic carcinoma is more common than malignant mesothelioma in asbestos-exposed individuals, as well as in the population at large. Asbestos exposure is also associated with pulmonary interstitial fibrosis and pleural reactions.

Bladder carcinoma (**choice A**) is associated with cigarette smoking and exposure to naphthalene dyes.

Lymphomas (**choice C**) and leukemias are often associated with chromosomal rearrangements (e.g., translocations) that alter the locations of proto-oncogenes (e.g., *c-myc*, *c-abl*, *bcl-1*, *bcl-2*).

The association between scrotal carcinoma (**choice E**) and hydrocarbon exposure was first noted by Percival Pott, who noticed an increased incidence of scrotal cancer in chimney sweeps in London.

34.  **The correct answer is B.** This patient has an autonomous neurogenic bladder, which is a type of "lower motor neuron" bladder. There are three types of lower motor neuron bladders: an autonomous neurogenic bladder (lesion to the sacral spinal cord centers involved in bladder function), a motor neurogenic bladder (**choice C**; lesion of motor and visceral efferents to the bladder), and a sensory neurogenic bladder (**choice D**; lesion of sensory afferents from the bladder). All these conditions are associated with a flaccid bladder that fills to capacity. Whereas a normal bladder typically empties at 300 mL, these bladders fill to about 1000 mL. These patients have overflow incontinence, which means the bladder expands completely. Because they cannot void, these patients dribble urine. These are the most dangerous neurogenic bladders, because uri-

**KAPLAN** MEDICAL

nary stasis predisposes patients to lower urinary tract infections, which may ascend to the kidneys, producing pyelonephritis.

An automatic neurogenic bladder (**choice A**) is a type of "upper motor neuron" bladder. This condition is caused by a lesion that disconnects the pontine micturition center (the center that is responsible for producing coordinated voiding) from the sacral spinal cord centers. The bladder is still able to void to some degree, but functions "on its own" without input from the brainstem center. As a result, the urethral sphincter does not relax when the detrusor muscle contracts, leading to urinary retention.

An uninhibited neurogenic bladder (**choice E**) is another type of "upper motor neuron" bladder. Normal adults have cortical control over their pontine micturition center, but when the corticopontine pathways are not functioning properly, the patient develops an uninhibited neurogenic bladder. In these patients, the act of voiding is well coordinated, but not under conscious control. This is seen in patients with frontal lobe lesions and in normal children prior to toilet training.

35. **The correct answer is B.** Osteoarthritis is characterized by mechanical, rather than inflammatory, damage to the joint. The damage usually begins as multiple small fractures of the cartilage tips of the involved bones, which can lead to wearing down of the cartilage to expose the underlying bone. In long-standing cases, the articular ends of the bones may develop a mushroom-like or flattened deformation.

Synovial proliferation with pannus formation (**choice A**) suggests chronic inflammatory joint disease, such as rheumatoid arthritis.

White flecks (**choice C**) in a joint suggest the crystals of gout or pseudogout.

The presence of pus (**choice E**) suggests an acute inflammatory (possibly infectious) etiology.

36. **The correct answer is E.** The tumor described is the linitis plastica form of gastric adenocarcinoma, in which individual mucin-producing tumor cells diffusely infiltrate the mucosa and muscularis propria to produce a rigid, thickened, "leather-bottle" gastric wall. This tumor is poorly differentiated and has a poor prognosis.

Keratohyalin granules (**choice A**) are a feature of squamous cell carcinoma, which does not usually occur in the stomach.

Melanosomes and premelanosomes (**choice B**) are observed with electron microscopy in melanocytic lesions, including melanoma.

Positive immunostaining for gastrin (**choice C**) would be a feature of gastrin-secreting carcinoids, which typically form small, yellow nodules composed of nests or cords of small cells with centrally located, round-to-oval, stippled nuclei.

Positive immunostaining for leukocyte common antigen (**choice D**) is associated with lymphoma, which can also affect the stomach, appearing similar to linitis plastica grossly. Microscopically, however, the individual malignant lymphocytes usually have centrally located nuclei and lack the large, clear, cytoplasmic vacuoles described in this question.

37. **The correct answer is C.** Cervical intraepithelial neoplasia (CIN) is associated with human papilloma virus (HPV) infection, particularly types 16 or 18. These papillomaviruses produce E6 and E7 proteins, which induce the expression of cellular p53 and p110$^{Rb}$ oncogenes, respectively.

EBNA proteins (**choice A**) are produced by the Epstein-Barr virus and are associated with hepatocellular carcinoma, Burkitt lymphoma, and carcinoma of the nasopharynx.

E1A and E1B proteins (**choice B**) are produced by adenoviruses 12, 18, and 31. They also bind to the p53 and p110$^{Rb}$ oncogenes, respectively.

Large tumor antigen (**choice D**) is produced by simian virus 40 (SV40), a papovavirus found in monkeys that is known to produce sarcoma in laboratory hamsters.

38. **The correct answer is E.** The testicular changes described are those observed in Klinefelter syndrome, most often due to 47,XXY genetics.

Testicular feminization syndrome (**choice A**) is due to a genetically determined unresponsiveness to testosterone that produces a phenotypic female in an individual with 46,XY chromosomes.

Trisomy 18 (**choice B**) is Edwards syndrome, characterized by facial features that are small and delicate.

Trisomy 21 (**choice C**) is Down syndrome, the most common trisomy. Characteristics include oblique palpebral fissures, epicanthal folds, endocardial cushion defects, simian creases, and a high-arched palate, among other anomalies.

Turner syndrome, 45,XO (**choice D**), produces a sterile but phenotypic female of short stature with webbing of the neck.

39. **The correct answer is E.** Congenital hypertrophic pyloric stenosis typically presents as described in the question stem and is more frequent in male infants. Physical examination reveals a palpable ovoid mass in the epigastrium;

surgical splitting of the hypertrophic pyloric muscle is curative. The etiology is not well understood.

Caroli disease (**choice A**) is a malformation that causes segmental dilatation of the intrahepatic biliary tree. Vomiting is not a prominent feature.

Cystic fibrosis (**choice B**) presents with malabsorption and/or pulmonary infection due to a global defect in chloride secretion.

Diaphragmatic hernia (**choice C**) is characterized by respiratory insufficiency at birth.

Gastric ulcers (**choice D**) would be quite unusual in an infant.

40. **The correct answer is D.** Hemosiderosis is due to increased total body iron content and is associated with the intracellular storage of excess iron as ferritin and hemosiderin. Iron may be found not only in the organs in which it is usually found but also in the pancreas, heart, kidneys, endocrine organs, and skin. This iron excess may be due to high levels of dietary iron or blood transfusion. Hemosiderin, a denatured form of ferritin, appears microscopically as yellow-brown granules in cytoplasm.

Although cells contain excess iron in hemosiderosis, they are not damaged by the accumulation. In contrast, hepatocytes are damaged by intracellular iron accumulation (**choice A**) in hemochromatosis, a much more severe form of iron overload than hemosiderosis. Hemochromatosis results from a hereditary abnormality of iron absorption.

Cells would exhibit intense staining with Prussian blue, not with methylene blue (**choice B**).

Storage of excess copper in hepatocytes (**choice C**) occurs in Wilson disease, not in hemosiderosis.

41. **The correct answer is B.** The patient has palmar fibromatosis, also known as Dupuytren contracture. This is a benign condition that may stabilize spontaneously or may require surgical excision. Incidence is highest in patients older than 40 who have chronic diseases (including diabetes and liver disease).

Desmoids (aggressive fibromatosis; **choice A**) are proliferations of fibrous tissue that biologically lie somewhere between exuberant reactive fibroproliferations and low-grade fibrosarcomas. They are often found in or near the abdomen.

Neurofibromas (**choice C**) produce tumors involving peripheral nerves.

Peyronie disease (**choice D**) is similar to Dupuytren contracture, but involves the penis.

Plantar fibromatosis (**choice E**) is similar to this patient's condition, but involves the foot.

42. **The correct answer is C.** A midsystolic click and a high-pitched heart murmur in a young woman is the classic presentation of mitral valve prolapse. Patients are usually asymptomatic, but may have dyspnea, tachycardia, chest pain, syncope, eventual congestive heart failure, or, rarely, sudden death. Prolapse may coincide with tricuspid or pulmonary valve disease or with psychiatric conditions such as anxiety or depression. Complications include atrial thrombosis, calcification, infective endocarditis, emboli to the brain, rupture of chordae, mitral regurgitation, arrhythmias, and premature ventricular contractions (PVCs).

Atrial fibrillation (**choice A**) may result from chronic mitral stenosis. This valvular disease is associated with an early diastolic opening snap.

Decreased peripheral pulse pressure (**choice B**) and slowed carotid upstroke (**choice D**) are seen in aortic valve stenosis. A systolic ejection click is associated with this valvular disease.

Wide pulse pressure (**choice E**) is seen clinically as bounding pulses. It is associated with aortic valve insufficiency.

43. **The correct answer is B.** These findings are characteristic of Conn syndrome (primary hyperaldosteronism), in which increased aldosterone secretion causes sodium retention, increased total plasma volume, increased renal artery pressure, and inhibition of renin secretion.

Bartter syndrome (**choice A**), or secondary hyperaldosteronism, is associated with juxtaglomerular hyperplasia and failure to thrive.

Empty sella syndrome (**choice C**) is due to atrophy of the pituitary. The sella is enlarged on skull x-ray and may mimic pituitary neoplasm. It is usually asymptomatic.

Kimmelstiel-Wilson syndrome (**choice D**) is a late complication of diabetes in which intercapillary glomerulosclerosis, hypertension, and edema occurs, accompanied by proteinuria. The syndrome develops approximately 20 years after the onset of diabetes.

Sheehan syndrome (**choice E**) is due to hemorrhagic or ischemic infarction of the pituitary following postpartum hemorrhage with excessive bleeding or shock. It may be present with failure to lactate in the postpartum period.

Waterhouse-Friderichsen syndrome (**choice F**) is characterized by adrenal apoplexy resulting from a massive, sudden adrenal hemorrhage, usually associated with meningococcal septicemia.

44.  **The correct answer is E.** This question first requires you to make the connection between cystic fibrosis (CF) and bleeding. The connection is that CF patients have problems with pancreatic exocrine secretions and therefore have fat malabsorption, which, in turn, results in malabsorption of the fat-soluble vitamins A, D, E, and K. Vitamin K is essential in the post-translational modification of factors II (prothrombin), VII, IX, X, and proteins C and S.

Factors V (**choice A**), VIII (**choice B**), and XII (**choice C**) are not vitamin K dependent.

Although protein C (**choice D**) and protein S are vitamin K dependent, these proteins are endogenous anticoagulants involved in clot lysis, not clot formation. Therefore, deficiency of protein C would cause thrombosis, not bleeding.

45.  **The correct answer is D.** Three pieces of information are needed to answer this question. First, a lesion of the right motor cortex leads to a left paresis or paralysis (immediately narrowing the choices to **D, E, or F**). Second, the leg is represented in the part of the motor cortex that is adjacent to the interhemispheric fissure. Third, the anterior cerebral artery supplies the medial surface of the hemisphere extending from the frontal pole to the parieto-occipital sulcus; this would include the motor and somatosensory cortices.

Blockade of the left anterior cerebral artery (**choice A**) would lead to a right leg paresis or paralysis and diminished sensation over the right leg.

The left middle cerebral artery (**choice B**) supplies the lateral convexity of the right hemisphere. Blockade would lead to a paresis or paralysis of the right face and arm. The middle cerebral artery is the most common location for stroke.

Blockade of the left posterior cerebral artery (**choice C**), which supplies the left occipital lobe, would lead to a right hemianopia with macular sparing.

The right middle cerebral artery (**choice E**) supplies the lateral convexity of the right hemisphere. Blockade would lead to paresis or paralysis of the left face and arm.

Blockade of the right posterior cerebral artery (**choice F**), which supplies the right occipital lobe, would lead to a left hemianopia with macular sparing.

46.  **The correct answer is A.** Hyperphosphatemia associated with renal failure is the likely cause for this patient's hypocalcemic state. Phosphate excretion is impaired, and metabolic phosphate production is often increased. High serum levels of phosphate can lead to the deposition of calcium phosphate in tissues, decreasing the plasma calcium concentration.

Hyponatremia (**choice B**) in acute renal failure (ARF) is generally due to ingestion of water or inappropriate administration of hypotonic IV solutions. It does not directly affect the levels of calcium in the plasma.

Decreased, rather than increased, sensitivity to 1,25-dihydroxyvitamin D (**choice C**) is typical of ARF. Again, increased sensitivity to 1,25-dihydroxyvitamin D could result in hypercalcemia, not in hypocalcemia.

Decreased, rather than increased, sensitivity to parathyroid hormone (**choice D**) is typical of ARF. Regardless, since parathyroid hormone acts to increase serum calcium, increased sensitivity to parathyroid hormone (PTH) could result in hypercalcemia, not in hypocalcemia.

Metabolic alkalosis (**choice E**) is rare in ARF, but may accompany vomiting or may be due to therapeutic administration of bicarbonate. Metabolic acidosis, which is much more common, results from the failure of the kidneys to excrete the organic acids derived from the metabolism of dietary protein.

47.  **The correct answer is D.** Removal of a lung, typically for treatment of lung cancer, has many physiologic consequences. The most obvious change is that the remaining lung fills the chest cavity (and typically displaces the heart across the midline). The volume of air that can be maximally inspired by the single lung is less than that inspired by two lungs. Another subtle change is that the pulmonary vascular bed is sufficiently large that it can accommodate the doubled blood flow at rest (by recruiting more alveolar wall capillaries), but there is not a sufficient reserve vascular bed to accommodate the larger blood flow produced during exercise.

Airway resistance (**choice A**) is decreased during exercise because of bronchodilation; this helps ventilate the lung.

Lung compliance (**choice B**) changes do not adversely affect blood flow during exercise.

Pulmonary vessels typically dilate, rather than constrict (**choice C**), during exercise.

Although the volume of the single lung (**choice E**) is less than that of two lungs, this would not account for an increase in pulmonary artery pressure.

48.  **The correct answer is B.** Chronic nonspecific lymphadenitis is a reactive lymph node hyperplasia that can take three distinct forms, seen in different clinical settings. In chronic bacterial infections, such as this patient's chronic tonsillitis, there is a stimulation of B cells that leads to prominence of germinal centers.

Acute nonspecific lymphadenitis (**choice A**), characterized by necrotic debris, prominent follicles, and, sometimes, a neutrophilic infiltrate, is seen as a response to acute, rather than chronic, infection.

This patient has a reactive, rather than neoplastic, etiology for lymph node enlargement (**choice C**).

Immunologic reactions induced by drugs such as phenytoin (Dilantin) produce reactive changes in the paracortical T cells, leading to expansion of cells outside the germinal centers (paracortical lymphoid hyperplasia; **choice D**).

Sinus histiocytosis (**choice E**) is seen in lymph nodes draining cancers (notably breast) and consists of lymphatic sinusoids packed with histiocytes.

49. **The correct answer is D.** Fibrocystic changes *per se* do not increase the risk of invasive cancer unless there is concomitant epithelial hyperplasia. This is defined as an increase in the number of epithelial cell layers in the terminal duct-lobular unit (TDLU). According to recommendations issued by the College of American Pathologists, patients with fibrocystic changes can be classified into three categories (1-3 below) with respect to the risk of developing invasive breast carcinoma:

    1. Fibrocystic changes with no or mild epithelial hyperplasia (<4 cell layers): no increased risk (compared with the normal population)
    2. Moderate or florid epithelial hyperplasia: 1.5 to 2 times the risk
    3. Atypical ductal or lobular hyperplasia: 5 times the risk
    4. *In situ* ductal or lobular carcinoma: 8 to 10 times the risk

    Apocrine metaplasia (**choice A**), calcification (**choice B**), cysts (**choice C**), and fibrosis (**choice E**) do not have any effect on the risk of cancer transformation, no matter how prominent or extensive these features appear. Such changes are nonetheless important in the diagnosis of fibrocystic changes. The cysts are also primarily responsible for the symptomatology, i.e., tenderness, pain, and discomfort often manifesting with a cyclical pattern. Aspiration of a large cyst may result in prompt relief of pain.

50. **The correct answer is C.** Hospital-acquired pneumonia (or *nosocomial* pneumonia) is defined as a pneumonia that manifests more than 48 hours after admission to the hospital. It more commonly affects patients who are in the ICU or are mechanically ventilated. The most frequent causative microorganisms are *Pseudomonas aeruginosa*, *Staphylococcus aureus*, *Klebsiella pneumoniae*, *Escherichia coli*, and Enterobacter. Pathologic features are those of acute bronchopneumonia, but the mortality rate is high, around 50%.

Anaerobic pneumonia (**choice A**) occurs in individuals predisposed to aspiration, i.e., those with depressed levels of consciousness, impaired deglutition, or tracheal/nasogastric tubes. Periodontal disease is an additional risk factor, as it leads to increased numbers of anaerobic bacteria in aspirated material. Necrotizing pneumonia, lung abscess, and pleural empyema are the most common pathologic lesions.

Community-acquired pneumonia (**choice B**) is usually caused by pneumococcus (*Streptococcus pneumoniae*) and results in homogeneous consolidation of an entire lobe. Microscopically, a fibrinopurulent exudate fills the alveolar spaces.

Lipid pneumonia (**choice D**) is characterized histologically by large numbers of lipid-laden macrophages. This form of pneumonia occurs in association with obstructive bronchial lesions or aspiration of mineral oils.

In primary atypical pneumonia (**choice E**) there is a lymphomonocytic infiltrate confined to interalveolar septa and interstitium. *Mycoplasma pneumoniae* is the most frequent etiologic agent.

# Pathology and Pathophysiology: **Test Five**

1. A 45-year-old woman presents with complaints of easy fatigability, anorexia, and weight loss. Blood tests reveal striking leukocytosis, with 100,000 leukocytes/mL, of which most are immature granulocytic precursors with less than 5% blasts. Cytogenetic studies demonstrate the presence of a reciprocal translocation between the long arms of chromosomes 9 and 22, giving rise to the Philadelphia chromosome. Which of the following is the most likely diagnosis?

   (A) Acute myelogenous leukemia (AML)

   (B) Chronic lymphocytic leukemia (CLL)

   (C) Chronic myelogenous leukemia (CML)

   (D) Leukemoid reaction

   (E) Myelofibrosis

2. Biopsy of the right femur in a 50-year-old man demonstrates irregularly shaped, thick, well-calcified, bony spicules with an abnormal arrangement of cement lines forming a mosaic pattern. This biopsy is most consistent with which of the following conditions?

   (A) Aneurysmal bone cyst

   (B) Chondrosarcoma

   (C) Osteomalacia

   (D) Osteoporosis

   (E) Paget disease

3. A 4-year-old girl with a history of a viral upper respiratory infection 3 weeks ago presents with mucous membrane bleeding. Physical examination is significant for petechiae. Laboratory studies reveal a platelet count of 15,000/mm$^3$. BUN and creatinine are normal. A peripheral blood smear exhibits large platelets. Which of the following is the most likely diagnosis?

   (A) Disseminated intravascular coagulation

   (B) Hemolytic uremic syndrome

   (C) Idiopathic thrombocytopenic purpura (ITP)

   (D) Thrombotic thrombocytopenic purpura (TTP)

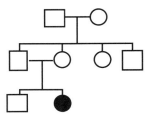

4. The patient shown in the pedigree above did poorly in school, then became increasingly forgetful and irrational. Over a period of years, he developed ataxia and began posturing. Eventually, he was demented and unable to care for himself. At autopsy, extensive cortical demyelination is observed. Microscopic examination of the areas of demyelination reveals numerous macrophages containing crystals that stain light brown with toluidine blue. This presentation is probably due to a deficiency of which of the following enzymes?

   (A) Arylsulfatase A

   (B) Galactocerebroside β-galactosidase

   (C) Glucocerebrosidase

   (D) Hexosaminidase A

   (E) Sphingomyelinase

5. Neurologic examination of a 34-year-old man reveals a direct and a consensual light reflex in his left eye, but neither a direct nor a consensual light reflex in his right eye. Which of the following signs is also likely to be found during his examination?

   (A) Abducted right eye

   (B) Absence of the right corneal reflex

   (C) Absence of touch sensation of the right face

   (D) Hyperacusis of the right ear

   (E) Inability to close the right eye

   (F) Visual field defect of the right eye

6. A 30-year-old, otherwise healthy woman presents to her physician with complaints of fatigue and dyspnea. Physical examination reveals normal breath sounds and the presence of third and fourth heart sounds. A chest x-ray film shows clear lung fields but right ventricular enlargement, main pulmonary artery enlargement, and "pruning" of the peripheral vasculature. An electrocardiogram shows right axis deviation and right ventricular hypertrophy. Left ventricular function appears normal on echocardiography. Serologic studies show antinuclear antibodies. Which of the following pathologic findings would this patient also show, either at autopsy or if an appropriate biopsy were taken?

(A) Mural thrombus of the right atrium

(B) Necrosis and scarring of the left ventricle

(C) Plexogenic pulmonary vasculopathy

(D) Pulmonary artery stenosis

(E) Severe pulmonary fibrosis

7. Patient A has carbon monoxide (CO) poisoning, and patient B has iron deficiency anemia. Assume that CO is binding 50% of the available $O_2$-binding sites on the hemoglobin, and that the anemic patient has 50% of the normal amount of hemoglobin. Patient A is more at risk of tissue hypoxia because CO causes

(A) arterial hypoxemia, while anemia does not

(B) a decrease in diffusing capacity

(C) a decrease in the $P_{50}$ of Hb for $O_2$

(D) a greater decrease in the concentration of arterial oxygen

(E) a reduced rate of $O_2$ binding to available Hb

8. A 27-year-old woman complains that she is constantly thirsty and has to urinate every 2 hours. Her plasma osmolality is 295 mOsmol/kg, and her urine osmolality is 100 mOsmol/kg. Her urine is negative for glucose. As part of a diagnostic workup, the patient is deprived of fluids for 3 hours. Her urine osmolality remains 100 mOsmol/kg. One hour after injection of arginine vasopressin (AVP), her urine osmolality becomes 400 mOsmol/kg. Which of the following is the most likely diagnosis?

(A) Diabetes mellitus

(B) Nephrogenic diabetes insipidus

(C) Neurogenic diabetes insipidus

(D) Primary polydipsia

(E) SIADH (syndrome of inappropriate antidiuretic hormone)

9. A 64-year-old man presents to his physician with vague complaints of fatigue. Physical examination is remarkable for splenomegaly without lymphadenopathy. The patient's hematocrit is 30%, his platelet count is 80,000/mm³, and his leukocyte count is 2500/mm³. Bone marrow biopsy shows "fried egg" cells expressing pan B-cell markers CD19 and CD20. Which of the following is the most likely diagnosis?

(A) Aplastic anemia

(B) Hairy cell leukemia

(C) Hereditary spherocytosis

(D) Hodgkin disease

(E) Sézary syndrome

10. A sports announcer reports that an older athlete will not be playing because he has a "ruptured" disc. Which of the following correctly describes the gross pathology of this condition?

(A) The anulus fibrosus protrudes anteriorly through a weakened nucleus pulposus

(B) The anulus fibrosus protrudes anteromedially through a weakened nucleus pulposus

(C) The anulus fibrosus protrudes posteriorly through a weakened nucleus pulposus

(D) The nucleus pulposus protrudes anteriorly through a weakened anulus fibrosus

(E) The nucleus pulposus protrudes posterolaterally through a weakened anulus fibrosus

11. A 4-year-old child develops a soft tissue mass in the orbit of his left eye, which on biopsy demonstrates a variety of cell geometries, including "strap" and "tadpole" eosinophilic cells. Bizarre mitotic figures are seen. This child most likely has which of the following conditions?

(A) Leiomyoma

(B) Leiomyosarcoma

(C) Lipoma

(D) Malignant fibrous histiocytoma

(E) Rhabdomyosarcoma

12. A 32-year-old man was revived after having been submerged underwater for 15 minutes. His physicians were concerned that he sustained hypoxic damage to his brain. Which of the following structures would most likely be damaged?

    (A) Claustrum

    (B) Layer 2 of the cerebral cortex

    (C) Mammillary bodies

    (D) Purkinje layer of the cerebellum

    (E) Subiculum

13. Laboratory studies return from a 67-year-old hospitalized patient. The serum BUN:Cr ratio is >20, urinary sodium is 17 mEq/L, fractional excretion percent of sodium is 0.7, and urine osmolality is 550 mOsm/kg. Which of the following is the most likely diagnosis?

    (A) Acute glomerulonephritis

    (B) Bladder tumor

    (C) Prostatic hyperplasia

    (D) Shock

    (E) Transplant rejection

14. A 73-year-old man with hepatitis C has a liver biopsy to evaluate the progress of his disease. While evaluating the biopsy specimen, the pathologist sees a lot of what she thinks is lipofuscin, but she is having difficulty differentiating this from hemosiderin. Histologic stains for which of the following substances would be most helpful in making this distinction?

    (A) Calcium

    (B) Iron

    (C) Lipid

    (D) Mucin

    (E) Sodium

15. A 50-year-old woman reports a sensation of "the room spinning" when she lies down from a sitting position. Her hearing is unaffected, and she is able to walk a straight line with her eyes closed. Her symptoms are caused by damage to the

    (A) cochlea

    (B) posterior inferior cerebellar artery

    (C) semicircular canals

    (D) utricle and saccule

    (E) vestibulocochlear nerve

16. A 70-year-old hypertensive man arrives at the emergency department complaining of shortness of breath. His history is significant for chronic hypertension, paroxysmal nocturnal dyspnea, and nocturia. Physical examination reveals evidence of pulmonary and peripheral edema. The patient is admitted, and furosemide is administered. A low-sodium diet is ordered. The purpose of this dietary restriction is to

    (A) decrease tubular reabsorption of sodium

    (B) increase extracellular water

    (C) increase intracellular water

    (D) reduce extracellular water

    (E) reduce intracellular water

17. A 14-year-old girl with a high fever and sore throat presents to the emergency department. A complete blood count with differential implies the presence of a viral infection. Which of the following best describes the cells that indicate a viral etiology to her illness?

    (A) They are basophilic with spherical dark-stained nuclei

    (B) They are precursors of osteoclasts and liver Kupffer cells

    (C) They contain a peripheral hyalomere and central granulomere

    (D) They have azurophilic granules and multilobed nuclei

    (E) They remain in the circulation approximately 120 days

18. A bronchial biopsy from a long-term smoker demonstrates focal areas where the normal respiratory epithelium is replaced by keratinizing squamous epithelium. The same change may occur as a pathologic response to deficiency of which of the following vitamins?

    (A) Vitamin A

    (B) Vitamin $B_{12}$

    (C) Vitamin C

    (D) Vitamin D

    (E) Vitamin E

19. A 65-year-old, fair-skinned man develops scaly erythematous papules that have a sandpaper texture on his forehead. A biopsy shows nuclear crowding, hyperchromasia, and pleomorphism of the basal keratinocytes, with alteration of the normal epidermal maturation. Hyperkeratosis is also present. Which of the following neoplasms may arise from this lesion?

    (A) Basal cell carcinoma

    (B) Melanoma

    (C) Merkel cell carcinoma

    (D) Mycosis fungoides

    (E) Squamous cell carcinoma

20. A 38-year-old woman comes to clinical attention because of chest pain of recent onset. Her blood pressure is 150/60 mm Hg, and auscultation reveals a diastolic murmur along the left sternal border. Laboratory studies are significant for a positive fluorescent treponemal antibody absorption test (FTA-ABS). Which of the following pathologic alterations is most likely associated with this clinical presentation?

    (A) Calcification of aortic cusps with stenosis of the aortic orifice

    (B) Fibrous thickening of mitral leaflets with commissural fusion

    (C) Intrachordal ballooning of mitral valve leaflets

    (D) Scarring of the ascending aorta with tree-barking appearance

    (E) Severe atherosclerosis of coronary arteries

21. A 60-year-old man presents with progressive weakness, recurrent fever, and night sweats. Physical examination reveals multiple enlarged lymph nodes in the lateral cervical region. A biopsy of one of these nodes demonstrates diffuse effacement of the nodal architecture by uniform sheets of large atypical lymphoid cells with frequent mitoses. Which of the following is the most likely diagnosis?

    (A) High-grade non-Hodgkin lymphoma

    (B) Hodgkin lymphoma

    (C) Low-grade non-Hodgkin lymphoma

    (D) Paracortical lymphoid hyperplasia

    (E) Reactive follicular hyperplasia

22. A 50-year-old man presents with renal colic. An IV pyelogram demonstrates "clumps" of contrast medium limited to the medulla, as well as multiple small stones. Blood chemistries are all within normal limits. Which of the following is the most likely explanation for these findings?

    (A) Adult polycystic renal disease

    (B) Horseshoe kidney

    (C) Infantile polycystic renal disease

    (D) Medullary sponge kidney

    (E) Renal dysplasia

23. A 30-year-old man presents to the dermatologist with silvery, scaling plaques on his elbows and knees. His mother had been afflicted with the same condition in the past. Which of the following is the most likely diagnosis?

    (A) Acne rosacea

    (B) Acne vulgaris

    (C) Pemphigus vulgaris

    (D) Pityriasis rosea

    (E) Psoriasis vulgaris

24. Testicular biopsy of an infertile man demonstrates a complete absence of sperm or sperm precursors in spermatic tubules that have a regular, round cross-section and are closely packed together. Which of the following is the most likely etiology of this condition?

    (A) Diabetes mellitus

    (B) Maturation arrest

    (C) Seminoma

    (D) Sertoli-only syndrome

    (E) Tuberculosis

25. When watching a routine immunization injection being given to her 2-year-old brother, a teenage girl suddenly complains of feeling faint and starts hyperventilating. A nurse has her sit on the floor and gives her a paper bag. What is the rationale for this therapy?

    (A) The higher $CO_2$ content of the bag will correct the patient's compensated respiratory acidosis

    (B) The higher $CO_2$ content of the bag will correct the patient's compensated respiratory alkalosis

    (C) The higher $CO_2$ content of the bag will correct the patient's uncompensated respiratory acidosis

    (D) The higher $CO_2$ content of the bag will correct the patient's uncompensated respiratory alkalosis

    (E) The paper bag is a placebo

26. A 30-year-old football player lacerates his face in a fall during practice. He is taken to a surgeon, who finds a clean wound with well approximated edges. There is little surrounding tissue damage. Which of the following stages of wound healing will occur first?

    (A) A thin, continuous epithelial cover will appear

    (B) Fibroblasts will lay down collagen fibers

    (C) Granulation tissue will fill the wound

    (D) Macrophages will appear

    (E) Neutrophils will line the wound edge

    (F) The wound will contract

27. A woman comes to the physician because of fatigue. Laboratory studies reveal leukemia with a translocation from the long arm of chromosome 22 to chromosome 9. The physician explains to the patient that this translocation finding is associated with a favorable prognosis in her condition. Which of the following is the most likely diagnosis?

    (A) Acute lymphoblastic leukemia

    (B) Acute myelogenous leukemia

    (C) Chronic lymphocytic leukemia

    (D) Chronic myelogenous leukemia

    (E) Hairy cell leukemia

28. A 65-year-old man with hyperlucent lung fields develops extreme shortness of breath over a period of about 15 minutes. A chest x-ray film shows shift of the mediastinum to the right, and the lung field on the left appears even more hyperlucent than before, with the exception of a white shadow near the heart border. Which of the following is the most probable cause of the patient's current problem?

    (A) Bronchogenic carcinoma

    (B) Pleural effusion

    (C) Pulmonary embolism

    (D) Rupture of an emphysematous bulla

    (E) Tuberculosis

29. Two bone marrow aspirates are studied under the microscope. One is taken from an adult with Hemoglobin SS disease (sickle cell anemia), and the other is from an adult with normal Hemoglobin A. The marrow aspirate from the patient with sickle cell anemia could be identified because of its increased

    (A) fat

    (B) iron stores

    (C) medullary bone

    (D) megakaryocytes

    (E) myeloid:erythroid ratio

30. A 16-year-old boy who plays on his high-school football team has dyspnea, chest pain, and a syncopal episode. Examination reveals an S4, a sustained apical impulse, and a systolic ejection murmur. An electrocardiogram shows left ventricular hypertrophy. Echocardiogram shows ventricular hypertrophy with asymmetric septal thickening. Which of the following is the most likely finding on microscopic examination of this patient's heart?

    (A) Aschoff bodies

    (B) Disorganization of myofibrils

    (C) Infiltration by inflammatory cells

    (D) Localized fibrous scarring

    (E) Structures resembling poorly formed vessels

31. An 18-year-old girl whose grandmother was recently diagnosed with breast cancer discovers a large, round, moveable nodule in her left breast. Concerned, she visits her primary care physician. Which of the following diagnoses should rank highest on the physician's differential?

    (A) Cystosarcoma phyllodes

    (B) Fibroadenoma

    (C) Fibrocystic breast disease

    (D) Infiltrating ductal carcinoma

    (E) Intraductal papilloma

32. A 38-year-old man has paroxysmal hypertension. He is subsequently found to have medullary carcinoma of the thyroid, pheochromocytoma, and mucosal neuromas. Parathyroid involvement is not noted. Which of the following is the most likely diagnosis?

    (A) Multiple endocrine neoplasia (MEN) type I

    (B) MEN type II

    (C) MEN type III

    (D) Sipple syndrome

    (E) Wermer syndrome

**KAPLAN) MEDICAL**

33. A biopsy of a very large neck mass shows a benign thyroid lesion composed of colloid-filled follicles separated by fibrous scars. Which of the following is the most likely diagnosis?

    (A) Diffuse nontoxic goiter

    (B) Multinodular goiter

    (C) Subacute thyroiditis

    (D) Thyroid adenoma

    (E) Thyroid cyst

34. A 20-year-old man is brought to the emergency department after being found unconscious on a local park bench. The police officer who found the patient hands the treating physician an empty syringe that was found on the bench. The patient has had multiple hospital admissions for heroin overdoses. Physical examination shows constricted pupils. When the patient's blood gases are checked, which of the following would be expected?

    (A) Metabolic acidosis

    (B) Metabolic alkalosis

    (C) Normal pH balance

    (D) Respiratory acidosis

    (E) Respiratory alkalosis

35. A 30-year-old woman presents to her physician with fever, night sweats, and weight loss. Physical examination reveals supraclavicular and lower cervical adenopathy. Lymph node biopsy reveals the presence of Reed-Sternberg cells with lacunae surrounding the nuclei of the cells. Which of the following variants of Hodgkin disease is most likely present?

    (A) Lymphocyte depletion

    (B) Lymphocyte predominance

    (C) Mixed cellularity

    (D) Nodular sclerosis

36. A patient presents with secondary amenorrhea. She reports that "things smell odd now." During the physical examination, papilledema is noted in one eye, and careful tests reveal loss of vision in some parts of the visual field. This patient should be carefully evaluated for a tumor in which of the following sites?

    (A) Falx cerebri

    (B) Hippocampus

    (C) Posterior fossa

    (D) Sphenoidal ridge

    (E) Suprasellar region

37. A 20-year-old black woman with a history of multiple small bowel resections for Crohn disease presents complaining of fatigue and dyspnea on exertion. Her physical examination is notable for pallor and a wide-based, unsteady gait. Her lab studies reveal a hemoglobin of 10.0 g/dL, with a mean corpuscular volume of 120 $\mu m^3$. Examination of the peripheral blood smear shows macrocytosis, anisocytosis, poikilocytosis, and neutrophils with 6 to 8 nuclear lobulations. Which of the following is the most likely cause of this patient's anemia?

    (A) Beta-thalassemia trait

    (B) Folate deficiency

    (C) Iron deficiency

    (D) Sickle cell trait

    (E) Vitamin $B_{12}$ deficiency

38. A 5-year-old boy with a 1-month history of fevers and lassitude is found to have severe anemia, moderate thrombocytopenia, and a white blood count of 12,000 cells per $mm^3$. A bone marrow biopsy would most likely reveal

    (A) acute lymphoblastic leukemia (ALL)

    (B) acute myeloblastic leukemia (AML)

    (C) chronic lymphocytic leukemia

    (D) chronic myeloid leukemia

    (E) hairy cell leukemia

39. A 55-year-old man develops a deep venous thrombosis that dislodges and travels to the left lung, completely blocking a branch of the left pulmonary artery. Which of the following is true about the partial pressure of oxygen in that area of the lung?

    (A) It is equal to arterial blood $P_{O_2}$

    (B) It is equal to atmospheric pressure $P_{O_2}$

    (C) It is equal to inspired $P_{O_2}$

    (D) It is equal to mixed venous blood $P_{O_2}$

    (E) It is less than mixed venous blood $P_{O_2}$

40. A 19-year-old man is rushed to the emergency department after being shot in the chest. He has lost a great deal of blood and appears very pale. His skin is cool and clammy, and his mental status is altered. On exam he is tachycardic and tachypneic, and the jugular veins are collapsed. Urinary output is minimal. Which of the following is most consistent with the patient's condition?

    |     | Preload | Cardiac Output | Vascular Resistance | Mixed Venous O$_2$ |
    | --- | --- | --- | --- | --- |
    | (A) | ↑ | ↑ | ↑ | ↓ |
    | (B) | ↑ | ↓ | ↓ | ↑ |
    | (C) | ↓ | ↓ | ↑ | ↓ |
    | (D) | ↓ | ↓ | ↓ | ↑ |
    | (E) | ↓ | ↓ | ↓ | ↓ |

41. A 12-year-old girl, with history of a streptococcal sore throat that occurred several weeks ago, presents to her physician with an erythematous macular skin rash in a "bathing suit" distribution. Which of the following signs would be necessary to make the diagnosis of rheumatic fever?

    (A) Elevated erythrocyte sedimentation rate

    (B) Leukocytosis

    (C) Migratory polyarthritis

    (D) Prolonged PR interval on EKG

    (E) Temperature greater than 100.4 F

42. A 53-year-old woman presents with a 6-month history of dysphagia, substernal pain, and melena. Her substernal pain is exacerbated when she eats large meals or goes to bed for the evening. Her symptoms are due to dysfunction of which of the following sphincters?

    (A) Ileocecal

    (B) Lower esophageal

    (C) Pyloric

    (D) Sphincter of Oddi

    (E) Upper esophageal

43. A patient with a pulmonary thromboembolism has blockage of the anterior branch of the right superior pulmonary artery, causing an infarct in the corresponding region of the right lung. Along with breathlessness, rapid respiration, and increased heart rate, the patient complains of chest pain, which is attributed to lack of blood supply to the pleura overlying the affected bronchopulmonary segment. Which nerve transmits pain sensation from the affected area of pleura?

    (A) Greater splanchnic nerve

    (B) Intercostal nerve

    (C) Phrenic nerve

    (D) Pulmonary plexus

    (E) Vagus nerve

44. A 69-year-old man with emphysema comes to the physician for a followup examination. He is on home oxygen therapy and has no new complaints at this time. He smoked one pack of cigarettes a day for 40 years but quit 7 years ago when his emphysema started to "slow" him down. Which of the following clinical observations is likely present in this patient and is directly related to the increased compliance caused by his disease?

    (A) Barrel chest

    (B) Chronic cough

    (C) Excessive mucus production

    (D) Long, slow, deep breathing pattern

    (E) Pink face

45. A 65-year-old woman with a long-standing disease has bone marrow fibrosis and increased bone remodeling, with bone resorption exceeding bone formation. She has a history of passing calcium-oxalate kidney stones. Which of the following laboratory result profiles would be expected in the serum of this patient?

|  | $Ca^{2+}$ | $PO_4^{3-}$ | PTH |
|---|---|---|---|
| (A) | ↓ | ↓ | ↑ |
| (B) | ↓ | ↑ | ↓ |
| (C) | ↓ | ↑ | ↑ |
| (D) | ↑ | ↓ | ↑ |
| (E) | ↑ | ↑ | ↑ |

46. A 24-year-old man has progressive, painless enlargement of neck lymph nodes. A routine chest film followed by CT scan demonstrates marked enlargement of mediastinal nodes. No nodules are seen in the liver or lungs. When evaluating the biopsy of one of the involved nodes, the pathologist should specifically look for which of the following?

(A) Abnormal plasma cells

(B) Giant platelets

(C) Immature neutrophil precursors

(D) Melanin pigment

(E) Reed-Sternberg cells

47. A concerned mother brings her 6-year-old child to the pediatric clinic for severe abdominal pain. The mother reports having found the child chewing on paint chips. Blood tests reveal microcytic hypochromic erythrocytes with basophilic stippling. Exposure to which of the following agents is the most likely cause of this child's presentation?

(A) Arsenic

(B) Carbon monoxide

(C) Cyanide

(D) Gold

(E) Lead

(F) Mercury

48. A 47-year-old man presents with a small, red, plaque-like lesion on the glans of his penis. A diagnosis of Bowen disease is made on biopsy examination. Which of the following changes of the uterine cervix is histopathologically equivalent to this patient's disease?

(A) Carcinoma *in situ*

(B) Chronic cervicitis

(C) Invasive squamous cell carcinoma

(D) Mild cervical dysplasia

(E) Nabothian cyst

49. A 25-year-old man presents with bilateral hearing loss. MRI reveals bilateral tumors within the cerebellopontine angles. Surgery is performed, and the tumors are removed. Both are found to be neurilemomas ("schwannoma"). Which of the following is the most likely diagnosis?

(A) Metastatic disease

(B) Multiple sclerosis

(C) Neurofibromatosis type 1

(D) Neurofibromatosis type 2

(E) Tuberous sclerosis

50. A 62-year-old man with a long history of cigarette smoking develops high blood pressure, a moon face, and central obesity. Serum ACTH is increased, but MRI studies of the pituitary and hypothalamus fail to demonstrate any tumors. A chest x-ray film reveals a small tumor in the right upper lobe, and a biopsy is performed. Histologically, the tumor is composed of sheets of anaplastic cells with a high nuclear/cytoplasmic ratio. The tumor is immunoreactive to antibodies directed against ACTH. Which of the following is the most likely diagnosis?

(A) Adenocarcinoma

(B) Carcinoid tumor

(C) Hamartoma

(D) Small cell carcinoma

(E) Squamous cell carcinoma

# Pathology and Pathophysiology Test Five: **Answers and Explanations**

## ANSWER KEY

| | | | |
|---|---|---|---|
| 1. | C | 26. | E |
| 2. | E | 27. | D |
| 3. | C | 28. | D |
| 4. | A | 29. | B |
| 5. | A | 30. | B |
| 6. | C | 31. | B |
| 7. | C | 32. | C |
| 8. | C | 33. | B |
| 9. | B | 34. | D |
| 10. | E | 35. | D |
| 11. | E | 36. | E |
| 12. | D | 37. | E |
| 13. | D | 38. | A |
| 14. | B | 39. | C |
| 15. | C | 40. | C |
| 16. | D | 41. | C |
| 17. | A | 42. | B |
| 18. | A | 43. | B |
| 19. | E | 44. | A |
| 20. | D | 45. | D |
| 21. | A | 46. | E |
| 22. | D | 47. | E |
| 23. | E | 48. | A |
| 24. | D | 49. | D |
| 25. | D | 50. | D |

1. **The correct answer is C.** Chronic myelogenous leukemia (CML) is one of the chronic myeloproliferative disorders, which develop from neoplastic transformation of a stem cell that may differentiate along erythrocytic, megakaryocytic, granulocytic, or monocytic lines. CML is characterized by the presence of the Philadelphia chromosome, arising from a balanced translocation involving 9q and 22q. This results in the formation of a bcr/abl fusion gene encoding a protein with tyrosine kinase activity.

Acute myelogenous leukemia (AML; **choice A**) is usually associated with a large number of blasts in peripheral blood, as well as in the bone marrow. Although the Philadelphia chromosome is absent, other chromosomal and genetic abnormalities define the various subtypes of AML. The most frequent form (with full myeloid maturation) is associated with t(8;21).

Chronic lymphocytic leukemia (CLL; **choice B**) and its lymphomatous counterpart—small lymphocytic lymphoma—derive from neoplastic proliferation of small well-differentiated lymphocytes. CLL is often associated with absolute lymphocytosis (up to 200,000/mL) in peripheral blood.

A leukemoid reaction (**choice D**) is an exuberant form of leukocytosis (with leukocyte counts up to 50,000/mL) that may follow infections. Sometimes it is difficult to distinguish between true leukemia and a leukemoid reaction, but the presence of the Philadelphia chromosome rules out the latter.

Myelofibrosis (**choice E**) is a chronic myeloproliferative disorder characterized by marrow fibrosis and widespread extramedullary hematopoiesis, resulting in massive splenomegaly. The Philadelphia chromosome is absent.

2. **The correct answer is E.** This is the microscopic pattern seen in Paget disease. This disorder is characterized by excessive bone resorption coupled with excessive formation of highly vascular bone with a rubbery consistency and increased susceptibility to fracture. Early on, osteolytic activity is greatest; later, osteoblastic activity becomes more marked. Eventually, the bone becomes sclerotic. The etiology of this condition is unknown. It usually occurs in adults older than 40, and may involve either a single site on one bone or many sites on multiple bones (particularly bones with marrow). Many cases are asymptomatic. In about 1% of the cases, osteosarcoma or other sarcomas may develop in the affected bone.

Aneurysmal bone cyst (**choice A**) produces a solitary, large, cystic space filled with blood, typically in the shaft of a long bone or vertebral body in children or adolescents.

Chondrosarcoma (**choice B**) is a malignant, cartilage-forming tumor composed of cells (sometimes with a bizarre appearance) that form variable amounts of poorly-to-well-formed neoplastic cartilage.

There is a decreased amount of well-calcified bone in both osteomalacia (**choice C**) and osteoporosis (**choice D**). In osteomalacia, the problem is a failure to calcify the bony matrix; in osteoporosis, active bone resorption produces thin bony spicules.

3. **The correct answer is C.** Idiopathic thrombocytopenic purpura (ITP) classically occurs acutely in children several weeks after a viral infection (a viral exanthem or upper respiratory infection in 70% of cases) and is the most common thrombocytopenic purpura of childhood. Physical examination findings usually include easy bruisability, mucous membrane bleeding, gastrointestinal or genitourinary bleeding, and petechiae. CNS bleeding may occur. The peripheral smear typically shows a few, large, young platelets. The other cell lines are normal.

Disseminated intravascular coagulation (**choice A**) is an acquired consumption deficiency of clotting factors and platelets, often resulting in fatal thrombosis and hemorrhage.

Hemolytic uremic syndrome (**choice B**) generally occurs in children following diarrhea due to *Shigella*, *Salmonella*, *Escherichia coli* O157:H7, or a virus. Patients typically present with renal failure (BUN and creatinine would be abnormal) along with bleeding and anemia. The disease is similar to thrombotic thrombocytopenic purpura (TTP; **choice D**).

TTP (**choice D**) is associated with fever, renal failure, neurologic changes, and microangiopathic hemolytic anemia. Platelet aggregation leads to the development of microthrombi throughout the vasculature. The peripheral smear shows few platelets, fragmented red blood cells (schistocytes), and helmet cells.

4. **The correct answer is A.** The presentation and autopsy findings are consistent with metachromatic leukodystrophy. The crystals in the macrophages that stained brown with toluidine blue are sulfatides, which accumulate in this disorder. The color shift seen in the toluidine blue stain is termed *metachromasia* (hence the term metachromatic leukodystrophy). The cause of metachromatic leukodystrophy is deficiency of arylsulfatase A.

Galactocerebroside β-galactosidase (**choice B**) deficiency produces Krabbe disease. In this disorder, multinucleated cells derived from macrophages (globoid cells) are seen around blood vessels. Electron microscopy of the macrophages reveals the presence of linear inclusions.

Glucocerebrosidase (**choice C**) deficiency results in Gaucher disease, characterized by accumulation of glucocerebrosides. Gaucher cells are distended with material that resembles crumpled tissue paper.

Hexosaminidase A (**choice D**) deficiency is associated with Tay Sachs disease, characterized by accumulation of $GM_2$ ganglioside in the central and autonomic nervous systems.

Sphingomyelinase deficiency (**choice E**) produces Niemann-Pick disease, in which sphingomyelin accumulates, especially in cells of the mononuclear phagocytic system.

5. **The correct answer is A.** Two pieces of information are necessary to answer this question. First, you need to determine which nerve is involved. Second, you need to know what other effects a lesion of that nerve would produce. The pupillary light reflex is assessed by shining a light in one eye and observing pupillary constriction in the same eye (direct response) and in the other eye (consensual response). The afferent limb of this reflex is the optic nerve (CN II), and the efferent limb is the oculomotor nerve (CN III). Clearly, the left CN II and left CN III are working because a direct response is seen in the left eye. Also, the right CN II must be working to produce a consensual response in the left eye. However, there must be a lesion of the right CN III because pupillary constriction is not observed under any circumstance in the right eye. CN III also innervates the medial rectus muscle of the eye. Absence of innervation of this muscle would result in unopposed action of the lateral rectus muscle, causing an outward deviation of the eye.

Absence of the right corneal reflex (**choice B**) would result from a lesion of the right trigeminal nerve (CN V; afferent limb) or the right facial nerve (CN VII; efferent limb).

Absence of touch sensation of the right face (**choice C**) would be the result of a lesion of the right CN V.

Hyperacusis of the right ear (**choice D**) could result from a lesion of the right CN V (which innervates the tensor tympani muscle) or the right CN VII (which innervates the stapedius muscle). Both of these muscles dampen sound through the middle ear.

Inability to close the right eye (**choice E**) would be produced by a lesion of the right CN VII. In fact, a CN III lesion would cause the eyelid to droop because the levator palpebrae muscle would be denervated.

A visual field defect of the right eye (**choice F**) would occur if the right CN II was lesioned, but because a consensual light response was elicited in the left eye, the right CN II must be functional.

6. **The correct answer is C.** The presentation described is classic for pulmonary hypertension and, more specifically, the primary idiopathic form of pulmonary hypertension. This rare condition is thought to be related to the collagen vascular diseases, since up to 50% of patients have antinuclear antibodies (despite the absence of frank presentation of other autoimmune disease). Also, a similar, known secondary form of pulmonary hypertension is sometimes seen in patients with a wide variety of collagen vascular diseases, including systemic lupus erythematosus, polymyositis, dermatomyositis, systemic sclerosis, and adult and juvenile forms of rheumatoid arthritis. A wide variety of other conditions have also been associated with secondary pulmonary hypertension, including shunts, left atrial hypertension, chronic hypoxia, pulmonary embolism, drug reaction, hepatic cirrhosis, and sickle cell disease. Both primary and secondary forms of pulmonary hypertension are associated with prominent changes in the pulmonary vasculature, which can include muscularization of smaller arterioles, concentric hypertrophy of the intima ("onion skinning"), and a distinctive plexiform lesion (plexogenic pulmonary vasculopathy) in which the smallest arterioles become markedly dilated with lumens partially occluded by endothelial (or possibly mesenchymal) cells and sometimes thrombus. The prognosis of untreated pulmonary hypertension is poor. However, the use of the vasodilator hydralazine with anticoagulation can slow the course (fatal in about 3 years in untreated patients). If the pulmonary hypertension is secondary, therapy of the primary disease can be helpful.

Unlike cor pulmonale, atrial fibrillation with mural thrombus formation (**choice A**) is uncommon in primary pulmonary hypertension.

The absence of left ventricular findings on echocardiography tends to exclude myocardial infarction as the source of the patient's findings (**choice B**).

The presence of enlargement of the main pulmonary artery excludes pulmonary artery stenosis (**choice D**).

The clear lung fields exclude severe pulmonary fibrosis (**choice E**).

7. **The correct answer is C.** The $P_{50}$ is defined as the partial pressure of oxygen necessary to bind 50% of available hemoglobin. CO will decrease the $P_{50}$ of Hb for $O_2$. Another way of stating this is that CO left-shifts the oxygen-hemoglobin dissociation curve. CO is deadly because it not only binds hemoglobin with a greater affinity than does $O_2$ (240 times better), it also left-shifts the curve, thereby making it more difficult to unload $O_2$ in peripheral tissues.

Neither of these conditions will cause arterial hypoxemia (**choice A**).

CO will not diminish the diffusing capacity of the lung (**choice B**); in fact, it is routinely used to measure diffusing capacity.

The concentration of oxygen in arterial blood will be approximately the same for both cases (**choice D**). If anything, the concentration will be slightly greater in the patient with CO poisoning because CO left-shifts the curve; therefore, the available binding sites of Hb for $O_2$ will be slightly more saturated.

CO does not change the rate of $O_2$ binding to Hb (**choice E**). It does, however, bind to hemoglobin with 240 times the affinity of oxygen.

8.  **The correct answer is C.** ADH (antidiuretic hormone, vasopressin) is normally released from the posterior pituitary in response to hypovolemia and increased osmotic pressure. It acts on the collecting duct of the nephron, increasing its permeability to water. This concentrates the urine and conserves water. Diabetes insipidus (DI) is a condition in which ADH function is absent.

    Two forms of DI exist: neurogenic and nephrogenic. Neurogenic DI (**choice C**) is due to absence of ADH secretion from the posterior pituitary; thus, serum ADH levels are always low, even in states of serious volume depletion. Nephrogenic DI (**choice B**) is due to complete or partial resistance to ADH; therefore, even though ADH levels are high, the hormone has no effect on renal water regulation.

    You are told in the question that the patient's urine did not concentrate on a water deprivation test. This immediately suggests DI. (Normally, when an individual is deprived of fluids for 3 hours, her kidneys respond by concentrating the urine and conserving water). Your task then becomes determining which type of DI the patient has. This is achieved by evaluating the results of the arginine vasopressin (AVP) suppression test. Patients with neurogenic DI readily respond to AVP by producing more concentrated urine. Patients with nephrogenic DI do not concentrate urine in response to AVP because of continued renal resistance.

    Although thirst is a common symptom of diabetes mellitus (**choice A**), the absence of glucosuria argues against this diagnosis.

    Primary polydipsia (**choice D**) usually occurs in patients taking antipsychotic drugs that cause dry mouth (e.g., phenothiazines), promoting the sensation of thirst. As a result, these patients drink large quantities of water. They excrete dilute urine, and eventually may dilute their serum as well, to the point of electrolyte imbalance. On water deprivation, however, their urine will concentrate normally.

    SIADH (syndrome of inappropriate antidiuretic hormone; **choice E**) occurs when there is oversecretion of ADH, for example by a small cell carcinoma of the lung or other ADH-producing neoplasm. One would expect test results opposite to those in this patient. In contrast to DI, the diagnosis of SIADH is usually made with a water-load test.

9.  **The correct answer is B.** Hairy cell leukemia is characterized by pancytopenia, often with massive splenomegaly. Lymphadenopathy is unusual. The proliferating cells express the pan B-cell markers CD19 and CD20 as well as monocyte markers. Histologically, the cells display fine, hairlike projections. A "fried-egg" appearance of bone marrow biopsies arises because of the fixation artifacts from the hairlike projections on many of the cells. Tartrate-resistant acid phosphatase (not mentioned in this question) is virtually diagnostic of hairy cell leukemia. Interferon-alfa is used for treatment.

    Aplastic anemia (**choice A**), or marrow aplasia, is also characterized by pancytopenia; however, the marrow would be hypocellular, with fatty replacement of hematopoietic cells.

    Hereditary spherocytosis (**choice C**) is due to a defect in the membrane of the red cells and would be accompanied by abnormal red cell morphology. Splenomegaly is typical, but other cell lines (white blood cells, platelets) are not affected. Remember that spherocytes exhibit increased osmotic fragility.

    Hodgkin disease (**choice D**) is a lymphoma characterized by the presence of Reed-Sternberg cells in a variable lymphocytic infiltrate.

    Sézary syndrome (**choice E**) is related to mycosis fungoides, a cutaneous T-cell (not B-cell) lymphoma. In both disorders, there is a characteristic "cerebriform" cell, which circulates in the blood in Sézary syndrome but remains confined to the skin in most cases of mycosis fungoides.

10. **The correct answer is E.** Herniated intervertebral discs, often called "slipped" or "ruptured" discs by lay people, occur when the weakened outer anulus fibrosus of the disc permits herniation of the centrally located nucleus pulposus. The defect typically occurs in a posterolateral direction, where it may compress an adjacent spinal nerve root, causing severe low back or leg pain.

    Hint on strategy: This was a question in which formulating your answer before looking at the choices would have prevented a lot of confusion and saved time.

11. **The correct answer is E.** The child has a rhabdomyosarcoma, which is the most common form of malignant soft-tissue tumor seen in infants and children. The characteristic strap and tadpole cells are immature forms of rhabdomyoblasts (and may be hard to find among many poorly differentiated cells). This child probably has embryonal rhabdomyosarcoma, which can also be seen in the genital urinary tract (where it may form "bunches of grapes"). Despite the prevalence in textbooks of dramatic photographs of genitourinary rhabdomyosarcomas in young children, these tumors actually occur more frequently in the head and neck region, particularly the orbit, nasopharynx, and middle ear.

   The presence of abnormal mitotic figures excludes the possibility of a benign tumor (**choices A and C**).

   Leiomyosarcoma (**choice B**) and malignant fibrous histiocytoma (**choice D**) are both malignant tumors, but would not be expected to contain strap and tadpole cells.

12. **The correct answer is D.** The Purkinje cell layer of the cerebellar cortex, pyramidal cells in the CA1 subfield of the hippocampus, and pyramidal cells in layers 3 and 5 of the cerebral cortex are all very sensitive to the effects of cerebral hypoxia and ischemia. The basis for this selective vulnerability may be NMDA-receptor mediated excitotoxic injury of these specific populations of neurons.

   The claustrum (**choice A**) is a thin sheet of gray matter located between the external capsule and the extreme capsule. It is not selectively targeted by hypoxic/ischemic injury to the brain.

   Layer 2 of the cerebral cortex (**choice B**) is the external granular layer, populated by closely packed granule cells. This layer is not affected by ischemia to the same extent as layers 3 and 5, the external and internal pyramidal cell layers.

   The mammillary bodies (**choice C**) are hypothalamic structures located at the base of the brain. They are damaged in Wernicke-Korsakoff syndrome, which is due to thiamine deficiency.

   The subiculum (**choice E**) lies medial and inferior to the hippocampus. The subiculum is not selectively vulnerable to hypoxia, in contrast to the nearby CA1 subfield of the hippocampus.

13. **The correct answer is D.** It is important to remember that not all oliguria is caused by intrinsic renal disease. Shock, of any etiology, is an example of a prerenal cause of oliguria in which poor renal perfusion leads to inadequate urine output. Other examples of prerenal causes include hepatorenal syndrome, postoperative oliguria, and dehydration. Postrenal causes of oliguria usually involve bilateral obstruction and may be due to disease of the ureters, bladder neck, or urethra.

   Acute glomerulonephritis (**choice A**) and transplant rejection (**choice E**) are examples of renal causes of oliguria.

   Bladder tumor (**choice B**) and prostatic hyperplasia (**choice C**) are examples of postrenal causes of oliguria.

14. **The correct answer is B.** Melanin, lipofuscin, and hemosiderin are all yellow-brown, granular pigments that may be difficult to distinguish microscopically. The S 100 stain helps identify melanocytes (such as occur in malignant melanoma), and an iron stain helps identify hemosiderin. No stain specifically identifies lipofuscin, which is consequently a diagnosis based on subtle morphologic features and, if necessary, the absence of staining by S 100 or iron stains.

   Stains for calcium (**choice A**) are used to identify bone tumors and dystrophic calcification.

   Stains for lipid (**choice C**) are used to identify intracellular fat.

   Stains for mucin (**choice D**) help distinguish between poorly differentiated adenocarcinomas and poorly differentiated squamous carcinomas.

   There are no available stains for sodium (**choice E**), which is a normal constituent of all tissues.

15. **The correct answer is C.** Each semicircular canal contains sensory areas that respond to movements of endolymph caused by motion of the head in the same plane as the duct. The posterior canal is implicated in backward motion of the head, as in the change from a sitting to a reclining position.

   The cochlea (**choice A**) contains receptors for the special sense of hearing.

   Insufficient blood flow to the posterior inferior cerebellar artery (**choice B**) would result in cerebellar symptoms, which include the inability to walk a straight line with the eyes closed.

   The utricle and saccule (**choice D**) react to acceleration and deceleration of the head rather than to rotary movement.

   Damage to the vestibulocochlear nerve (**choice E**) would result in disturbances of both equilibrium and hearing.

16. **The correct answer is D.** This hypertensive patient has symptoms and signs of congestive heart failure (paroxysmal nocturnal dyspnea, nocturia, and pulmonary and peripheral edema), for which dietary sodium restriction is

recommended to reduce water retention. Most of the sodium in the body exists in locations outside cells, such as plasma, interstitial fluid, cerebrospinal fluid, intraocular fluid, semen, peritoneal fluid, and pleural fluid. The concentration of sodium in these fluids is tightly regulated by the kidney's action on blood plasma. When dietary sodium is severely restricted, the losses in the kidney (and small losses in sweat) exceed the intake, and the total body sodium is decreased. The body then tries to maintain serum sodium concentration by excreting more water via the kidneys. Most of the water comes from the extracellular fluid rather than the intracellular fluid (**choice E**), since sodium ion is not a quantitatively important component of intracellular fluid. Decreased dietary sodium will increase tubular reabsorption of sodium rather than decreasing it (**choice A**).

17. **The correct answer is A.** This question is really asking you two things. First, it tests whether you know that lymphocytosis is associated with viral infection. Second, it tests your knowledge of the lymphocytes' histologic appearance. Note that these cells are generally small and normally constitute 25 to 33% of leukocytes. Two types of lymphocytes have been distinguished: T cells (involved in cell-mediated immunity) and B cells (involved in humoral immunity).

Monocytes are precursors of osteoclasts and liver Kupffer cells (**choice B**) and also give rise to tissue macrophages and alveolar macrophages.

Platelets contain a peripheral hyalomere and central granulomere (**choice C**).

Neutrophils have azurophilic granules and multilobed nuclei (**choice D**). They increase in number in response to bacterial infection.

Erythrocytes remain in the circulation for about 120 days (**choice E**).

18. **The correct answer is A.** The histopathologic change described here is *squamous metaplasia*, which may be induced by vitamin A deficiency in different types of epithelial membranes, including conjunctiva, respiratory airways, and urinary tract. This change is probably related to the fact that vitamin A and retinoids play an important role in regulating epithelial differentiation.

Vitamin $B_{12}$ deficiency (**choice B**) results in megaloblastic anemia and degeneration of the posterolateral tracts of the spinal cord.

Vitamin C deficiency (**choice C**) causes scurvy, a syndrome characterized by vascular fragility and bleeding diathesis, with resultant recurrent hemorrhage in the gums, skin, and joints.

Vitamin D deficiency (**choice D**) results in two different clinical pictures depending on the patient's age, i.e., rickets in children and osteomalacia in adults.

Vitamin E (**choice E**) is a major free radical scavenger. For obscure reasons, deficiency of vitamin E results in degeneration of the ascending axons in the posterior spinal column and spinocerebellar tract.

19. **The correct answer is E.** The lesion described is *actinic keratosis*, which is frequent on sun-exposed areas of people of fair complexion. It is related to progressive dysplastic changes triggered by the carcinogenic action of ultraviolet light. Actinic keratosis is a premalignant change, but only a small number of untreated lesions will eventually progress to invasive squamous cell carcinoma.

Basal cell carcinoma (**choice A**) is a common skin neoplasm with minimal metastatic potential. It is also most frequent on sun-exposed areas, but actinic keratosis is not a precursor.

As with squamous cell and basal cell carcinomas, sunlight is an important predisposing condition for the development of skin melanomas (**choice B**), but actinic keratosis is not. Besides sunlight, pre-existing nevi, genetic factors, and possibly chemical carcinogens play a pathogenetic role.

Merkel cell carcinoma (**choice C**) is a rare neoplasm that is morphologically identical to small cell carcinoma of the lung. It originates from the epidermal Merkel cells. No premalignant precursor is known for this cancer.

Mycosis fungoides (**choice D**) is a malignant T-cell lymphoma that arises from the skin manifesting with scaly patches, plaques, and nodules. Malignant lymphocytes accumulate underneath the epidermis and infiltrate the overlying epidermis.

20. **The correct answer is D.** This patient has syphilis. In its tertiary stage, syphilis may affect the ascending aorta causing an *obliterative endarteritis* of the vasa vasorum. This results in scarring of the media with wrinkling of the intima, producing the characteristic tree-barking appearance. The aortic ring becomes dilated and the coronary ostia narrowed, leading to aortic regurgitation and myocardial ischemia. Hence, the murmur and the chest pain. Note the typically high systolic pressure and low diastolic pressure accompanying aortic insufficiency.

Calcification of aortic cusps with stenosis of the aortic orifice (**choice A**) is found in elderly patients with clinically evident aortic stenosis. This would lead to an ejection systolic murmur.

Fibrous thickening of mitral leaflets with commissural fusion (**choice B**) is characteristic of chronic rheumatic heart disease and is associated with mitral stenosis. A diastolic murmur is heard at the apex, but this is not associated with a wide difference between systolic and diastolic pressure.

Intrachordal ballooning of mitral valve leaflets (**choice C**) refers to the ballooning of mitral valve leaflets secondary to mitral valve prolapse. This condition may cause mitral valve regurgitation with a systolic murmur.

Severe atherosclerosis of coronary arteries (**choice E**) would be highly unusual in a young patient and would not explain signs of aortic insufficiency. However, cardiovascular syphilis leads to development of secondary atherosclerosis of the ascending aorta.

21. **The correct answer is A.** The presence of atypical lymphocytes, frequent mitoses, and effacement of the lymph node architecture clearly indicates that this is a highly malignant neoplastic process. High-grade non-Hodgkin lymphomas are characterized by markedly atypical cells with usually brisk mitotic activity. The large size of the cells and diffuse pattern of growth suggest *diffuse large cell lymphoma*, the most frequent aggressive non-Hodgkin lymphomas affecting adult patients.

Hodgkin lymphoma (**choice B**) also leads to effacement of the nodal architecture, but it is characterized by the presence of *Reed-Sternberg cells* within a polymorphic cellular background including small lymphocytes, histiocytes, plasma cells, and eosinophils.

Low-grade non-Hodgkin lymphoma (**choice C**) may present with a follicular pattern that mimics the normal follicular architecture of lymph nodes or a diffuse pattern. In both cases, neoplastic lymphocytes are well differentiated (i.e., similar to their normal counterpart), and mitotic activity is scanty.

Paracortical lymphoid hyperplasia (**choice D**) and follicular reactive hyperplasia (**choice E**) represent normal reactive patterns of the T-cell and B-cell dependent areas, respectively. In both forms, the lymph node architecture is preserved.

22. **The correct answer is D.** This is a classic presentation for medullary sponge kidney, which has a male predominance and typically presents at 40 to 60 years of age. Histologically, medullary sponge kidney shows multiple small cysts lined by columnar or cuboidal epithelium localized to the medullary collecting tubules. The cysts can contain laminated concretions of calcium phosphates. Renal failure is rare in patients with medullary sponge kidney, and the pathogenesis for the lesion has not been clarified. The rare uremic medullary sponge kidney, unlike the more common form, occurs in 20- to 30-year-olds, is associated with salt-losing nephropathy, and progresses to renal failure.

The kidney of adult polycystic disease (**choice A**) is massively enlarged and filled throughout with round cysts of varying sizes. Adult polycystic kidney disease often presents with hypertension rather than renal failure or stones.

Horseshoe kidney (**choice B**) involves fusion of the upper or lower (most common) pole of the kidney. It is fairly common (as high as 1:500) and is typically an incidental finding at autopsy.

Infantile polycystic kidney (**choice C**) produces a small kidney with round medullary cysts and "radiating" linear cortical cysts.

Renal dysplasia (**choice E**) can also cause cystic change in a kidney but typically involves only the medulla and cortex of part of the kidney.

23. **The correct answer is E.** Psoriasis vulgaris usually appears on the nails, knees, elbows, and scalp. It does not generally affect the mucous membranes. Lesions are well-demarcated, coral-colored plaques with a white or silvery scale (classic clue). Histologically, epidermal hyperplasia causing thickening and lengthening of the rete ridges is apparent, as is thinning of the epidermis over the dermal papillae. There is a recognized genetic component to this condition. Peak incidence is at age 30.

Acne rosacea (**choice A**) affects the central face. Erythema, telangiectasias, acneform lesions (papules, cysts, pustules), and rhinophyma (telangiectasias and hyperplasia of nasal soft tissue) are found in various combinations. It is common from ages 30 to 50. Women are affected three times more frequently than men, but the syndrome is more severe in the latter.

Acne vulgaris (**choice B**) causes comedones, papules, and cysts. It may be related to hormones, drugs, diet, irritants, and genetic factors. Allergy to *Propionibacterium acnes* has been found to contribute to this condition.

Pemphigus vulgaris (**choice C**) starts with small vesicles, usually on the oral or nasal mucosa, then spreads to other parts of the body. Bullae are delicate and flaccid. The condition is due to autoantibodies to intercellular junctions between keratinocytes. Nikolsky's sign (production of blistering by light stroking or rubbing of the skin) is positive. Pemphigus is most common from ages 40 to 60.

Pityriasis rosea (**choice D**) presents first with a red, scaling, "herald patch" approximately 4 cm in diameter. It is followed within days by eruption in a "short-sleeve turtleneck" distribution. The classic clue to the diagnosis is the appearance of crops of small, pink, oval patches in a "fir tree configuration" on the flexural lines.

**KAPLAN) MEDICAL**

24. **The correct answer is D.** All of the conditions listed can cause infertility because of a low or absent sperm count. Only in Sertoli-only syndrome is there a complete absence of sperm precursors in an undamaged tubule. There is no known method to correct Sertoli-only syndrome (or maturation arrest) that is not due to a treatable chronic disease.

    Chronic diseases, such as diabetes mellitus (**choice A**) or tuberculosis (**choice E**), can arrest the maturation of sperm but do not usually show a complete absence of sperm precursors.

    In maturation arrest (**choice B**), mature sperm are absent, but precursors are found.

    Tumors such as seminomas (**choice C**) cause infertility by occluding the flow of semen or by replacing the seminiferous tubules. Sampling of a seminiferous tubule not replaced by tumor would probably still demonstrate sperm.

25. **The correct answer is D.** Hyperventilation can be triggered by emotional stress, and the resulting rapid breathing tends to "blow off" more $CO_2$ from the lung than usual. Since $CO_2$ is carried in the serum principally as bicarbonate plus hydrogen ion, blowing off $CO_2$ shifts the balance so that less bicarbonate and less hydrogen ion are present in the blood. Less hydrogen ion translates to higher blood pH, i.e., alkalosis, which in this case is of respiratory origin. It is an uncompensated respiratory alkalosis, since renal compensation takes several days to occur. Re-breathing air, which is easily accomplished by breathing into a paper bag, will slow the rate of $CO_2$ loss and quickly correct the alkalosis. The manifestations of the type of mild respiratory alkalosis seen in emotional hyperventilation include light headaches, paresthesias, and sometimes syncope. Severe respiratory alkalosis (not seen in this setting) can also cause cramps, tetany, seizures, and cardiac arrhythmias.

26. **The correct answer is E.** Neutrophils line the wound edge within 24 hours of injury.

    A thin, continuous epithelial cover appears (**choice A**) 24 to 48 hours after injury. Soon after, macrophages replace the neutrophils (**choice D**), while granulation tissue fills the wound (**choice C**). By day 5, fibroblasts lay down collagen fibers (**choice B**) along fibrin and fibronectin matrices formed across the site of incision. Full maturation of the scar requires up to 1 year.

    Wound contraction (**choice F**), mediated by myofibroblasts, characterizes healing by secondary union by second intention, which occurs when the two skin edges of a wound are not in contact. During the healing process, large amounts of granulation tissue are formed and slowly fill the defect.

27. **The correct answer is D.** The presence of the Philadelphia chromosome, a translocation from the long arm of chromosome 22 to chromosome 9 [t(9;22)], is associated with a more favorable prognosis in patients with chronic myelogenous leukemia.

    Acute lymphoblastic leukemia (ALL; **choice A**) is the most common cause of leukemia in children. The presence of the Philadelphia chromosome is associated with a worse prognosis for the patient. This form of leukemia is also associated with a B-ALL translocation of the c-*myc* proto-oncogene of chromosome 8 to chromosome 14 [t(8;14)(q24;q32)].

    Acute myelogenous leukemia (AML; **choice B**) is the most common acute leukemia in adults. The M2 subtype is associated with the t(8;21) translocation, and the M3 subtype is associated with the t(15;17) translocation.

    More than half the patients with chronic lymphocytic leukemia (**choice C**) display one of several chromosomal abnormalities. This includes trisomy 12 (involves the h-*ras* proto-oncogene), translocation t(11;14) (involves k-*ras* and *bcl-1* proto-oncogenes), and deletion (14q-) or inversion (14q) (involves immunoglobulin heavy chain gene).

    Hairy cell leukemia (**choice E**) is associated with the expression of tartrate-resistant acid phosphatase (TRAP) on the surface of B cells.

28. **The correct answer is D.** The patient's initially hyperlucent lung fields strongly suggest the presence of emphysema. The radiologic findings after the increase in shortness of breath are consistent with free air in the chest, which has collapsed the left lung and caused a shift in the location of the mediastinum. Such air might have been introduced by rupture of a bulla. Small pneumothoraces are usually well tolerated, but larger ones may require decompression (the needle from a syringe is sometimes used), or even surgical correction if bullae continue to leak air.

    Bronchogenic carcinoma (**choice A**) would be expected to produce a mass lesion.

    Pleural effusion (**choice B**) usually develops slowly and causes a whitening of lung fields when fluid is present.

    Pulmonary embolism (**choice C**) can cause sudden shortness of breath but would not cause an increase in the lucency of the lung fields.

    Tuberculosis (**choice E**) would be expected to produce a mass lesion in the lung.

29. **The correct answer is B.** Adults with sickle cell disease have undergone decades of accelerated RBC formation and destruction, leading to accelerated erythropoiesis in the bone marrow. Consequently, the bone marrow

becomes hyperplastic, with marked increases in the number of normoblasts (erythroblasts) at the expense of marrow fat and marrow bone (**choices A and C**). Although the white cell and megakaryocyte lines are undiminished (**choices D and E**), there is a marked increase in RBC precursors and iron stores. Iron storage increases as a consequence of both chronic transfusions and increased dietary absorption; these increased iron stores can be appreciated with a Prussian blue stain.

30. **The correct answer is B.** Microscopic examination of heart muscle from a patient with hypertrophic cardiomyopathy would reveal short, thick myofibrils arranged in circular patterns admixed with normal tissue. On electron microscopy, myofibrils and myofilaments appear disarrayed.

    Aschoff bodies (**choice A**) appear in rheumatic myocarditis and consist of degenerating material and leukocytes. These occur along with Anitschkow myocytes, which contain "ribbon-like" nuclei and eosinophilic cytoplasm.

    Infiltration by inflammatory cells (**choice C**) would be expected in association with an infectious process, such as acute bacterial endocarditis.

    Localized fibrous scarring (**choice D**) is associated with myocardial healing after infarction.

    Structures resembling poorly formed vessels (**choice E**) are found in cardiac myxoma, the most common primary tumor of the heart. The tumor cells are derived from primitive multipotent mesenchymal cells. They may be sessile or pedunculated masses.

31. **The correct answer is B.** Fibroadenoma is the most common benign breast tumor. It occurs in women of reproductive age, generally before age 30, and may be related to increased estrogen sensitivity. It presents as a single, movable breast nodule, not fixed to the skin. Surgical excision is required for definitive diagnosis.

    Cystosarcoma phyllodes (**choice A**) is a fibroadenoma-like tumor that has become large, cystic, and lobulated. It may contain malignant elements.

    Fibrocystic breast disease (**choice C**) is the most common breast disorder. It usually affects women older than 35. It involves a distortion of the normal breast changes associated with the menstrual cycle. Patients often have lumpy, tender breasts, especially during the several days prior to menstruation.

    Infiltrating ductal carcinoma (**choice D**) is the most common type of breast cancer. It occurs most frequently after age 40. Other risk factors include nulliparity, family history, early menarche, late menopause, previous history of breast cancer, obesity, and high-fat diet.

Intraductal papilloma (**choice E**) is associated with bloody or serous nipple discharge. It is most common in women aged 20 to 50.

32. **The correct answer is C.** Multiple endocrine neoplasia type III (MEN III), also known as MEN IIb, is characterized by medullary thyroid carcinoma, pheochromocytoma, and mucosal neuromas.

    Wermer syndrome, also called MEN type I (**choices A and E**), is characterized by pancreatic (insulinoma), pituitary, and parathyroid involvement.

    Sipple syndrome, or MEN type II (**choices B and D**), is similar to MEN III, but it has parathyroid involvement (tumor or adenoma) as opposed to neuromas.

33. **The correct answer is B.** Multinodular goiters can produce the most extreme enlargements of any of the benign thyroid diseases. The multinodular goiters are composed of nodules created by colloid-filled or hyperplastic follicles separated by fibrous scars. Focal hemorrhage, hemosiderin deposition, calcifications, and microcyst formation may also be present. Multinodular goiters often arise from smaller simple goiters, but the trigger for development of multinodularity is poorly understood. Like simple goiters, most cases in endemic areas are related to iodine deficiency, whereas sporadic cases may have multifactorial causes.

    The other conditions listed in the answers can also cause thyroid enlargement, but the degree of enlargement is usually much less.

34. **The correct answer is D.** Opioids, such as heroin, depress respiration centrally by reducing the responsiveness of brainstem respiratory centers to $CO_2$. The resulting hypoventilation leads to $CO_2$ retention because of the inability of the patient to "blow off" the $CO_2$. This increases the production of carbonic acid ($H_2CO_3$) by carbonic anhydrase present in red blood cells (which converts $CO_2$ to carbonic acid). Dissociation of carbonic acid to bicarbonate ($HCO_3^-$) and protons produces a respiratory acidosis.

    Metabolic acidosis (**choice A**) is caused by a primary decrease in $HCO_3^-$, which can occur after tissue hypoxia (which increases levels of lactic acid) or in uncontrolled diabetes mellitus.

    Metabolic alkalosis (**choice B**) is caused by an increase in $HCO_3^-$, which can occur subsequent to ingestion of alkali or a loss of gastric acid (vomiting).

    Normal pH balance (**choice C**) might be anticipated if the respiratory acidosis persists, allowing time for the kidneys to compensate for the altered pH by conserving $HCO_3^-$. However, renal compensation takes several days (this patient had an acute heroin overdose) and is rarely complete.

Respiratory alkalosis (**choice E**) is caused by a decrease in $P_{CO_2}$, which can occur with hyperventilation.

35. **The correct answer is D.** The nodular sclerosis variant of Hodgkin disease is more common in women and is associated with the presence of lacunar cells (Reed-Sternberg [RS] cells with nuclei surrounded by a clear space) and fibrous bands in the lymph nodes. It has a good prognosis.

Lymphocyte depletion (**choice A**) is associated with scarcity of lymphocytes, multiple RS cells, fibrosis, and necrosis. It has a poor prognosis.

Lymphocyte predominance (**choice B**) is the least common form of Hodgkin disease. It is associated with an abundance of lymphocytes and histiocytes and scant RS cells.

Mixed cellularity (**choice C**) is the most common form of Hodgkin disease. It is associated with the presence of neutrophils, lymphocytes, eosinophils, plasma cells, and histiocytes. Many classic RS cells may be identified.

36. **The correct answer is E.** A large tumor involving the suprasellar region and adjacent base of the brain can produce the deficits noted. Examples of such tumors include craniopharyngiomas and large pituitary adenomas that have outgrown the pituitary fossa. The patient's amenorrhea is due to pituitary destruction. The loss of vision is due to involvement of the optic nerve or chiasm, and the optic disc changes are related to pressure from behind pressing on the optic nerve and disc. The olfactory changes are related to involvement of cranial nerve I.

A tumor of the falx (**choice A**) or the parasagittal meninges typically produces sensory or motor dysfunction of the leg.

A tumor of the hippocampus (**choice B**) might produce memory problems or seizures.

A tumor of the posterior fossa (**choice C**) produces unilateral deafness, tinnitus, vertigo, and, sometimes, sensory loss in the distribution of cranial nerves V or VII.

A tumor of the sphenoidal ridge (**choice D**) can cause cranial nerve palsies involving III, IV, V, or VI.

37. **The correct answer is E.** The patient has a macrocytic anemia with hypersegmented neutrophils. This picture is consistent with either folate or vitamin $B_{12}$ deficiency. The history of small bowel resections and the presence of neurologic signs on physical examination tip the diagnosis to $B_{12}$ deficiency.

Beta-thalassemia trait (**choice A**) and iron deficiency (**choice C**) cause a microcytic, not a macrocytic, anemia.

Folate deficiency (**choice B**) causes a similar picture on peripheral blood smear but is not associated with neurologic signs and symptoms.

Sickle cell trait (**choice D**) does not cause anemia and is associated with a normal peripheral blood smear under usual physiologic conditions.

38. **The correct answer is A.** Acute lymphoblastic leukemia (ALL) is primarily a disease of children, with peak incidence at 4 years of age. Approximately 80% of childhood leukemias are of the ALL type. Other features in this scenario that further support an acute leukemia are fevers and anemia without marked elevations of the white blood cell count.

Acute myeloblastic leukemia (AML; **choice B**) would present in a similar fashion—acute symptoms and anemia with thrombocytopenia. Bone marrow biopsy is needed to definitively differentiate ALL and AML, but AML represents only 20% of childhood leukemias. AML is primarily a disease of adolescents and young adults.

The chronic leukemias (**choices C and D**) are diseases of adulthood that present with nonspecific symptoms and are typically diagnosed when white counts are markedly elevated. Chronic myeloid leukemia (**choice D**), a neoplasm of a pluripotent stem cell, also may present with thrombocytosis, rather than thrombocytopenia.

Hairy cell leukemia (**choice E**) is a relatively rare leukemia of older men. It infiltrates the spleen early in its course and tends to present with pancytopenia due to bone marrow failure and splenic sequestration.

39. **The correct answer is C.** Even though blood flow is interrupted to a portion of the lung, the lung will still continue to ventilate. There will be no gas exchange, and the $P_{O_2}$ and $P_{CO_2}$ of alveolar gas will approach that of inspired air ($P_{O_2} = 150$ mm Hg, and $P_{CO_2} = 0$ mm Hg).

**Choice A** indicates the normal situation.

The $P_{O_2}$ of the lung will always be less than the $P_{O_2}$ of the atmosphere (**choice B**) because air is warmed and moistened in the airways, so water vapor pressure must be accounted for. $P_{O_2}$ in the atmosphere is approximately 160 mm Hg ($0.21 \times 760$ mm Hg); $P_{O_2}$ in the lung is approximately 150 mm Hg (760 mm Hg $-$ 47 mm Hg) $\times$ 0.21 = 150 mm Hg (atmospheric pressure = 760 mm Hg; water vapor pressure = 47 mm Hg).

$P_{O_2}$ of the lung would approximate mixed venous blood (**choice D**) if ventilation were blocked.

$P_{O_2}$ of the lung cannot be less than that of mixed venous blood (**choice E**).

40. **The correct answer is C.** This case depicts a classic picture of hypovolemic shock due to hemorrhage. When blood volume is low, less blood fills the ventricles during diastole, corresponding to reduced preload. Consequently, cardiac output is decreased because of the diminished stroke volume. Vascular resistance is increased to compensate for volume loss. Mixed venous oxygen levels are reduced because of the increased tissue demand of oxygen and the loss of hemoglobin.

The remaining choices are inconsistent with hemorrhagic shock.

41. **The correct answer is C.** This patient's macular skin rash in a "bathing suit" distribution is also known as erythema marginatum, one of the five major Jones criteria for diagnosing rheumatic fever. The other four major criteria are migratory polyarthritis, Sydenham chorea, subcutaneous nodules, and pancarditis. In context of prior streptococcal infection, the presence of two of five major criteria or one major plus two minor criteria (**choices A, B, C, D**) is sufficient to establish the diagnosis. Other minor criteria include previous rheumatic fever and elevated C-reactive protein.

A mnemonic for the major criteria is "CANCER" (not pleasant, but easy to remember): Chorea, Arthritis, Nodules, Carditis, Erythema marginatum, Rheumatic fever diagnosis.

42. **The correct answer is B.** This patient has reflux esophagitis due to an incompetent lower esophageal sphincter (which separates the esophagus from the stomach). Her symptoms arise from the reflux of gastric contents back into the esophagus, leading to inflammation of the esophageal mucosa. Her symptoms are exacerbated by large meals, which lead to increased gastric acid secretion, and lying in bed, a position that allows more of the gastric contents to pass back through the incompetent lower esophageal sphincter.

The ileocecal sphincter (**choice A**), also called the ileocecal valve, separates the small intestine from the large intestine. Relaxation of this sphincter is modulated by the presence of food within the stomach (gastroileal reflex), which increases peristalsis and facilitates the transfer of the contents of the small intestine to the large intestine.

The pyloric sphincter (**choice C**) separates the stomach from the duodenum. Pyloric stenosis results in a palpable mass that obstructs gastric outflow and leads to projectile vomiting. Congenital pyloric stenosis is three to four times more prevalent in males than in females.

The sphincter of Oddi (**choice D**) is a band of circular muscle fibers that envelops the openings of the bile duct and the main pancreatic duct into the duodenum. Relaxation of this sphincter is stimulated by cholecystokinin.

The upper esophageal sphincter (**choice E**) separates the pharynx from the esophagus. It is voluntarily relaxed at the time of swallowing to allow passage of the food bolus from the pharynx to the esophagus.

43. **The correct answer is B.** The costal parietal pleura is supplied by intercostal nerves. Visceral pleuritic pain is referred to the area of skin representing the cutaneous distribution of the intercostal nerves over the affected bronchopulmonary segment.

The greater splanchnic nerve (**choice A**) is composed of the preganglionic sympathetic fibers from the sympathetic trunk that bypass the sympathetic chain ganglia, run in the thorax against the bodies of thoracic vertebrae, pierce the diaphragm, and innervate sympathetic ganglia in the abdomen.

The phrenic nerve (**choice C**) provides motor innervation to the diaphragm. Although it does carry sensory fibers from the diaphragm, pericardium, and mediastinal pleura, it would not be involved with the pleura adjacent to the anterior bronchopulmonary segment.

The pulmonary plexus (**choice D**) is where the vagal preganglionics synapse with the parasympathetic postganglionics to the smooth constrictor muscles of the bronchial tree.

The vagus nerve (**choice E**) in the chest carries only preganglionic parasympathetic fibers, which are visceral motor in function.

44. **The correct answer is A.** A barrel chest with increased anterior/posterior diameter is commonly observed in patients with long-standing, severe emphysema. This change in chest shape occurs because these patients, who have high compliance of the lung proper, tend to function with their lungs to some degree "over-inflated" compared with people who have normal lung compliance. This over-inflation limits their ability to take further deep breaths. (The "balloon" of emphysematous lung remains compliant, but the "box" of the chest wall is not very compliant and limits the volume of air that can be inhaled.) Patients with moderately severe emphysema are able to maintain an adequate lung ventilation by taking many short breaths (compare with **choice D**); this physiology is sometimes expressed by describing these patients as "pink puffers" (**choice E**).

Chronic cough (**choice B**) in emphysema patients is not directly related to the change in compliance.

Excessive mucus production (**choice C**) is more characteristic of chronic bronchitis than of emphysema.

45. **The correct answer is D.** This is one of those questions for which having a good idea of what you are looking for before exploring the answer choices will certainly save you valuable time. The answers all look alike, and you could have been easily confused if you were not confident of the answer before approaching the choices.

This patient has long-standing hyperparathyroidism (*elevated PTH*), which predisposes to the development of osteitis fibrosa, her bone disease. PTH acts initially on osteocytes of bone tissue (osteocytic osteolysis) and subsequently on osteoclasts (osteoclastic resorption) to resorb calcium from bone matrix and make it available to the circulation. This *increases plasma calcium* levels. PTH also causes decreased phosphate reabsorption in the proximal renal tubule, yielding *hypophosphatemia*. Hypercalciuria is another sequela of excess PTH production, which predisposes the patient to the formation of calcium oxalate stones.

Choices **A** and **E** correspond to neither hyper- nor hypoparathyroid states.

**Choice B** is the profile of hypoparathyroidism. You should have quickly eliminated this choice since the PTH was decreased, and you were looking for a profile consistent with *hyper*parathyroidism.

**Choice C** is the profile of secondary hyperparathyroidism. This occurs when the parathyroid overproduction is due to a nonparathyroid cause. By far, the most common cause is chronic renal failure. In such cases, there is decreased calcium absorption, since the kidneys are involved in the conversion of $25(OH)D_3$ to the active form $1,25(OH)D_3$. The decreased calcium ion level stimulates the parathyroid, leading to elevated PTH levels. Hyperphosphatemia results from diminished renal synthesis of 1,25-dihydroxyvitamin $D_3$, creating further calcium-phosphate imbalance and enhanced PTH production.

46. **The correct answer is E.** This is a classic presentation of Hodgkin disease, which is a form of lymphoma characterized by neoplastic proliferation of Reed-Sternberg cells admixed with variable numbers of reactive lymphocytes, neutrophils, and eosinophils. The cell of origin of the Reed-Sternberg cells is still disputed. These cells have a distinctive appearance with a large double nucleus that contains paired, large, nucleoli that are often red in hematoxylin and eosin stains, producing an "owl's eye" effect.

Abnormal plasma cells (**choice A**) would be a feature of multiple myeloma or some B-cell leukemias and lymphomas, which are not as likely in this patient.

Giant platelets (**choice B**) are a feature seen in several myeloproliferative disorders (notably essential thrombocytopenia), which do not cause lymphadenopathy.

Immature neutrophil precursors (**choice C**) would most likely be a feature of a myeloid leukemia, which would not cause a lymphadenopathy.

Melanin pigment (**choice D**) would be a feature of malignant melanoma, which would probably have caused lung or liver metastases if it were at such an advanced stage as to have caused massive lymphadenopathy.

47. **The correct answer is E.** This is a classic case of lead poisoning: chewing on paint chips, abdominal pain, and red blood cells with basophilic stippling. A related physical finding you would expect is lead lines at the gingival margins. X-ray films of the long bones would reveal increased radiodensity at the epiphyses.

Arsenic poisoning (**choice A**) acutely causes hemorrhagic gastroenteritis, fluid loss, and hypotension. Nausea, vomiting, abdominal pain, seizures, or coma may occur. The breath may exhibit a garlicky odor.

Carbon monoxide poisoning (**choice B**) causes hypoxia and bright red fingernails (cherry red cyanosis).

Cyanide poisoning (**choice C**) causes death within minutes. Generalized petechiae and a bitter almond smell are characteristic.

Gold toxicity (**choice D**) causes erythema and pruritus, as well as damage to hematopoietic organs.

Mercury toxicity (**choice F**) acutely causes lassitude, anorexia, and gastrointestinal symptoms. Chronic exposure produces emotional lability, memory loss and excitability (Mad Hatter disease), and polyneuropathies.

48. **The correct answer is A.** Bowen disease is one of three different clinical designations that produce the same histopathologic change of the penis, i.e., carcinoma *in situ*. Erythroplasia of Queyrat and bowenoid papulosis are the other two forms of carcinoma *in situ* of the penis. All these conditions are strongly associated with human papillomavirus (HPV), especially type 16. Carcinoma *in situ* refers to a malignant epithelial neoplasm confined within the basement membrane, without invasion of the underlying stroma. Once carcinoma *in situ* breaks through the basement membrane, invasive carcinoma (**choice C**) is diagnosed. Both carcinoma *in situ* of the penis and carcinoma *in situ* of the cervix have a strong propensity to invade the underlying stroma and transform into invasive squamous cell carcinoma.

Chronic cervicitis (**choice B**) is a very common chronic condition characterized by lymphocytic and, to a lesser extent, neutrophilic infiltration of the cervix. Some degree of chronic cervicitis can be found in any woman. Unless associated with infectious agents, such as *Chlamydia*, gonococcus, *Mycoplasma,* or herpesvirus, chronic cervicitis does not have clinical importance and *is not* associated with an increased frequency of dysplasia.

Mild cervical dysplasia (**choice D**) refers to the presence of dysplasia involving the lower third of the squamous epithelium of the cervix. Most cases spontaneously regress, but some progress to more severe degrees of dysplasia and, eventually, carcinoma.

Nabothian cysts (**choice E**) derive their name from the surgeon Martin Naboth (Leipzig, 1675-1721), who first described these small, mucus-containing cysts in the lower cervix. Nabothian cysts represent a normal effect of the *transformation zone*. After menarche, the simple columnar epithelium of the exposed endocervical epithelium is replaced by squamous epithelium advancing from the ectocervix. This process leads to obstruction of the endocervical crypts, with subsequent accumulation of mucus and formation of cystlike spaces. Nabothian cysts are therefore *normal* histologic features.

49. **The correct answer is D.** Neurofibromatosis type 2 is an autosomal dominant condition caused by mutations of a gene on chromosome 22 coding for a cytoskeleton-related protein called *merlin.* Much less common than neurofibromatosis type 1, it manifests with multiple CNS tumors, the most frequent of which are schwannomas of the 8th cranial nerve and meningiomas. Bilateral schwannomas are virtually pathognomonic (i.e., diagnostic) of neurofibromatosis type 2.

Metastases to the CNS (**choice A**) are often multiple and usually involve the gray-white matter junction. Besides the unusual location, the young age would make this diagnosis highly improbable.

Multiple sclerosis (**choice B**) is a chronic remitting/relapsing demyelinating disease. It manifests with focal neurologic deficits caused by well circumscribed areas of myelin loss in the white matter of the brain (usually periventricular), brainstem, spinal cord, or optic nerves. It is not associated with an increased incidence of any type of brain tumor.

Neurofibromatosis type 1 (**choice C**) is also autosomal dominant and is caused by mutations of a gene on chromosome 17 coding for *neurofibromin*, a protein involved in signal transduction. The most characteristic clinical features include café-au-lait spots, neurofibromas (tumors of peripheral nerves different from

schwannomas), Lisch nodules (pigmented nodules of the iris), and CNS tumors, but not schwannomas.

Tuberous sclerosis (**choice E**), like neurofibromatosis, is a "neurocutaneous syndrome," i.e., a condition characterized by concomitant neurologic and skin lesions. Tuberous sclerosis is caused by mutations in two loci, either TS1 or TS2. Multiple hamartomas of the brain (cortical "tubers") and other organs, shagreen patches, ash-leaf patches, and other skin lesions constitute the clinical findings in this disorder.

50. **The correct answer is D.** Small cell carcinoma of the lung is composed of extremely undifferentiated (i.e., anaplastic) cells, with high nuclear/cytoplasmic ratio. This neoplasm is very aggressive and tends to metastasize so early in its course that even small tumors are considered inoperable by the time of clinical diagnosis. One of the most interesting characteristics of this type of tumor is the frequent association with paraneoplastic syndromes, the most common of which is due to ectopic production of ACTH. Paraneoplastic syndromes also occur with other types of lung tumors.

Adenocarcinomas of the lung (**choice A**) are composed of mucin-producing neoplastic cells arranged in a glandular pattern. Its histologic features make this tumor easily distinguishable from small cell carcinoma.

Carcinoid tumors of the lung (**choice B**) are histologically similar to carcinoid tumors of the gastrointestinal tract. They are composed of cords and islands of uniform cuboidal cells. Carcinoid syndrome may be produced because of the ability of the tumor to produce and release serotonin.

A hamartoma (**choice C**) is not a true neoplasm, but rather a malformative lesion consisting of normal lung tissues arranged in haphazard manner. Hamartomas are often discovered incidentally on chest x-ray films as "coin lesions" and contain cartilage, smooth muscle, and cystlike spaces lined by bronchial epithelium.

Squamous cell carcinomas (**choice E**) are characterized by neoplastic squamous epithelium with evidence of extracellular and/or intracellular keratin production. The most frequent paraneoplastic syndrome accompanying pulmonary squamous cell carcinomas is hypercalcemia.

Finally, remember that cigarette smoking is a strong risk factor for all types of lung cancer, especially squamous cell carcinoma and small cell carcinoma.

# Pharmacology: **Test One**

1. A 67-year-old man presents to the emergency department with shaking chills and a temperature of 38.0 C (101 F). Laboratory examination reveals a hematocrit of 23%, and urine tests are positive for blood. The patient states that he is taking only one medication for his "irregular heartbeat." Which of the following drugs most likely caused the appearance of these signs and symptoms in this patient?

   (A) Digoxin
   (B) Hydralazine
   (C) Propranolol
   (D) Quinidine
   (E) Verapamil

2. A 41-year-old diabetic woman presents to her physician complaining of gastrointestinal distress and heartburn, particularly after meals. Which of the following drugs should her physician prescribe to relieve her symptoms?

   (A) Omeprazole
   (B) Diphenoxylate
   (C) Famotidine
   (D) Prochlorperazine
   (E) Sucralfate

3. A 58-year-old woman arrives at her physician's office complaining of moderate anxiety. Which of the following drugs will help relieve her anxiety, with a minimum of unwanted sedative side effects?

   (A) Buspirone
   (B) Chlordiazepoxide
   (C) Lorazepam
   (D) Trazodone
   (E) Zolpidem

4. A 55-year-old woman is receiving chemotherapy for non-Hodgkin lymphoma. Several days after a treatment, she notices blood in her urine. Which of the following antineoplastic drugs is most likely responsible for this side effect?

   (A) Bleomycin
   (B) Cisplatin
   (C) Cyclophosphamide
   (D) Doxorubicin
   (E) Plicamycin
   (F) Vincristine

5. The pharmacokinetic properties of a new drug are being studied in normal volunteers during phase I clinical trials. The volume of distribution and clearance determined in the first subject are 80 L and 4 L/hr, respectively. The half-life of the drug in this subject is approximately

   (A) 0.03 hours
   (B) 14 hours
   (C) 78 hours
   (D) 139 hours
   (E) 222 hours

6. A 45-year-old man presents to the emergency department with severe pneumonia. He recently returned from a business trip, and has a history of smoking and alcohol use. An x-ray film shows extensive consolidation affecting portions of each lung lobe. Culture on charcoal yeast extract medium grows out a small gram-negative bacterium. Which of the following antibiotics is the most appropriate treatment for this patient?

   (A) Ceftriaxone

   (B) Chloramphenicol

   (C) Clindamycin

   (D) Erythromycin

   (E) Metronidazole

   (F) Penicillin V

   (G) Pentamidine

   (H) Trimethoprim-sulfamethoxazole

   (I) Vancomycin

7. A 46-year-old woman visits her podiatrist to have several bunions removed from her right foot. She chooses conscious sedation rather than general anesthesia for this procedure. She is given IV midazolam to supplement the local anesthetics that are injected into her foot. Midway through the surgery, she suddenly becomes agitated and combative and exhibits involuntary movements. The anesthesiologist determines that she is having a paradoxical reaction to the midazolam and immediately administers

   (A) flumazenil

   (B) glucagon

   (C) naloxone

   (D) nitrite

   (E) protamine

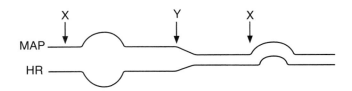

8. Mean arterial blood pressure (MAP) and heart rate (HR) measurements were recorded during the IV administration of two different drugs (see above figure). Select the most likely drugs given at the indicated points.

   | | X | Y |
   |---|---|---|
   | (A) | Acetylcholine | phentolamine |
   | (B) | Epinephrine (low dose) | hexamethonium |
   | (C) | Isoproterenol | propranolol |
   | (D) | Metaproterenol | propranolol |
   | (E) | Norepinephrine | hexamethonium |
   | (F) | Phenylephrine | phentolamine |

9. A 55-year-old diabetic man is brought to the emergency department in an unresponsive state. The following laboratory values are obtained:

   $P_{CO_2}$: 19 mm Hg

   Bicarbonate: 11 mEq/L

   pH: 6.9

   Which of following is the most appropriate immediate treatment for this patient?

   (A) Administration of bicarbonate

   (B) Administration of insulin and glucose

   (C) Administration of an oral hypoglycemic agent

   (D) Close observation only

10. A 62-year-old woman is being prepared for cardiac bypass surgery. Before she is intubated, she is given a skeletal muscle relaxant that causes her to have muscle fasciculations prior to muscle relaxation. Which of the following drugs was most likely administered?

   (A) Atracurium

   (B) Succinylcholine

   (C) Pancuronium

   (D) Rocuronium

   (E) Vecuronium

11. A 62-year-old white man complains of left thigh and leg pain and swelling that are exacerbated by walking. One week earlier, the patient underwent cardiac catheterization. The patient is currently vacationing and has spent the past 28 hours in a car. Which of the following drugs, which might be prescribed in this instance, works by inhibiting the enzyme epoxide reductase?

    (A) Acetylsalicylic acid

    (B) Dipyridamole

    (C) Heparin

    (D) Streptokinase

    (E) Tissue-type plasminogen activator (tPA)

    (F) Warfarin

12. A 58-year-old man presents with difficulty initiating movements and a resting tremor. On physical examination, his face appears expressionless and he has a slow shuffling gait. He is started on selegiline. Which of the following is the mechanism of action of this drug?

    (A) It inhibits degradation of dopamine by MAO type B

    (B) It inhibits dopa decarboxylase

    (C) It is an agonist at dopamine receptors

    (D) It is a precursor of dopamine

    (E) It blocks catechol-*O*-methyltransferase (COMT)

13. A 34-year-old man with a long history of asthma is referred to a pulmonologist. The physician decides to prescribe zileuton. The mechanism of action of this drug is to

    (A) antagonize $LTD_4$ receptors

    (B) inhibit 5-lipoxygenase

    (C) inhibit phosphodiesterase

    (D) inhibit phospholipase $A_2$

    (E) stimulate beta$_2$ receptors

14. A 60-year-old hypertensive woman presents to her physician with visual changes. Transient ischemic attack is ruled out. She is then referred to an ophthalmologist, who prescribes a medication that subsequently causes drowsiness and tingling in her arms. Laboratory evaluation reveals hyperchloremic metabolic acidosis. Which of the following drugs was most likely prescribed?

    (A) Acetazolamide

    (B) Demeclocycline

    (C) Ethacrynic acid

    (D) Furosemide

    (E) Hydrochlorothiazide

    (F) Spironolactone

15. A patient was administered mecamylamine during surgery. This drug will most likely cause which of the following responses?

    (A) Accommodation

    (B) Hypertension

    (C) Peristalsis

    (D) Pupillary constriction

    (E) Tachycardia

16. A 70-year-old man complains of chronic heartburn. It is painful for him to bend over, and he sleeps on a wedge-shaped pillow to try to reduce the burning sensation. Which of the following agents would be the most efficacious in reducing his symptoms?

    (A) Bisacodyl

    (B) Cimetidine

    (C) Magnesium hydroxide

    (D) Omeprazole

    (E) Promethazine

17. An 82-year-old woman presents to her physician complaining of difficulty sleeping and problems coping throughout the day since the recent death of her husband. She requests a medication that will help her through this time of her life. Her physician prescribes oxazepam. The most likely rationale behind prescribing this drug is that oxazepam

    (A) does not deplete liver glutathione

    (B) does not have first pass metabolism

    (C) does not require phase I metabolism

    (D) does not require phase II metabolism

    (E) induces cytochrome P450

**KAPLAN) MEDICAL**

18. A continuous IV infusion of lidocaine is given to a 70-kg patient with cardiac arrhythmias. The pharmacokinetic parameters for lidocaine are as follows: clearance (CL) = 9 mL/min/kg, volume of distribution ($V_d$) = 70 L, half-life = 2 hours. How long will it take for drug levels to reach 87.5% of steady state?

    (A)  1.75 hours

    (B)  3.5 hours

    (C)  5.5 hours

    (D)  6.0 hours

    (E)  8.0 hours

19. A 5-year-old boy with no previous medical history is brought to the emergency department by his mother because he accidentally ingested a large dose of rat poison. He is conscious but appears quite agitated. On physical examination, his blood pressure is 110/70 mm Hg and pulse is 90/min. Laboratory results are significant for an elevated prothrombin time (PT) but a normal partial prothrombin time (PTT). Which of the following is the most appropriate pharmacotherapy?

    (A)  Atropine

    (B)  Flumazenil

    (C)  N-acetylcysteine

    (D)  Protamine

    (E)  Vitamin K

20. A pharmacology professor is teaching his class about the actions of different drugs on vessels. A certain drug produces vasodilation by increasing cGMP in the smooth-muscle cells of arterioles. Which of the following drugs has this mechanism of action?

    (A)  Bethanechol

    (B)  Isoproterenol

    (C)  Metaproterenol

    (D)  Nifedipine

    (E)  Phentolamine

    (F)  Phenylephrine

21. A 74-year-old woman with multiple myeloma is being treated with high doses of doxorubicin (Adriamycin). She has also received cyclophosphamide and prednisone recently. During an examination, the physician should check the patient for which of the following?

    (A)  Abdominal tenderness

    (B)  Bladder distention

    (C)  Limitation of movement

    (D)  Papilledema

    (E)  Pulmonary rales

22. A 48-year-old smoker with deep venous thrombosis is given heparin. Heparin achieves its anticoagulant activity by binding to which of the following substances?

    (A)  $Alpha_2$ antiplasmin

    (B)  $Alpha_2$ macroglobulin

    (C)  Antithrombin III

    (D)  Factor VIII

    (E)  Factor IX

    (F)  Factor X

    (G)  Prothrombin

23. An elderly man presents with complaints of ringing in his ears, blurred vision, and upset stomach. He is taking multiple medications. His wife states that he has had a few episodes of confused, delirious behavior over the past few weeks. Which of the following agents might be responsible for this man's symptoms?

    (A)  Allopurinol

    (B)  Hydralazine

    (C)  Niacin

    (D)  Quinidine

    (E)  Spironolactone

24. A patient is administered a skeletal muscle relaxant prior to abdominal surgery. The patient soon begins to exhibit hypotension, bronchospasm, and excessive bronchial and salivary secretions. Which of the following skeletal muscle relaxants did this patient most likely receive?

    (A) Atracurium

    (B) Baclofen

    (C) Dantrolene

    (D) Tubocurarine

    (E) Vecuronium

25. Genetic analysis of a female infant with a broad, enlarged neck demonstrates an XO karyotype. When the child reaches puberty, hormone replacement therapy should be started with which of the following agents?

    (A) Estrogen only

    (B) Estrogen and progestin

    (C) Insulin

    (D) Progestin only

    (E) Thyroid hormone

26. A former drug abuser visits his physician to ask for pain medication for a legitimate back pain. The physician takes the history of drug abuse into account. Which of the following medications has the greatest potential for abuse?

    (A) Codeine

    (B) Dextromethorphan

    (C) Loperamide

    (D) Meperidine

    (E) Nalbuphine

    (F) Pentazocine

    (G) Propoxyphene

27. A 48-year-old type 2 diabetic patient on daily extended-release glipizide presents with complaints of polyuria and polydipsia. Laboratory evaluation reveals a blood glucose of 192 mg/dL. She states that her diabetes had been well controlled and that she had been symptom-free for the past 8 years. Recently, however, she began taking medication for hypertension. Which of the following antihypertensive drugs is she most likely taking?

    (A) Diltiazem

    (B) Enalapril

    (C) Hydrochlorothiazide

    (D) Methyldopa

    (E) Terazosin

28. A 33-year-old with a history of asthma is being treated for symptoms of hypertension. Which of the following beta-blockers would be an appropriate therapy for this patient?

    (A) Isoproterenol

    (B) Labetalol

    (C) Metoprolol

    (D) Propranolol

    (E) Timolol

29. A patient with essential hypertension is starting diuretic therapy. He has a history of calcium oxalate renal stones. Which of the following diuretics would be most appropriate for this patient?

    (A) Acetazolamide

    (B) Furosemide

    (C) Hydrochlorothiazide

    (D) Spironolactone

    (E) Triamterene

30. A 64-year-old man presents to his family physician complaining of difficulty urinating and "dribbling" at the end of urination. The physician diagnoses benign prostatic hyperplasia. Which of the following drugs would be most appropriate for treating this man's condition?

    (A) Finasteride
    (B) Leuprolide
    (C) Mifepristone
    (D) Pergolide
    (E) Tamoxifen

31. Drug X has a $t_{1/2}$ of 4 hours and is renally eliminated. After elimination of one kidney, how long (in hours) would it take for Drug X to reach steady state?

    (A) 10
    (B) 20
    (C) 30
    (D) 40
    (E) 60

32. A 30-year-old woman with a history of tonic-clonic seizures complains of double vision, thickened gums, and growth of facial hair since starting a new medication. Which of the following anticonvulsant medications is most likely responsible for her symptoms?

    (A) Carbamazepine
    (B) Ethosuximide
    (C) Phenobarbital
    (D) Phenytoin
    (E) Valproic acid

33. A 32-year-old woman who is 36 weeks pregnant is told during a prenatal appointment that her fetus is in a breech presentation. An external cephalic version (manually turning the fetus from the outside) is scheduled for the following week. For this procedure, the uterus must be relaxed. Which of the following drugs would be most appropriate for achieving this result?

    (A) Clomiphene
    (B) Phenylephrine
    (C) Progesterone
    (D) Propranolol
    (E) Ritodrine

34. A 26-year-old woman undergoing surgery is given an inhalant anesthetic. She is also given an IV dose of succinylcholine. Within minutes, she develops a heart rate of 124/min and increasing core body temperature. Which of the following is the mechanism of action of the drug of choice for this patient's condition?

    (A) It interferes with the release of $Ca^{2+}$ from the sarcoplasmic reticulum
    (B) It is a competitive antagonist of ACh at the motor end plate
    (C) It is a GABA receptor agonist that enhances inhibition of nerve impulses
    (D) It uncouples oxidative phosphorylation, thereby preventing heat formation

35. A neurophysiologist is studying the consequences of diminished brain perfusion in an experimental animal. The carotid artery is occluded, and brain function is monitored by positron emission tomography. Which of the following drugs would be most effective in reversing the change in heart rate produced by the experimental occlusion?

    (A) Atropine
    (B) Metaproterenol
    (C) Neostigmine
    (D) Phenoxybenzamine
    (E) Propranolol

36. A 33-year-old man receiving chemotherapy for testicular carcinoma develops signs of renal tubular damage. Which of the following drugs is most likely responsible for this nephrotoxicity?

    (A) Bleomycin
    (B) Cisplatin
    (C) Cyclophosphamide
    (D) Vinblastine
    (E) Vincristine

37. A new antibiotic is being tested in clinical trials. The following pharmacokinetic parameters have previously been determined:

Clearance = 100 mL/min

Volume of distribution ($V_d$) = 50 L

Half-life = 3 hours

Assuming that the drug is being administered intravenously, what loading dose (LD) should be given to a patient to quickly obtain a plasma concentration of 10 mg/L?

(A) 5 mg

(B) 25 mg

(C) 100 mg

(D) 500 mg

(E) 1000 mg

38. A 24-year-old migrant farm worker is rushed to a nearby emergency department after an accidental exposure to parathion. He is in respiratory distress and is bradycardic. Which of the following drugs can be given to increase the activity of his acetylcholinesterase?

(A) Atropine

(B) Deferoxamine

(C) Dimercaprol

(D) N-acetylcysteine

(E) Physostigmine

(F) Pralidoxime

39. A 48-year-old vagrant with a history of alcoholism ingests a bottle of antifreeze and presents to the emergency department obtunded but with intact vision. Which of the following is the most appropriate pharmacotherapy?

(A) Amyl nitrite

(B) Atropine

(C) Ethanol

(D) Glucagon

(E) Naloxone

(F) Oxygen

(G) Pyridoxine

(H) Sodium bicarbonate

40. A man is taking phenelzine for atypical depression. He goes to a party and consumes a few bottles of beer and some aged cheese and crackers. Later that evening, he develops a headache so severe he needs to go to the hospital. He is found to have a blood pressure of 210/100 mm Hg. The emergency room physician explains to him that because he is taking this medication, he should not have consumed those particular foods at the party because they contain which of the following types of substances?

(A) A direct-acting sympathomimetic

(B) A false transmitter

(C) A muscarinic agonist

(D) A neuronal uptake inhibitor

(E) An indirect-acting sympathomimetic

41. A 47-year-old man presents with acute pain in his big toe. Laboratory tests reveal a uric acid level of 10 mg/dL. He is started on medication (Drug 1). Several days after the resolution of the acute attack, he is started on a second medication (Drug 2). Drug 2 decreases both the serum and urine levels of uric acid. Which of the following is Drug 2?

(A) Allopurinol

(B) Colchicine

(C) Indomethacin

(D) Probenecid

(E) Sulfinpyrazone

42. A 57-year-old smoker with a long history of chronic obstructive lung disease presents to the physician with a blood pressure of 150/95 mm Hg. Which of the following antihypertensives is *contraindicated* in this patient?

(A) Acebutolol

(B) Atenolol

(C) Esmolol

(D) Metoprolol

(E) Nadolol

43. To help learn the effects of medications on different organs, a group of medical students put together a quiz show for the class. They draw the following diagram on the chalkboard:

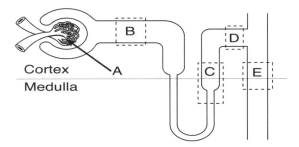

The first question on the quiz show is: Ethacrynic acid would act at which of the above areas?

(A) A

(B) B

(C) C

(D) D

(E) E

44. A worried mother complains to her pediatrician that both she and her 6-year-old son's teacher have noticed that the child has become inattentive. She states that her son frequently stops what he is doing and "stares blankly into space" before resuming his activities. Electroencephalography reveals a 3/second spike and slow wave pattern of discharges. Which of the following agents would most effectively treat this child's disorder?

(A) Carbamazepine

(B) Diazepam

(C) Ethosuximide

(D) Methylphenidate

(E) Phenytoin

45. Two alpha-adrenergic antagonists (Drugs A and B) decrease blood pressure by the same amount following IV administration at the following doses:

Drug A: 120 mg

Drug B: 15 mg

This information implies that Drug A

(A) has a higher therapeutic index than Drug B

(B) has a lower bioavailability than Drug B

(C) has a shorter half-life than Drug B

(D) is less efficacious than Drug B

(E) is less potent than Drug B

46. A 33-year-old woman goes to the physician for a minor outpatient procedure. The physician wants to use a long-duration ester for a local anesthetic. Which of the following agents should be used?

(A) Bupivacaine

(B) Cocaine

(C) Lidocaine

(D) Procaine

(E) Tetracaine

47. A 24-year-old woman attempts suicide by ingesting 50 acetaminophen tablets. She is rushed to the emergency department. Which of the following treatments would the attending physician most likely order?

(A) Alkalinization of urine

(B) $Ca^{2+}$/EDTA chelation

(C) Deferoxamine

(D) N-acetylcysteine

(E) Protamine sulfate

48. A 52-year-old man with peptic ulcer disease has been on drug therapy for 3 months and has noticed changes in his bowel habits, increasing headaches, dizziness, skin rashes, loss of libido, and gynecomastia. Which of the following drugs is most likely responsible for these side effects?

(A) Cimetidine

(B) Famotidine

(C) Metronidazole

(D) Omeprazole

(E) Sucralfate

49. A medical professor is cleaning out her files and comes across an old case report about a 56-year-old man with hypertension who had been treated with reserpine for many years. On a routine blood pressure check, the patient was found to have an increase in blood pressure. When told about this finding, the patient reported that since his last visit he had taken an additional medication, and he admitted to recreational drug use. Which of the following medications was most likely responsible for his increase in blood pressure?

    (A) Amphetamine

    (B) Bethanechol

    (C) Cocaine

    (D) Guanethidine

    (E) Phenylephrine

50. A 53-year-old man comes to the physician because of tingling in his feet and recurrent blurry vision. He is an obese man who rarely exercises and who eats an excessive amount of fatty, high-caloric food. He takes no medications. A fasting plasma glucose level is 169 mg/dL on this visit and 172 mg/dL on a subsequent visit. Which of the following drugs used in the treatment of his condition has no effect on the secretion of insulin?

    (A) Acetohexamide

    (B) Chlorpropamide

    (C) Glyburide

    (D) Metformin

    (E) Tolbutamide

# Pharmacology Test One: **Answers and Explanations**

## ANSWER KEY

| | | | |
|---|---|---|---|
| 1. | D | 26. | D |
| 2. | D | 27. | C |
| 3. | A | 28. | C |
| 4. | C | 29. | C |
| 5. | B | 30. | A |
| 6. | D | 31. | B |
| 7. | A | 32. | D |
| 8. | E | 33. | E |
| 9. | B | 34. | A |
| 10. | B | 35. | E |
| 11. | F | 36. | B |
| 12. | A | 37. | D |
| 13. | B | 38. | F |
| 14. | A | 39. | C |
| 15. | E | 40. | E |
| 16. | D | 41. | A |
| 17. | C | 42. | E |
| 18. | D | 43. | C |
| 19. | E | 44. | C |
| 20. | A | 45. | E |
| 21. | E | 46. | E |
| 22. | C | 47. | D |
| 23. | D | 48. | A |
| 24. | D | 49. | E |
| 25. | B | 50. | D |

1. **The correct answer is D.** Hemolytic anemia is a disorder in which red blood cell survival is decreased, either episodically or continuously. Although the bone marrow has the ability to increase erythroid production, this type of anemia is typically seen when the bone marrow is unable to compensate for the marked hemolysis of red blood cells. Since red blood cells typically survive for 120 days, the hematocrit will fall at a rate of 1% per day, in the absence of red blood cell production. The mechanism for the hemolytic anemia in this patient is related to the formation of an immune complex between a circulating red blood cell and quinidine, a medication used in the treatment of premature atrial, AV-junctional, and ventricular contractions, as well as various other arrhythmias. Since the immune complex is viewed as foreign, the red blood cell in this complex is lysed by the complement system. The quinidine molecule then dissociates from the lysed red blood cell and binds to another red blood cell to repeat the process. This recycling of drug-antibody complex accounts for the dramatic decrease in the hematocrit.

   Digoxin (**choice A**) is typically used to treat atrial fibrillation, atrial flutter, and paroxysmal atrial tachycardia. Digoxin is not associated with the development of hemolytic anemia.

   Hydralazine (**choice B**) is a vasodilator used in the treatment of essential hypertension. Although it is not associated with the development of hemolytic anemia, it has been known to cause a lupus-like syndrome.

   Neither propranolol (**choice C**), a beta-blocker, nor verapamil (**choice E**), a calcium channel blocker, is associated with the development of hemolytic anemia.

2. **The correct answer is D.** Prochlorperazine (**choice D**) is an antiemetic agent that acts as a $D_2$-receptor antagonist at the chemoreceptor trigger zone in the medulla. Although this woman's heartburn may cause her to feel nauseous, this symptom would be relieved by treating the underlying motility problem.

   Patients with diabetes may have damage to the nerves innervating their viscera, resulting in gastroparesis (loss of motility of the esophagus and stomach). This loss of motility causes delayed gastric emptying, bloating, and nausea, and gastroesophageal reflux disease (GERD). Dopamine antagonists, such as metoclopramide, enhancer lower esophageal sphincter (LES) tone and prevent symptoms and complications of GERD (i.e., Barrett esophagitis).

   Omeprazole (**choice A**) is a proton pump inhibitor used for the treatment of ulcers.

   Diphenoxylate (**choice B**), which is structurally related to meperidine, is an antidiarrheal agent. By diminishing gastric motility even further, diphenoxylate would likely exacerbate this woman's symptoms.

   Famotidine (**choice C**) is an $H_2$-receptor antagonist that inhibits histamine-induced gastric acid secretions. Excessive gastric acid secretion does not underlie this patient's problems.

   Sucralfate (**choice E**), or aluminum sucrose sulfate, is a poorly soluble agent that polymerizes in the acid environment of the stomach. The polymer then binds to ulcerated tissue and protects it from pepsin-mediated protein hydrolysis and damage by acid. It also binds bile salts, which are thought to play a role in the pathogenesis of gastric ulcers. However, there is no indication that this woman has ulcer disease.

3. **The correct answer is A.** Buspirone is a nonbenzodiazepine anxiolytic that is devoid of the sedative (or anticonvulsive and muscle relaxant) properties typically associated with the benzodiazepines. It is a partial agonist at $5-HT_{1A}$ receptors.

   Chlordiazepoxide (**choice B**) and lorazepam (**choice C**) are benzodiazepines. Although they are useful anxiolytics, they produce sedation.

   Trazodone (**choice D**) is a very sedating atypical antidepressant.

   Zolpidem (**choice E**) is a nonbenzodiazepine hypnotic used for the treatment of insomnia.

4. **The correct answer is C.** Step 1 questions related to antineoplastic agents are most likely going to ask you about mechanism of action, cell cycle specificity, or side effects. Bone marrow suppression, nausea, vomiting, ulcers, and alopecia are common side effects; however, you are probably more likely to be asked about the unique side effects of certain drugs. In this case, cyclophosphamide has the unique side effect of hemorrhagic cystitis, which could cause hematuria. Note that cyclophosphamide is also consistent with the fact that the patient is being treated for non-Hodgkin lymphoma.

   All the other answer choices have unique, USMLE-worthy side effects:

   Bleomycin (**choice A**) is notable for its pulmonary toxicity. Although bleomycin can be used to treat lymphoma, you are more likely to see it as part of the treatment regimen (with vinblastine and cisplatin) for testicular tumors.

   Cisplatin (**choice B**) is notable for its nephrotoxicity and ototoxicity. It is used in the treatment of testicular and lung cancers. It would not be used in a patient with lymphoma.

   Doxorubicin (**choice D**) is also called Adriamycin. It is an antibiotic agent used in the treatment of many cancers, including lymphomas, sarcomas, and many carcinomas. Its unique side effect is its cardiotoxicity.

You might have been tempted by plicamycin (**choice E**) if you recalled that it can cause a hemorrhagic diathesis. You could have eliminated this answer, however, because plicamycin is not used in the treatment of lymphoma. It is used in the treatment of testicular cancer and cases of hypercalcemia.

Vincristine (**choice F**) is notable for its dose-limiting neurotoxicity. It is used as part of the MOPP regimen for Hodgkin disease. It is also used for the treatment of acute lymphocytic leukemia (ALL), lymphoma, CNS tumors, sarcoma, and Wilms tumor.

5. **The correct answer is B.** The half-life of a drug can be determined using the following equations:

*1)* $CL = k \times Vd$
$4 \text{ L/h} = k \times 80 \text{ L}$
or
$k = 4/80 = 1/20 \text{ h}^{-1}$

*2)* $t_{1/2} = 0.7/k$
$t_{1/2} = 0.7 \times 20 \text{ h}$
$t_{1/2} = 14 \text{ h}$

6. **The correct answer is D.** This patient has Legionnaires disease, an acute, and sometimes fatal, pneumonia. It is caused by *Legionella pneumophila*, a facultative intracellular parasite that can be grown on charcoal yeast agar; erythromycin is the treatment of choice. *Legionella* is acquired from inhaling an infectious aerosol produced from sources such as air conditioning systems of large buildings (e.g., hotels) or respiratory therapy equipment. Legionnaires disease affects men more often than women, and is more common in individuals older than 40. The disease is more severe in smokers, alcoholics, diabetics, and immunosuppressed patients.

Ceftriaxone (**choice A**) is a third-generation cephalosporin. It is a broad-spectrum antibiotic and is the drug of choice for *Neisseria gonorrhoeae* infections.

Chloramphenicol (**choice B**) is a broad-spectrum antibiotic that is rarely used in the U.S. because of the risk of aplastic anemia, a rare but fatal side effect. In developing nations, it is the drug of choice for typhoid fever.

Clindamycin (**choice C**) is a broad-spectrum antibiotic active against gram-positive cocci and anaerobic bacteria. It is the most common agent associated with antibiotic-induced pseudomembranous colitis due to *Clostridium difficile*.

Metronidazole (**choice E**) is active against many obligate anaerobes, certain protozoa (*Amoeba, Trichomonas,*

*Giardia*), and *Helicobacter pylori*. It is also used to treat pseudomembranous colitis due to *Clostridium difficile* infection.

Penicillin V (**choice F**) is a natural penicillin that is active against many gram-positive microorganisms, including beta-hemolytic streptococci, pneumococci, some gram-negatives (including *Neisseria meningitidis*), and spirochetes.

Pentamidine (**choice G**) is used to treat *Pneumocystis carinii* pneumonia in patients either allergic or resistant to trimethoprim-sulfamethoxazole.

Trimethoprim and sulfamethoxazole (**choice H**) are broad-spectrum antibiotics that are folate antagonists. The combination is active against many gram-positives (except *Streptococcus* species) and many gram-negatives (except anaerobes and *Pseudomonas*). The combination is also active against *Pneumocystis carinii*.

Vancomycin (**choice I**) is slowly bactericidal for many gram-positive bacteria, but has no activity against gram-negative bacteria. It is the drug of choice for treating methicillin-resistant *Staphylococcus aureus* and penicillin-resistant *Streptococcus pneumoniae*.

7. **The correct answer is A.** Flumazenil is a benzodiazepine antagonist and has been approved to hasten the recovery from benzodiazepines used in anesthetic and diagnostic settings and to reverse the CNS depressant effects following an overdose with benzodiazepines. Flumazenil can be used only for benzodiazepines or benzodiazepine-receptor agonists, such as zolpidem and zaleplon; it is not useful in reversing the effects of other CNS depressants, such as barbiturates and ethanol.

Glucagon (**choice B**) is an antidote for beta-blocker overdose.

Naloxone (**choice C**), an opioid receptor antagonist, is an antidote for opioid overdose.

Nitrite (**choice D**), or sodium nitrite, is an antidote for cyanide poisoning.

Protamine (**choice E**) is an antidote for heparin overdose.

8. **The correct answer is E.** Several strategies are useful in solving drug tracing problems: *1) Always* look at blood pressure first and heart rate second. Blood pressure changes will be the direct result of the administered drug; heart rate changes may be a direct effect or they may result from a baroreceptor reflex. *2)* Assume that when an agonist effect is gone, so is the agonist; however, also assume that an antagonist stays on board for the entire trace. *3)* Eliminate as many options as possible by examining the initial agonist effect.

The only two agonists that would be expected to raise blood pressure to this degree are norepinephrine (alpha$_1$, alpha$_2$, and beta$_1$ agonist), phenylephrine (alpha$_1$ agonist), and epinephrine at high doses. Thus, **choices A, C,** and **D** can be eliminated immediately.

Drug Y lowers blood pressure and raises heart rate. Hexamethonium (ganglionic blocker) would lower blood pressure and increase heart rate by blocking the predominant tone of the arterioles (sympathetic) and the heart (parasympathetic). Phentolamine (alpha antagonist) would lower blood pressure by blocking arteriolar alpha$_1$ receptors. The increase in heart rate would be a baroreceptor reflex.

The second administration of Drug X causes an increase in both blood pressure and heart rate. Only the combination of norepinephrine and hexamethonium could do this. Norepinephrine would still increase blood pressure by stimulating end organ receptors; however, the baroreceptor reflex would be blocked by hexamethonium. The ability of norepinephrine to increase heart rate by stimulating cardiac beta$_1$ receptors is now revealed.

**Choice A:** Acetylcholine would cause a decrease in blood pressure by stimulating noninnervated muscarinic receptors present on arterioles. Heart rate would increase because of a baroreceptor reflex. Phentolamine would cause a decrease in blood pressure and an increase in heart rate (baroreceptor reflex). It should have no effect on a subsequent administration of acetylcholine.

**Choice B:** Low-dose epinephrine would cause a small increase in mean blood pressure, but not enough to elicit a baroreceptor reflex. So, an increase in heart rate would be seen as a result of beta$_1$ stimulation of the heart. Hexamethonium would cause a decrease in blood pressure and an increase in heart rate. Hexamethonium should not affect subsequent epinephrine administration because a baroreceptor reflex was not initially produced.

**Choice C:** Isoproterenol (beta$_1$ and beta$_2$ agonist) would cause a decrease in blood pressure (by stimulating arteriolar beta$_2$ receptors) and an increase in heart rate (a combination of cardiac beta$_1$ receptor stimulation and baroreceptor reflex). Phenoxybenzamine (alpha antagonist) would cause a decrease in blood pressure and increase in heart rate (baroreceptor reflex). Phenoxybenzamine should not have an effect on subsequent administration of isoproterenol.

**Choice D:** Metaproterenol (beta$_2$ agonist) would decrease blood pressure (by stimulating arteriolar beta$_2$ receptors) and increase heart rate (baroreceptor reflex). Propranolol (beta$_1$ and beta$_2$ antagonist) would decrease blood pressure and increase heart rate. It

would completely block subsequent administration of metaproterenol.

**Choice F:** Phenylephrine would increase blood pressure and decrease heart rate (baroreceptor reflex). Phentolamine would decrease blood pressure and increase heart rate (baroreceptor reflex). Phentolamine would completely block subsequent administration of phenylephrine.

9. **The correct answer is B.** This patient is in a diabetic ketoacidotic coma. The goals in treating such a patient are to increase the rate of glucose utilization by insulin-dependent tissues, to reverse ketonemia and acidosis, and to replenish fluids.

Treatment with bicarbonate (**choice A**) would result in only a transient elevation of pH.

Oral hypoglycemic agents (**choice C**) are commonly prescribed for the maintenance of patients with type 2 diabetes and would not be appropriate in an acute setting.

Since this is a life-threatening condition, monitoring the patient without treatment (**choice D**) is unacceptable.

10. **The correct answer is B.** This patient was given succinylcholine, a depolarizing neuromuscular blocker. It initially causes fasciculations because it stimulates the nicotinic acetylcholine receptors on skeletal muscle ($N_M$) and causes depolarization of the skeletal muscle. Muscle fasciculations can be observed before the muscle goes into depolarization block, at which time the patient will have flaccid paralysis.

All the other drugs listed are nondepolarizing, or competitive, skeletal muscle relaxants. These drugs act by competitively blocking the $N_M$ receptors. Patients receiving these drugs would exhibit flaccid paralysis immediately.

11. **The correct answer is F.** This patient has deep venous thrombi (DVT). He has several risk factors for the development of DVT, including a recent hospitalization that likely included catheterization in the femoral region and a recent period of prolonged stasis. The enzyme epoxide reductase is responsible for converting vitamin K into its active quinone form. The drugs that inhibit epoxide reductase are the vitamin K antagonists such as warfarin. Clotting factors II, VII, IX, and X and proteins C and S are all dependent on vitamin K, which acts as a cofactor for carboxylation reactions. Carboxylation makes factors II, VII, IX, and X better able to interact with calcium and thus able to participate in thrombosis.

Acetylsalicylic acid (**choice A**) acts as a platelet aggregation inhibitor by decreasing thromboxane A$_2$ production, which under normal circumstances causes platelet aggregation.

Dipyridamole (**choice B**) is also a platelet aggregation inhibitor that increases cAMP levels by inhibiting cyclic nucleotide phosphodiesterase. This causes inhibition of thromboxane $A_2$ production in platelets and may potentiate the effects of prostacyclin, causing decreased platelet adhesion to thrombogenic surfaces. Dipyridamole may be used in combination with warfarin, in contrast to acetylsalicylic acid, which may cause an unpredictable potentiation of warfarin anticoagulation.

Heparin (**choice C**) is used in emergency management of DVT but is limited to parenteral use because it does not readily cross membranes. It acts by potentiating the activity of antithrombin III, which is a suicide inhibitor of thrombin and factors IXa, Xa, XIa, and XIIa.

Streptokinase (**choice D**) is also used in cases of DVT but it is limited to IV, intra-arterial, and intracoronary use. It is a protein produced by beta hemolytic streptococci that converts plasminogen to plasmin, which is involved in digesting fibrin clots.

tPA (**choice E**) is also a thrombolytic agent used intravenously. Its mechanism of action is similar to that of streptokinase. tPA has the advantage of not being rapidly inactivated by antibodies from a previous streptococcal infection (as streptokinase can be) because it is a recombinant human enzyme. It is very expensive.

12. **The correct answer is A.** This question allows us to review the various mechanisms of action of the antiparkinsonian drugs.

Selegiline inhibits the degradation of dopamine by MAO type B (**choice A**).

Carbidopa works by inhibiting dopa decarboxylase (**choice B**). Carbidopa is unable to cross the blood-brain barrier; therefore, it prevents the conversion of levodopa (L-dopa) to dopamine in the periphery, but this conversion still occurs in the brain. This significantly reduces the dosage of L-dopa required to achieve an effect and is generally used in combination with L-dopa.

Bromocriptine and pergolide are dopaminergic receptor agonists (**choice C**). Bromocriptine is typically administered in combination with levodopa. It is also useful in end-stage Parkinson disease, when L-dopa loses its effectiveness because of progressive degeneration of the nigrostriatal neurons.

L-dopa is a precursor of dopamine (**choice D**). At higher doses, it has many side effects and is therefore often used in combination with carbidopa or bromocriptine. Tolcapone is a COMT inhibitor that increases the efficacy of L-dopa.

Note that muscarinic antagonists (e.g., benztropine, biperiden, procyclidine, trihexyphenidyl) are also used as adjuncts to the dopaminergic agents in the treatment of parkinsonism. Recall that dopaminergic neurons have an inhibitory effect on striatal cholinergic interneurons. So, if there is a decrease in dopaminergic activity (e.g., as in Parkinson disease), there will be an increase in striatal ACh. Therefore, administration of these anticholinergics aids in maintaining a dopamine/acetylcholine balance in the striatum.

13. **The correct answer is B.** Zileuton is a recently approved oral inhibitor of 5-lipoxygenase, the first enzyme in the pathway from arachidonic acid to leukotrienes. Leukotrienes are synthesized in many inflammatory cells in the airways, such as mast cells, macrophages, eosinophils, and basophils. $LTC_4$ and $LTD_4$ are thought to be responsible for many of the symptoms of asthma, including bronchoconstriction, increased bronchial reactivity, hypersecretion of mucus, and mucosal edema. In addition, $LTB_4$ is a potent chemotactic agent for neutrophils. Zileuton and similar agents are efficacious in the treatment of asthma because they inhibit leukotriene production.

Zafirlukast is another drug that is used to interrupt the leukotriene pathway. This drug acts as an $LTD_4$ antagonist (**choice A**); it is taken orally.

Methylxanthines, such as theophylline, inhibit phosphodiesterase (**choice C**), thus increasing intracellular levels of cAMP and resulting in smooth muscle relaxation. At therapeutic doses, methylxanthines also block adenosine receptors.

Corticosteroids prevent the release of arachidonic acid from cell membranes by inhibiting phospholipase $A_2$ (**choice D**). This reduces the production of both leukotrienes and prostaglandins. Corticosteroids also inhibit the production of cytokines, which are thought to play an important role in initiating the inflammatory cascade provoked by antigen inhalation and viral infection. Examples of corticosteroids include beclomethasone, budesonide, flunisolide, fluticasone, and triamcinolone.

$Beta_2$ agonists (**choice E**), such as albuterol, terbutaline, metaproterenol, and bitolterol, cause smooth muscle relaxation by increasing intracellular levels of cAMP.

14. **The correct answer is A.** This patient's visual changes may be attributed to glaucoma, for which she was given acetazolamide. Side effects of acetazolamide (a carbonic anhydrase-inhibiting diuretic used primarily for treating glaucoma) include paresthesias and drowsiness. The drug can cause a hyperchloremic metabolic acidosis, with decreased serum bicarbonate, increased

serum chloride, and decreased serum pH. Renal stones may also occur. Hepatic encephalopathy may appear in patients with hepatic impairment.

Demeclocycline (**choice B**), an antidiuretic hormone (ADH) antagonist and a tetracycline, causes bone and teeth abnormalities in children younger than 8 years. Demeclocycline can be used in the treatment of SIADH.

Ethacrynic acid (**choice C**) and furosemide (**choice D**) are loop diuretics that can cause hypovolemia and cardiovascular complications. They can also induce a hypokalemic metabolic alkalosis and ototoxicity. Furosemide, a sulfonamide, may also cause sulfonamide allergy.

Hydrochlorothiazide (**choice E**), a thiazide diuretic, can cause hyponatremia, an uncommon but potentially dangerous early side effect. Potassium wasting can occur with chronic use. Thiazides are sulfonamides and can cause sulfonamide allergy.

Spironolactone (**choice F**), a potassium-sparing diuretic, can cause hyperkalemia. It can also cause various endocrine side effects, such as anti-androgen effects and gynecomastia.

15. **The correct answer is E.** Mecamylamine is a ganglionic blocker that is sometimes administered during surgery to maintain controlled hypotension and to minimize blood loss. The trick to determining the effect of a ganglionic blocker is to first know the predominant tone of the end organ in question. The blocker will produce the opposite effect of the predominant tone. The vessels, arterioles, and veins are predominantly under sympathetic tone. Most everything else is under parasympathetic tone. The heart is under predominantly parasympathetic control. Parasympathetic stimulation of the heart causes bradycardia. Removal of this tone with trimethaphan would result in tachycardia.

The eye is predominantly under parasympathetic control. Parasympathetic stimulation causes the eye to accommodate (focus for near vision, **choice A**). Removal of this tone with trimethaphan would prevent accommodation.

Arterioles are predominantly under sympathetic control. Sympathetic stimulation produces vasoconstriction and possibly hypertension (**choice B**). Removal of this tone with trimethaphan would produce vasodilation and hypotension.

The gut is predominantly under parasympathetic control, which increases gut motility (**choice C**). Removal of parasympathetic tone with trimethaphan would diminish gut motility.

The eye is predominantly under parasympathetic control. Parasympathetic stimulation causes the pupil to constrict (**choice D**). Removal of this tone with trimethaphan would prevent miosis.

16. **The correct answer is D.** Omeprazole is an irreversible inhibitor of $H^+/K^+/ATPase$ of the parietal cell. It is used in the treatment of peptic ulcer disease, reflux esophagitis, and Zollinger-Ellison syndrome. Omeprazole can reduce daily gastric acid secretion by more than 95%. This drug is of particular value to patients who do not respond sufficiently to $H_2$ antagonists. Because of the profound reduction in gastric acid secretion, patients can develop modest hypergastrinemia. In laboratory rats, the increased gastrin causes hyperplasia of oxyntic mucosal cells and carcinoid tumors. Although there has been concern that the hyperplasia could also occur in humans, this has not been substantiated to date.

Bisacodyl (**choice A**) is a stimulant laxative.

Cimetidine (**choice B**) is an $H_2$-receptor antagonist that would block histamine-induced acid secretion. It is not as efficacious as omeprazole.

Magnesium hydroxide (**choice C**) is an antacid. It would help relieve the heartburn but would not be as efficacious as omeprazole.

Promethazine (**choice E**), a dopamine-receptor antagonist, is an antiemetic.

17. **The correct answer is C.** Phase I metabolism, which is accomplished largely by cytochrome P450, becomes less efficient with age. Phase II metabolism, which conjugates drugs to yield polar, inactive metabolites, is not generally affected by age. Oxazepam is a benzodiazepine that does not require phase I metabolism; it simply undergoes conjugation, making it a useful drug for elderly individuals. Lorazepam is the other benzodiazepine that undergoes only phase II metabolism. These two drugs are also useful for patients with liver failure; phase I metabolism can be severely affected by liver failure.

18. **The correct answer is D.** It takes one half-life to reach 50% of steady state, two half-lives to reach 75% of steady state, three half-lives to reach 87.5% of steady state, and four half-lives to reach 93.75% of steady state. Each successive half-life brings the level of the drug closer to 100%, but by a smaller amount (half of the previous increase) in each case. In this case, it should take three half-lives to reach 87.5% of steady state, or $2 \times 3 = 6$ hours. Note: The clearance and volume of distribution were not necessary to answer this question!

19. **The correct answer is E.** As you might have guessed from his elevated PT, the active ingredient in rat poison is warfarin. It acts as an anticoagulant by interfering with the normal hepatic synthesis of the vitamin K–dependent clotting factors II, VII, IX, and X. The most important adverse effect of warfarin is bleeding. The action of warfarin can be reversed with vitamin K.

Atropine (**choice A**) is used as an antidote for anticholinesterase toxicity (e.g., ingestion of organophosphates).

Flumazenil (**choice B**) is used as an antidote for benzodiazepine toxicity (e.g., diazepam).

N-acetylcysteine (**choice C**) is used as an antidote for acetaminophen toxicity.

Protamine (**choice D**) is used as an antidote for heparin overdose. Note that heparin enhances the activity of antithrombin III, augmenting its anticoagulant effect. Heparin toxicity would have resulted in an elevated PTT.

20. **The correct answer is A.** Muscarinic agonists stimulate noninnervated muscarinic (M3) receptors located on the endothelium of blood vessels. These receptors activate phospholipase C (via $G_q$), thereby raising levels of inositol triphosphate ($IP_3$) and diacylglycerol (DAG). $IP_3$ produces an increase in intracellular calcium, which activates nitric oxide synthase and thus produces nitric oxide. Nitric oxide, in turn, diffuses to the smooth muscle cells of arterioles and raises cGMP by activating guanylate cyclase. cGMP causes vasodilatation, by dephosphorylating myosin light chain, thus preventing the interaction of myosin with actin.

Isoproterenol (**choice B**), a nonselective beta agonist, causes vasodilatation by activating $beta_2$ receptors located in the smooth muscle of arterioles. $Beta_2$ receptors activate adenylate cyclase, thus raising levels of cAMP. cAMP activates cAMP-dependent protein kinase (protein kinase A), which phosphorylates myosin light chain kinase (MLCK), rendering this enzyme inactive. MLCK can no longer phosphorylate the myosin light chain, an essential step in smooth muscle contraction.

Metaproterenol (**choice C**), a $beta_2$ agonist, causes vasodilatation by the same mechanism as isoproterenol.

Nifedipine (**choice D**) blocks L-type calcium channels in both smooth and cardiac muscle. Increased blocking of calcium channels in the smooth muscle cells of arterioles prevents the activation of MLCK. MLCK can no longer phosphorylate the myosin light chain, an essential step in smooth muscle contraction.

Phentolamine (**choice E**) causes vasodilatation by blocking alpha receptors on arteriolar smooth muscle cells.

Alpha$_1$ receptors cause constriction by $IP_3$-induced increases in intracellular calcium. Phentolamine therefore prevents the increase in intracellular calcium, thereby causing less activation of MLCK.

Phenylephrine (**choice F**), an alpha$_1$ agonist, causes vasoconstriction, not vasodilatation. Interestingly, alpha$_1$ receptors are linked to the same G protein ($G_q$) as the M3 receptor, but have the opposite effect because they are located on smooth muscle cells rather than endothelial cells. Alpha$_1$ receptor stimulation leads to an $IP_3$-dependent increase in intracellular calcium. The calcium binds to calmodulin, which leads to the activation of MLCK. MLCK phosphorylates the myosin light chain, leading to smooth muscle contraction.

21. **The correct answer is E.** Doxorubicin (Adriamycin) is an anthracycline antibiotic. When given in high doses ($>550$ mg/m$^2$), it can produce cardiomyopathy leading to congestive heart failure, accompanied by pulmonary edema and rales. This complication is especially likely if the patient is older than 70 years of age, has received cardiac irradiation, has underlying heart disease or hypertension, or has received cyclophosphamide.

Abdominal tenderness (**choice A**), bladder distention (**choice B**), limitation of movement (**choice C**), and papilledema (**choice D**) are not typically associated with administration of doxorubicin. Doxorubicin does, however, cause alopecia and suppress the bone marrow.

22. **The correct answer is C.** Heparin, a highly negatively charged molecule, binds to the coagulation inhibitor antithrombin III, increasing its activity 100 to 1000 times.

Alpha$_2$-antiplasmin (**choice A**) binds plasmin. Plasmin functions to break down clots, and the binding of alpha$_2$-antiplasmin to plasmin acts to inhibit clot lysis.

Alpha$_2$-macroglobulin (**choice B**) is a circulating antiprotease macromolecule that assists in preventing blood clotting by inhibiting the action of proteolytic coagulation factors.

The remaining answer choices are all clotting factors. They do not interact with heparin.

23. **The correct answer is D.** The collection of symptoms described above—tinnitus, blurred vision, gastrointestinal upset, and delirium—is known as cinchonism, a side effect of quinidine toxicity. EKG changes, such as prolongation of the QT and QRS intervals, may also occur. Quinidine is an antiarrhythmic used for the treatment of ventricular arrhythmias and atrial fibrillation.

Allopurinol (**choice A**) is used in the treatment of gout. Its side effects include rash and fever.

Hydralazine (**choice B**) is a vasodilator used for the treatment of hypertension. Side effects include tachycardia, headache, nausea, and a lupus-like syndrome in slow acetylators.

Niacin (**choice C**) is used in the treatment of hyperlipidemia. Its side effects include cutaneous flushing and pruritus.

Spironolactone (**choice E**) is a potassium-sparing diuretic that blocks the effect of aldosterone at its receptor. Side effects include hyperkalemia and gynecomastia.

24. **The correct answer is D.** The symptoms described were caused by drug-induced histamine release. Of all the drugs listed, only tubocurarine produces a substantial amount of histamine release.

Atracurium (**choice A**) would also be appropriate for this procedure. However, it results in much less histamine release than tubocurarine.

Baclofen (**choice B**) is an antispasmodic but would not be used for this procedure. In addition, it does not cause histamine release.

Dantrolene (**choice C**) is a skeletal muscle relaxant but would not be used for this procedure; it is instead used in the treatment of malignant hyperthermia. In addition, it does not cause histamine release.

Vecuronium (**choice E**) would also be appropriate for this procedure. However, it does not cause histamine release.

25. **The correct answer is B.** The infant has Turner syndrome, in which only one sex chromosome, the X chromosome, is present as a result of chromosomal loss early after fertilization of the egg. The chromosome loss can occur either in all cells, or only in part of the body, because of random X-chromosome inactivation, producing the variant known as a Turner mosaic. Affected infants often have a prominent "webbed" neck related to lymphatic stasis in the neck, sometimes producing a frank cystic hygroma (large cystic mass composed of dilated lymphatic channels). Edema of the dorsum of the hands and feet caused by similar mechanisms is also seen in these infants. An infant with these clinical features should have a chromosomal analysis. Affected infants should also be carefully checked for cardiac anomalies (notably preductal coarctation of the aorta and aortic stenosis with endocardial fibroelastosis), since congenital heart disease can cause early death. By puberty, the neck and extremity edema generally has resolved, but careful physical examination often reveals residual redundant skin of the neck and shoulders, producing the mature form of webbed neck. Mosaic

patients and patients with partial deletions of one X chromosome may present only at puberty with the combination of short stature and primary amenorrhea. The ovaries (usually not biopsied in obvious cases) lose all their oocytes by 2 years of age ("menopause before menarche") and become atrophic fibrous strands without ova or follicles ("streak ovaries"). Hormonal replacement in Turner patients should include both estrogens and progestins, since unopposed estrogens (**choice A**) can cause atypical adenomatous hyperplasia of the endometrium.

Insulin (**choice C**) replacement is not required in these patients.

Replacement of progestin alone (**choice D**) is not recommended.

Thyroid hormone (**choice E**) replacement is not required in these patients.

26. **The correct answer is D.** The drug that is most likely to be abused is that which causes the greatest euphoric effect. Euphoria is mediated by mu opioid receptors, and meperidine is the only drug listed that is a full mu agonist.

Codeine (**choice A**) is a moderately effective agonist at the mu receptor and therefore has less abuse potential than meperidine.

Dextromethorphan (**choice B**) is an over-the-counter antitussive agent with limited abuse potential.

Loperamide (**choice C**) is an over-the-counter antidiarrheal agent with very limited abuse potential.

Nalbuphine (**choice E**) is a mixed agonist/antagonist (also called a partial agonist) with antagonist actions at the mu receptor. As a result, it has less abuse potential than meperidine.

Pentazocine (**choice F**) is a mixed agonist/antagonist (also called a partial agonist). It is either a weak agonist or an antagonist at the mu receptor. As a result, it has less abuse potential than meperidine.

Propoxyphene (**choice G**) is a weak agonist at the mu receptor, and would therefore have less abuse potential than meperidine.

27. **The correct answer is C.** The fact that the patient had well-controlled diabetes until the addition of an antihypertensive medication suggests that the new agent is responsible for increasing the blood glucose level. Hydrochlorothiazide is a thiazide diuretic that is known to increase fasting blood glucose in diabetic patients. Dosage adjustments of both oral hypoglycemic agents, like glipizide, and insulin may be required to maintain euglycemia. None of the other agents would directly

increase the blood glucose level in this patient. Thus, all these agents are considered to be safe and effective for the treatment of hypertension in diabetic patients.

Diltiazem (**choice A**), a calcium channel blocker, and enalapril (**choice B**), an ACE inhibitor, can both be used in the treatment of hypertension in diabetic patients. Because these agents have favorable side effect profiles, their use in the initial treatment of hypertension would be recommended, particularly the ACE inhibitor because it protects against nephropathy.

Both methyldopa (**choice D**), a centrally acting alpha receptor agonist, and terazosin (**choice E**), a peripherally acting alpha receptor blocking agent, can be used to treat hypertension in diabetic patients. Because of their side effect profiles, however, these agents should be used after other more tolerable agents have been attempted.

28. **The correct answer is C.** If the patient has asthma, you should select a drug that blocks $beta_1$-receptors without affecting the $beta_2$-receptors found in the respiratory smooth muscle. Therefore, a selective $beta_1$-blocker (such as metoprolol) would be appropriate.

Isoproterenol (**choice A**) is a (nonselective) beta agonist, not antagonist.

Labetalol (**choice B**) is a mixed alpha and nonselective beta antagonist used for chronic hypertension and hypertensive emergencies.

Propranolol (**choice D**) is a nonselective beta antagonist. It would block both $beta_1$ and $beta_2$ receptors and would therefore be contraindicated in a patient with asthma.

Timolol (**choice E**) is also a nonselective beta-antagonist that is used topically in the treatment of glaucoma.

29. **The correct answer is C.** A thiazide diuretic would be the drug of choice for this patient because it is the only class of diuretic that decreases urinary secretion of calcium. Thiazide diuretics, like hydrochlorothiazide, inhibit the $Na^+/Cl^-$ cotransporter in the distal convoluted tubule and promote the reabsorption of calcium.

Acetazolamide (**choice A**), a carbonic anhydrase inhibitor, and furosemide (**choice B**), a loop diuretic, induce diuresis at the expense of all three major cationic electrolytes ($Na^+$, $K^+$, and $Ca^{2+}$), which are secreted in increased amounts.

Spironolactone (**choice D**) and triamterene (**choice E**), so-called potassium-sparing diuretics, block $Na^+/K^+$ exchange in the collecting duct. Although they decrease $K^+$ secretion, they elevate $Na^+$ and $Ca^{2+}$ secretion.

30. **The correct answer is A.** Finasteride, an inhibitor of 5-alpha-reductase, prevents the conversion of testosterone to dihydrotestosterone (DHT). Because dihydrotestosterone is essential for the normal growth and development of the prostate gland, finasteride is an effective treatment for benign prostatic hyperplasia, which is a DHT-dependent process. (A better choice would have been an alpha-blocking agent, but none was available as an answer.)

Leuprolide (**choice B**) is a gonadotropin-releasing hormone (GnRH) analog. It is used at times for the palliative treatment of advanced prostate carcinoma.

Mifepristone (**choice C**), also known as RU486, is a competitive inhibitor at progesterone receptors. It has been used as a contraceptive or as an abortifacient to terminate early pregnancy.

Pergolide (**choice D**), a synthetic ergoline, is a direct agonist at dopamine $D_1$ and $D_2$ receptors. It has been used in association with levodopa in the therapy of Parkinson disease.

Tamoxifen (**choice E**) is a competitive antagonist at estrogen receptors located in the breast. This drug is used in reducing the recurrence of estrogen-receptor-positive breast cancer, particularly in postmenopausal women.

31. **The correct answer is B.** It takes 4 to 5 $t_{1/2}$ to reach steady state, or 16 to 20 hours under normal conditions. If one kidney is removed, the elimination of Drug X is halved. Elimination and $t_{1/2}$ are inversely related. So the new $t_{1/2}$ for Drug X is 8 hours, and the new time to reach steady state is 32 to 40 hours.

32. **The correct answer is D.** Diplopia, gingival hyperplasia, and hirsutism are classic side effects of phenytoin. Other side effects include nystagmus, sedation, ataxia, and enzyme induction. Phenytoin is used in the treatment of grand mal and tonic-clonic seizures. It is not used for absence seizures.

Carbamazepine (**choice A**) does produce diplopia, but not the other symptoms in this vignette. It can also produce ataxia, enzyme induction, and blood dyscrasias. It is useful in tonic-clonic and partial seizures and in tic douloureux.

Ethosuximide (**choice B**) causes gastrointestinal distress, headache, and lethargy. It is used exclusively for absence seizures.

Phenobarbital (**choice C**) is used for grand mal and partial seizures. It causes sedation, enzyme induction, and dependence.

Valproic acid (**choice E**) causes gastrointestinal distress, hepatotoxicity, and inhibition of drug metabolism. It can be used for all seizure types but is particularly useful in myoclonic and petit mal seizures.

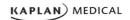

33. **The correct answer is E.** Stimulation of beta$_2$ receptors causes uterine relaxation. Ritodrine is a beta$_2$ agonist. Terbutaline is also sometimes used.

Clomiphene (**choice A**) is a nonsteroidal estrogen used in the treatment of infertility. In women, it can improve follicular development and induce ovulation. In men, it can improve spermatogenesis.

Phenylephrine (**choice B**) is an alpha$_1$ agonist; alpha$_1$ stimulation causes contraction in the pregnant uterus.

Progesterone (**choice C**) is used in oral contraceptives and in the treatment of dysmenorrhea, dysfunctional uterine bleeding, and endometriosis.

Beta$_2$ stimulation causes uterine relaxation; propranolol (**choice D**) is a nonspecific beta antagonist.

34. **The correct answer is A.** This is a three-step question. First you need to figure out the diagnosis, then you need to determine the drug of choice for this condition, and, finally, you need to remember the mechanism of action of that drug. The clinical picture presented suggests malignant hyperthermia. The treatment for this condition (a USMLE favorite) is dantrolene. Dantrolene prevents the release of $Ca^{2+}$ from the sarcoplasmic reticulum, thereby reducing skeletal muscle contractions. Side effects include muscle weakness and hepatotoxicity (if used chronically). Other uses include spasticity, multiple sclerosis, and cerebral palsy.

Nondepolarizing blockers competitively inhibit the activity of acetylcholine at the neuromuscular junction (**choice B**). Examples include curare, atracurium, and vecuronium.

Baclofen is a GABA$_B$ receptor agonist that is inhibitory at synapses in the spinal cord (**choice C**).

Uncouplers of oxidative phosphorylation (**choice D**) include dinitrophenol and thermogenin and would increase heat production.

35. **The correct answer is E.** The first thing that you have to know is the effect that carotid occlusion will have on this animal. A carotid occlusion blocks blood flow to the carotid baroreceptors, thereby simulating a low blood pressure. The animal's response will be to initiate a baroreceptor response, which will increase sympathetic output and decrease parasympathetic output. The net result will be an increase in blood pressure and heart rate. The second thing to determine is which drug will oppose this increase in heart rate. Propranolol, a nonspecific beta antagonist, will prevent norepinephrine from acting on the beta$_1$ receptors on the heart following an increase in sympathetic output, thus opposing the reflex increase in heart rate.

Atropine (**choice A**), a muscarinic antagonist, might further increase heart rate. However, because part of the baroreceptor reflex involves withdrawing parasympathetic output, the effect of atropine would be negligible.

Metaproterenol (**choice B**), a beta$_2$ agonist, does not have much of a direct effect on heart rate because the predominant adrenergic receptor on the heart is beta$_1$. Metaproterenol decreases blood pressure by producing vasodilatation in the skeletal muscle vasculature, which is sensed at the aortic arch baroreceptors. This in itself elicits a baroreceptor reflex that is additive to the reflex produced by the carotid occlusion.

Neostigmine (**choice C**), a carbamylating acetylcholinesterase inhibitor, may slow the heart slightly. However, because parasympathetic output is withdrawn during a carotid occlusion, there is not a sufficient amount of acetylcholine present even if its metabolism is prevented by a cholinesterase inhibitor.

Phenoxybenzamine (**choice D**), an alpha-adrenergic antagonist, does not affect heart rate directly because there are no alpha-adrenergic receptors in the heart. It acts to decrease blood pressure by blocking alpha receptors in the vasculature. This true decrease in blood pressure is sensed by the aortic arch baroreceptors, contributing further to the baroreceptor reflex initiated by the carotid occlusion and further increasing heart rate.

36. **The correct answer is B.** Cisplatin is an antineoplastic drug used in the treatment of carcinoma of the testes (along with bleomycin and vinblastine), ovaries, bladder, and lung (especially small cell). Along with the typical side effects of nausea, vomiting, and bone marrow suppression, cisplatin is notable for its dose-limiting nephrotoxicity and ototoxicity.

The other answer choices also have unique, USMLE test-worthy side effects:

Bleomycin (**choice A**) is very effective against testicular tumors and is used in combination with cisplatin and vinblastine. The most noteworthy side effect of bleomycin is pulmonary toxicity that can progress to pulmonary fibrosis.

Cyclophosphamide (**choice C**) is a commonly used chemotherapeutic that is effective in the treatment of lymphomas, multiple myeloma, lymphoblastic leukemias, carcinomas (e.g., breast, ovary, lung, cervix), mycosis fungoides, and neuroblastoma. Note that it is not used in the treatment of testicular cancer. In addition, its most notable side effect is hemorrhagic cystitis (not nephrotoxicity).

Vinblastine (**choice D**) is used for the treatment of testicular tumors. It is also used for Hodgkin disease, lymphomas, and Kaposi sarcoma. Vinblastine is notable for its dose-limiting bone marrow suppression.

Vincristine, also known as Oncovin (**choice E**), is used as part of the MOPP (mechlorethamine, Oncovin, procarbazine and prednisone) regimen for the treatment of Hodgkin disease. It is also used in the treatment of acute lymphocytic leukemia (ALL), sarcoma, CNS tumors, and Wilms tumor. Vincristine's noteworthy side effect is its dose-limiting neurotoxicity.

37.  **The correct answer is D.** The object of a loading dose (LD) is to "load up" the volume of distribution in order to quickly achieve the desired plasma concentration. You can calculate it by the following equation:

$$LD = V_d \times C_p$$

($V_d$ = volume of distribution; $C_p$ = plasma concentration)

In this case, LD = (50 L) × (10 mg/L) = 500 mg

38.  **The correct answer is F.** Pralidoxime (2-PAM) is an acetylcholinesterase (AChE) reactivating agent. It is useful only for counteracting AChE inhibitors that act by phosphorylating the enzyme (organophosphates). Pralidoxime can remove the phosphate group from AChE, thus regenerating the enzyme. This must be done in a timely fashion because normally after the phosphate group is bound to the enzyme, it undergoes a chemical reaction known as "aging." Once this bond ages, pralidoxime will no longer be effective.

Atropine (**choice A**) is a nonselective muscarinic antagonist. Although atropine would be an appropriate agent for this patient, it acts by preventing the excess ACh from stimulating muscarinic receptors rather than altering the activity of AChE.

Deferoxamine (**choice B**) is a chelator used for iron poisoning.

Dimercaprol (**choice C**) is a chelator used alone for arsenic, mercury, and gold poisoning. It is also used in conjunction with edetate calcium disodium (EDTA) to treat severe lead poisoning.

N-acetylcysteine (**choice D**) is used to treat acetaminophen overdose.

Physostigmine (**choice E**) is a carbamylating acetylcholinesterase inhibitor that can be used to treat antimuscarinic overdose. This drug would certainly exacerbate this patient's symptoms.

39.  **The correct answer is C.** Ethanol is the appropriate treatment for patients who have ingested methanol or ethylene glycol. This therapy is effective because ethanol competes for the same enzyme (alcohol dehydrogenase)

that is required for methanol/ethylene glycol breakdown. Methanol can cause blindness; ethylene glycol (a component of antifreeze) does not. Therefore, the patient probably ingested ethylene glycol. Ethylene glycol is a CNS depressant; ingestion produces obtundation and unresponsiveness to painful stimuli.

Amyl nitrite (**choice A**) is the appropriate antidote for cyanide poisoning; sodium nitrite is also used.

Atropine (**choice B**) is the appropriate antidote for carbamate-type or organophosphate-type acetylcholinesterase insecticide poisoning. It acts by blocking muscarinic receptors. 2-Pyridine aldoxime methiodide (2-PAM, pralidoxime) can also be given early in the course of organophosphate poisoning to help regenerate the enzyme.

Glucagon (**choice D**) is the approved therapy for treating beta-adrenergic blocker overdose, helping to restore blood glucose levels.

Naloxone (**choice E**) is the approved treatment for overdose of opioids. It is an antagonist at opioid receptors.

Oxygen (generally hyperbaric oxygen; **choice F**) is the approved therapy for the treatment of carbon monoxide poisoning. Oxygen under high pressure competes with carbon monoxide for hemoglobin binding sites.

Pyridoxine (**choice G**) can ameliorate the symptoms associated with isoniazid toxicity.

Sodium bicarbonate (**choice H**) is the treatment for acidosis produced by overdose of tricyclic antidepressants (or many other drugs).

40.  **The correct answer is E.** These foods contain tyramine, which is an indirect-acting sympathomimetic. Tyramine is broken down by monoamine oxidase in the liver. If this is inhibited, tyramine causes the release of norepinephrine, which leads to increased blood pressure. This patient is taking a monoamine oxidase inhibitor. Foods containing tyramine, such as aged cheese, dark beer, wine, overripe fruits, chicken liver, and smoked meat products, should be avoided.

Direct-acting sympathomimetic agents (**choice A**) stimulate postsynaptic adrenergic receptors themselves. They do not need to be taken up and released by the nerve terminal in order to act. An example of this is norepinephrine.

False transmitters (**choice B**) mimic adrenergic neurotransmitters, but they have little or no postsynaptic receptor activity. An example of this is octopamine, which is a breakdown product of tyramine.

Muscarinic agonists (**choice C**) act at postganglionic parasympathetic receptors and produce a cholinergic response. Pilocarpine is an example.

**KAPLAN** MEDICAL

Neuronal uptake inhibitors (**choice D**) prevent the uptake of catecholamines into the nerve terminal. They are used to terminate the action of catecholamines. An example is tricyclic antidepressants.

41. **The correct answer is A.** This is a simple drug mechanism question made somewhat more difficult by the additional information presented in the stem. First, the diagnosis of gout should have been easily made. (Other "classic clues" for gout include negatively birefringent needle-shaped crystals and the presence of tophi.) The only crucial information in the question is that Drug 2 decreases uric acid in both the serum and the urine. Allopurinol inhibits the formation of uric acid by blocking the conversion of hypoxanthine to xanthine and xanthine to uric acid by xanthine oxidase (allopurinol is an analog of hypoxanthine). If uric acid synthesis is decreased, you would expect to see a decrease in both the serum and urine levels. Note that allopurinol is used in the treatment of severe hyperuricemia, whether or not it is related to gout. Also note that in acute attacks of gout, therapy with allopurinol should be delayed until after the acute episode has resolved and the patient is on maintenance doses of colchicine (probably Drug 1 in this vignette).

Colchicine (**choice B**) works by interfering with microtubule polymerization, thereby preventing granulocyte migration to the inflammatory site and decreasing metabolic and phagocytic activity of granulocytes. Colchicine has no effect on uric acid levels and is not an analgesic. Colchicine is used to treat acute attacks of gout and is also given prophylactically to prevent recurrent episodes.

Indomethacin (**choice C**) is a nonsteroidal anti-inflammatory drug (NSAID) that works by inhibiting both cyclooxygenase and the motility of polymorphonuclear leukocytes. Although indomethacin can be used in the treatment of acute gout, it affects neither the serum nor the urine levels of uric acid.

Both probenecid (**choice D**) and sulfinpyrazone (**choice E**) increase urinary excretion of uric acid (uricosuric). As such, you would expect increased, not decreased, urine levels of uric acid in patients taking either drug (serum levels would be decreased).

42. **The correct answer is E.** The point of this question is that nonselective beta-blockers are contraindicated in patients with lung disease. These agents will cause bronchoconstriction by blocking the beta$_2$ receptors responsible for promoting bronchial smooth muscle relaxation (recall that beta$_2$ agonists are a mainstay of asthma therapy). Acebutolol (**choice A**), atenolol (**choice B**), esmolol (**choice C**), and metoprolol (**choice D**) are all cardioselective beta$_1$ blockers that could be used in a patient with lung/airway disease. Another cardioselective blocker that is not listed is betaxolol. As for nadolol (**choice E**), it is a nonselective beta-blocker and should *not* be used in a patient with lung disease.

43. **The correct answer is C.** Ethacrynic acid is a loop diuretic and acts by inhibiting the Na$^+$/K$^+$/2Cl$^-$ transporter located in the ascending loop of Henle.

Only vasodilators like caffeine and the new ANF receptor agonists act at the glomerulus (**choice A**).

Carbonic anhydrase inhibitors, such as acetazolamide, inhibit sodium bicarbonate reabsorption from the proximal tubule (**choice B**).

Thiazide diuretics inhibit the Na$^+$/Cl$^-$ transporter in the early segment of the distal convoluted tubule (**choice D**).

Potassium-sparing diuretics act as antagonists of the intracellular aldosterone receptor located in the collecting tubule (**choice E**). By doing so, they decrease the expression of the genes for sodium channels and the Na$^+$/K$^+$ ATPase.

44. **The correct answer is C.** The child has absence seizures. The age of onset is typically from 3 to 7 years; seizures may continue into adolescence, but generally subside before adulthood. These seizures have been known to occur up to 100 times a day. Ethosuximide is indicated for this type (but no other type) of seizure. Other drugs used in the treatment of absence seizures are valproic acid, clonazepam, and lamotrigine.

Carbamazepine (**choice A**) is used in the treatment of tonic-clonic (grand mal) and partial (focal) seizures.

Diazepam (**choice B**) has long been the drug of choice for status epilepticus. Recently, lorazepam (a shorter acting benzodiazepine) has also been accepted as a drug for this condition. IV phenytoin is used if prolonged therapy is required. Phenobarbital has also been used, especially in children. If the status epilepticus is very severe and does not respond to these measures, general anesthesia may be used.

Methylphenidate (Ritalin; **choice D**) is a stimulant used to treat children with attention deficit disorder. This child has no history of hyperactivity, and the underlying cause of his "inattentiveness" is his seizure disorder.

Phenytoin (**choice E**) is effective in all seizure types except for the one in this question (absence). Note that phenytoin has some idiosyncratic, test-worthy side effects, including hirsutism and gingival hyperplasia.

45. **The correct answer is E.** Both drugs produce exactly the same effect, but Drug B achieved the blood pressure response with one-eighth the dosage of Drug A. This means that Drug A is 8 times less potent than Drug B.

    A high therapeutic index (**choice A**) means that the drug is relatively safe. However, the safety of a drug is not necessarily related to its potency.

    Differences in bioavailability (**choice B**) between these two drugs cannot be determined because both of these drugs were administered intravenously. Bioavailability is the fraction of a (typically orally administered) drug that reaches the systemic circulation. Bioavailability is by definition 1 (100%) when drugs are administered intravenously.

    The half-life (**choice C**) is the amount of time it takes for the concentration of a drug to fall to 50% of a previous measurement. There is no information provided to determine the half-lives of these drugs.

    Efficacy (**choice D**), which is a measurement of the drug's maximal response, is given by the maximal height of the dose-response curve. At these doses, each drug produced the same effect, but there is no information provided to determine what the maximal effect of each drug would be. In addition, potency and efficacy are not related.

46. **The correct answer is E.** Tetracaine is a long-duration ester local anesthetic.

    Bupivacaine (**choice A**) is a long-duration amide.

    Cocaine (**choice B**) is a medium-duration ester and an uptake blocker.

    Lidocaine (**choice C**) is a medium-duration amide and an antiarrhythmic.

    Procaine (**choice D**) is a short-duration ester.

47. **The correct answer is D.** N-acetylcysteine is the drug of choice for treatment of overdose of acetaminophen, the active ingredient in Tylenol.

    Alkalinization of urine (**choice A**) is a reasonable strategy for salicylate poisoning, e.g., due to aspirin overdose, or for other poisonings with weak acid drugs.

    $Ca^{2+}$/EDTA (**choice B**) and/or dimercaprol are chelators used in cases of lead poisoning.

    Deferoxamine (**choice C**) is an effective chelator for poisoning with iron salts.

    Protamine sulfate (**choice E**) is administered to reverse the anticoagulant effects of heparin overdose.

48. **The correct answer is A.** Cimetidine, an $H_2$-receptor antagonist, can produce all the side effects exhibited when taken in high doses over a long period of time. In addition, cimetidine can alter the hepatic metabolism of several drugs by inhibiting CYP450 enzyme.

Famotidine (**choice B**) is also an $H_2$-receptor antagonist, but it does not have the side effects of cimetidine.

Metronidazole (**choice C**) is an antibacterial and antiprotozoal drug that may present with the adverse effects of headaches, dizziness, diarrhea, and rashes, but not gynecomastia.

Omeprazole (**choice D**) is a proton-pump inhibitor, and sucralfate (**choice E**) is a physical barrier to gastric acid. Neither has been associated with effects on sexual function or breast development.

49. **The correct answer is E.** Reserpine acts by blocking vesicular uptake of monoamine neurotransmitters (norepinephrine, dopamine, serotonin), thus making the neurotransmitter vulnerable to the catabolic effects of monoamine oxidase (MAO) present in the nerve terminal. High doses of reserpine can even destroy synaptic vesicles. Chronic administration of reserpine causes depletion of norepinephrine. Therefore, for a drug to raise blood pressure after norepinephrine depletion, it must act directly on the alpha$_1$ adrenergic receptors present on arterioles. Phenylephrine, a direct alpha$_1$ agonist, is such a drug.

    Amphetamine (**choice A**) is an indirect-acting sympathomimetic. It raises blood pressure by causing the release of endogenous norepinephrine.

    Bethanechol (**choice B**), a muscarinic agonist, decreases blood pressure by stimulating the noninnervated muscarinic receptors present on arterioles.

    Cocaine (**choice C**) is an indirect-acting sympathomimetic that raises blood pressure by blocking the reuptake of norepinephrine.

    Guanethidine (**choice D**) is an adrenergic neuron blocker that acts by blocking the release of norepinephrine.

50. **The correct answer is D.** Metformin is often used in conjunction with oral hypoglycemic agents for the treatment of type 2 diabetes. Its mechanism of action is twofold: *1)* it decreases the production of glucose in the liver; and *2)* it increases the uptake of glucose in the liver. Metformin has no effect on the secretion of pancreatic insulin.

    Acetohexamide (**choice A**), chlorpropamide (**choice B**), glyburide (**choice C**), and tolbutamide (**choice E**) are oral hypoglycemic agents that are sulfonylurea derivatives. These agents stimulate secretion of insulin from the pancreas.

# Pharmacology: **Test Two**

1. A 74-year-old man has not been able to pass urine today, but had been able to do so normally the previous 2 days. Physical examination is remarkable for a blood pressure of 175/90 mm Hg. Laboratory examination reveals a serum creatinine of 4.5 mg/dL and a blood urea nitrogen of 115 mg/dL. Urinalysis reveals a specific gravity of 1.01 mg/dL and an occasional white blood cell per high-powered field. Which of the following could be used to ameliorate the patient's symptoms?

   (A) Benazepril

   (B) Doxazosin

   (C) Furosemide

   (D) Hyoscyamine

   (E) Phenazopyridine

2. A 21-year-old college senior comes to the university health clinic to discuss contraception options. She is in a monogamous relationship with her boyfriend of 2 years and would like a prescription for oral contraceptive pills. She does not smoke and has no medical conditions. Her blood pressure is 110/70 mm Hg. Physical examination is unremarkable. After the patient is counseled about safe-sex practices, she says that she does not want to get pregnant and is curious about the availability of medications to induce abortion. She should be told that which of the following eicosanoids is available as a vaginal suppository to induce abortion?

   (A) $LTA_4$

   (B) $PGD_2$

   (C) $PGE_2$

   (D) $PGF_2$

   (E) $PGG_2$

   (F) $PGH_2$

   (G) $PGI_2$

   (H) $TXA_2$

3. Several hospitals are participating in a study to test the efficacy of a newly developed drug prior to its release. This drug is designed to lower cholesterol levels. Of the 1000 patients who are involved in this study, half receive the drug and half receive a placebo. Neither the physicians in charge of the study nor the patients are permitted to know what the patients have received. Which of the following steps in the drug development process does this scenario most closely describe?

   (A) Investigational New Drug (IND) Application

   (B) New Drug Application (NDA)

   (C) Phase I

   (D) Phase II

   (E) Phase III

   (F) Phase IV

4. A patient has been given an anticoagulant. Which of the following findings suggests that he was given warfarin, not heparin?

   (A) Anticoagulation is being monitored by measuring the prothrombin time (PT)

   (B) Anticoagulation was achieved within 1 hour of drug administration

   (C) The anticoagulant's effects are reversed by administering protamine sulfate

   (D) The anticoagulant was administered intravenously

5. A 64-year-old man presents to his physician with aching, burning pain after meals. He had been self-medicating with antacids for several months but has found this to be increasingly ineffective. His physician decides to take him off the antacids and instead places him on a combination of ranitidine and sucralfate. Why is this combination a bad idea?

   (A) Ranitidine increases the toxicity of sucralfate

   (B) Ranitidine inhibits the action of sucralfate

   (C) Sucralfate and ranitidine coprecipitate

   (D) Sucralfate increases the toxicity of ranitidine

   (E) Sucralfate inhibits the action of ranitidine

6. A young white man presents with febrile illness and productive cough with green sputum hemoptysis. A chest x-ray reveals patchy opacification of both lung fields. This patient's history is significant for cystic fibrosis. Which of the following drug combinations match the treatment for his likely condition?

   (A) Amoxicillin plus ampicillin

   (B) Amoxicillin plus aminoglycosides

   (C) Amoxicillin plus clavulanic acid

   (D) Ticarcillin plus aminoglycosides

   (E) Vancomycin and aminoglycosides

7. A 55-year-old man with hypertension and a past medical history of myocardial infarction is prescribed atenolol. This medication will lower his blood pressure by

   (A) blocking catecholamine release

   (B) blocking the conversion of angiotensin I to angiotensin II

   (C) decreasing cardiac output

   (D) decreasing intravascular volume

   (E) increasing renin release from the kidney

8. A 24-year-old woman presents to her physician with a rasping cough. The physician gives her a sample of an antitussive drug that is neither addicting nor constipating. Which of the following drugs was she mostly likely given?

   (A) Codeine

   (B) Dextromethorphan

   (C) Diphenoxylate

   (D) Levorphanol

   (E) Oxycodone

9. A 68-year-old man presents with complaints of chronic fatigue, exertional and nocturnal dyspnea, orthopnea, and a chronic nonproductive cough. On examination, respiratory wheezing and rhonchi are noted. Cardiac examination reveals a diminished first heart sound and an S3 gallop. The patient indicates that he was recently treated for hypertension and vasospastic angina. On the basis of his initial presentation, which of the following agents was most likely prescribed?

   (A) Amlodipine

   (B) Captopril

   (C) Furosemide

   (D) Hydralazine

   (E) Verapamil

10. A patient with Graves disease is scheduled for a subtotal thyroidectomy. Propylthiouracil is used to control her hyperthyroidism until surgery. The enzyme inhibited by this drug is involved in which of the following reactions?

    (A) Conversion of iodide to iodine at the apex of the follicular cell

    (B) Iodide uptake at the base of the follicular cell

    (C) Iodination of thyroglobulin in the colloid

    (D) Proteolysis of iodinated thyroglobulin into monoiodotyrosine (MIT) and diiodotyrosine (DIT)

    (E) Reuptake of iodinated thyroglobulin from the follicular lumen

11. A 48-year-old woman is being treated for breast carcinoma. Over the past few days, she has been complaining of dysuria and frequency. Laboratory examination reveals the presence of microscopic hematuria. The next day the patient develops gross hematuria. Which of the following drugs could be used to treat the side effect from the antineoplastic medication taken by this patient?

    (A) Cyclophosphamide

    (B) Mitomycin

    (C) Mesna

    (D) Tamoxifen

    (E) Vincristine

12. A 24-year-old man underwent treatment for Hodgkin lymphoma 1 year ago. He presents with increasing dyspnea and cough. Physical exam is remarkable for rales bilaterally. Arterial blood gases show hypoxia, and bilateral pulmonary infiltrates are seen on chest x-ray. Which of the following chemotherapeutic agents most likely produced these side effects?

    (A) Bleomycin

    (B) Cyclophosphamide

    (C) Doxorubicin

    (D) Etoposide

    (E) 5-Fluorouracil

    (F) Streptozocin

    (G) Vincristine

13. A new antibiotic is being tested in phase III clinical trials. The following pharmacokinetic parameters had been determined in earlier trials:

    $V_d$ (volume of distribution) = 60 L

    CL (clearance) = 30 mL/min

    F (bioavailability) = 50%

    $t_{1/2}$ (half-life) = 23 hours

    This antibiotic is administered orally, and the target plasma concentration ($C_p$) is 2 mg/L. What is the appropriate loading dose for this drug?

    (A) 15 mg

    (B) 30 mg

    (C) 60 mg

    (D) 120 mg

    (E) 240 mg

14. A 27-year-old drug abuser ingested 15 10-mg dextroamphetamine tablets 5 hours ago, and is brought to the emergency department in an agitated state. Which of the following agents can hasten the elimination of the drug from this patient?

    (A) Acetazolamide

    (B) Ammonium chloride

    (C) Penicillamine

    (D) Probenecid

    (E) Sodium bicarbonate

15. A 30-year-old pregnant woman has a history of rheumatoid arthritis, which has been managed successfully with NSAIDs. However, she has recently visited her general practitioner complaining of burning epigastric pain worsened by food intake. Which of the following ulcer medication is most likely contraindicated in this patient?

    (A) Cimetidine

    (B) Famotidine

    (C) Misoprostol

    (D) Omeprazole

    (E) Ranitidine

16. A 65-year-old patient has experienced several transient ischemic attacks over the past few months. Because his general health is poor, he is not considered an appropriate candidate for carotid endarterectomy. The decision is made to treat him medically. Which of the following agents would be most appropriate for his therapy?

    (A) Aspirin

    (B) Coumadin

    (C) Dipyridamole

    (D) Heparin

    (E) Sulfinpyrazone

17. A 24-year-old man presents to the emergency department with hypertension, tachycardia, an elevated body temperature, diaphoresis, mydriasis, and severe agitation. His mother reports that he uses illicit drugs, although she is not sure which kind. Which of the following agents is the most appropriate therapy for this patient?

    (A) Atropine

    (B) Flumazenil

    (C) Fluoxetine

    (D) Labetalol

    (E) Naloxone

    (F) Physostigmine

18. A 59-year-old man with a history of myocardial infarction presents to his physician complaining of shortness of breath. On examination, his heart rate is 110/min and respiratory rate is 22/min. He has rales in both lung fields, a normal sinus rhythm with an S3 gallop, and 2+ pitting ankle edema. A chest x-ray film reveals cardiomegaly, and his ejection fraction on echocardiogram is calculated at 37%. Which of the following medications would alleviate this patient's symptoms by significantly reducing both the preload and afterload on the heart without affecting its inotropic state?

    (A) Digoxin

    (B) Diltiazem

    (C) Enalapril

    (D) Furosemide

    (E) Propranolol

19. A 24-year-old woman is diagnosed with cancer. Her oncologist wants to use a chemotherapy agent specific for the M phase of the cell cycle in her regimen. Which of the following drugs meets the criteria?

    (A) Cytarabine

    (B) Daunorubicin

    (C) Hydroxyurea

    (D) Mechlorethamine

    (E) Vincristine

20. A 35-year-old woman with systemic lupus erythematosus abruptly stops taking her glucocorticoids because "she is well now and does not want to get fat." Several days later, the woman goes to the emergency department because she "feels terrible." If serum studies are performed on this patient, which of the following findings would be expected?

    (A) Elevated ACTH

    (B) Elevated cortisol

    (C) Hypernatremia

    (D) Hypoglycemia

    (E) Hypokalemia

21. A 33-year-old newlywed presents to her physician with a sharp, burning epigastric pain. She had recently begun a regimen of nonsteroidal anti-inflammatory drugs (NSAIDs) to help relieve pain caused by rheumatoid arthritis. Her physician recommends misoprostol to relieve her gastric distress. Before prescribing this drug, the physician should first obtain the results of a(n)

    (A) antinuclear antibody test

    (B) barium swallow

    (C) esophageal manometry

    (D) osmotic fragility test

    (E) pregnancy test

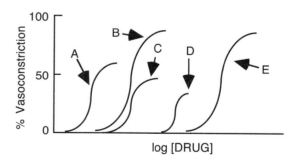

22. A researcher is studying the interaction of drugs X and Y. Drug X is an agonist and is represented by curve B. Drug Y is a noncompetitive antagonist. Which of the above curves would be obtained from a combination of drugs X and Y?

    (A) A

    (B) B

    (C) C

    (D) D

    (E) E

    (F) F

23. A 45-year-old woman is brought to the hospital after collapsing on the sidewalk in front of the hospital. Her friend reports that the patient has no known medical conditions. Initial evaluation reveals severe hypotension, and she is given intravenous norepinephrine. Which of the following drugs antagonizes both the vascular and cardiac actions of the given medication?

    (A) Atenolol

    (B) Esmolol

    (C) Carvedilol

    (D) Metaproterenol

    (E) Prazosin

24. A 19-year-old girl accompanies her 21-year-old boyfriend into the emergency department after a party. He is agitated and diaphoretic, and has dilated pupils. He resists efforts to subdue him, stating, "there are ants crawling up my arm." The girl recalls seeing her boyfriend and others at the party heating "something on aluminum foil" with a cigarette lighter and inhaling the fumes. Which of the following substances did he most likely inhale?

    (A) Heroin

    (B) Jimson weed

    (C) Lysergic acid diethylamide (LSD)

    (D) Methamphetamine

    (E) Model airplane glue

25. A 75-year-old pharmacologist comes to the emergency department because of chest pain and shortness of breath. She has a history of hypertension. She says that she takes an aspirin daily and a diuretic that "acts at the distal tubule of the nephron." She cannot remember the name of the diuretic. Considering her description, which of the following is the most likely diuretic?

    (A) Ethacrynic acid

    (B) Furosemide

    (C) Hydrochlorothiazide

    (D) Mannitol

    (E) Spironolactone

26. A 10-year-old asthmatic is prescribed a cromolyn sodium inhaler to be administered prior to vigorous activity to prevent an attack. Which of the following is the mechanism of action of this drug?

    (A) It blocks muscarinic receptors

    (B) It inhibits the degranulation of mast cells

    (C) It reduces bronchial inflammation and edema

    (D) It selectively stimulates beta$_2$ receptors

    (E) It stimulates all beta receptors

27. A 49-year-old alcoholic businessman complains of 2 days of severe worsening pain with redness and swelling of his first metatarsophalangeal joint. He has no history of injury or trauma. He is afebrile with no constitutional symptoms. Which of the following drugs is the most appropriate pharmacotherapy?

    (A) Allopurinol

    (B) Indomethacin

    (C) Colestipol

    (D) Pravastatin

    (E) Probenecid

28. A 32-year-old man is spraying malathion on the plum trees in his backyard. While taking a break, he reaches down to grab his drink and accidentally takes a swig of malathion instead. His girlfriend immediately takes him to a nearby emergency department. Which of the following drugs could be given to induce emesis?

    (A) Apomorphine

    (B) Loperamide

    (C) Metoclopramide

    (D) Ondansetron

    (E) Ranitidine

29. An airplane pilot working for a major commercial airline suffers from hay fever. Which of the following drugs would be most suitable for the pilot during working hours?

    (A) Chlorpheniramine

    (B) Diphenhydramine

    (C) Fexofenadine

    (D) Meclizine

    (E) Pyrilamine

30. A patient who is being treated for a hypertensive crisis that occurred 2 hours ago is medicated with IV nitroprusside. Which of the following is the expected action of this drug?

    (A) Constriction of arterioles alone

    (B) Constriction of both arterioles and venules

    (C) Constriction of venules alone

    (D) Dilatation of arterioles alone

    (E) Dilatation of arterioles and venules

31. A 72-year-old man with prostate cancer is treated with leuprolide. Which of the following is the mechanism of action of this drug?

    (A) It inhibits 5α-reductase

    (B) It is a competitive antagonist at androgen receptors

    (C) It is a competitive inhibitor of LH

    (D) It is a synthetic analog of GnRH

    (E) It is a testosterone agonist

32. A 50-year-old man with moderate familial hypertriglyceridemia is treated with gemfibrozil. Which of the following is the primary mechanism of action of this drug?

    (A) Binding of bile acids in the intestine

    (B) Inhibition of hepatic VLDL secretion

    (C) Inhibition of HMG-CoA reductase

    (D) Stimulation of HDL production

    (E) Stimulation of lipoprotein lipase

33. A 58-year-old man with a history of atrial fibrillation is prescribed warfarin to prevent clot and embolism formation. His prothrombin time (PT) is regularly monitored. Administration of which of the following drugs would result in an increase in his PT and require readjustment of his warfarin dosage?

    (A) Amobarbital

    (B) Carbamazepine

    (C) Ketoconazole

    (D) Phenytoin

    (E) Rifampin

34. If phenylephrine and tropicamide were instilled as eye drops together in the same eye, what would be the most likely resulting effect?

    (A) Miosis with no effect on accommodation

    (B) Miosis and cycloplegia

    (C) Mydriasis and cycloplegia

    (D) No change in pupil size or in accommodation

    (E) No change in pupil size but cycloplegia

35. A patient admitted to the emergency department with chest pain is diagnosed with myocardial infarction. On discharge, the patient is prescribed aspirin but develops an allergic hypersensitivity reaction. Ticlopidine is prescribed instead as a maintenance anticoagulant. Which of the following is the mechanism of action of this drug?

    (A) It binds to the active site of cyclo-oxygenase via acetylation

    (B) It blocks the binding of plasmin to fibrin

    (C) It hinders the production of thromboxane $A_2$

    (D) It prevents fibrinogen from binding to platelets

    (E) It stimulates platelet adenylyl cyclase

36. A patient with severe systemic lupus erythematosus is receiving long-term glucocorticoid therapy. She should consequently receive supplemental therapy with which of the following?

    (A) Calcium

    (B) Carotene

    (C) Folate

    (D) Iron

    (E) Vitamin $B_{12}$

37. A 65-year-old man is in the severe burn unit of a clinic for third-degree burns over 80% of his body following a house fire. He now suffers a multidrug-resistant gram-positive infection acquired in the hospital. He is given a prescription for imipenem. Which of the following has to be coadministered with imipenem in this patient?

    (A) Cilastatin

    (B) Clavulanic acid

    (C) Para-aminobenzoic acid (PABA)

    (D) Sulbactam

    (E) Trimethoprim

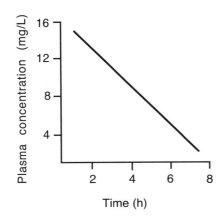

38. A pharmacologist is examining a new drug with potential sedative properties. He begins by analyzing the pharmacokinetic properties of the drug. Studies of the drug's rate of elimination yield the above data. Which of the following drugs has similar kinetics to the drug being studied?

    (A) Carbamazepine

    (B) Cimetidine

    (C) Ethanol

    (D) Ketoconazole

    (E) Phenobarbital

39. Four subjects are involved in a study of the effects of autonomic drugs on blood pressure. Each of the subjects had one pretreatment regimen as listed below.

    1. No pretreatment

    2. Atropine

    3. Phentolamine

    4. Propranolol

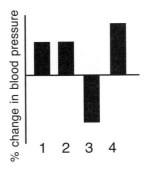

Following pretreatment, the same drug was given intravenously to each of the subjects. The results are summarized in the figure above. Which of the following drugs was most likely given to these subjects?

    (A) Acetylcholine (low dose)

    (B) Acetylcholine (high dose)

    (C) Epinephrine

    (D) Isoproterenol

    (E) Norepinephrine

    (F) Phenylephrine

40. A 24-year-old woman on her honeymoon presents to the cruise ship physician with a dilated right eye and complains that she could not read the lunch menu with the same eye. Which of the following drugs is most likely responsible for her symptoms?

    (A) Phenylephrine

    (B) Physostigmine

    (C) Pilocarpine

    (D) Scopolamine

    (E) Tetrahydrozoline

    (F) Timolol

41. On a routine annual examination, a previously healthy 59-year-old woman is found to have high blood pressure. Her high blood pressure is confirmed on three subsequent visits. She tries to control it with diet and exercise, but 1 year later it is still elevated and so she is given a prescription for a diuretic. She returns for a followup visit, and laboratory studies show an elevation of her potassium levels. She was most likely prescribed which of the following diuretics?

    (A) Acetazolamide

    (B) Furosemide

    (C) Hydrochlorothiazide

    (D) Metolazone

    (E) Triamterene

42. A 50-year-old woman with urinary incontinence is diagnosed with detrusor instability on urodynamic evaluation. Stimulation of which of the following results in contraction of this muscle?

    (A) Alpha-adrenergic receptors

    (B) Beta-adrenergic receptors

    (C) Muscarinic receptors

    (D) Nicotinic receptors

43. A pharmacy fellow is trying to determine the plasma concentration of an experimental antiarrhythmic agent (Drug X) at steady-state. A continuous IV infusion of the agent began 6 hours earlier at a rate of 3 mg/min. Drug X has a half-life of 3 hours, a volume of distribution of 120 L, and a clearance of 0.6 L/min. If the rate of infusion remains constant, what will the plasma concentration be at steady-state?

    (A) 0.005 mg/L

    (B) 0.4 mg/L

    (C) 2 mg/L

    (D) 5 mg/L

    (E) 40 mg/L

    (F) 200 mg/L

44. A 20-year-old female college athlete develops irregular menstrual cycles, acne, a deepening voice, and recent growth of facial hair. Lab values are significant for elevated liver transaminases. She is not on oral contraceptives. Which of the following drugs could be responsible for her presentation?

    (A) Ethinyl estradiol

    (B) Flutamide

    (C) Medroxyprogesterone

    (D) Megestrol acetate

    (E) Nandrolone

45. A 46-year-old woman comes to the emergency department complaining of light-headedness and confusion. She has no chronic medical conditions and takes no medications. An electrocardiogram shows third-degree atrioventricular block. She is started on intravenous isoproterenol. The reflex change in heart rate in response to this medication would likely be enhanced by which of the following drugs?

    (A) Dobutamine

    (B) Esmolol

    (C) Hexamethonium

    (D) Phenylephrine

    (E) Pirenzepine

46. A healthy 46-year-old man comes to the emergency department because of chest pain and shortness of breath for the past 2 hours. He has no prior medical history and takes no medications. Evaluation reveals elevated cardiac enzymes and troponin and new Q waves on an electrocardiogram. Tissue plasminogen activator (tPA) is administered. Which of the following is the advantage of this agent over streptokinase for fibrinolytic therapy?

    (A) It can be used in the setting of acute myocardial infarction

    (B) It cannot cause hemorrhage

    (C) It is less expensive

    (D) It is not likely to produce an allergic reaction

    (E) It results in the activation of plasminogen

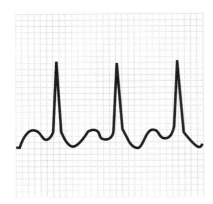

47. A 57-year-old woman with coronary artery disease is brought to the emergency department after a syncopal episode. She is alert and able to tell the staff that she also suffers from palpitations and light-headedness. An electrocardiogram is shown. Which of the following drugs will increase AV conduction and is therefore *contraindicated* in this patient?

    (A) Digoxin

    (B) Propranolol

    (C) Quinidine

    (D) Verapamil

48. A patient with congestive heart failure, hypertension, diabetes, and glaucoma receives multiple drugs in his disease management. During a routine urine and blood sample analysis, the following electrolyte disturbances are noted: decreased sodium, increased chloride, decreased potassium in the blood, increased calcium, phosphate and bicarbonate in the urine. Which of the following drugs most likely caused these electrolyte disturbances?

    (A) Acetazolamide

    (B) Captopril

    (C) Furosemide

    (D) Hydrochlorothiazide

    (E) Spironolactone

49. A 22-year-old woman develops secondary amenorrhea and galactorrhea, and MRI of the head reveals a small intrasellar tumor. Which of the following is the most appropriate pharmacologic treatment for this patient's condition?

    (A) Cholinesterase inhibitors

    (B) Dopamine agonists

    (C) Dopamine antagonists

    (D) Drugs enhancing GABAergic transmission

    (E) Serotonin reuptake inhibitors

50. A 32-year-old man, infected with HIV, is diagnosed with Hodgkin lymphoma. If the patient's CD4 count is 505/mm$^3$, which of the following agents would be suitable for the treatment of this patient's lymphoma without further compromising his immune system?

    (A) Busulfan

    (B) Cisplatin

    (C) Cyclophosphamide

    (D) Paclitaxel

    (E) Vincristine

# Pharmacology Test Two: **Answers and Explanations**

## ANSWER KEY

| | | | |
|---|---|---|---|
| 1. | B | 26. | B |
| 2. | C | 27. | B |
| 3. | E | 28. | A |
| 4. | A | 29. | C |
| 5. | B | 30. | E |
| 6. | D | 31. | D |
| 7. | C | 32. | E |
| 8. | B | 33. | C |
| 9. | E | 34. | C |
| 10. | A | 35. | D |
| 11. | C | 36. | A |
| 12. | A | 37. | A |
| 13. | E | 38. | C |
| 14. | B | 39. | C |
| 15. | C | 40. | D |
| 16. | A | 41. | E |
| 17. | D | 42. | C |
| 18. | C | 43. | D |
| 19. | E | 44. | E |
| 20. | D | 45. | A |
| 21. | E | 46. | D |
| 22. | C | 47. | C |
| 23. | C | 48. | A |
| 24. | D | 49. | B |
| 25. | C | 50. | E |

1. **The correct answer is B.** Prostatic hypertrophy in elderly men is very common; therefore, it should be considered as a primary cause of renal insufficiency until proven otherwise. The patient's signs and symptoms are consistent with obstructive uropathy; there is a history of high urine output followed by periods of almost no urine output. This pattern leads to the accumulation of urine in the collecting system, which creates a high pressure system. The high pressure is then "transmitted" back to the kidney and results in renal insufficiency. Since the patient's obstructive uropathy is most likely caused by prostatic hypertrophy, doxazosin should be used to treat the cause of these signs and symptoms. Doxazosin is a peripherally acting alpha1-adrenergic blocking agent indicated for the treatment of urinary outflow obstruction secondary to benign prostatic hyperplasia (BPH). It is also indicated for the treatment of hypertension, especially in men with BPH. Therefore, the use of this agent will correct the obstructive uropathy and treat his hypertension.

   Benazepril (**choice A**) is an ACE inhibitor used in the treatment of hypertension; however, it is known to cause azotemia and oliguria, especially in those with renal insufficiency. Therefore, this agent would be contraindicated.

   Furosemide (**choice C**) is a loop diuretic used to increase urine output in patients without a urinary tract obstruction.

   Hyoscyamine (**choice D**) is used in the treatment of gastrointestinal disorders caused by spasm and hypermotility. Since this agent is a potent anticholinergic, it would not be recommended in a patient with urinary obstruction. Remember, anticholinergic agents cause urinary retention.

   Phenazopyridine (**choice E**) is a urinary tract analgesic used to decrease the dysuria associated with urinary tract infections. The use of this agent in patients with renal insufficiency is not recommended because phenazopyridine can accumulate, resulting in renal stones and transient renal failure.

2. **The correct answer is C.** $PGE_2$ is available clinically as dinoprostone. It can be used to induce abortion, evacuate a missed abortion, or treat a benign hydatidiform mole.

   $LTA_4$ (**choice A**) is the first leukotriene produced by the lipoxygenase pathway. (Note that 5-HPETE is produced by the direct action of lipoxygenase on arachidonic acid; 5-HPETE is then converted to either 5-HETE or $LTA_4$.) On Step 1, you might be asked about $LTC_4$ or $LTD_4$ since they form the slow-reacting substance of anaphylaxis (SRS-A) and are potent bronchoconstrictors.

   $PGD_2$ (**choice B**) causes both vasodilatation and vasoconstriction, depending on the vascular bed.

   $PGF_2$ (**choice D**), which is also vasoactive, increases cardiac output, constricts bronchial smooth muscle, initiates uterine contractions, and causes contraction of gastrointestinal longitudinal muscle.

   $PGG_2$ (**choice E**) and $PGH_2$ (**choice F**) are unstable and are isomerized to form $PGD_2$ (**choice B**), $PGE_2$, or $PGF_2$ (**choice D**). Note that both $PGG_2$ and $PGH_2$ do not have any known physiologic effects of importance.

   $PGI_2$ (**choice G**), also called prostacyclin, is a potent inhibitor of platelet aggregation. It is produced by the vascular endothelia and opposes the effects of $TXA_2$ (thromboxane, **choice H**), which is produced (from the same precursor, $PGH_2$) by the platelets and promotes platelet aggregation.

3. **The correct answer is E.** Phase III trials consist of large, double-blind, controlled studies using patients for whom the drug is targeted. Typically, 500 to 5,000 patients participate in the study, which is designed to determine whether the drug is more efficacious than placebo and to compare it with older therapies. Drug toxicity is also monitored; infrequent toxicities have a greater likelihood of appearing in this phase (because of the greater number of subjects) than the previous two phases.

   For human testing to commence, an IND Application (**choice A**) must be submitted by the manufacturer to the Food and Drug Administration (FDA). This application includes chemical and manufacturing information about the drug, data from animal testing, and designs for clinical testing.

   The NDA (**choice B**), which contains the results of the clinical studies, must be submitted following human testing to gain approval for general marketing of a drug for prescription use.

   Phase I trials (**choice C**) are the first phase of clinical testing. Approximately 20 to 30 normal volunteers are used to determine the safety and pharmacokinetic properties of a new drug. Occasionally, patients are used in this phase (e.g., cancer patients who are tested with new chemotherapeutic agents).

   Phase II trials (**choice D**) test a new drug on a small group of selected patients (100-300) with regard to therapeutic efficacy, dose range, kinetics, and metabolism.

   Phase IV (**choice F**) is the post-marketing surveillance phase, which is not regulated by the FDA and essentially consists of physicians reporting toxic side effects to the FDA. This phase hopefully detects drugs with infrequent side effects that could not be determined with the limited number of subjects used in clinical testing. If it is determined that a drug does exhibit toxic side effects, and that its benefits do not outweigh its costs, the drug can be pulled from the market. (Incidentally, this is how the diet drug fenfluramine was removed from the market.)

4. **The correct answer is A.** The following chart summarizes the differences between heparin and warfarin:

| Heparin | Warfarin |
|---|---|
| Increased effect of antithrombin III on thrombin | Interferes with synthesis of vitamin K clotting factors |
| Monitored by PTT | Monitored by PT |
| Given IV or SQ | Given orally |
| Toxicity treated with protamine sulfate | Toxicity treated with vitamin K and fresh frozen plasma |
| Rapid anticoagulation | 2 to 3 days before anticoagulation |
| Can be used in pregnancy | Can't be used in pregnancy |

5. **The correct answer is B.** Sucralfate is a promising drug that is not currently in widespread use because it is incompatible with $H_2$ antagonists, such as cimetidine, ranitidine, famotidine, and nizatidine. Sucralfate is aluminum sucrose sulfate, a sulfated disaccharide, which polymerizes and binds to ulcerated tissue. It forms a protective coating against acid, pepsin, and bile, giving the tissue a chance to heal. Unfortunately, a low gastric pH is required for polymerization, meaning that sucralfate is incompatible with drugs that reduce gastric acidity, such as $H_2$ blockers and antacids. The moral of the story is that you cannot assume that two medications that are individually helpful in a medical condition will be synergistic. Learning the mechanisms by which the drugs work will help you spot potential interactions and earn you points on the USMLE.

6. **The correct answer is D.** This patient with a history of cystic fibrosis and a classic bronchopneumonia to *Pseudomonas* would best be treated with an antipseudomonal penicillin (ticarcillin) and possibly combined with aminoglycosides because of the synergy between the two.

Amoxicillin plus ampicillin (**choice A**) uses two similar penicillins with no added benefits.

Amoxicillin plus aminoglycosides (**choice B**) may not be as good as an antipseudomonal as ticarcillin, but there is synergy with aminoglycosides.

The combination of amoxicillin plus clavulanic acid (**choice C**) is very effective for beta-lactamase-producing strains.

The combination of vancomycin plus aminoglycosides (**choice E**) is effective for enterococci; if possible, vancomycin is reserved for methicillin-resistant *Staphylococcus aureus* and enterococci infections, not *Pseudomonas*.

7. **The correct answer is C.** Atenolol is a beta-adrenergic receptor blocking agent used in the treatment of hypertension. Medications in this drug class lower blood pressure by reducing both cardiac output and decreasing renin release from the kidney (to a lesser extent).

Blocking catecholamine release from peripheral sympathetic nerves (**choice A**) is the antihypertensive effect seen with peripherally acting adrenergic neuron blockers (e.g., guanethidine and bretylium).

Angiotensin converting enzyme (ACE) inhibitors block the conversion of angiotensin I to angiotensin II (**choice B**).

Diuretics decrease intravascular volume (**choice D**), which ultimately leads to a reduction in blood pressure.

Increasing renin release from the kidney (**choice E**) would increase, not decrease, blood pressure.

8. **The correct answer is B.** Dextromethorphan is a synthetic morphine derivative that acts centrally to suppress coughing by an opioid receptor-independent mechanism. It does not produce significant addiction, constipation, analgesia, respiratory depression, or euphoria. It is therefore available as an over-the-counter medication (e.g., Robitussin DM™).

Codeine (**choice A**), or methylmorphine, is a more effective antitussive than dextromethorphan, but it has abuse liability and is constipating.

Diphenoxylate (**choice C**) is an oral antidiarrheal agent that is a derivative of meperidine. This drug exhibits typical opioid effects at high doses and is prescribed only in combination with atropine.

Levorphanol (**choice D**) is a potent analgesic used for severe pain and has the typical side effects of opioids: euphoria, respiratory depression, and constipation. It has substantial abuse liability. Although levorphanol would suppress cough, it is not prescribed for this purpose.

Oxycodone (**choice E**) is a morphine derivative used for moderate-to-severe pain. It produces typical opioid effects, including constipation and dependence.

Although oxycodone would suppress cough, it is not prescribed for this purpose.

9. **The correct answer is E.** The patient is presenting with classic signs and symptoms of congestive heart failure: chronic fatigue, exertional and nocturnal dyspnea, orthopnea, a chronic nonproductive cough, respiratory wheezing, and rhonchi, as well as a diminished first heart sound and an S3 gallop. Verapamil is a calcium channel blocker used to treat both hypertension and vasospastic angina. However, it has a strong negative inotropic effect on the heart that can cause signs and symptoms of heart failure. Furthermore, some clinical studies have shown that congestive heart failure can develop in a small percentage of individuals taking verapamil.

Amlodipine (**choice A**) is also a calcium channel blocker used in the treatment of both hypertension and vasospastic angina. However, it does not have a negative inotropic effect on the heart and does not cause signs and symptoms of heart failure. Furthermore, amlodipine is generally well tolerated in heart failure patients.

Captopril (**choice B**) is an ACE inhibitor used in the treatment of both hypertension and congestive heart failure. Therefore, this agent would not potentiate signs and symptoms of congestive heart failure.

Furosemide (**choice C**) is a diuretic commonly used to treat the congestion and edema associated with heart failure. It can also be used to treat hypertension.

Hydralazine (**choice D**) is a vasodilator used primarily to treat signs and symptoms associated with hypertension. The use of this agent in patients with angina is not recommended because it can potentiate the angina through reflex tachycardia.

10. **The correct answer is A.** Propylthiouracil inhibits thyroid peroxidase, the enzyme that allows the iodide taken up at the base of the thyroid follicular cell to be oxidized to iodine at the apex of the cell. Thyroid peroxidase also catalyzes the oxidative coupling of two diiodotyrosine (DIT) molecules into $T_4$ and of one DIT and one monoiodotyrosine (MIT) into $T_3$. Note: if you knew that thyroid peroxidase was involved in oxidations, then you probably could have arrived at choice A by the process of elimination.

Iodide uptake at the base of the follicular cell (**choice B**) occurs via an active transport mechanism; thyroid peroxidase is not involved.

Iodination of thyroglobulin in the colloid (**choice C**) into DIT and MIT does not involve thyroid peroxidase.

Proteolysis of the iodinated thyroglobulin into MIT and DIT (**choice D**) occurs in the follicular cell and is catalyzed by lysosomal enzymes, not by thyroid peroxidase.

Reuptake of iodinated thyroglobulin from the follicular lumen (**choice E**) occurs via endocytosis and does not involve thyroid peroxidase.

11. **The correct answer is C.** Mesna traps acrolein, a byproduct of cyclophosphamide therapy. Cyclophosphamide is metabolized to acrolein, which is excreted in the urine. If the patient's urine is concentrated, this toxic metabolite may cause severe bladder damage. Early symptoms of bladder toxicity include dysuria and frequency. This can be distinguished from a urinary tract infection, since there is no bacteriuria with cyclophosphamide-induced bladder toxicity. However, microscopic hematuria is often present on urinalysis. In severe hemorrhagic cystitis, large segments of the bladder mucosa may be shed, which can lead to prolonged, gross hematuria. The incidence of cyclophosphamide-induced hemorrhagic cystitis can be decreased by ensuring that the patient maintains a high fluid intake. Cyclophosphamide is an alkylating agent used in the treatment of breast carcinoma, malignant lymphoma, multiple myeloma, and adenocarcinoma of the ovary, as well as various other forms of cancer. The major toxic reactions commonly seen with this agent include mucositis, nausea, hepatotoxicity, sterile hemorrhagic and non-hemorrhagic cystitis, leukopenia, neutropenia, and interstitial pulmonary fibrosis.

Mitomycin (**choice B**) is an antibiotic, antineoplastic agent used in the treatment of breast carcinoma and adenocarcinoma of the pancreas and stomach, as well as various other forms of cancer. The major toxic reactions commonly seen with this agent include bone marrow depression, nausea, hepatotoxicity, acute bronchospasm, thrombocytopenia, and interstitial pneumonitis.

Paclitaxel (**choice C**) is an antineoplastic agent primarily used in the treatment of ovarian and breast cancer. The major toxic reactions commonly seen with this agent include bone marrow depression, nausea, hepatotoxicity, bronchospasm, thrombocytopenia, and neutropenia.

Tamoxifen (**choice D**) is an antineoplastic hormone primarily used in the palliative treatment of estrogen-receptor positive breast cancer patients. The major toxic reactions commonly seen with this agent include depression, dizziness, thrombosis, mild leukopenia, and thrombocytopenia.

Vincristine (**choice E**) is a mitotic inhibitor antineoplastic agent used in the treatment of breast cancer, Hodgkin disease, non-Hodgkin lymphoma, advanced testicular cancer, and various other types of cancer. The major toxic reactions commonly seen with this agent include mental depression, hemorrhagic enterocolitis, bone marrow depression, nausea, thrombocytopenia, and leukopenia.

12. **The correct answer is A.** Pulmonary toxicity (characterized by interstitial pneumonitis that may progress to pulmonary fibrosis) is a dosage-related complication seen with the administration of bleomycin, an antibiotic chemotherapeutic agent. Other agents associated with pulmonary toxicity include methotrexate and busulfan.

Cyclophosphamide (**choice B**) is an alkylating agent used in the treatment of numerous cancers (e.g., breast, testicular), leukemia, and Hodgkin lymphoma. It is also used as a conditioning agent for bone marrow transplant. Hemorrhagic cystitis, which can be severe and even fatal, can develop. The mechanism is thought to be secondary to irritation from the toxic cyclophosphamide metabolite acrolein.

Doxorubicin (**choice C**) is an antibiotic chemotherapeutic that acts by intercalating between DNA and inducing DNA strand breaks via topoisomerase II. Irreversible cardiotoxicity is an important adverse reaction. This includes EKG changes and congestive heart failure.

Etoposide (**choice D**) interferes with topoisomerase, inducing DNA strand breaks, and is used to treat testicular and lung cancers. Adverse reactions include stomatitis, erythema, and bone marrow suppression.

5-Fluorouracil (**choice E**) is an $S/G_1$ phase-specific antimetabolite that is a widely used antineoplastic agent used systemically to treat solid tumors and topically to treat skin cancers. Adverse reactions include alopecia, bone marrow suppression, dermatitis, stomatitis, and gastrointestinal distress.

Streptozocin (**choice F**) is a DNA alkylating agent used to treat metastatic testicular, ovarian, and bladder cancer. Adverse reactions include myelosuppression, ototoxicity, and renal toxicity manifested by proteinuria, increased blood urea nitrogen, increased phosphorus, and renal tubular acidosis.

Vincristine, (**choice G**), a Vinca alkaloid that binds to the microtubule protein of the mitotic spindle, is often associated with a dosage-limiting peripheral neuropathy. Other adverse effects include alterations in mental status, constipation, ileus, and, rarely, SIADH.

13. **The correct answer is E.** To achieve the desired drug plasma level rapidly, a loading dose can be given to "load" the volume of distribution. Therefore, the only necessary information to answer this question is the volume of distribution, the desired plasma concentration, and how well the drug is absorbed into the body (bioavailability). The equation to calculate loading dose is as follows:

$$\text{Loading dose} = C_p \times \frac{V_d}{F}$$

In this case, $2 \text{ mg/L} \times \dfrac{60 \text{ L}}{0.5} = 240 \text{ mg}$

Note that clearance is important to calculate maintenance dose. To maintain target plasma levels, it is important to administer the amount of drug that is being cleared by the patient.

14. **The correct answer is B.** Ammonium chloride acidifies the urine (ascorbic acid could also be used) and hastens the elimination of weak bases, such as amphetamine. This occurs because basic drugs are not charged in their nonionized, free base form, and can easily diffuse out of the urine across tubular epithelial cells, back into the bloodstream. Ionizing the drug (in this case by lowering the urine pH) prevents it from leaving the filtrate, and the drug is excreted in the urine.

Acetazolamide (**choice A**) is a carbonic anhydrase inhibitor. It is used to alkalinize the urine in patients with hyperuricemia to increase the solubility of uric acid in the urine. It would tend to delay the elimination of the ingested amphetamine.

Penicillamine (**choice C**) is effective in chelating lead in cases of poisoning by that metal. It also chelates copper and is used in treatment of Wilson disease.

Probenecid (**choice D**) blocks renal tubular acid transport. It is used as a uricosuric.

Sodium bicarbonate (**choice E**) would alkalinize the urine, thus delaying the elimination of the ingested amphetamine.

15. **The correct answer is C.** Although misoprostol would be best indicated in NSAID-induced ulcers, prostaglandin analogs are abortifacient and are contraindicated during pregnancy.

Famotidine (**choice B**) is an $H_2$-blocker that does not affect liver metabolism.

Misoprostol (**choice C**) is a prostaglandin $E_1$ analog used in peptic ulcer disease. It does not affect hepatic metabolism.

Omeprazole (**choice D**) is a proton-pump inhibitor used to decrease acid production in patients with peptic ulcer disease or reflux. It does not affect drug metabolism by the liver.

Ranitidine (**choice E**) is another $H_2$-blocker. It does not inhibit liver enzymes as strongly as cimetidine does.

16. **The correct answer is A.** Although treatment of transient ischemic attacks (actually prophylaxis against stroke) remains a controversial area, you should be aware of current recommendations. Daily aspirin therapy has been shown in prospective, randomized studies to reduce the incidence of stroke and death in patients with transient ischemic attacks. If alternative therapy is needed, either because the patient cannot tolerate aspirin or because aspirin therapy has failed, the antiplatelet agent ticlopidine can be used.

Anticoagulation with Coumadin (**choice B**) does not decrease the risk of stroke and death but does increase the risk of intracerebral hemorrhage.

Despite the antiplatelet activity of dipyridamole (**choice C**), therapeutic trials have not shown efficacy in the prophylaxis of stroke.

Anticoagulation with heparin (**choice D**) does not decrease the risk of stroke and death but does increase the risk of intracerebral hemorrhage.

Despite the antiplatelet activity of sulfinpyrazone (**choice E**), therapeutic trials have not shown efficacy in the prophylaxis of stroke.

17. **The correct answer is D.** The patient described is probably under the influence of a CNS stimulant, such as methamphetamine. Labetalol is a nonselective alpha- and beta-antagonist that blocks many of the dangerous peripheral side effects of CNS stimulants, such as hypertension and cardiac stimulation. Other appropriate medications include antipsychotic agents (to control the agitation and psychotic symptoms) and diazepam (to control possible seizures). Supportive care should be given as needed to control the hyperthermia and to maintain respiration.

Atropine (**choice A**), which is a muscarinic antagonist, would be an appropriate therapy for an acetylcholinesterase inhibitor overdose. Patients presenting with an acetylcholinesterase inhibitor overdose would not be expected to have an elevated body temperature or hypertension. Their eyes would be miotic, not mydriatic. Bradycardia, not tachycardia, would be expected. They would, however, have diaphoresis because of increased cholinergic tone at the sweat glands, which are innervated by sympathetic cholinergics.

Flumazenil (**choice B**) is a benzodiazepine receptor antagonist. It is specifically useful in the case of a benzodiazepine overdose.

Fluoxetine (**choice C**) is a selective serotonin reuptake inhibitor (SSRI) type of antidepressant. It would not be indicated in the case of CNS stimulant overdose.

Naloxone (**choice E**), which is an opioid receptor antagonist, would be an appropriate therapy for an opiate (e.g., heroin or morphine) overdose. A patient would appear sleepy, lethargic, or comatose, depending on the degree of overdose. Pupils would be miotic, not mydriatic. Blood pressure and heart rate would usually be decreased. Respiration would be depressed.

Physostigmine (**choice F**), which is an acetylcholinesterase inhibitor, might be used for overdose of an antimuscarinic drug, such as atropine, scopolamine, or Jimson weed. An antimuscarinic overdose can look similar to a CNS stimulant overdose, with at least one important exception. The hyperthermia seen with an antimuscarinic overdose is accompanied by *hot and dry skin* (because of blockade of the sympathetic cholinergics to the sweat glands). Stimulant overdose is often characterized by *profuse sweating*. Tachycardia, hypertension, hyperthermia, mental changes, and mydriasis are common to both.

18. **The correct answer is C.** Everything in this case points to congestive heart failure (CHF): dyspnea, elevated heart rate, S3, peripheral edema, and reduced ejection fraction. A drug that will alleviate the symptoms by decreasing both preload and afterload is necessary.

Enalapril is an angiotensin-converting enzyme (ACE) inhibitor. ACE inhibitors (captopril, enalapril, lisinopril) work by blocking the conversion of angiotensin I to angiotensin II in the lungs. Angiotensin II is both a potent vasoconstrictor and a stimulator of aldosterone production. Aldosterone acts by promoting sodium (and thus water) reabsorption by the kidney. An ACE inhibitor will therefore promote vasodilatation (reducing afterload), as well as reduce intravascular volume (decreasing preload). It does not affect the heart's inotropic state.

Although digoxin (**choice A**) is a mainstay in the therapy of CHF, it has no effect on either preload or afterload. Instead, it works by having a positive inotropic effect on the heart. The mechanism involves inhibition of $Na^+/K^+$ ATPase and a consequent increase in intracellular calcium, which, in turn, increases the heart's contractile force.

Diltiazem (**choice B**) is a calcium-channel blocker. As their name implies, calcium-channel blockers block the influx of calcium (via specific calcium channels) into the cell from the extracellular fluid; this interferes with excitation-contraction coupling in cardiac muscle, producing a negative inotropic effect. Although these drugs can be used in the treatment of hypertension and angina (they inhibit the contraction of the vascular smooth muscle and thereby decrease peripheral vascular resistance/afterload), they are contraindicated in patients with CHF because of their negative inotropic effect.

Furosemide (**choice D**) is a loop diuretic. It decreases intravascular volume (and hence, preload), but at typical doses has no significant effect on either afterload or inotropic state. Diuretics are often used in the treatment of CHF, and furosemide is used for the immediate relief of pulmonary congestion.

Propranolol (**choice E**) is a beta-blocker. It has a negative inotropic effect on the heart and is therefore contraindicated in patients with CHF.

19.  **The correct answer is E.** Vincristine (and vinblastine) are Vinca alkaloids that bind to tubulin, a component of cellular microtubules. This leads to disruption of the mitotic spindle apparatus and results in metaphase arrest because the chromosomes are unable to segregate. Since these drugs interfere with mitosis, they are considered cell-cycle specific for the M phase.

Cytarabine (**choice A**) belongs to the class of antineoplastics that are antimetabolites. This drug class interferes with normal metabolic pathways by competing for enzymatic sites. Specifically, cytarabine (Ara-C) is a pyrimidine nucleoside analog. It interrupts DNA synthesis and function by inhibiting DNA polymerase and incorporating into the DNA or RNA of the cell. As you would expect, this drug is cell-cycle specific for the S phase.

Daunorubicin (**choice B**) is one of the antibiotic antineoplastic agents (others include dactinomycin, doxorubicin, bleomycin, plicamycin, and mitomycin). These agents work by disrupting DNA functioning. Daunorubicin binds to DNA between base pairs on adjacent strands, resulting in uncoiling of the helix and destruction of the DNA template. Although this drug has its maximal effect during the S phase, it is not cell-cycle specific. (Note: the only antibiotic that is cell-cycle specific is bleomycin.)

Hydroxyurea (**choice C**) works by interfering with ribonucleoside diphosphate reductase, the enzyme responsible for generating the deoxyribonucleotides needed for DNA synthesis. It is S-phase specific.

Mechlorethamine (**choice D**) is a nitrogen mustard. The nitrogen mustards (mechlorethamine, cyclophosphamide, melphalan, chlorambucil) belong to the larger class of alkylating agents. These agents work by alkylating DNA (along with RNA and proteins). The alkylating agents are generally NOT cell-cycle specific.

20.  **The correct answer is D.** Long-term, particularly daily, use of exogenous systemic corticosteroids causes pituitary/adrenal suppression, and abrupt cessation may induce an Addison-like crisis characterized by hypotension, hypoglycemia, and sometimes (if mineralocorticoid function is suppressed as well) hyponatremia (opposite of **choice C**) and hyperkalemia (opposite of **choice E**). Decreased ACTH (opposite of **choice A**) and low cortisol (opposite of **choice B**) would also be expected. Treatment is with IV steroids, and, if the patient is in shock, IV saline. The patient should also be examined for other conditions (such as infection) that may have contributed to the acute adrenal crisis.

21.  **The correct answer is E.** Misoprostol, a methyl analog of prostaglandin $E_1$, is approved for the prevention of ulcers caused by the administration of NSAIDs. Because this drug is a potential abortifacient, it should not be given to pregnant women, or to women who are attempting to conceive.

Antinuclear antibodies (**choice A**) are associated with autoimmune diseases, such as systemic lupus erythematosus, scleroderma, Sjögren syndrome, and inflammatory myopathies. The test would be of no value in this case.

A barium swallow (**choice B**) is not indicated prior to the administration of misoprostol.

Esophageal manometry (**choice C**) is used to evaluate the competency of the lower esophageal sphincter and to assess esophageal motor activity.

The osmotic fragility test (**choice D**) is performed by placing erythrocytes into a low-salt solution. An increased susceptibility to osmotic lysis is found in hereditary spherocytosis.

22.  **The correct answer is C.** Noncompetitive, or irreversible, antagonists block receptors in several different ways. They can bind covalently at the active site, or can bind either covalently or noncovalently at other sites on the receptor (allosteric effect). Either way, adding more agonist does not reverse the effects of the antagonist. Noncompetitive antagonists essentially decrease the number of working receptors by binding to them. Any receptors that do not bind the noncompetitive antagonist behave normally. This can be depicted graphically by a downward shift in the dose-response curve. The efficacy is decreased, but the potency remains the same. In this example, **curve B** is the original agonist dose-response curve, and **curve C** is the same agonist in the presence of a noncompetitive antagonist.

Competitive antagonists bind reversibly to the agonist binding site of a receptor, and their effects can be surmounted if a sufficient amount of agonist is present. This is graphically depicted as a parallel right shift of the curve. In this example, **curve B** represents the agonist alone. **Curve E** represents the agonist in the presence of a competitive antagonist. Thus, one can achieve the same response, but a greater concentration of agonist is required.

The other curves represent drugs with greater and lesser efficacy and potency than Drug B:

**Curves A and D** represent drugs that have a lower efficacy than Drug B; **Curve F** represents a drug with a greater efficacy than Drug B.

**Curve A** represents a drug that is more potent than Drug B. **Curve D** represents a drug that is less potent than Drug B.

23. **The correct answer is C.** Norepinephrine (NE) is an agonist at $\alpha_1$, $\alpha_2$, and $\beta_1$ receptors. NE exerts is vascular actions via alpha (predominantly alpha$_1$) receptors and its cardiac actions via $\beta_1$ receptors. Carvedilol is a nonselective antagonist at alpha and beta receptors and therefore could prevent all actions of NE.

Atenolol (**choice A**) and esmolol (**choice B**) are selective $\beta_1$ antagonists and therefore would block only the cardiac effects of NE.

Metaproterenol (**choice D**) is a selective $\beta_2$ agonist and so would not block NE's effects.

Prazosin (**choice E**) is a selective $\alpha_1$ antagonist and would therefore block most of NE's actions in the vasculature, but would not antagonize other effects.

24. **The correct answer is D.** The patient was probably smoking methamphetamine hydrochloride from aluminum foil. This practice can swiftly produce very high blood levels of the drug, since the vaporized methamphetamine is absorbed efficiently from the lungs and goes directly into the systemic circulation. The symptoms are classic for psychostimulant toxicity (agitation, diaphoresis, dilated pupils), including the delusional perception of insects crawling on or in the skin ("formication").

Heroin (**choice A**) could be smoked from aluminum foil but would produce miosis, respiratory depression, and sedation.

Jimson weed (from Datura species; **choice B**) contains potent antimuscarinic agents, such as atropine and scopolamine. It might produce delirium and agitation but would not produce diaphoresis (instead, the skin would be dry and warm). Also, Jimson weed is typically brewed as a tea, rather than smoked.

LSD (**choice C**) generally produces brightly colored hallucinations with a clear sensorium, and is unlikely to produce a sensation of bugs crawling on the skin. LSD is ingested, rather than smoked.

Model airplane glue (**choice E**) contains toluene and/or ketones that produce a narcotic-like "high" if inhaled, rather than symptoms of stimulant overdose. These agents are not typically heated on aluminum foil, as they are very flammable and are sufficiently volatile to be inhaled at room temperature.

25. **The correct answer is C.** The thiazide diuretics (e.g., hydrochlorothiazide, chlorothiazide, benzthiazide) promote diuresis by inhibiting reabsorption of NaCl, primarily in the early distal tubule.

Ethacrynic acid (**choice A**) and furosemide (**choice B**) are loop diuretics. They act by inhibiting electrolyte reabsorption in the thick ascending loop of Henle. If you didn't know where these agents act, but did know that they both belong to the same class of diuretics, you could have eliminated them as possibilities since there can't be more than one correct answer choice.

Mannitol (**choice D**) is an osmotic diuretic. It is freely filtered at the glomerulus and is not reabsorbed. Its primary action occurs at the proximal tubule.

Spironolactone (**choice E**) is a potassium-sparing diuretic. It acts on the collecting tubule to inhibit the reabsorption of $Na^+$ and the secretion of $K^+$. Spironolactone is a structural analog of aldosterone that binds to its receptor. (Triamterene and amiloride are also potassium-sparing diuretics but are not aldosterone antagonists.)

26. **The correct answer is B.** Cromolyn sodium inhibits the degranulation of mast cells, thereby preventing the release of histamine and other bronchoconstrictive autacoids. It is administered by inhalation and is used prophylactically to prevent an asthma attack (especially in children). It has no direct bronchodilator, adrenergic, antihistaminic, or anti-inflammatory actions.

The remaining answer choices relate to some of the other major categories of drugs available for the treatment of asthma:

Muscarinic antagonists (**choice A**) work by inhibiting acetylcholine-induced bronchoconstriction. Atropine and other belladonna alkaloids used to be first-line drugs for the treatment of asthma, but with little success. The newer agent, ipratropium, is a quaternary amine designed for aerosol use. It is a much more successful agent than the earlier muscarinic blockers and has limited side effects because it is minimally absorbed.

Corticosteroids are useful in asthma because they reduce inflammation and edema (**choice C**). They also potentiate the bronchodilating effects of the adrenergic agonists. Their use is limited by their many systemic side effects, and they are typically used only in cases of severe or acute bronchospasm or in the treatment of status asthmaticus. Fewer systemic side effects occur in aerosolized preparations such as beclomethasone dipropionate.

Selective beta$_2$ agonists (**choice D**) include metaproterenol, albuterol, and terbutaline. These drugs are the mainstay in the treatment of acute asthma. They work by stimulating beta$_2$-mediated bronchodilation (bronchial smooth muscle relaxation) without the cardiac side effects of nonselective beta agonists (**choice E**), such as isoproterenol. Note that new long-acting beta agonists have been developed (salmeterol and formoterol) for prophylactic use.

27. **The correct answer is B.** This patient is experiencing an acute attack of gout. The association of gout with alcoholism is well documented. Gout is caused by overproduction or underexcretion of uric acid. Precipitation of sodium urate (uric acid is ionized at body pH) in joint fluid causes an acute inflammatory synovitis with synovial edema and leukocytic infiltrate. It usually affects the joints of the lower extremity, most commonly, the large toe. Formation of tophi (urate deposits surrounded by inflammatory cells, including foreign body giant cells) is pathognomonic.

Nonsteroidal anti-inflammatory drugs (NSAIDs), such as indomethacin (**choice B**), can be used in the treatment of acute gout. They are as efficacious as colchicine and less toxic.

Allopurinol (**choice A**) is an anti-gout drug indicated for the treatment of chronic gout. Allopurinol functions to inhibit the enzyme xanthine oxidase, which results in decreased production of uric acid from its immediate precursor, xanthine. It lowers both serum and urinary concentrations of uric acid.

Colestipol (**choice C**) is a bile acid sequestrant that is useful in lowering cholesterol levels in familial hyperlipidemias. It is not used for the treatment of gout.

Pravastatin (**choice D**) is a hydroxymethylglutaryl-CoA (HMG-CoA) reductase inhibitor useful in the treatment of familial hyperlipidemias. It is not used for the treatment of gout.

Probenecid (**choice E**) is indicated for the treatment of chronic gout. Probenecid inhibits uric acid reabsorption and therefore increases the urinary excretion of uric acid.

28. **The correct answer is A.** Apomorphine is a dopamine and opioid agonist that stimulates the chemoreceptor trigger zone in the medulla of the brainstem to induce vomiting. It must be administered parenterally and, because it is a respiratory depressant, it should not be given to patients with compromised respiration. If necessary, the apomorphine-induced respiratory depression can be reversed by naloxone.

Loperamide (**choice B**) is an over-the-counter antidiarrheal.

Metoclopramide (**choice C**) is a dopamine receptor antagonist used to stimulate upper gastrointestinal motility. Because it is a dopamine antagonist, it also acts as an antiemetic used in chemotherapy.

Ondansetron (**choice D**), a 5HT$_3$ antagonist, is an antiemetic.

Ranitidine (**choice E**), an H$_2$ antagonist, reduces histamine-induced gastric acid release.

29. **The correct answer is C.** Fexofenadine, which belongs to the piperidine drug class, is the only drug listed that does not cross the blood-brain barrier and therefore does not cause sedation (a bad thing for someone flying an airplane). Other drugs from the same class include cetirizine and levocabastine. Terfenadine and astemizole were also members of this second generation of antihistamines but have since been removed from the U.S. market because their metabolism was easily inhibited (by ketoconazole, itraconazole, macrolide antibiotics, and even by grapefruit juice), resulting in high concentrations that could lead to a lethal arrhythmia (torsade de pointes).

All the other choices have some degree of sedation as a side effect and therefore would not be recommended for someone who is flying an airplane or operating any kind of machinery.

30. **The correct answer is E.** Nitroprusside is somewhat tricky to use, but is a very useful IV agent that causes dilatation of both arterioles and venules. It has a very rapid onset of action and is typically used in an emergency department or intensive care unit situation. The typical setting is a patient with acute or chronic low cardiac output and high ventricular filling pressures due to poor systolic left ventricular function. Underlying causes for the poor ventricular function may be diverse: malignant hypertension, dilated cardiomyopathy, acute myocardial infarction, chronic coronary heart disease, or aortic or mitral incompetence. Nitroprusside can improve perfusion of vital organs and reduce the workload of the heart. Problems sometimes encountered with this drug include hypotension (best avoided by starting with a low dose and continuously monitoring systemic arterial and pulmonary capillary wedge pressures) and accumulation of toxic metabolites of cyanide in patients with liver or renal failure. Many physicians prefer to use IV nitrate rather than nitroprusside because of its lesser toxicity.

31. **The correct answer is D.** Leuprolide is a GnRH analog. Given long-term in a continuous fashion, it will inhibit FSH and LH release, thereby decreasing testosterone production and exacting a chemical castration in men. It can be used in the treatment of prostate cancer, polycystic ovary syndrome, uterine fibroids, and endometriosis.

    Inhibition of 5α-reductase (**choice A**) is the mechanism of action of finasteride. It thereby inhibits the production of dihydrotestosterone. It is used in the treatment of benign prostatic hyperplasia (BPH).

    Flutamide is another drug used in the treatment of prostate cancer. It is a competitive antagonist at androgen receptors (**choice B**).

    Since LH activates interstitial cells to secrete testosterone, a synthetic analog of LH (**choice C**) would not be appropriate treatment for prostatic cancer. The same goes for a testosterone analog (**choice E**).

    Here is a brief chart that will aid you in remembering the actions of these similar sounding drugs:

    | Drug | Action | Indication |
    | --- | --- | --- |
    | Leuprolide | GnRH analog | Prostate CA |
    | Flutamide | Competitive androgen antagonist | Prostate CA |
    | Finasteride | 5α-reductase inhibitor | BPH |

    Remember, "loo"-prolide and "floo"-tamide are both used for prostate cancer. Finasteride is used for BPH.

32. **The correct answer is E.** Gemfibrozil (as well as clofibrate) works by increasing the activity of lipoprotein lipase, leading to increased clearance of VLDLs, which are elevated in familial hypertriglyceridemia. This question gives us the opportunity to review the mechanisms of action of the drugs used in the treatment of hyperlipidemia:

    Binding of bile acids (**choice A**) is the mechanism of action of resins such as cholestyramine. They cause the liver to use cholesterol for the synthesis of new bile acids.

    Inhibition of hepatic VLDL secretion (**choice B**) is the mechanism of action of niacin.

    Inhibition of HMG-CoA reductase (**choice C**) is the mechanism of action of lovastatin and simvastatin.

    Stimulation of HDL production (**choice D**) may occur with both gemfibrozil and niacin, but it is not the main mechanism of action.

33. **The correct answer is C.** This question is testing a favorite USMLE concept—the relationship between the hepatic cytochrome P-450 system and the metabolism of drugs. Certain drugs can affect the metabolism of other drugs by either inducing or inhibiting hepatic microsomal enzyme activity. In this case, you are told that the PT of this patient increases with the administration of the second drug. This means that the amount of circulating warfarin increased and that you are looking for a drug that inhibits the P-450 system (thereby decreasing warfarin metabolism). Of the drugs listed, only ketoconazole inhibits the P-450 system. Other important inhibitors include cimetidine and isoniazid.

    You should study all the other choices in this question because they are all inducers of the P-450 system and would require an increased dose of warfarin to achieve the same level of anticoagulation.

34. **The correct answer is C.** Phenylephrine, an alpha-1 antagonist, will constrict radial muscle and cause mydriasis. It will have no effect on accommodation because ciliary muscle has no alpha-1 receptors. Tropicamide, an M antagonist, will prevent sphincter M contraction, prevent miosis, and result in sympathetic dominance, with observation of a mydriasis. Tropicamide will also block M receptors of ciliary muscle, resulting in paralysis of accommodation called cycloplegia. If the drugs are used together, there will be an additive effect on pupillary dilation (mydriasis) and lack of accommodation from tropicamide only (cycloplegia).

    Miosis with no effect on accommodation (**choice A**) is incorrect because muscarinic agonists or alpha-1 receptors would causes miosis. Muscarinic receptors would also cause a spasm of accommodation.

    Miosis and cycloplegia (**choice B**) is incorrect because of the reasons listed for choice A, and cycloplegia would have needed a blocker of M receptors.

    No change in pupil size or in accommodation (**choice D**) and no change in pupil size but cycloplegia (**choice E**) are also incorrect because these effects would have required drugs with opposite effects on pupillary tone, such as an M agonist with an alpha-1 agonist or an M blocker with an alpha-1 blocker.

35. **The correct answer is D.** Ticlopidine is an antiplatelet drug that interacts with platelet glycoprotein IIb/IIIa, a fibrinogen receptor that links platelets together and leads to plug formation. Thus, the drug prevents fibrinogen from binding to platelets. The drug is useful both for patients with coronary disease and for those with cerebrovascular disease such as stroke. Of course, hemorrhagic stroke should first be ruled out before it is

deemed safe to use any anticoagulant. Ticlopidine is particularly indicated for stroke prophylaxis after a transient ischemic attack.

Aspirin irreversibly acetylates cyclo-oxygenase at or near the active site (**choice A**) and thus hinders the production of thromboxane $A_2$ (**choice C**).

Aminocaproic acid strongly inhibits fibrinolysis. It blocks the binding of plasmin to fibrin (**choice B**) by attaching to lysine binding sites on plasmin and plasminogen.

Dipyridamole is a phosphodiesterase inhibitor that also blocks the reuptake of adenosine, which acts on the platelets to stimulate adenylyl cyclase (**choice E**).

36. **The correct answer is A.** Long-term corticosteroid use can cause osteopenia with vertebral compression factors. This can be minimized with oral calcium supplementation. If the patient is a post-menopausal woman, estrogen therapy is also useful. More controversial is the use of vitamin D, thiazide diuretics, calcitonin, and diphosphonates. Weight-bearing exercise, in moderation, may stimulate bone formation.

Carotene (**choice B**) is an antioxidant and has no role in the amelioration of bone loss due to long-term corticosteroid treatment.

Some patients with lupus develop hemolytic anemia, and extra-nutritional support with folate (**choice C**) or iron (**choice D**) may be helpful. However, the anemia is a feature of the disease itself, rather than of the steroid therapy.

Supplementation with vitamin $B_{12}$ (cobalamin; **choice E**) is not indicated with glucocorticoid therapy.

37. **The correct answer is A.** Imipenem is a broad-spectrum (including activity against *Pseudomonas*), synthetic, beta-lactam antibiotic that is currently the *most potent* and *broadest* spectrum beta-lactam available. It is given in combination with cilastatin, which limits imipenem's toxicity by blocking renal dipeptidase, thereby minimizing accumulation of nephrotoxic metabolites. It is used in severe nosocomial infections.

Clavulanic acid (**choice B**) covalently reacts with bacterial penicillinase (beta-lactamase), thereby inhibiting the enzyme that cleaves the beta-lactam ring of penicillins, such as amoxicillin and ticarcillin.

Para-aminobenzoic acid (PABA; **choice C**) is a folic acid precursor. Sulfonamides are structural analogs of PABA, and thus interfere with folate synthesis in bacteria.

Sulbactam (**choice D**) is a penicillinase (beta-lactamase) inhibitor used with parenteral ampicillin.

Trimethoprim (**choice E**) is an antibiotic that is usually given in conjunction with sulfamethoxazole, because

the two drugs block sequential steps in bacterial folate synthesis.

38. **The correct answer is C.** The graph presented is classic for zero-order elimination; the graph is a straight line using standard graphic coordinates. Note that the plasma concentration of the drug diminishes linearly with time. Zero-order elimination means that the rate of elimination is constant and is independent of the drug plasma concentration. Another way of saying this is that a constant *amount* of drug is cleared per unit time. There are very few drugs that exhibit zero-order elimination; examples include alcohol, phenytoin, and aspirin (at high concentrations).

The vast majority of drugs exhibit first-order elimination kinetics, which means that a constant *fraction* of the drug is cleared per unit time. Thus, elimination is proportional to the drug plasma concentration. This can be graphically depicted in several different ways. Using standard graphic coordinates, an exponential decrease in the concentration of the drug is seen. If a semi-logarithmic scale is used, the graph will appear as a straight line, similar to the graph in this question.

39. **The correct answer is C.** The best way to approach this question is to eliminate as many choices as you can, as quickly as possible. Note that the drug, when given alone, increases blood pressure. Acetylcholine (by stimulating muscarinic receptors on vascular endothelium) and isoproterenol (by stimulating $beta_2$ receptors on vascular smooth muscle) both decrease blood pressure, so **choices A, B, and D** can be immediately eliminated.

This leaves epinephrine, norepinephrine, and phenylephrine. Epinephrine (**choice C**; a nonselective alpha and beta adrenergic agonist), when administered alone, produces a modest rise in blood pressure by activating $alpha_1$ receptors in arterioles and $beta_1$ receptors in the heart. (The increase in blood pressure is not especially large because it also stimulates $beta_2$ receptors, which dilate the vasculature.) This would not be affected by atropine pretreatment. In contrast, pretreatment with phentolamine, a nonselective alpha antagonist, would permit epinephrine to bind only to $beta_1$ and $beta_2$ receptors. This would cause epinephrine to function like a beta agonist, such as isoproterenol. Although epinephrine usually has a pressor effect, in the presence of phentolamine it has a depressor effect. This classic drug interaction is called *epinephrine reversal*. Propranolol would block epinephrine's actions on beta receptors, causing it to function like an alpha agonist. Epinephrine would then have a greater pressor effect with propranolol pretreatment than without it, because the vasodilatory $beta_2$ actions would be blocked.

**KAPLAN) MEDICAL**

Norepinephrine (**choice E**) produces an increase in blood pressure by activating alpha$_1$ receptors in arterioles and beta$_1$ receptors in the heart. Atropine would have no effect on this. Phentolamine would block most of the effects of norepinephrine on blood pressure by blocking its action on arterioles. It would not, however, make norepinephrine a depressor. Propranolol would be expected to prevent (rather than increase) part of the pressor effects of norepinephrine by blocking its actions on the heart.

Phenylephrine (**choice F**), an alpha$_1$ agonist, can be easily eliminated because the drug's effect is not blocked by phentolamine. In addition, propranolol should have no effect on the actions of phenylephrine.

40. **The correct answer is D.** The question is asking for a drug that dilates the pupil (mydriasis) and prevents accommodation by paralyzing the ciliary muscle (cycloplegia). Scopolamine would produce both of these actions by blocking muscarinic acetylcholine receptors on the pupillary constrictor muscle (leading to mydriasis) and on the ciliary muscle (producing cycloplegia). An additional hint to arrive at this answer is the fact that she is on a cruise ship. Scopolamine patches are used to prevent motion sickness. The woman most likely applied the patch and subsequently rubbed her eye.

Phenylephrine (**choice A**), an alpha$_1$-adrenergic agonist, could produce mydriasis by acting on receptors present on the radial dilator muscle. This would constrict the radial dilator muscles without affecting the ciliary muscles, which have muscarinic receptors (and a few beta-adrenergic receptors) and therefore have no accommodation effects.

Physostigmine (**answer B**) is an intermediate-acting carbamylating inhibitor of acetylcholinesterase; it would increase cholinergic tone to the pupillary constrictor muscle, producing miosis, and cause ciliary muscle contraction to focus for near vision. It is used in the treatment of glaucoma.

Pilocarpine (**answer C**) is a nonspecific muscarinic agonist and would therefore produce miosis and contraction of the ciliary muscle to focus for near vision. It is used in the treatment of glaucoma.

Tetrahydrozoline (**answer E**) is an alpha$_1$-adrenergic agonist and is the active ingredient in Visine™. It "gets the red out" by vasoconstricting vessels of the eye. It could cause some mydriasis by acting on alpha-receptors on the radial dilator muscle; however, it would not have an effect on the ciliary muscle.

Timolol (**choice F**) is a nonspecific beta-adrenergic antagonist. It is used in chronic open angle glaucoma because it diminishes aqueous humor production from the ciliary body. It is well tolerated because it does not affect one's ability to focus. It also would not affect pupil size.

41. **The correct answer is E.** Triamterene is grouped in the category of potassium-sparing diuretics. Along with spironolactone and amiloride, these diuretic agents may cause excess renal retention of potassium. In this manner, use of these drugs may increase potassium levels and cause hyperkalemia.

Acetazolamide (**choice A**) is a carbonic anhydrase inhibitor that initially causes a moderate amount of potassium loss. This would predispose the patient to hypokalemia.

Furosemide (**choice B**) is a loop diuretic that causes a moderate to severe loss of potassium.

Hydrochlorothiazide and metolazone (**choices C and D**) are thiazide diuretics that cause moderate amounts of potassium loss.

42. **The correct answer is C.** Stimulation of muscarinic receptors (cholinergic parasympathetic) causes contraction of the detrusor muscle, which is located in the wall of the bladder and is responsible for bladder emptying. Detrusor instability, resulting in incontinence, can therefore be effectively treated with anticholinergic medications, such as oxybutynin (Ditropan). Note that this is also why drugs with anticholinergic activity (e.g., tricyclic antidepressants) can result in urinary retention.

Alpha-adrenergic stimulation, specifically alpha$_1$ (**choice A**), causes contraction of the trigone of the bladder and smooth muscle of the urethra (including the internal urethral sphincter). Alpha agonists are therefore useful for treating stress incontinence, which results from an incompetent sphincter. Alpha antagonists, which relax the sphincter, are useful for treating overflow incontinence resulting from bladder outlet obstruction.

Beta-adrenergic stimulation, specifically beta$_2$ (**choice B**), of the detrusor muscle causes relaxation, not contraction, of the structure.

Stimulation of nicotinic cholinergic receptors (**choice D**) causes contraction of the external urethral sphincter, which consists of skeletal muscle.

43. **The correct answer is D.** This is actually a fairly straightforward question. The most difficult aspect is to determine which values given in the stem are necessary to answer this question. The patient is given a constant IV infusion (infusion rate [k$_o$]) of a drug, and the clearance is known. This is all that is necessary to determine the plasma concentration at steady-state.

The equation to use is:

$$C_{ss} = \frac{k_o}{CL}$$

where    $C_{ss}$ = plasma concentration at steady-state

   CL = clearance

   $k_o$ = infusion rate

$$C_{ss} = \frac{3 \text{ mg/min}}{0.6 \text{ L/min}}$$

$$= 5 \text{ mg/L}$$

44.   **The correct answer is E.** Nandrolone is an anabolic steroid. The clue in this question is that the woman competes in athletic events. The other signs (facial hair, menstrual irregularity, and acne) support the supposition that this woman is taking androgenic steroids.

Ethinyl estradiol (**choice A**) is a synthetic steroidal estrogen used for oral contraception.

Flutamide (**choice B**) is a nonsteroidal anti-androgen used in the treatment of prostate carcinoma.

Medroxyprogesterone and megestrol acetate (**choices C and D**) are synthetic progestins. They are also used in oral contraception, in combination with estrogens.

45.   **The correct answer is A.** The first thing you need to know to answer this question is what effect isoproterenol has on blood pressure. Isoproterenol, a nonselective beta agonist, decreases blood pressure primarily because of $beta_2$-induced vasodilation. This would lead to a reflex increase in heart rate by stimulating the sympathetic nervous system and inhibiting the parasympathetic nervous system. The next step is to determine which drug would enhance this increase in heart rate. Of all the drugs listed, only dobutamine would increase heart rate. Dobutamine is a $beta_1$ agonist that increases heart rate by stimulating cardiac receptors; it is typically given intravenously in a hospital setting.

Esmolol (**choice B**) is a $beta_1$ antagonist. This would prevent some of the reflex increase in heart rate by blocking $beta_1$ receptors on the heart.

Hexamethonium (**choice C**) is a ganglionic blocker that acts by blocking nicotinic receptors at peripheral ganglia. This would prevent any baroreceptor reflexes by blocking all sympathetic and parasympathetic outflow.

Phenylephrine (**choice D**) is an $alpha_1$-selective agonist. This would not have a direct effect on the heart and, if anything, would diminish the isoproterenol-induced baroreceptor reflex because it would cause peripheral vasoconstriction.

Pirenzepine (**choice E**) is a selective muscarinic$_1$ ($M_1$) antagonist. This would not have an effect on the heart because $M_2$ receptors are the subtype of muscarinic receptor that reside on the heart. Atropine, a nonselective muscarinic antagonist, would enhance the reflex increase in heart rate.

46.   **The correct answer is D.** Tissue plasminogen activator is produced by and secreted from endothelial cells. Since it is not a foreign protein like streptokinase (derived from hemolytic streptococci), tPA is not allergenic.

Both drugs can be used in the setting of acute myocardial infarction (**choice A**).

Both drugs can result in hemorrhage (**choice B**), especially during prolonged therapy for treatment of pulmonary embolism or venous thrombosis.

tPA is as much as 10 times more expensive (**choice C**) than streptokinase.

Both drugs result in the activation of plasminogen (**choice E**).

47.   **The correct answer is C.** This patient has atrial flutter (AF), as determined by the "sawtooth" pattern on EKG. This arrhythmia is associated with a regular, rapid (250-350/min) arrhythmia originating in the atria, often resulting from a wave of depolarization that propagates continuously within a closed circuit. The goal of treatment of AF is to decrease ventricular rate. This is accomplished by decreasing AV nodal conduction, using digoxin (**choice A**), propranolol (**choice B**), or verapamil (**choice D**). Quinidine increases AV nodal conduction and is therefore contraindicated.

48.   **The correct answer is A.** Acetazolamide, a carbonic anhydrase inhibitor, causes loss of bicarbonate, rendering urine alkaline and resulting in metabolic acidosis. Less sodium is retained (diuretic effect). This forces adaptation from the kidney, which reabsorbs more chloride instead of bicarbonate (hyperchloremia) and loses more potassium distally (hypokalemia). Alkaline urine precipitates calcium phosphate, increasing their excretion and the risk of renal stones.

Captopril (**choice B**), an ACE inhibitor, would have caused hyperkalemia from aldosterone secretion inhibition.

Furosemide (**choice C**) does not increase bicarbonate losses; rather, it causes severe hypocalcemia and hypomagnesemia.

Hydrochlorothiazide (**choice D**) causes hypercalcemia.

Spironolactone (**choice E**) causes hyperkalemia.

49. **The correct answer is B.** Whenever secondary amenorrhea develops in association with galactorrhea, hyperprolactinemia should be suspected. A prolactin-secreting pituitary adenoma is the most frequent cause of this condition, which can be treated either pharmacologically or surgically. Prolactin secretion (as any anterior pituitary hormone) is regulated by factors released by the hypothalamus. In this case, prolactin secretion is inhibited by *dopamine*. Thus, drugs such as bromocriptine or pergolide, which act as agonists on dopamine receptors, will inhibit prolactin release. In contrast, dopamine antagonists (**choice C**), such as most antipsychotic drugs, may increase prolactin secretion and cause amenorrhea-galactorrhea syndrome.

Cholinesterase inhibitors (**choice A**) that cross the blood-brain barrier, such as tacrine, are used to enhance cholinergic neurotransmission in Alzheimer disease, but they have no effect on pituitary physiology.

Drugs enhancing GABAergic transmission (**choice D**) include compounds such as benzodiazepines, valproic acid, and gabapentin, which potentiate GABA inhibitory action through different mechanisms. These drugs are used in the treatment of epilepsy.

Serotonin reuptake inhibitors (**choice E**) are used to treat mental depression (see, for example, fluoxetine and sertraline). They prolong the action of serotonin in serotoninergic pathways, which are involved in mood regulation.

50. **The correct answer is E.** Bone marrow suppression, diarrhea, and alopecia are the most common side effects seen with cancer chemotherapy regimens. Vincristine, a mitotic inhibitor, is a chemotherapeutic agent that is not associated with the development of bone marrow suppression and would be the most appropriate agent to use in this patient. Vincristine is effective in the treatment of acute lymphoblastic leukemia and other leukemias, Hodgkin disease, lymphosarcoma, neuroblastoma, and various other types of cancer. Bleomycin is another antineoplastic agent that does not cause bone marrow suppression.

Busulfan (**choice A**) is an alkylating agent primarily used in the palliative treatment of chronic myelogenous leukemia; it is known to cause severe bone marrow suppression. As a general rule, the alkylating agents typically produce severe immunosuppressive effects.

Cisplatin (**choice B**) is another alkylating agent indicated for the treatment of metastatic testicular and ovarian tumors in combination with other agents. This agent can also cause profound bone marrow suppression.

Cyclophosphamide (**choice C**) is classified as a nitrogen mustard, a subcategory of the alkylating agents. It is primarily used to treat breast, testicular, and other solid tumors, as well as leukemia and lymphoma. This drug suppresses bone marrow.

Paclitaxel (**choice D**) is an antimicrotubule agent typically used in the treatment of ovarian and breast cancer. Profound neutropenia is typically seen with this agent.

# Behavioral Science and Biostatistics: **Test One**

1. A 48-year-old man is brought to the psychiatric emergency department after an attempted suicide. He claims to hear voices telling him to kill himself. The patient's family notes that he has been on several different kinds of antipsychotic medications, with no improvement of his symptoms. The attending psychiatrist places the patient on a new medication and admits him. One week after therapy has begun, a routine blood test reveals profound depletion of polymorphonuclear leukocytes. Which of the following drugs is most likely responsible for these symptoms?

   (A) Chlorpromazine

   (B) Clozapine

   (C) Fluoxetine

   (D) Haloperidol

   (E) Imipramine

   (F) Phenelzine

2. After a bout of aseptic meningitis, a patient is unable to recall a surgical procedure he underwent before the infection. He is, however, able to register and recall present events. The patient most likely has which of the following conditions?

   (A) Anterograde amnesia

   (B) Proactive inhibition

   (C) Retroactive inhibition

   (D) Retrograde amnesia

   (E) Transient global amnesia

3. A 9-year-old boy has been caught stealing the lunches of his classmates on three separate occasions. He sleeps in class and usually does not participate in the educational process. The boy is small for his age and generally does not interact with his classmates except when they hit him. When his fourth-grade teacher tries to contact the parents for a conference, she discovers that they have no telephone and the address given to the school is a post office box. Which of the following is most likely cause of this child's behavior?

   (A) Antisocial personality

   (B) Child abuse

   (C) Mental retardation

   (D) Oppositional defiant disorder

   (E) Thyroid dysfunction

4. A city has a population of 250,000. Of these, 10,000 have disease X, which is incurable. There are 1000 new cases and 400 deaths each year from this disease. There are 2500 deaths per year from all causes. The prevalence of this disease is given by

   (A) 400/250,000

   (B) 600/250,000

   (C) 1000/250,000

   (D) 2500/250,000

   (E) 10,000/250,000

5. A 64-year-old man is brought to the emergency department by the police after he is discovered wandering in a local park late one evening. When examined, the man is able to give his name but appears confused and asks repeatedly where he is and how he got there. He is, however, able to accurately answer questions about the current year and president. Level of consciousness and attention span are both normal on the mental status exam. Subsequent investigation shows that the man was reported missing several days ago by his relatives who live some 300 miles away in a different city. Which of the following is the most likely preliminary diagnosis?

   (A) Delirium

   (B) Dementia

   (C) Fugue

   (D) Somnambulism

   (E) Stupor

6. A 30-year-old heterosexual man repeatedly cross-dresses to achieve sexual excitement but is content with his biologic gender. Which of the following is the most likely diagnosis?

   (A) Exhibitionism

   (B) Transsexualism

   (C) Transvestic fetishism

   (D) Voyeurism

7. In a medical class of 147 students, the distribution of scores on a biochemistry final examination has a mean equal to 67, a median equal to 76, a mode equal to 80, a standard deviation equal to 5.5, and a variance equal to 30.25. Three students were unable to take the test on the scheduled date and were given a different form of the exam one week later. Which parameter is most likely to be the least biased estimator of central tendency for this distribution of biochemistry test scores?

   (A) Mean

   (B) Median

   (C) Mode

   (D) Standard deviation

   (E) Variance

8. A 27-year-old man believes that he lives on a planet circling the star Alpha Centauri. His speech is rambling, he giggles frequently at inappropriate times, and he does not make sense when talking with others, He exhibits purposeful behaviors that do not accomplish an end and often "hears voices." The first episode of this behavior occurred when he was 18 years old. Which of the following is the most likely diagnosis?

   (A) Catatonic schizophrenia

   (B) Disorganized schizophrenia

   (C) Paranoid schizophrenia

   (D) Residual schizophrenia

   (E) Undifferentiated schizophrenia

9. A 5-year-old boy is taken to a dermatologist to remove a suspicious-looking lesion from his back. He is extremely afraid of receiving an injection and of the procedure in general. The best way to alter his pain perception threshold would be to

   (A) allow his parents to be present during the procedure

   (B) divert his attention away from the procedure

   (C) encourage him to vent his emotions

   (D) explain sensory pain pathways to him

   (E) have him focus on and examine the nature of the pain

10. A 64-year-old woman is hospitalized for an acute exacerbation of schizophrenia. The medications that she is prescribed cause some immediate adverse effects, but she tolerates them and continues to be compliant. A few years pass and she begins to develop neurologic abnormalities. These include involuntary, repetitive movement of the lips and tongue, as well as of her trunk and extremities. Which of the following medications should now be prescribed to this patient?

   (A) Chlorpromazine

   (B) Clozapine

   (C) Fluphenazine

   (D) Haloperidol

   (E) Metoclopramide

   (F) Thioridazine

11. A 27-year-old woman reveals to her gynecologist that her last three miscarriages were caused by spousal abuse while she was pregnant. Her husband also abuses her at times when she is not pregnant. When the husband is confronted with this report, he does not deny it. The husband's behavior is most likely explained by which of the following?

    (A) Being the first-born child

    (B) Concern about financial security

    (C) Dislike of children

    (D) Feelings of inadequacy

    (E) Wanting out of the marriage

12. A 25-year-old actress tends to behave seductively and with exaggerated charm to obtain continuous attention. She often puts on an overdramatized display of emotion but lacks genuine deep feelings. She craves control in her interpersonal relationships, often causing them to disintegrate. This patient most likely has which of the following personality disorders?

    (A) Histrionic

    (B) Narcissistic

    (C) Paranoid

    (D) Passive-aggressive

    (E) Schizotypal

13. A 57-year-old woman is diagnosed with pancreatic cancer. After a complete workup, she is informed that she has between 6 months and 1 year to live. Kubler-Ross' stages of dying are listed below:

    1. Acceptance
    2. Anger
    3. Bargaining
    4. Denial
    5. Sadness/depression

    Which of the following correctly expresses the order in which she will most likely experience these stages?

    (A) 1-2-4-5-3

    (B) 2-5-3-1-4

    (C) 3-2-4-1-5

    (D) 4-2-3-5-1

    (E) 5-3-4-1-2

14. A 32-year-old man reports difficulty maintaining an erection during intercourse with his wife. This has developed gradually over the past 3 years. He had experienced no such difficulty prior to marriage. He reports full morning erections with wakening. He had a sexual experience on a recent business trip and noted no difficulty on that occasion. He looks embarrassed as he gives his history. Although there is no evidence for anger when speaking about his wife, evidence of anxiety is prominent. Which of the following is the most likely diagnosis?

    (A) Adjustment disorder with anxious mood

    (B) Hypoactive sexual desire disorder, psychogenic

    (C) Inhibited male orgasm, psychogenic

    (D) Latent ego-dystonic homosexuality

    (E) Male erectile disorder, psychogenic

15. An 88-year-old man complaining of abdominal pain enters the emergency department with his wife. A mini-mental status exam reveals pronounced forgetfulness and confusion. The patient is discovered to have acute appendicitis requiring immediate surgery. He is unable to understand the situation and cannot provide informed consent. Which of the following further actions must the physician take?

    (A) Do not perform surgery

    (B) Have another physician confirm the necessity of surgery

    (C) Obtain a court order to perform surgery

    (D) Obtain consent from his wife to perform surgery

    (E) Try to persuade the patient to consent to surgery

16. A 37-year-old man is referred to a psychiatrist for evaluation for sexual reassignment. He states that from as early as he can remember, he has been sexually attracted only to other men. However, he always feels enormous guilt after a sexual liaison with a man. While he has functioned adequately with women, he has no emotional or physical affinity for them. He is requesting sexual reassignment because he wants to have a husband and a normal heterosexual life. Which of the following is the most likely diagnosis?

    (A) Ego-dystonic gender identity disorder

    (B) Ego-dystonic homosexuality

    (C) Ego-syntonic gender identity disorder

    (D) Ego-syntonic homosexuality

    (E) Paraphilia

**KAPLAN) MEDICAL**

17. An 18-month-old child is brought to a pediatrician by his 17-year-old mother because the child weighs only 14 lb. His birth weight was 7.25 lb. The mother states the infant never "ate right." Observation reveals a hypokinetic child who is dull and listless with a poverty of spontaneous activity. He appears sad and miserable but visually tracks the physician. Examination suggests malnourishment. His muscle tone is poor, and his skin is cool and more mottled than expected. There are no signs of physical trauma. The mother spends a great deal of time talking to the pediatrician about her own problems. Which of the following is the most likely diagnosis?

   (A) Autistic disorder

   (B) Möbius syndrome

   (C) Reactive attachment disorder of infancy

   (D) Rett syndrome

   (E) Tay-Sachs disease

18. A 43-year-old man is sitting on the examining table with his shoulders slumped. His head and eyes are downcast. His eyes are red. He looks up slowly and, after a deep sigh, says "I am sorry to bother you, Doctor, but I have to talk to someone. I have been so discouraged and so depressed for over 2 years, and I can't take it anymore." Which of the following is the most likely diagnosis?

   (A) Dysthymic disorder

   (B) Major depressive disorder

   (C) Organic affective syndrome

   (D) Schizoaffective disorder

   (E) Uncomplicated bereavement

19. A 30-year-old woman sees a psychiatrist three times a week. She is having an extremely hard time dealing with a death in her family, but at the moment she is concerned about the length of time that she has been feeling this way. She is somewhat comforted when the psychiatrist tells her that the grief and bereavement process typically takes the longest to resolve after the death of this family member. Which of the following family members most likely died?

   (A) Child

   (B) Grandparent

   (C) Parent

   (D) Sibling

   (E) Spouse

20. A 73-year-old woman has difficulty concentrating and demonstrates some mild immediate-memory problems. She has a poor appetite and has lost 24 lb in 6 weeks. She resists participation in recreational activities, and she wakes up at 4:00 AM everyday and is unable to get back to sleep. Her condition is worsening on a daily basis. Which of the following is the most likely diagnosis?

   (A) Alcohol-related delirium

   (B) Dementia of the Alzheimer type

   (C) Hypothyroidism

   (D) Normal pressure hydrocephalus

   (E) Pseudodementia

21. A pharmaceutical researcher is examining the ulcerogenic potential of a new nonsteroidal anti-inflammatory drug. He gives 20 rats a single subcutaneous injection of the drug every day for 1 week, and gives a similarly matched group of 20 animals daily saline injections for 1 week. Twenty-four hours after the final injection, the investigator sacrifices the rats, removes their stomachs, and examines them to determine whether any ulcers were produced. He obtains the following data:

|  | Ulcers present | Ulcers absent |
|---|---|---|
| Drug | 12 | 8 |
| No Drug | 8 | 12 |

   Which of the following tests would be most appropriate for determining whether administration of the drug increased the incidence of stomach ulcers?

   (A) Analysis of variance (ANOVA)

   (B) Chi-squared ($\chi^2$) test

   (C) Linear regression

   (D) Paired $t$-test

   (E) Pearson correlation coefficient

22. A 29-year-old man reveals to his psychiatrist that he has been hearing voices telling him to kill his girlfriend. Which of the following principles requires that the physician inform the girlfriend that she is in danger?

   (A) Good Samaritan law

   (B) Irresistible Impulse rule

   (C) McNaughten rule

   (D) Tarasoff I decision

   (E) Tarasoff II decision

23. A disgruntled surgical technician who is being treated for depression with phenelzine takes an analgesic he found on the drug cart in the surgical suite. Several hours later, he arrives at the emergency department in a delirious state and has a temperature of 105.0 F. Soon after his arrival, he begins having convulsions. Which of the following analgesics did he most likely take?

    (A) Buprenorphine
    (B) Codeine
    (C) Meperidine
    (D) Pentazocine
    (E) Propoxyphene

24. A child psychiatrist would like to evaluate the intellectual ability of a 3-year-old patient. Which of the following is the most appropriate test for him to use?

    (A) Denver Developmental Scale
    (B) Stanford-Binet Scale
    (C) WAIS-R
    (D) WISC III
    (E) WPPSI

25. The parents of a 7-year-old boy divorce. The boy lives with the mother and sees his father every-other weekend. During these visits, the boy is alternately sullen and angry with the father, but when it is time to return home, he clings to the father and cries in a desperate manner while saying "I'm sorry! I want you and mom to live together again." Which of the following is the most helpful statement that the father can make to the son?

    (A) "Big boys don't cry."
    (B) "I left your mother, I didn't leave you."
    (C) "I'll see you in 2 weeks."
    (D) "You're the man of the house now."
    (E) "Your mother was too hard to live with."

26. At the Academy Awards ceremony, a very successful movie star becomes loud and agitated when she does not win in the category in which she had been nominated. She states to those around her that her performance was superior to that of the winner, that the Academy clearly does not appreciate her genius and acting skills and that there should be a separate category for persons of her extraordinary abilities. She further states that she did not win because the Academy members are envious of her skills. This person most likely has which of the following disorders?

    (A) Antisocial personality disorder
    (B) Histrionic personality disorder
    (C) Narcissistic personality disorder
    (D) Paranoid personality disorder
    (E) Schizophrenia, paranoid type

27. A group of patients with lung cancer is matched to a group of patients without lung cancer. Their smoking habits over the course of their lives is compared. On the basis of this information, researchers compute the rate of lung cancer in patients who smoke versus those who never smoked. This is an example of a

    (A) case-control study
    (B) cohort study
    (C) cross-sectional study
    (D) longitudinal study
    (E) randomized control study

28. A research study investigating the effects of three variables (age, sex, and ethnicity) on the efficacy of a new malaria vaccine reports a significant ($p < 0.001$) analysis of variance (ANOVA) result. There is a significant two-way interaction. Regarding these variables, which of the following is the best interpretation of these results?

    (A) Any of the three variables alone affects the vaccine's efficacy
    (B) The interaction suggests the vaccine has no efficacy
    (C) The three variables all work together to produce the vaccine's efficacy
    (D) The three variables interact together and have no affect on the vaccine's efficacy
    (E) Two of the three variables affect the vaccine's efficacy

29. A 42-year-old man has just been informed that he has poorly differentiated small cell carcinoma of the lung. When asked whether he understands the serious nature of his illness, the patient proceeds to tell his physician how excited he is about renovating his home. Which of the following defense mechanisms is this patient exhibiting?

    (A) denial

    (B) displacement

    (C) projection

    (D) rationalization

    (E) reaction formation

    (F) sublimation

30. A new test is being designed to diagnose cervical *Chlamydia trachomatis* infections. Which of the following epidemiologic parameters would directly affect the positive predictive value of this test?

    (A) Incidence of the disease

    (B) Odds ratio for contracting the disease

    (C) Prevalence of the disease

    (D) Relative risk for contracting the disease

31. A 91-year-old woman with Alzheimer disease is hospitalized because of multiple injuries caused by elder abuse. She has a fractured humerus and a healing burn mark on her forearm. She has ecchymoses in various stages of resolution on her upper arms, buttocks, back, and legs. Which of the following best describes the attributes of the individual who committed this abuse?

    (A) They are concerned caretakers of the abused person

    (B) They expect nothing in return from the abused person

    (C) They have lived with the abused person for a long period of time

    (D) They have no history of being abused

    (E) They occasionally use alcohol/drugs in a recreational manner

32. A 44-year-old man has completed college, has had a good work history, and has never had difficulty with the authorities. However, he has few friends and attends meetings of persons who share telepathic interests and "abilities." When his coworkers attempt to talk to him about these meetings, he is quiet and vague regarding what is done at the meetings and where they are held. His only close associations are with his relatives. He is more likely than the average person to have a relative with a diagnosis of

    (A) anxiety disorder

    (B) bipolar disorder, type II

    (C) factitious disorder

    (D) major depressive disorder

    (E) schizophrenia

33. A 52-year-old white man who had been found wandering the streets is brought into the hospital by police. On initial physical examination, his motor behavior is notable for bradykinesia and a 4- to 6-Hz hand tremor at rest. He is kept under observation in the psychiatric ward but is not medicated. Over the next few days, his motor symptoms start to abate, but he becomes increasingly paranoid and confused and insists that he is the President of the United States. Which of the following conditions best describes the patient at the time of admission?

    (A) Alcoholic experiencing acute symptoms of withdrawal

    (B) Chronic amphetamine user experiencing drug-induced psychosis

    (C) Chronic schizophrenic experiencing tardive dyskinesia

    (D) Parkinsonian patient overmedicated with L-dopa

    (E) Schizophrenic overmedicated with haloperidol

34. A 60-year-old man has had difficulty falling asleep for the past several weeks and asks his physician for advice. The patient has no underlying psychopathology. Which of the following is the most appropriate nonpharmaceutical treatment for this patient?

    (A) Increasing fluid intake during the 3 hours prior to sleep

    (B) Retiring for sleep at the same time each day

    (C) "Sleeping in" if the time of retiring has been delayed

    (D) Staying in bed until sleep is attained

    (E) Strenuous exercise 1 hour before retiring

35. Medical students at a major teaching hospital are routinely assigned to observe obstetric patients and to assist during delivery. When a male medical student introduces himself to an obstetric patient, the patient becomes agitated and requests that no students be present during her delivery. The patient had been informed, prior to admission, that this was a teaching hospital and that a student would be assigned to her case. When informed of the patient's refusal, the attending physician in charge should

    (A) ask the patient's husband for his consent

    (B) assign a female medical student to observe

    (C) do not allow any medical students to observe this patient

    (D) have the patient's nurse seek permission

    (E) have the student approach the patient again and explain the necessity for student observation

    (F) have the student observe in the background as a part of the health care team

    (G) meet with the patient and discuss the value of observation in medical training

36. Eight research scientists are brought into the hospital by paramedics. The scientists are experiencing diaphoresis, blurred vision, palpitations, and hallucinations with brilliant colors. Police suspect that the coffee at their lab meeting was laced with a psychoactive substance. Which of the following substances is most likely to be found in the coffee pot?

    (A) Lysergic acid diethylamide (LSD)

    (B) Methadone

    (C) Phencyclidine (PCP)

    (D) Phenobarbital

    (E) Tetrahydrocannabinol (THC)

37. A patient comes to the physician for a periodic health maintenance examination. The patient has no specific complaints at this time; however, many friends of this patient have recently been diagnosed with HIV, and the patient is very concerned about contracting the disease. The patient reveals his/her sexual orientation and admits to having unprotected sex. The physician reassures the patient that s/he is within the sexually active group with the lowest risk of contracting HIV. Which of the following most likely describes this patient?

    (A) Female heterosexual

    (B) Female homosexual

    (C) Male heterosexual

    (D) Male homosexual

    (E) Male transsexual

38. A 27-year-old, rather plain-appearing woman, fabricates a story that she was raped in the restroom at her child's school. She inflicts wounds on her body with a pair of scissors, gives herself a mild concussion by hitting her head on the sink, and describes the attacker and the episode in great detail when the emergency care persons arrive and take her to the hospital. Later she admits that there was no attack and that she produced the signs and symptoms herself. She states that she did it to get more attention from her husband. If she has a personality disorder, the most likely diagnosis would be

    (A) antisocial personality disorder

    (B) borderline personality disorder

    (C) dependent personality disorder

    (D) histrionic personality disorder

    (E) narcissistic personality disorder

39. A child is in psychotherapy that is financially supported by the parents. Which of the following is the best way to avoid breaching the child's confidentiality while the parents are legally responsible for the child's welfare?

    (A) Give parents information only after they agree not to discuss the information with the child

    (B) Give parents information only if it has been so ordered by the court

    (C) Inform the child that parents have the right to any and all information since they are the responsible party

    (D) Invite the child to attend all parent meetings in which the child is discussed

    (E) Make a blanket rule to hold all information coming from the child as off-limits to the parents

40. A neuropsychologist is studying the effects of drug A and drug B on cognitive performance in Alzheimer patients. He administers a memory test to two groups of subjects (those taking drug A and those taking drug B) and compares their mean scores. Which of the following statistical tests would be most appropriate for this purpose?

    (A) Analysis of variance (ANOVA)

    (B) Chi-squared test

    (C) Fisher exact test

    (D) Multiple linear regression

    (E) Paired $t$-test

    (F) Pearson product-moment correlation formula

    (G) Pittman Welch permutation test

    (H) Simple linear regression

    (I) Spearman rank order formula

    (J) Student $t$-test

41. A second-year medical student falls asleep during a lecture. The instructor observes that the instant the student falls asleep, his eyes make rapid lateral movements under his closed eyelids. Which of the following is the most likely diagnosis?

    (A) Dysthymic disorder

    (B) Major depressive disorder

    (C) Narcolepsy disorder

    (D) Sleep-deprived hypersomnia disorder

    (E) Substance-induced sleep disorder

42. A previously healthy 32-year-old woman comes to the physician for a routine examination. She reports that she has been "very down" and has had trouble sleeping. She has also lost weight, even though she has not been trying to diet. For the last few months, she has been staying home at night and on weekends, despite friends' efforts to take her out. Physical examination and laboratory studies are normal. The physician recommends cognitive therapy. This therapy is based on the theory that her disorder is caused by

    (A) anger toward others that is turned on the self

    (B) distorted negative beliefs and self-talk that reinforces those beliefs

    (C) fluctuating neurotransmitter levels

    (D) genetic predisposition

    (E) significant object loss in the first 3 years of life

43. In a study, a group of people are exposed to an environmental toxin but are not treated. Instead, they are observed over time on a standard set of measures to ascertain the potential effects of the toxin. This type of study design is called

    (A) Clinical trial

    (B) Double-blind

    (C) Longitudinal

    (D) Prospective

    (E) Retrospective

44. A man is distraught because he has to sell his car and move from his house to a one-room apartment. He no longer has extra spending money, and he has difficulty covering his weekly grocery bills. He cannot afford to eat out in restaurants and has been unable to buy new clothes in years. He used to have enough money to cover all of these expenses. Which of the following is the most likely reason for this "downward move" in socioeconomic status?

    (A) Disabling physical problems

    (B) Disabling psychiatric problems

    (C) Inability to defer gratification

    (D) Lack of education

    (E) Unwillingness to work

45. A husband comes to the family physician to discuss his wife's sleep behavior. During the past 2 months, she has been kicking and hitting him in her sleep. She does not remember these occurrences the next morning or if he wakens her in the night. He is concerned that she has developed some anger toward him, which she is unwilling or unable to discuss. Which of the following is the most likely diagnosis?

    (A) Narcolepsy

    (B) Night terrors

    (C) Non-REM sleep disorder

    (D) Rapid eye movement (REM) sleep disorder

    (E) Sleep apnea disorder

46. A 60-year-old man hospitalized with metastatic colon cancer signs a DNR order. This means that the medical staff treating him is required to

    (A) discontinue narcotic pain medication

    (B) not attempt CPR in case of cardiac arrest

    (C) refrain from prescribing future medications

    (D) withhold parenteral nutrition and IV fluid hydration

47. A patient comes to the physician because of sexual dysfunction. After a thorough evaluation and a trial of conservative therapy, the patient is scheduled for surgery. Which of the following is the most likely cause of this patient's sexual dysfunction?

    (A) Dyspareunia

    (B) Premature ejaculation

    (C) Primary impotence

    (D) Secondary orgasmic dysfunction in females

    (E) Vaginismus

48. A group of researchers mistakenly concludes from a poorly designed experiment that acetaminophen cures the common cold. These researchers have committed which of the following types of error?

    (A) 1-β

    (B) Alpha

    (C) Beta

    (D) Type 1

    (E) Type 2

49. A girl is brought to the pediatrician for a well-child visit. The mother reports no problems with her daughter. Physical examination is unremarkable, and the child is up to date on her immunizations. Further evaluation reveals that the girl understands that the volume of a liquid poured out of a narrow glass remains the same when poured into a wider glass. This child is at which of Piaget's stages of intellectual development?

    (A) Concrete operations

    (B) Formal operations

    (C) Preoperational

    (D) Sensorimotor

50. In a restaurant, the parents of a 4-year-old child are talking with each other and not with the child. The child first says "Mommy"; when the mother does not respond, the intensity of the word "Mommy" increases. The child then begins to drop her eating utensils. When the parents still do not respond, the child knocks over her glass of milk. The parents then scold the child and busy themselves cleaning up the spilled milk and getting more for the child. This scenario is repeated three times before the parents angrily take the child from the restaurant. This entire scene is an example of which of the following types of learning?

    (A) Classical conditioning

    (B) Cognitive learning

    (C) Imprinting

    (D) Operant conditioning

    (E) Social learning

# Behavioral Science and Biostatistics Test One:
## Answers and Explanations

## ANSWER KEY

| | | | |
|---|---|---|---|
| 1. | B | 26. | C |
| 2. | D | 27. | A |
| 3. | B | 28. | E |
| 4. | E | 29. | A |
| 5. | C | 30. | C |
| 6. | C | 31. | C |
| 7. | B | 32. | E |
| 8. | B | 33. | E |
| 9. | B | 34. | B |
| 10. | B | 35. | C |
| 11. | D | 36. | A |
| 12. | A | 37. | B |
| 13. | D | 38. | B |
| 14. | E | 39. | D |
| 15. | D | 40. | J |
| 16. | B | 41. | C |
| 17. | C | 42. | B |
| 18. | A | 43. | C |
| 19. | A | 44. | A |
| 20. | E | 45. | D |
| 21. | B | 46. | B |
| 22. | D | 47. | A |
| 23. | C | 48. | D |
| 24. | B | 49. | A |
| 25. | B | 50. | D |

1.  **The correct answer is B.** The antipsychotic drug clozapine has been shown to cause agranulocytosis, an acute condition characterized by profound leukopenia, with marked reduction in polymorphonuclear leukocytes ($<500$ cells/mm$^3$). Infected ulcers are likely to form in the throat, intestinal tract, and other mucous membranes, as well as on the skin. Other side effects caused by clozapine include orthostatic hypotension, sinus tachycardia, hypersalivation, temperature elevation, lowered seizure threshold, and constipation. Clozapine is generally prescribed only after several other alternative neuroleptic medications have failed, because of the possibility of agranulocytosis and the drug's prohibitive cost.

    Chlorpromazine (**choice A**) is an antipsychotic drug that has antimuscarinic side effects, such as dry mouth and constipation. It can also cause orthostatic hypotension, sedation, and tardive dyskinesia. It does not cause agranulocytosis.

    Fluoxetine (**choice C**) is a selective serotonin reuptake inhibitor (SSRI), an antidepressant drug that can cause anxiety and insomnia, altered appetite and weight loss, activation of mania or hypomania, seizures, and cognitive motor impairment.

    Haloperidol (**choice D**) is an antipsychotic drug that has less antimuscarinic side effects than does chlorpromazine, but has more extrapyramidal effects, such as acute dystonia (face, neck, and back spasms, and abnormal posture), parkinsonism, neuroleptic malignant syndrome (catatonia, rigidity, stupor, fever, dysarthria, fluctuating BP), and akathisia (restlessness). It can also cause tardive dyskinesia. It does not cause agranulocytosis.

    Imipramine (**choice E**) is a tricyclic antidepressant drug that can cause orthostatic hypotension, anticholinergic effects, antihistamine effects, and hypomania. It does not cause agranulocytosis.

    Phenelzine (**choice F**) is a MAO inhibitor that can cause orthostatic hypotension (once the body adapts to higher basal levels of catecholamines, it is no longer able to further vasoconstrict in response to stress), hepatotoxicity, and hypomania. It does not cause agranulocytosis. Remember, there is a risk of developing a hypertensive crisis when an individual taking an MAO inhibitor consumes tyramine-containing foods, such as wine and aged cheeses.

2.  **The correct answer is D.** Retrograde amnesia is characterized by an inability to remember events prior to the onset of disease, with preservation of the ability to form new memories.

    Anterograde amnesia (**choice A**) is characterized by an inability to register and form lasting memories of new or present events.

    Proactive inhibition (**choice B**) is when something newly learned interferes with previously learned information. New material inhibits old material.

    Retroactive inhibition (**choice C**) is when previously learned material interferes with the ability to acquire new information. Old material inhibits new material.

    Transient global amnesia (**choice E**) is characterized by confusion and impairment of recent memory. It often occurs in elderly people and resolves without sequelae.

3.  **The correct answer is B.** This is a case of child abuse of the neglect type. The family fits the pattern of social isolation often found in child abuse. The boy's sleepiness in class suggests lack of appropriate rest at home, often caused by turmoil in the home or unsupervised late night activity, or lack of appropriate nutrition in the morning.

    Antisocial personality disorder (**choice A**) is not correct because a person must be 18 years of age to be so classified.

    Mental retardation (**choice C**) is not correct because this boy is advancing appropriately in school. He is 9 years old and in the fourth grade.

    Oppositional defiant disorder (**choice D**) is not correct since these children usually act out in a defiant and rebellious manner to authority figures.

    Thyroid dysfunction (**choice E**) is not correct because these conditions usually produce agitated behavior of some type along with cognitive-emotional dysfunction, regardless of whether there is hypo- or hyperthyroidism.

4.  **The correct answer is E.** The prevalence of a disease is defined as the number of cases of the disease at a given time divided by the total population. In this case, it would be 10,000/250,000.

    The disease-specific mortality rate is the number of deaths per year from a specific disease divided by the population; in this case, 400/250,000 (**choice A**).

    The rate of increase of a disease is given by the number of new cases per year, minus the number of deaths (or cures) per year, divided by the total population. In this case, $(1000 - 400)/250,000 = 600/250,000$ (**choice B**).

    The incidence of a disease is given by the number of new cases in a given period divided by the total population. This gives 1000/250,000 (**choice C**).

    The crude mortality rate is given by the number of deaths from all causes, divided by the population; in this case, 2500/250,000 (**choice D**).

5. **The correct answer is C.** Psychogenic fugue is one of the class of dissociative disorders and is defined by the combination of amnesia plus travel. The patient typically regains awareness after traveling to a different locale but retains no memory of the trip on the decision to embark on it. When they emerge from the fugue state, the patient is often confused and may be scared.

   In delirium (**choice A**), the patient passes in and out of conscious awareness of his surroundings over a period of days or weeks. Onset is generally acute and rapid, orientation to time and place may be impaired, recent memories will contain gaps, and attention span will be very short. The sleep-wake cycle is disrupted, and alterations of consciousness can be accompanied by visual hallucinations.

   Dementia (**choice B**) is a chronic condition with a generally insidious onset lasting months or years. The level of consciousness remains normal, but the person may be disoriented in terms of time, place, and person. Extended travel would be difficult for the patient suffering from dementia. Note that most dementias are not reversible.

   Somnambulism (**choice D**) or "sleep walking" is a disorder of Stage 4 sleep. The sleeping individual may become ambulatory and even speak but appears disconnected to the world around him or her. When woken, the patient displays the same confusion and disorientation displayed by most people when roused from a deep sleep. Somnambulism episodes usually last for less than an hour.

   In stupor (**choice E**), alcohol or drugs degrades the person's mental and physical abilities and may foreshadow a complete loss of consciousness. The stuporous individual evidences a pronounced decrease in movements and increased impulsive behavior. Someone in a stupor lacks the mental and physical capacity to complete the sort of travel suggested in this question.

6. **The correct answer is C.** Do not confuse transvestic fetishism with transsexualism (**choice B**). Transsexuals might cross-dress, but they do so because of persistent discomfort with their anatomic sex. Transvestic fetishism involves no such discomfort.

   Exhibitionism (**choice A**) refers to exposing one's genitals to unsuspecting strangers for sexual excitement.

   Voyeurism (**choice D**) refers to observing unsuspecting people, generally strangers, who are naked, undressing, or engaged in sexual activity, for sexual excitement.

7. **The correct answer is B.** In any normal distribution, the mean is conventionally used to represent central tendency. Recall that in a normal distribution, the mean (arithmetic average), median (the most common score), and mode (the most common score) are all the same value. This means that the distribution described in this question is not normal, but negatively skewed. We can tell that the distribution is negatively skewed because the mean is less than the median (mean < median). Because the mean (**choice A**) is overly sensitive to extreme values, in a skewed distribution the median is a better representation of central tendency than the mean.

   The mode (**choice C**) is generally only used to represent central tendency when the distribution is excessively skewed, such as when close to 50% of the students received the same score.

   The standard deviation (**choice D**) provided an assessment of variation or spread of the distribution and is of no help in defining central tendency.

   The variance (**choice E**) is computed by taking the square of the standard deviation. Like the standard deviation, it is a measure of variation, not central tendency.

8. **The correct answer is B.** The disorganized type of schizophrenia is characterized by disorganized speech, disorganized behavior, and an inappropriate affect. This patient's rambling speech, inappropriate giggling, and purposeful behavior illustrate these issues.

   Catatonic schizophrenia (**choice A**) is characterized by movement disorders, peculiarities like posturing or stereotyped behaviors, and echolalia.

   Paranoid schizophrenia (**choice C**) is characterized by manifest delusions and hallucinations involving persecution or grandeur.

   Residual schizophrenia (**choice D**) is diagnosed when there is a clear schizophrenic problem; however there are no prominent delusions or hallucinations, and the person's behavior and speech are not disorganized (as seen in this patient).

   Undifferentiated schizophrenia (**choice E**) has characteristics of all the above types; however, they are too fluid to place into a specific diagnostic category.

9. **The correct answer is B.** Diverting the child's attention with such things as talk, games, television, and virtual reality is a very effective mechanism for pain control.

   Allowing parents to be present (**choice A**) will often only intensify the child's reaction because parents might display their own fears and concerns.

   Encouraging the child to vent his emotions (**choice C**) can be of some assistance. However, because of the child's limited cognitive structures, this is not a recommended procedure.

The young child does not yet have the cognitive structures to control pain mentally; therefore, neither explaining sensory pathways (**choice D**) nor having the child focus on and examine pain sensations (**choice E**) will be effective.

10. **The correct answer is B.** A serious side effect of the antipsychotics is tardive dyskinesia, which has been seen with virtually every neuroleptic (e.g., chlorpromazine [**choice A**], fluphenazine [**choice C**], haloperidol [**choice D**], and thioridazine [**choice F**]). Usually, the symptoms of tardive dyskinesia appear late in treatment and consist of involuntary, repetitive movements of the lips, tongue (e.g., tongue thrusting, lip smacking), and, not infrequently, the extremities and trunk. Patients older than 60 and those with pre-existing CNS pathology are at a higher risk for this disorder (up to 70%), but other risk factors have not been confirmed. Clozapine is called an atypical antipsychotic medication because of its lack of extrapyramidal side effects, including tardive dyskinesia, and would be an appropriate medication for a patient who is developing tardive dyskinesia. Metoclopramide (**choice E**) is a centrally acting antiemetic that has been shown to cause tardive dyskinesia as well.

11. **The correct answer is D.** Abusive husbands usually use the abuse to bully and humiliate their wives in order to build up their own self-esteem. They often view their behavior as an attempt to communicate.

    Being the first-born child (**choice A**) is incorrect because there has never been a birth-order effect established in spousal abuse.

    Concern about financial security (**choice B**) is incorrect because spousal abuse occurs in all socioeconomic groups, and fiscal concerns have not been demonstrated to be etiologic.

    A dislike of children (**choice C**) is incorrect because it is the spouse who is being abused, not a child. Disliking children would be more likely to result in some permanent form of birth control.

    Wanting out of the marriage (**choice E**) is incorrect because the abuse itself is an attempt to pull the spouse closer and control her, not to separate from the spouse and give her freedom.

12. **The correct answer is A.** This is a typical description of histrionic personality disorder. Clues are seductive behavior, exaggerated charm, need for attention, overdramatized emotions, shallowness of feelings, and craving control.

Narcissistic personality disorder (**choice B**) is characterized by the word "entitlement." These individuals have a grandiose but unstable sense of self-importance that often alternates with feelings of unworthiness.

Paranoid personality disorder (**choice C**) is characterized by suspiciousness, excessive vigilance toward the environment, mistrust of others, and a concern with hidden meanings or motivations.

Passive-aggressive personality disorder (**choice D**) is associated with difficulties in assertiveness and the appropriate expression of anger. People with this disorder may act out their anger indirectly, presenting a resistant stance in situations involving social or occupational functioning.

People with schizotypal personality disorder (**choice E**) are emotionally cold and aloof like schizoids, but display magical thinking as well (e.g., beliefs that others can sense their thoughts or feelings). They may have ideas of reference, recurrent perceptual illusions, depersonalization, or suspiciousness.

13. **The correct answer is D.** If you understand the thought process behind these stages, you are unlikely to forget the progression. Patients first experience denial that they are dying. Once aware, they become angry at their lot and proceed to "bargain" for a more favorable outcome. When this proves futile, they become depressed. Then, they finally accept the truth. The mnemonic is DABSA.

14. **The correct answer E.** This patient has male erectile disorder, psychogenic. It is defined by the DSM IV as the persistent inability to attain or maintain adequate erection for completion of sexual activity. It causes distress and interpersonal difficulties. The disorder may be due to psychologic factors if it occurs only with specific partners or during certain situations. This patient's dysfunction occurs only with his wife, implying no physiologic etiology to his problem.

    An adjustment disorder (**choice A**) requires there be a stressor as the etiologic factor; no such event is noted in the history.

    Since the patient can attain an erection and is emotionally distressed by the situation with his wife, he does not have hypoactive sexual desire disorder (**choice B**).

    There is no mention of orgasmic problems, and erection is not necessary for orgasm. Therefore, inhibited male orgasm, psychogenic (**choice C**) is unlikely.

    There is nothing in the history to suggest a homosexual orientation; therefore, latent ego-dystonic homosexuality (**choice D**) is not the best diagnosis.

15. **The correct answer is D.** In cases in which an emergency exists, the patient is incompetent to give consent, and the withholding of treatment would be potentially life-threatening, the physician must obtain consent from a close relative of the patient. The physician should proceed with treatment, assuming the patient would concur had he or she understood the situation.

Not performing surgery (**choice A**) could cost the patient's life.

Having another physician confirm the necessity of surgery (**choice B**) is favorable (if done immediately) but not mandatory and does not change the patient's consent status.

Obtaining a court order (**choice C**) is not necessary with the patient's wife immediately accessible.

Trying to persuade the patient to consent to surgery (**choice E**) would not only waste time and prove futile but might agitate the patient as well.

16. **The correct answer is B.** This man is basically homosexual; however, his homosexuality causes him to experience feelings of guilt if he participates in homosexual physical activity (therefore, his homosexuality is ego-dystonic, rather than ego-syntonic, **choice D**).

The man does not have a gender identity disorder (syntonic, **choice C** or dystonic, **choice A**) because he does not have a female gender identity and has not described any feelings of abhorrence regarding his genitalia.

He does not have a paraphilia (**choice E**), which is the general term for a diagnosable sexual disorder in which the person conceals the behaviors from others, the behaviors exclude or harm others, and the behaviors disrupt the potential for bonding between persons.

17. **The correct answer is C.** Reactive attachment disorder of infancy is caused by severe interruption in the parent-child bond, with the parent being unable to supply the nurturing needed for adequate development of the infant. The description of this child is classic, and unless the underlying pathologic bonding process is addressed, the child may die. Sometimes this syndrome is seen in children who have had multiple care takers (e.g., orphanages and foster homes) or, as in the case described here, a young, immature, and inadequate mother (and/or father).

This is not autistic disorder (**choice A**) because the child visually tracks the pediatrician. Children with autistic disorder do not interact socially with others.

In Möbius syndrome (**choice B**), or congenital facial diplegia, the face is expressionless, and ocular palsy may be present. Frequently, this is accompanied by clubfoot and syndactyly, and patients may be mentally retarded. None of these symptoms are described in this patient.

Rett syndrome (**choice D**) is characterized by normal development in the first 6 months of life followed by a precipitous deterioration. This child's development has never been normal.

Tay-Sachs disease (**choice E**) is an autosomal-recessive inborn error of metabolism that results in mental retardation, macular changes, seizures, and spasticity. None of these are described in this child.

18. **The correct answer A.** Dysthymic disorder is the most likely diagnosis. The patient is severely depressed by his own assessment; however, it is not of psychotic proportion. The patient has recognized the severity of his symptoms and taken appropriate action by going to the doctor. He has also indicated that this is not a new event for him (supporting the diagnosis of dysthymic disorder, which tends to be chronic, lasting longer than 2 years). Note that dysthymic patients tend to cry a lot, explaining this patient's red eyes.

Major depressive disorders (**choice B**) are characterized by depressed mood, diminished interest in activities, weight loss without change in diet or exercise, sleep disturbances, fatigue, feelings of worthlessness, decreased ability to concentrate, and thoughts about death. This patient does not report such concrete symptoms and therefore does not qualify for the diagnosis of major depressive disorder.

Organic affective syndrome (**choice C**) and uncomplicated bereavement (**choice E**) require trigger etiologies that are not implied in this case.

There is no thought disorder or other psychotic symptoms, ruling out the diagnosis of schizoaffective disorder (**choice D**).

19. **The correct answer is A.** The natural order in which one comes to expect losses (through social learning) is chronologic. That is, grandparents (**choice B**) die first, parents (**choice C**) die next, then siblings and spouses, and finally one's children. When this natural order is inverted, there is a much more severe and protracted grief reaction than for the loss of an older relative.

20. **The correct answer is E.** Pseudodementia is more appropriately described as major depression in an elderly person. She has all the symptoms of depressive disorder (sleep difficulties, appetite and weight problems, concentration problems, lack of interest in pleasurable activities) but none of the hallmarks of an organic condition.

Delirium (**choice A**) is associated with fluctuation of consciousness. This patient's memory problems are mild and confined to immediate memory difficulties. If she were demented, she would demonstrate more recent and long-term memory problems.

**KAPLAN) MEDICAL**

Alzheimer disease (**choice B**) is associated with more recent and long-term memory impairment.

Hypothyroidism (**choice C**) is associated with wider mood swings, from depressive affect to manic-like episodes, as well as with more indices of psychotic level disturbance (e.g., hallucinations and paranoia).

Normal pressure hydrocephalus (**choice D**) is associated with depressive symptomatology; however, it is also characterized by the diagnostic triad of progressive dementia, gait disturbance, and urinary incontinence, none of which is present in this woman.

21. **The correct answer is B.** The most commonly used method for calculating p values from a two-by-two contingency table is the chi-squared test. This test is used for frequency data (such as those above) rather than for comparison of means. Since the investigator scored the stomachs as either containing ulcers or not containing ulcers, without attempting to quantify the number of ulcers, the data represent frequencies rather than means. Chi-squared is calculated as the sum for all cells of (Observed − Expected)$^2$/Expected. The p value for this value of chi-squared is obtained from a table using degrees of freedom equal to (number of rows − 1) × (number of columns − 1).

ANOVA (**choice A**) is used to determine whether the difference between two or more groups is significantly different. This method is not applicable to raw frequency data.

Linear regression (**choice C**) is the process of fitting a straight line to a set of correlational data points by minimizing the sum of squares of the vertical distances from the points to the line. This method would not be suitable for the above data.

A paired *t*-test (**choice D**) is used to compare the means of two groups. It is not used to compare raw frequency data.

Correlation is used when two variables are simultaneously measured in a sample. The Pearson correlation coefficient (**choice E**) is used when both the independent and dependent variables are continuous. In this case, the independent variable is not continuous (since the drug is either given or not given), and the dependent variable is also not continuous (the ulcers are either present or absent).

22. **The correct answer is D.** The Tarasoff I decision requires that physicians warn a potential victim if they truly believe the patient will cause harm to that person. The Tarasoff II decision (**choice E**) states that even though physicians must warn a potential victim, they must also protect the patient from harm from that person.

The Good Samaritan law (**choice A**) states that stopping at the scene of an accident to render care is not required but that once physicians initiate such care they must practice within their confidence and may not abandon the patient.

The Irresistible Impulse rule (**choice B**) is involved in insanity defenses in criminal prosecution. It considers whether a person's actions were under voluntary control or resulted from an uncontrollable passion.

The McNaughten rule (**choice C**) is also involved in insanity defenses. It acknowledges that people may not realize the nature and consequences of their actions because of mental illness.

23. **The correct answer is C.** The combination of an MAO inhibitor (such as phenelzine) and meperidine produces a severe drug reaction. Many types of reactions have been reported, including delirium, hyperpyrexia, convulsions, and hypertension. Other patients react as if they have had an overdose of meperidine and present with severe respiratory depression, cyanosis, hypotension, and coma. Meperidine is contraindicated in patients who have taken MAO inhibitors during the previous 14 days.

Interactions with MAO inhibitors and other opioid analgesics, such as buprenorphine (**choice A**), codeine (**choice B**), pentazocine (**choice D**), and propoxyphene (**choice E**), have not been observed.

24. **The correct answer is B.** The Stanford-Binet scale is best for younger children (aged 2-4 years), since it does not rely exclusively on language.

The Denver Developmental Scale (**choice A**) is used to assess the attainment of developmental milestones in children younger than 2 years.

The WAIS-R (Wechsler Adult Intelligence Scale; **choice C**) is used for individuals aged 17 and older. (Just think, the WAIS-R is rated "R").

The WISC III (Wechsler Intelligence Scale for Children; **choice D**) is useful for evaluating children aged 6 to 16 years.

The WPPSI (Wechsler Preschool and Primary Scale of Intelligence; **choice E**) is used for children aged 4 to 6 years.

25. **The correct answer is B.** This statement from the father would reflect his understanding of the egocentric nature of school-aged children. That is, the child is assuming that he is responsible for the divorce between his parents. The anger and withdrawal reflect the child's frustration with the situation, but the tears and apology suggest the child's fear and assumed responsibility for the breakup.

"Big boys don't cry" (**choice A**) is a demeaning and belittling statement.

"I'll see you in 2 weeks" (**choice C**) ignores the child's felt responsibility for the divorce.

"You're the man of the house now" (**choice D**) places too much responsibility on a 7-year-old child.

"Your mother was too hard to live with" (**choice E**) places all the blame and responsibility for the divorce on the parent with whom the boy lives on a daily basis. It ignores the reality that divorce is usually due to difficulties that both parents have with each other.

26. **The correct answer is C.** In narcissistic personality disorder, the person feels "entitled" to recognition, admiration, and privileges. In addition, they often believe they are so special that others are envious of their talents. They do not tolerate perceived rejection well.

    People with antisocial personality disorder (**choice A**) commit behaviors that are against societal rules. They commit criminal offenses against others and property.

    People with histrionic personality disorder (**choice B**) are overly dramatic and exhibit seductive behavior.

    People with paranoid personality disorder (**choice D**) believe others are out to harm them. They tend to be secretive in their thoughts, fearing that others will use information against them, and they are concerned with fidelity in intimate relations with others. Although this patient displays thoughts of envy from others, this is secondary to the non-recognition of her "specialness" rather than a malevolent intent.

    There is no evidence of a psychotic level thought disorder such as schizophrenia (**choice E**); there are no hallucinations or disorganized emotions or behaviors.

27. **The correct answer is A.** Case-control studies are retrospective and are as described in the question stem. Case-control studies allow researchers to compute an odds ratio.

    In cohort studies (**choice B**), subjects are assembled on the basis of some common experience (such as attending medical school) and are then monitored for a specified amount of time at regular intervals (e.g., taking USMLE Steps 1, 2, and 3; see also longitudinal studies below), until they develop the outcome of interest (they become practicing physicians) or the followup time ends. The cohort study minimizes many of the biases evident in case-control designs and is the definitive observational clinical study. Cohort studies allow researchers to compute a relative risk.

    Cross-sectional studies (**choice C**) usually have more modest goals than those of case-control and cohort studies. A variable or group of variables is measured in a sample of a larger population to get an idea of the distribution and interrelationships of those variables in that population.

    Longitudinal studies (**choice D**) identify individual subjects and follow them over a given period of time. For example, the study of cholesterol-lowering drugs on cardiovascular events requires that the same subject is observed over a significant period of time (e.g., 10 years).

    A randomized controlled trial (**choice E**) is considered the most rigorous and powerful approach to answering a clinical question in which two treatments, strategies, or therapies are compared or when one therapy is compared with placebo. In this type of study, subjects are assigned treatments on a randomized basis.

28. **The correct answer is E.** The term "two-way interaction" indicates that two of the three variables in the study affect the efficacy of the vaccine. For example, persons of a given sex and age group benefit the most from the vaccine, regardless of ethnic group.

    A one-way interaction (**choice A**) indicates that any of the three variables in isolation can affect the vaccine's efficacy.

    The vaccine has efficacy (compare with **choice B**), as evidenced by the positive results ($p < 0.001$) in the study.

    A three-way interaction (**choice C**) indicates that only people of a given ethnic group, age, and sex benefit from the vaccine.

    The three variables would have no effect on the efficacy (**choice D**) only if there were no interaction effect at all.

29. **The correct answer is A.** This patient is in denial about his serious illness. By talking about something totally unrelated, he is trying to avoid the bad news he has just received.

    Displacement (**choice B**) involves the transferring of feelings to an inappropriate person, situation, or object (e.g., a man who has been yelled at by his boss takes out his anger on his wife).

    Projection (**choice C**) is the attribution of one's own traits to someone else (e.g., a philandering husband accuses his wife of having an affair).

    Rationalization (**choice D**) involves creating explanations for an action or thought, usually to avoid self-blame.

    Reaction formation (**choice E**) is the unconscious changing of a feeling or idea to its opposite (e.g., a man acts very friendly toward a coworker when in fact he is unconsciously jealous).

    Sublimation (**choice F**) involves turning an unacceptable impulse into an acceptable one (e.g., someone with very aggressive impulses becomes a professional boxer).

30. **The correct answer is C.** Of the choices listed, only prevalence, the total number of cases of a disease in a given period of time, directly affects the positive predictive value of a test (which equals true positives/all positives).

    Incidence (**choice A**) is the number of new cases of a disease in a given period of time.

    The odds ratio (**choice B**), which may be calculated from case-control studies, approximates relative risk.

    Relative risk (**choice D**) can reflect the incidence of a disease in a treated group divided by the incidence of a disease in a placebo group.

31. **The correct answer is C.** Persons who abuse elderly people usually have lived with the elderly person for some time. There has been opportunity for idiosyncratic behavior on the part of the elderly person to create resentment in the caretaker. Elder abuse is usually not the expression of a momentary impulse; rather, it develops over some time.

    Abusers tend to want their needs to be met by the abused person (unlike **choice B**), have a history of having been abused themselves (the opposite of **choice D**), are unwilling caretakers (often fiscal conditions necessitate the living arrangement; the opposite of **choice A**), and usually abuse drugs, not just use them occasionally (**choice E**).

32. **The correct answer is E.** The description of this man is consistent with the diagnosis of schizotypal personality disorder. Persons with this condition have a higher incidence of schizophrenia among their biologic relatives. There is also a higher incidence of the disorder in monozygotic vs. dizygotic twins, suggesting an underlying biologic foundation in which there is significant impairment in the social interaction skills.

    No such correlation exists between schizotypal personality disorder and anxiety disorder (**choice A**), bipolar disorder, type II (**choice B**), factitious disorder (**choice C**), or major depressive disorder (**choice D**).

33. **The correct answer is E.** The patient is a schizophrenic overmedicated with haloperidol. When the patient was first brought into the hospital, he was experiencing parkinsonian motor symptoms that are a significant side effect of many neuroleptics (particularly haloperidol). Over the next few days, he remained unmedicated, and the effects of haloperidol began to wear off, which relieved his motor symptoms but led to the reappearance of his psychotic symptoms.

    Although alcohol withdrawal (**choice A**) can produce delirium tremens, it would not explain the initial presentation with parkinsonian symptoms.

    Chronic amphetamine use (**choice B**) can result in an amphetamine-induced psychosis that resembles an acute schizophrenic attack. However, these attacks abate within a few days after drug use ceases. This patient's psychosis surfaced after a few days without medication.

    Chronic schizophrenics (**choice C**) with an extensive history of neuroleptic use can develop tardive dyskinesia, which is characterized by involuntary jaw and tongue movements.

    A parkinsonian patient overmedicated with L-dopa (**choice D**) may have visual and auditory hallucinations, as well as involuntary movements. These symptoms are the result of increased activity in the dopamine system and would be expected to abate after several days without treatment. Parkinsonian motor symptoms suppressed by L-dopa would be expected to reemerge as the drug is cleared from the system.

34. **The correct answer is B.** In the treatment of "normal" insomnia (the patient has no underlying psychopathology), it is important to establish a routine that does not vary. Therefore, the person should retire and rise at the same time each day.

    While some may think that increasing fluid intake (**choice A**) will assist sleep by precluding awakening from thirst, it actually encourages sleep interruption by pressure from a full bladder.

    One should not sleep in (**choice C**), since it disrupts the routine.

    Since it is important not to classically condition the bed to wakefulness, if one does not fall asleep within 20 minutes, one should arise and perform a nonstimulating activity, such as reading a book, rather than staying in bed until sleep is attained (**choice D**).

    Strenuous exercise before retiring (**choice E**) does not "wear the person out." Instead, it stimulates the autonomic nervous system and drives wakefulness. Exercise should not be done during the 2 to 3 hours before sleep.

35. **The correct answer is C.** The patient has the right to decide who will or will not be present during her care. This includes the right to refuse to be a part of a student's educational experience. The desires of the patient, not the physician or training facility, come first. If the patient does not want a medical student present during the delivery, respect the patient's wishes.

    **Choice A** is incorrect because the patient's consent, not her husband's, is required. The husband cannot give consent for an alert, competent patient.

    **Choice B** is incorrect because the patient is not rejecting male students, but all students.

    **Choice D** is incorrect because the patient has already refused. Sending the nurse to get permission suggests that the physician is not respecting her expressed wishes.

**Choice E** is incorrect because the patient has already refused. Having the student go back and ask again will only make the student uncomfortable and may make the patient angry.

**Choice F** is incorrect because sneaking the student in to observe in the background is a direct contradiction of the patient's wishes.

**Choice G** is incorrect because meeting with the patient to discuss the value of teaching encounters suggests putting pressure on the patient to change her mind. The purpose of the medical encounter is to seek the greatest benefit for the patient, not seek the best educational experience for the student. The patient's wishes predominate here.

36. **The correct answer is A.** These eight researchers are probably under the influence of LSD, which causes hallucinations notable for their brilliant colors. LSD also shows activity at serotonin receptors and can activate the sympathetic nervous system, resulting in symptoms such as diaphoresis, blurred vision (due to pupil dilation), and palpitations.

Methadone (**choice B**) is a synthetic opiate used to treat heroin addiction. It has analgesic properties but does not ordinarily induce hallucinations.

PCP (**choice C**) can cause hallucinations marked by alterations of body image and distortions of space and time. PCP can also cause a dissociative anesthesia and analgesia. Common side effects of PCP use include hypersalivation, muscular rigidity, hypertension, and nystagmus. Highly colored visual hallucinations are not as commonly seen with PCP intoxication as with LSD intoxication.

Phenobarbital (**choice D**) is a long-acting barbiturate that acts as a CNS depressant. It is used in the long-term management of seizure disorders.

THC (**choice E**) is found in marijuana and produces a euphoric high followed by subsequent relaxation and sleepiness. Marijuana use can result in visual hallucinations, delusions, and a toxic psychosis, but generally only at extremely high doses.

37. **The correct answer is B.** The key to this question rests on the basic fact that HIV transmission occurs through the exchange of bodily fluids. Lesbian sexual activity mainly involves oral and digital contact and body friction. The likelihood of contaminated bodily fluid transmission is minimal with these practices.

Female heterosexual transmission (**choice A**) is very high, as is male homosexual (**choice D**) and male transsexual (**choice E**) transmission, because transference of seminal fluid during receptive intercourse is common.

Male heterosexuals (**choice C**) have the second lowest risk of acquiring HIV since they are not routinely exposed to contaminated fluids for an extended period of time after intercourse.

38. **The correct answer is B.** The lives of persons with borderline personality disorder are filled with very unstable interpersonal relations. They usually demand a great deal of attention and care from others. They frequently mutilate themselves, with the motivation being to elicit caring and closer relations with the other persons in their lives.

Individuals with antisocial personality disorder (**choice A**) tend to hurt others, not themselves, and they do not have interest in closer relations with anyone.

People with dependent personality disorder (**choice C**) characteristically subjugate themselves to others in order to get their dependency needs met. They would not report an attack; rather, they would try to cling to the attacker.

The central feature of histrionic personality disorder (**choice D**) is a flamboyant, overly dramatic presentation of everything, including physical appearance. However, these individuals tend to not sexualize actual physical relations. They are seductive everywhere except the bedroom.

The central issue in narcissistic personality disorder (**choice E**) is "entitlement" and self-importance. These individuals would not mutilate themselves, because they perceive themselves as too important to self-inflict bodily injury.

39. **The correct answer is D.** This is a difficult situation since the parents do have a legal responsibility for the child, and the child needs to trust the therapist to respect his or her innermost thoughts and feelings. Generally the parents know most of the child's behaviors and worries; however, they may not know the child's extensive and deep rooted concerns. The best way to approach this is to invite the child to attend all parent meetings in which the child is discussed. Given this scenario, the parents are unlikely to request extremely personal data, and the child can build a trust in the therapist to not violate intimate details.

**Choice A** aligns the therapist in a conspiracy of silence with the parents and is not recommended.

**Choice B** is not recommended because it sets up a comparable but opposite scenario as **choice A**. That is, it aligns the therapist with the child against the parents.

**Choice C** will reliably result in the child withholding sensitive information with which he or she is struggling.

**Choice E** can place the therapist in an untenable position if the child is self-destructive and needs parental intervention. Remember, only parents and courts can legally detain a child; a physician cannot. This choice also works against the therapist-patient-parent alliance, which is necessary for good outcomes in psychotherapy with a child.

40. **The correct answer is J.** The Student *t*-test is used to compare two means derived from two samples.

    Analysis of variance (ANOVA; **choice A**) is used when the means of a continuous variable are being compared in three or more groups or when the independent variable responsible for a difference in means is being sought.

    The chi-squared test (**choice B**) is commonly used to compare noncontinuous data in two groups.

    The Fisher exact test (**choice C**) and the Pittman Welch permutation test (**choice G**) consider all possible permutations of the data and compare them with the values actually observed.

    Multiple linear regression (**choice D**) is used to consider the impact of more than one independent variable on the dependent variable.

    The paired *t*-test (**choice E**) is typically used when an observation is made twice on a sample.

    The Pearson product-moment correlation formula (**choice F**) can be used for ranked data that have no intrinsic numeric value, where the ranking system represents equal intervals between measurement units.

    Simple linear regression (**choice H**) is a process by which the data collected are fitted to the best straight line.

    The Spearman rank order formula (**choice I**) produces a correlation coefficient—a numeric way of describing the direction and strength of the linear relationship between two variables. This particular formula is used for data that are continuous and based on ranking.

41. **The correct answer is C.** Narcolepsy is defined as recurrent intrusions of elements of rapid eye movement (REM) sleep into the transition between sleep and wakefulness.

    Although affective disorders (**choices A and B**) are associated with sleep abnormalities, they are not characterized by sudden onset of REM.

    Likewise, sleep deprivation hypersomnia (**choice D**) and substance-induced sleep disorders (**choice E**) do not present with sudden onset of REM.

42. **The correct answer is B.** Cognitive therapy is based on the theory that depressed persons have acquired negative cognitions about themselves, reinforcing these cognitions with self-talk that is often not verbalized. The goal of therapy is to identify the negative cognitions, question the validity of the beliefs, and substitute more positively reinforcing self-talk for the aversive self-criticism.

Internalized anger (**choice A**) and early loss of significant love objects (**choice E**) are psychodynamic explanations for depression.

Neurotransmitter (**choice C**) and genetic (**choice D**) underpinnings are biologic explanations for depression.

43. **The correct answer is C.** In a longitudinal study, the same group is followed over a long period of time. Generally, no active intervention is instituted after the initial event. Note that the event may be either negative or positive.

    Clinical trials (**choice A**) are predicated on some treatment being administered to the persons in the study. In the described situation, nothing is done to this group except observation and evaluation.

    In a double-blind study (**choice B**), neither the subject nor the experimenter knows whether the subject is getting a treatment or a placebo.

    In a prospective study (**choice D**), subjects are identified and followed over time; the outcome has not yet occurred when the study begins.

    A retrospective study (**choice E**) looks backward in subjects' histories to see whether a particular event or events occurred.

44. **The correct answer is A.** Contrary to popular impressions, the most common reason for a significant downward shift in socioeconomic status (SES) is the presence of serious health problems, which both use up financial resources and prevent a person from working full-time at a high-paying job, or from working at all in some cases.

    Significant psychiatric illness (**choice B**) is a cause of decline in SES, but is quantitatively less important than physical problems.

    Inability to defer gratification (**choice C**), lack of education (**choice D**), and unwillingness to work (**choice E**) can all contribute to a decline in SES, but are not numerically as important as disabling physical problems.

45. **The correct answer is D.** In rapid eye movement (REM) sleep disorder, the normal paralysis of muscles during REM sleep is not present, and the person "acts out" the dream they are experiencing. This often results in injury to oneself or to others with whom the person is sleeping. In addition, the content of the dreams associated with this sleep problem is often violent or aggressive.

    Night terrors (**choice A**) typically have their onset in childhood; in some persons, however, they persist into adulthood. During night terrors, the person exhibits terrified behavior, such as screaming during sleep. They do not involve an organized attack on another person.

Narcolepsy (**choice B**) is characterized by the sudden onset of REM sleep at inappropriate times (e.g., while driving), during which there is loss of muscle tone.

Non-REM sleep disorder (**choice C**) encompasses both night terrors and sleepwalking. People do not act out dreams in either of these conditions. Rather, their behavior is autonomous and not aggressive toward others.

Sleep apnea disorder (**choice E**) is a breathing problem during sleep in which the person stops regular breathing. It is not associated with acting out behavior.

46.  **The correct answer is B.** The DNR (do not resuscitate) order means that the patient asks that his or her life not be prolonged by artificial means. It does not mean that the patient wishes to forgo palliative therapy, such as current narcotic pain medication (**choice A**), future medications (**choice C**), and nutrition and hydration (**choice D**). Limitations on such interventions might be specified on living wills or advance directives, however.

47.  **The correct answer is A.** Relaxation of uterine ligaments or endometriosis can produce dyspareunia. These conditions can be corrected by surgical intervention.

Premature ejaculation (**choice B**) is addressed by behavior modification techniques such as the "squeeze" technique to teach the male how to voluntarily control the ejaculatory response.

Primary impotence (**choice C**) is diagnosed in a patient who has always had difficulty attaining and maintaining an erection. That is, the problem has existed ever since the male became sexually active.

Secondary orgasmic dysfunction (**choice D**) is addressed by resolving the traumatic issue that precipitated the symptoms.

Graduated dilators are the treatment for vaginismus (**choice E**).

48.  **The correct answer is D.** Type 1 errors occur when researchers reject the null hypothesis when they should not have. In other words, they conclude a significant result when in actuality it does not exist. This is a particularly dangerous error to make, as it could lead to the administration of an ineffective drug to patients in need of life-preserving treatment.

The term "$1-\beta$ error" (**choice A**) is not used, but $1-\beta$ does correspond to a meaningful value. It reflects the power of a study, which equals the probability of rejecting the null hypothesis when it is false, or in other words, the probability of discovering a true relationship (e.g., concluding that acetaminophen has antipyretic action).

The term "alpha error" (**choice B**) is not used, but alpha values do correspond to a meaningful concept. Alpha is the probability of committing a type 1 error (explained above). Alpha corresponds to the $p$ value ($<0.05$) commonly used in statistical analysis.

The term "beta error" (**choice C**) is not used, but beta values do correspond to a meaningful concept. Beta is the probability of committing a type 2 error. Type 2 errors (**choice E**) occur when researchers accept the null hypothesis when it is false, thereby failing to detect a true relationship (e.g., concluding that acetaminophen has no antipyretic action).

A good mnemonic for distinguishing type 1 and type 2 errors is as follows: Type 1 kills everyone. Type 2 makes professors blue (because they can't publish their statistically insignificant results).

49.  **The correct answer is A.** The concrete operational period (ages 7-11 years) is defined by the child's awareness of the conservation of volume, which demonstrates that the child is able to reason in a logical way in terms of the physical world. Note that the child does not develop understanding of abstract concepts until he or she has reached the formal operational stage (**choice B**), at age 11 to adulthood.

The preoperational stage (**choice C**), ages 2 to 7 years, is associated with significant language development. However, the child has not yet developed the ability to take the perspective of others; thus, the child's thinking tends to remain egocentric.

The sensorimotor stage (**choice D**) corresponds to ages 0 to 2 years and is characterized by the infant developing increasingly sophisticated sensorimotor skills and behavior patterns.

50.  **The correct answer is D.** This is a case of operant conditioning, or learning by reinforcement. In this example, the child's behavior is the operant, which is being reinforced by the parents. That is, the child wants parental attention and is rewarded by the parents only when her disruptive behavior escalates to the point at which the parents must pay attention. The parents are using a "fixed-ratio" of reinforcement, since every time the child gets to the truly disruptive point, they reinforce the behavior.

Classical conditioning (**choice A**) is the type of associative learning in which a stimulus that did not originally elicit a given response now does. This occurs secondary to association of the stimulus with a behavior that previously did elicit the response. For example, a cat does not normally come to its owner if the owner rings a bell. However, if the bell is rung while the cat is eating, the cat associates the bell with food and learns to come to the owner when the bell is rung.

Cognitive learning (**choice B**) requires full attention and purposeful intent to acquire the information.

Imprinting (**choice C**) forms the basis of bonding between an infant and the mothering figure. This form of attachment is learned by association during the immediate postnatal period.

Social learning (**choice E**) involves modeling or imitation. For instance, a child learns familial values by modeling the parental example.

# Behavioral Science and Biostatistics: **Test Two**

1. A 25-year-old man is brought to the psychiatric emergency department by his wife, who reports that he has been acting strangely. He recently has spent thousands of dollars on a new sports car, has become uncharacteristically promiscuous, and has been working and speaking at a frantic pace. History is significant for an episode of major depression last year. Urine toxicology screen is negative. He is prescribed a medication that effectively alleviates his symptoms. Which of the following is a well established side effect of the drug of choice for his condition?

   (A) Agranulocytosis

   (B) Akathisia

   (C) Diabetes insipidus

   (D) Hyperprolactinemia

   (E) Urinary retention

2. A 55-year-old woman was diagnosed with schizophrenic disorder, paranoid type at age 23. She has been on neuroleptic medications for the majority of time since diagnosis. Which of the following conditions would be most likely to appear at this time as a consequence of her treatment?

   (A) Akathisia

   (B) Anticholinergic symptoms

   (C) Dystonia of the laryngeal muscles

   (D) Neuroleptic malignant syndrome

   (E) Tardive dyskinesia

3. A 34-year-old man presents to the hospital complaining of weight loss, nausea, vomiting, and lethargy. There is no evidence of edema, orthostatic hypotension, or dehydration. Blood samples show hyponatremia, but his urine is highly concentrated. A water-load test is performed, in which the patient is instructed to drink a large volume of water and five hourly samples of urine are analyzed. All samples show concentrated urine. Which of the following drugs could have caused this condition?

   (A) Baclofen

   (B) Carbamazepine

   (C) Dantrolene

   (D) Phenelzine

   (E) Phenytoin

   (F) Tranylcypromine

4. A 22-year-old model worries about her job security when a more experienced model is hired. She begins to throw temper tantrums and continuously makes negative statements about the new employee behind her back to her boss. Which of the following defense mechanisms is the model exhibiting?

   (A) Reaction formation

   (B) Regression

   (C) Repression

   (D) Splitting

   (E) Sublimation

5. A 15-year-old boy presents at his family physician's office with a chief complaint of burning on urination. A purulent urethral discharge is noted on physical examination; a Gram stain of the smear is consistent with gonorrhea. The patient explains that he had sexual intercourse with a female friend about 7 days earlier. The physician may treat the patient

   (A) but must have both parents' consent

   (B) but must inform the parents

   (C) with one parent's consent

   (D) without a parent's consent or informing the parents

   (E) without informing parents, but must inform the court

6. A businessman whose work entails much traveling complains to his physician that he has sleep difficulties after returning home from long trips. His lack of sleep has affected his productivity on the job. Which of the following drugs would be most appropriate for treating this patient's jet lag?

   (A) Alprazolam

   (B) Diazepam

   (C) Flurazepam

   (D) Prazepam

   (E) Triazolam

7. A mother brings her child to the pediatrician, concerned that the child is not yet toilet-trained. The mother reports that she has been chatting with other mothers on the Internet, and their children, who are younger than this woman's child, are already toilet-trained. The physician should inform her that which of the following is the earliest age at which toilet training is likely to be successful?

   (A) 10 months

   (B) 13 months

   (C) 16 months

   (D) 19 months

   (E) 22 months

8. An experimental serologic test is developed to detect the presence of HIV antibody. Epidemiologic analysis reveals the results shown below.

   | | People with HIV antibody | People without HIV antibody |
   |---|---|---|
   | Positive test | 100 | 50 |
   | Negative test | 20 | 950 |

   Which of the following is the sensitivity of this test?

   (A) 11%

   (B) 67%

   (C) 83%

   (D) 95%

   (E) 98%

9. A 10-year-old boy is sent home from school for hitting younger children and taking things from them by force. The parents meet with the school principal. During the conference, the father says to the principal, "Just wait till I get home. He's going to get his butt whipped." The father's disciplinary technique, with the resultant behavior in the son, is an example of which type of learning?

   (A) Classical conditioning

   (B) Cognitive learning

   (C) Imprinting

   (D) Operant conditioning

   (E) Social learning

10. A 35-year-old night watchman has few close relationships with family or friends because they find him cold and aloof. He has no particularly odd behaviors except for his preference for being alone. This patient most likely has which of the following personality disorders?

    (A) Antisocial

    (B) Avoidant

    (C) Borderline

    (D) Dependent

    (E) Schizoid

11. A 16-year-old girl is pregnant and seeking an abortion. She does not want her parents to know either that she is pregnant or that she wants an abortion. The physician may perform the abortion

    (A) but must have at least one parent's consent

    (B) but must have both parents' consent

    (C) but must inform the parents

    (D) without parental consent only in certain states

    (E) without telling the parents

12. A trial comparing coronary bypass surgery with medical treatment for coronary artery disease is conducted at a hospital specializing in cardiothoracic surgery. Which of the following types of biases should be considered in evaluating the results of this trial?

    (A) Ascertainment bias

    (B) Detection bias

    (C) Proficiency bias

    (D) Recall bias

    (E) Referral bias

    (F) Susceptibility bias

13. A 34-year-old woman is telling her friend that she is very pleased with her health care system. She is able to select the physician that she would like to see, and the federal government pays the physician on a fee-for-service basis. This type of health care is guaranteed to all persons. She is most likely referring to which of the following health care systems?

    (A) The British system

    (B) The Canadian system

    (C) The Indian health service system

    (D) The U.S. system

    (E) The Veterans Administration system

14. A 23-year-old woman visits a primary care physician complaining of recurrent nausea and generalized abdominal pain, which has distressed her and compromised her functioning for the past several months. Thorough evaluations by a gynecologist and gastroenterologist have revealed no abnormalities. She was referred to a neurologist for headaches and has been taking acetaminophen for her "joint pains." The primary care physician completes a thorough physical exam; the results are normal. Which of the following is the most likely diagnosis?

    (A) Body dysmorphic disorder

    (B) Conversion disorder

    (C) Factitious disorder

    (D) Malingering

    (E) Somatization disorder

15. A 19-year-old man describes episodes in which he feels as if he's "floating out of his body" and observing himself from a place about 2 feet over his head. He is aware of everything going on around him and can respond to others. Which of the following terms most accurately describes what this patient is experiencing?

    (A) Delirium tremens

    (B) Delusion

    (C) Dementia

    (D) Depersonalization

    (E) Derealization

    (F) Hallucination

    (G) Illusion

16. A physician enters an examination room where a 31-year-old woman is sitting on a chair with tears running down her face. After the physician introduces herself, which of the following is the most appropriate first statement to get the most correct information from the patient in the least amount of time?

    (A) "Are you depressed?"

    (B) "How are you feeling?"

    (C) "What is scaring you?"

    (D) "You seem to be sad."

    (E) "You seem to be upset."

17. A new mother is surprised by all of the reflexes her child has. The pediatrician explains that during development a child exhibits many types of reflexes. Of the following reflexes present in a neonate, which is most critical to its immediate survival?

    (A) Grasp
    (B) Plantar
    (C) Rooting
    (D) Startle
    (E) Tonic neck

18. A researcher publishes new results on the efficacy of a procedure using transplanted embryonic cells to correct a diabetic condition induced in experimental animals by chemical ablation of pancreatic beta cells. At another institution, a different researcher attempts to reproduce the findings, but cannot. This disparate finding calls into question the first study's

    (A) accuracy
    (B) power
    (C) reliability
    (D) sensitivity
    (E) validity

19. A patient comes to the urologist to discuss an "embarrassing issue." The patient asks that the medical student leave the room. Once the doctor and patient are alone, and after much reassurance, the patient finally admits to sexual problems. The physician performs a thorough evaluation. Later, in discussing the case with the medical student, the physician says that this patient's type of sexual dysfunction is the most difficult to treat. Which of the following is the most likely cause of this patient's sexual dysfunction?

    (A) Dyspareunia
    (B) Premature ejaculation
    (C) Primary ejaculatory incompetence in a male
    (D) Secondary orgasmic dysfunction in a female
    (E) Vaginismus

20. A 45-year-old woman is brought to the emergency department by ambulance after a car accident that caused injuries resulting in a significant loss of blood. The patient is conscious and informs the attending physician that her religion forbids a blood transfusion. She has an identification card in her purse that verifies her religious affiliation and her wishes not to undergo transfusion. Although the physician explains that without the transfusion she is likely to die, she still refuses the procedure. Which of the following actions should the physician take?

    (A) Declare an emergency and transfuse against the patient's wishes
    (B) Declare the patient incompetent and transfuse
    (C) Make the patient comfortable, but not transfuse
    (D) Request the hospital chaplain try to persuade the patient
    (E) Transfuse when the patient becomes comatose

21. A 34-year-old woman is brought to her family physician by her brother. He states that the patient's husband ran away with another woman the previous day. After discovering this, the patient arrived at her brother's home in a "dazed state," was unable to function appropriately the remainder of the evening, and slept fitfully all night. Early in the morning she began to talk to people who were not present, and debated whether to kill her children and herself. He denies anything like this ever happening before. Which of the following is the most likely diagnosis?

    (A) Bipolar disorder
    (B) Brief psychotic disorder
    (C) Schizoaffective disorder
    (D) Schizophrenic disorder
    (E) Schizophreniform disorder

22. A mother brings her 6-week-old infant to the pediatrician because she is concerned that her child is not babbling in response to her stimulation. Which of the following is the most likely diagnosis?

    (A) Autism
    (B) Hearing impairment
    (C) Mental retardation
    (D) Visual impairment
    (E) Within normal limits

23. A 20-year-old woman sees her baby cousin for the first time. As she attempts to play with the infant, he begins to cry incessantly. Which of the following is the most likely age of this infant?

    (A) 1 to 4 months
    (B) 5 to 8 months
    (C) 9 to 12 months
    (D) 13 to 16 months
    (E) 17 to 20 months

24. A woman's 11-year-old son is injured in an automobile accident and requires a blood transfusion. The mother refuses to consent to the transfusion for the boy on the grounds of her religious belief system. The physician should

    (A) declare an emergency and perform the transfusion against the mother's wishes
    (B) discharge the mother and son from the hospital
    (C) make the patient comfortable, but not transfuse
    (D) request the hospital chaplain try to persuade the mother to allow the transfusion
    (E) seek a court order to perform the transfusion, but do nothing until the court rules

25. A 38-year-old woman successfully commits suicide. Her best friend claims to be very surprised by what happened because her friend was a married, wealthy woman with no history of major affective disorder and had no previous suicide attempts. Which of the following variables in this woman's history is associated with a higher risk for successfully committing suicide?

    (A) Age younger than 45
    (B) Female gender
    (C) High socioeconomic status
    (D) Married
    (E) No history of major affective disorder
    (F) No previous suicide attempts

26. A 27-year-old swimmer who feels insecure about her athletic abilities harshly criticizes her teammates' techniques. Which of the following ego defense mechanisms is she displaying?

    (A) Displacement
    (B) Projection
    (C) Reaction formation
    (D) Repression
    (E) Sublimation

27. A 27-year-old man is brought into the emergency department by the police, who found him walking aimlessly and shouting the names of former presidents. Urine toxicology is negative, and the man appears to be oriented with respect to person, place, and time. He has had five similar admissions over the past year. Attempts to interview the patient are fruitless, as he seems easily distracted and unable to concentrate. A phone call to a friend listed in the chart provides the additional information that the man is homeless and unable to care for himself. This patient is exhibiting the signs and symptoms of

    (A) schizoaffective disorder
    (B) schizoid personality disorder
    (C) schizophrenia
    (D) schizophreniform disorder
    (E) schizotypal personality disorder

28. While performing a mental status examination on a hospitalized 54-year-old woman, a medical student finds that there is a disruption in the sensorium section of the exam. This is the first interview with this patient, and the student does not know anything about the case. On the basis of the exam findings, the medical student should explore which of the following etiologic areas?

    (A) Educational/deprivation
    (B) Familial/child-rearing
    (C) Organic/neurologic
    (D) Psychological/learned
    (E) Social/cultural

29. A couple visits their primary care physician because of sleep difficulties. The wife reports that she cannot fall asleep at night because of her obese husband's loud snoring. He complains of feeling drowsy during the day and falling asleep while driving home from work. Which of the following conditions does the husband most likely have?

    (A) Central sleep apnea
    (B) Obstructive sleep apnea
    (C) Narcolepsy
    (D) Pavor nocturnus
    (E) Somnambulism

**KAPLAN) MEDICAL**

30. An adolescent male is referred for drug abuse. He confides to the therapist that he has been taking large amounts of "reds" (secobarbital sodium) for some time and that they make him feel confident and calm. He would like to stop but says he would prefer to "do it on his own," without additional medication. The therapist should advise the patient to detoxify with medical assistance because of the danger of

    (A) insomnia

    (B) rebound anxiety

    (C) recidivism

    (D) respiratory depression

    (E) seizures

31. An urban health department reports the infant mortality rate of the city in the past year. This value corresponds to which of the following?

    (A) The number of deaths during the past year from all causes divided by the total population

    (B) The number of deaths occurring after the first 4 weeks of life and before the first birthday divided by the total number of live births

    (C) The number of deaths occurring until the first birthday divided by the total number of live births

    (D) The number of deaths occurring within the first 4 weeks of life divided by the total number of births

    (E) The number of deaths occurring within the first 4 weeks of life divided by the total number of live births

32. A 19-year-old woman, who recently moved from her family's home in another state, is hospitalized for attempting suicide by taking an overdose of antidepressant medications. On the third day of her hospital stay, she insists, under threat of a lawsuit, that her medications be stopped and that she be discharged from the hospital so she "can go home and finish the job." Her sensorium is clear. Her physician should

    (A) discharge her against medical advice (AMA)

    (B) honor her request and release her immediately

    (C) obtain an emergency order of detention

    (D) release her to go back to her parents' home

    (E) sedate her

33. A female patient presents to a physician with the isolated symptom of pulling out all the hair on her head and face. She reports that there is a build up of "pressure" or tension inside her, and the hair extraction reduces the pressure/tension feeling. Which of the following is the most appropriate medication for this condition?

    (A) Clozapine

    (B) Diazepam

    (C) Fluvoxamine

    (D) Lithium

    (E) Verapamil

34. A 23-year-old man arrives at the emergency department at 11:30 PM complaining of flank pain and blood in his urine. He requests Demerol™ to control the pain. The physician requests a urine sample, and the patient goes to the restroom, removes a pin from under his shirt collar, pricks his finger, and holds the dripping blood in the stream of urine. He returns the urine to the physician and intensifies his complaints of pain, which he now says has migrated to his ipsilateral testicle. Which of the following is the most likely diagnosis?

    (A) Antisocial personality disorder

    (B) Factitious disorder

    (C) Malingering disorder

    (D) Schizotypal personality disorder

    (E) Somatization disorder

35. White coat hypertension is defined as an elevation of blood pressure resulting from the apprehension associated with visiting a physician. It is thought that the patient associates the physician's white coat with distressing experiences (e.g., being vaccinated as a child), resulting in transient hypertension. This may be viewed as a physiologic manifestation of which of the following phenomena?

    (A) Classical conditioning

    (B) Extinction

    (C) Habit hierarchies

    (D) Negative reinforcement

    (E) Operant conditioning

36. A 10-year-old girl who is a suspected victim of child abuse is referred to a psychologist for evaluation. As part of her workup, the patient is asked to construct a story using pictures. Which of the following psychometric measures was used?

    (A) Minnesota Multiphasic Personality Inventory (MMPI)
    (B) Myers-Briggs Personality Inventory
    (C) Rorschach Test
    (D) Thematic Apperception Test
    (E) Type A and B Behavior Patterns Test

37. A 32-year-old man is being treated for impulsive aggression. He has been incarcerated several times and now is required to undergo intensive therapy. In trying to understand what he is going through, the man asks if there is any biochemical component to his disorder. Which of the following neurotransmitter systems has been most strongly linked to his disorder?

    (A) Dopamine
    (B) Endorphin
    (C) Epinephrine
    (D) Gamma-amino butyric acid
    (E) Serotonin

38. A young mother wishes to teach her 3-year-old son to pick up his toys when he is finished playing. A friend advises her to reward her child for completing this task. Though the approach is effective for about 1 week, the little boy returns to his previous untidy behavior. Which of the following patterns of reinforcement did she likely use?

    (A) Continuous
    (B) Fixed interval
    (C) Fixed ratio
    (D) Variable interval
    (E) Variable ratio

39. A 47-year-old man is hospitalized with acute pancreatitis. His history reveals a history of episodic binge alcohol consumption. When the physician meets with the patient to discuss the condition, the patient asks: "Doctor, what caused this?" Which of the following is the most appropriate response to this question?

    (A) "I'm not sure."
    (B) "Probably a consequence of alcohol consumption."
    (C) "Probably your alcoholism."
    (D) "We need to talk about where we go from here in your long-term care."
    (E) "What do you think?"

40. An oncologist tells his patient that her laboratory results support a diagnosis of advanced malignant melanoma with multiple metastases to the liver and brain. He also advises her that the prognosis is poor. Which of the following is most likely to be the first statement that the patient will make?

    (A) "Can you keep me alive until my daughter graduates from medical school?"
    (B) "Damn you doctor, you should have caught this earlier!"
    (C) "Doctor, you must be wrong."
    (D) "I think it is time that I make a will and say good-bye to everyone."
    (E) "It's no use, I always lose and get the short end of the stick."

41. A 45-year-old woman has just given birth to her fifth child. She wishes to undergo a tubal ligation. The physician should

    (A) convince the patient to use alternative contraception until she reaches menopause
    (B) discuss the benefits and risks of the procedure with both the patient and her husband
    (C) explain to the patient that her chances of becoming pregnant are very low at her age
    (D) maintain strict confidentiality and not disclose the patient's wishes to her husband

42. A man brings his 45-year-old wife to the emergency department. He states she has been ill for 3 days and has had a temperature of 99.8 to 100.5 F. Today she is having difficulty staying awake, is talking to persons who are not there, and at times appears to be frightened of something. She is restless and somewhat combative when restrained. What is the most likely diagnosis?

    (A) Acute stress disorder
    (B) Bipolar I disorder, manic type
    (C) Brief psychotic disorder
    (D) Delirium
    (E) Dementia

43. A 40-year-old man visits a crisis counselor after a devastating explosion. Which of the following would be most likely to predispose this patient to developing emotional problems after the disaster?

    (A) Having been physically injured and trapped under rubble for 24 hours
    (B) Having lived all his life in the area where the disaster occurred
    (C) Having a previous diagnosis of post-traumatic stress disorder
    (D) Having recently been widowed
    (E) Having worked 15 miles from the site of the explosion

44. A new drug with in vitro activity against HIV is tested on a population of patients with Western-blot confirmed HIV infections. Out of the 200 individuals in the patient population, 100 individuals are chosen by lottery to receive the drug. The drug, which is tasteless, is administered in a cup of orange juice; the other patients receive pure orange juice. Neither the nurses, doctors, nor patients know which patients receive the drug. At the end of the study period, the number of CD4+ T cells is determined for all of the subjects. This is an example of a

    (A) case-control study
    (B) case report
    (C) cohort study
    (D) cross-sectional study
    (E) double-blind randomized clinical trial

45. Which of the following is the highest level of functioning that a 27-year-old person with an Intelligence Quotient (IQ) of 53 could be reasonably expected to achieve?

    (A) Live alone, work at a semi-skilled job, and maintain a totally independent lifestyle
    (B) Work in a sheltered workshop situation and maintain a totally independent lifestyle
    (C) Work in a sheltered workshop situation and be assisted during times of mild social or economic stress
    (D) Live in a controlled environment and be partially self-maintained
    (E) Live in a nursing home environment

46. There were no new cases of Ebola virus in the United States from January 1, 1997 through January 1, 1998. Which of the following epidemiologic terms does this statement describe?

    (A) Incidence
    (B) Lifetime expectancy
    (C) Lifetime prevalence
    (D) Period prevalence
    (E) Point prevalence

47. The data presented below compare the results of a diagnostic test in the presence and absence of a disease.

| | Disease present | Disease absent |
|---|---|---|
| Positive test | 40 | 5 |
| Negative test | 10 | 95 |
| Total | 50 | 100 |

Which of the following is the specificity of this test?

    (A) 0.05
    (B) 0.40
    (C) 0.80
    (D) 0.90
    (E) 0.95

48. A 33-year-old woman is brought into the emergency department by ambulance. She has been diagnosed as having schizophrenic disorder, disorganized type, since the age of 17. She has been on antipsychotic medications since that time, which have controlled her symptoms well. Physical examination reveals a well nourished woman with a temperature of 103.2 F, blood pressure of 180/99/mm Hg, pulse of 97/min, and copious perspiration. She is mute, has muscular rigidity, and appears to be obtunded. Which of the following is the most likely diagnosis?

    (A) Acute dystonia
    (B) Akathisia
    (C) Neuroleptic malignant syndrome
    (D) Parkinsonism
    (E) Tardive dyskinesia

49. A 34-year-old woman complains of early morning awakenings and loss of interest in everyday activities. She is diagnosed with major depressive disorder and given fluoxetine, but does not improve. Tricyclic antidepressants and MAO inhibitors are subsequently tried without effect, and electroconvulsive therapy (ECT) is recommended. Which of the following represents the most serious side effect of ECT?

    (A) Extrapyramidal symptoms
    (B) Hearing loss
    (C) Mania
    (D) Retrograde amnesia
    (E) Rhabdomyolysis

50. A 35-year old woman lives alone. She has never been married, has a Masters of Business Administration, and has been employed as a stock broker. She was fired from her present firm because on three separate occasions over the past 2 years, without authorization from her clients, she sold all the securities in their accounts and invested the money in securities that had glossy portfolios but were worthless. On these three occasions she worked 22 to 24 hours per day for 10 days at a time, gorged herself on "junk food," and drank alcohol excessively. Which of the following is the most likely diagnosis?

    (A) Bipolar disorder, type I
    (B) Bipolar disorder, type II
    (C) Cyclothymic disorder
    (D) Schizophrenic disorder, paranoid type
    (E) Substance-induced delirium

# Behavioral Science and Biostatistics Test Two:
# Answers and Explanations

## ANSWER KEY

| | | | |
|---|---|---|---|
| 1. | C | 26. | B |
| 2. | E | 27. | C |
| 3. | B | 28. | C |
| 4. | B | 29. | B |
| 5. | D | 30. | E |
| 6. | E | 31. | C |
| 7. | D | 32. | C |
| 8. | C | 33. | C |
| 9. | E | 34. | C |
| 10. | E | 35. | A |
| 11. | D | 36. | D |
| 12. | C | 37. | E |
| 13. | B | 38. | A |
| 14. | E | 39. | B |
| 15. | D | 40. | C |
| 16. | B | 41. | B |
| 17. | C | 42. | D |
| 18. | C | 43. | A |
| 19. | C | 44. | E |
| 20. | C | 45. | C |
| 21. | B | 46. | A |
| 22. | E | 47. | E |
| 23. | B | 48. | C |
| 24. | A | 49. | D |
| 25. | C | 50. | A |

1. **The correct answer is C.** This patient has bipolar disorder and is experiencing a manic episode. The drug of choice for this condition, lithium, can cause nephrogenic diabetes insipidus at therapeutic drug levels. Other side effects include tremor, ataxia, aphasia, and sedation.

   Agranulocytosis (**choice A**) is a side effect of clozapine, which is used for schizophrenic patients with symptoms refractory to traditional antipsychotic therapy. Unlike the standard antidopaminergics (e.g., haloperidol), clozapine rarely produces extrapyramidal side effects. Note that lithium administration causes leukocytosis, rather than leukopenia, in most cases.

   Akathisia (**choice B**), which is characterized by uncontrollable restlessness, is an extrapyramidal side effect of antidopaminergic medications used to treat schizophrenia.

   Hyperprolactinemia (**choice D**) is typically associated with antidopaminergic medications (antipsychotics), rather than with lithium.

   Urinary retention (**choice E**) is a classic anticholinergic side effect of tricyclic antidepressants.

2. **The correct answer is E.** Tardive dyskinesia is a result of long-term treatment with neuroleptic medications and is seen more frequently in older women. The condition presents with abnormal choreoathetoid movements, often involving the face and mouth in adults and the limbs in children. Once tardive dyskinesia develops, there is no known treatment to mitigate the symptoms.

   Akathisia (**choice A**), also known as restless leg syndrome, is usually well controlled by reduction of the dose of antipsychotic medication and the addition of beta-adrenergic receptor antagonists or anticholinergic drugs and benzodiazepines. It can occur early in the course of treatment.

   Anticholinergic symptoms (**choice B**), such as dry mouth, blurred vision, or constipation, usually appear early in the course of treatment, and the patient becomes tolerant to these effects.

   Dystonia of the laryngeal muscles (**choice C**) is an acute condition that is well managed with medications such as benztropine or diphenhydramine.

   Neuroleptic malignant syndrome (**choice D**) is a life-threatening condition that can occur at any point in treatment. It is characterized by muscle rigidity, hyperpyrexia, and increased blood pressure. Bromocriptine and dantrolene are used to treat this disorder.

3. **The correct answer is B.** The patient has the syndrome of inappropriate secretion of ADH (SIADH). When ADH (vasopressin) is secreted in excessive amounts, or at inappropriate times, it can cause hyponatremia as well as symptoms of nausea, vomiting, anorexia, and lethargy. Excessive release of vasopressin also results in the excretion of a concentrated urine (with a urinary osmolality usually greater than 300 mOsmol/kg) despite a subnormal plasma osmolality and serum sodium concentration. SIADH can be caused by many factors, such as ectopic ADH production and release from neoplastic tissue (small cell carcinoma of lung, pancreatic carcinoma, lymphosarcoma, Hodgkin disease, reticulum cell sarcoma, thymoma, and carcinoma of duodenum or bladder) or by drugs that release or potentiate the action of ADH, such as carbamazepine, vincristine, vinblastine, cyclophosphamide, chlorpropamide, general anesthetics, and tricyclic antidepressants.

   Baclofen (**choice A**) is a spasmolytic agent. Baclofen has not been shown to be associated with the release of ADH.

   Dantrolene (**choice C**) is a spasmolytic agent and is also used to treat malignant hyperthermia. Dantrolene has not been shown to be associated with the release of ADH.

   Phenelzine (**choice D**) and tranylcypromine (choice F) are MAO inhibitors. MAO inhibitors have not been shown to be associated with the release of ADH.

   Phenytoin (**choice E**) is an antiseizure drug and has not been shown to be associated with the release of ADH.

4. **The correct answer is B.** The model is exhibiting regression, an automatic retreat to a less mature level of behavior in times of stress (e.g., throwing temper tantrums and tattletaling).

   Reaction formation (**choice A**) involves turning a repressed impulse or unconscious wish to its opposite.

   Repression (**choice C**) occurs when conflict-provoking thoughts or feelings are hidden from the person's awareness.

   Splitting (**choice D**) refers to the unconscious inability to see an important person as having both good and bad characteristics. The characteristics are "split," such that the person is perceived as either wonderful or terrible.

   Sublimation (**choice E**) is a very mature defense mechanism that involves consciously turning socially unacceptable impulses into acceptable or more benign forms to allow their expression.

**5. The correct answer is D.** No states specifically mandate parental involvement for a minor to obtain contraception, prenatal care and delivery services, diagnosis and treatment of an STD, outpatient alcohol and/or drug treatment, or outpatient mental health services. In these situations, the physician may go ahead and treat; informing the parents is the physician's option, not a requirement.

**6. The correct answer is E.** Short-acting benzodiazepines (BZD) are the most appropriate pharmaceutical therapy for acute insomnia, including jet lag. Triazolam is the only short-acting BZD listed. It has the added benefit of not having many adverse actions (e.g., hangover effect) when taken in low doses. Higher doses, however, predispose to transient anterograde amnesia.

Alprazolam (**choice A**) is an intermediate-acting BZD used primarily for panic attacks.

Diazepam (**choice B**) is effective for status epilepticus and muscle spasticity. Note that lorazepam is also effective for status epilepticus.

Flurazepam (**choice C**) is a long-acting BZD that can cause drowsiness or ataxia, rendering it a less desirable choice. It is not used as an anxiolytic, unlike many other BZDs.

Prazepam (**choice D**) is a long-acting BZD unsuitable for the treatment of sleep disorders.

**7. The correct answer is D.** Toilet training is not possible before the age of 18 months because the long nerve fibers have not yet myelinated and sphincter control is not possible. Toilet training should be completed by 4 years of age.

**8. The correct answer is C.** Sensitivity is defined as the ability of a test to detect the presence of a disease in those who truly have the disease. It is calculated as the number of people with a disease who test positive (true positive) divided by the total number of people who have the disease (true positive + false negative). In this case, sensitivity equals the number of people with HIV antibody who test positive (100) divided by the total number of people who have HIV antibody (120). This yields 100/120 = 83% (not a very sensitive test).

11% (**choice A**) corresponds to the prevalence of the disease in the tested population, which in this case equals the total number of people with HIV antibody (true positive + false negative = 100 + 20 = 120) divided by the total number of people tested (100 + 20 + 50 + 950 = 1120). This yields 120/1120 = 11%.

67% (**choice B**) corresponds to the positive predictive value of the test, which equals the number of people with the disease who test positive (true positives = 100)

divided by the total number of people testing positive (all positives = 50). This yields 100/150 = 67%.

95% (**choice D**) corresponds to the specificity of the test, which equals the number of people without HIV antibody who test negative (950) divided by the total number of people without HIV antibody (1000). This yields 950/1000 = 95%.

98% (**choice E**) corresponds to the negative predictive value of the test, which equals the number of people without HIV antibody who test negative (950) divided by the total number of people testing negative (970). This yields 950/970 = 98%.

An easy way to remember these concepts is:

Sensitivity = true positives/all diseased

Specificity = true negatives/all normal

PPV = true positives/all positives

NPV = true negatives/all negatives

Prevalence = all diseased/total population

If you prefer charts and formulas:

| | (Diseased) People with HIV antibody | (Normal) People without HIV antibody |
|---|---|---|
| Positive test | a, true pos. | b, false pos. |
| Negative test | c, false neg. | d, true neg. |

Sensitivity = a/(a + c)

Specificity = d/(b + d)

PPV = a/(a + b)

NPV = d/(c + d)

Prevalence = (a + c)/(a + b + c + d)

**9. The correct answer is E.** This is an example of social learning. That is, the father is providing the example that "big people" get their way with "little people" by using force. The son is simply modeling his father's example.

Classical conditioning (**choice A**) is the type of associative learning in which a stimulus that did not originally elicit a given response now does. This is done by associating the stimulus with a behavior that previously did elicit the response. In this question, the child may learn to fear the principal's office because of the punitive consequences.

Cognitive learning (**choice B**) is a type of learning that requires full attention and purposeful intent to acquire the information. This boy may learn better social interactive skills if the principal required him to write an essay on how he feels when "big people" beat up on him.

Imprinting (**choice C**) forms the basis of bonding between an infant and the mothering figure. This form of attachment is learned by association during the immediate postnatal period.

Operant conditioning (**choice D**) is learning by reinforcement of a given behavior. If the father had said to his son: "Good boy. You have to take what you want in this world," the son would be reinforced for his antisocial behavior.

10. **The correct answer is E.** This is a typical description of schizoid personality disorder. Classic clues are "night watchman" and "cold and aloof" without odd behaviors or beliefs.

Antisocial personality disorder (**choice A**) is characterized by disregard for and violation of the rights of others, deceitfulness, impulsiveness, recklessness, irresponsibility, and a lack of remorse.

People with avoidant personality disorder (**choice B**) have a fear of rejection in interpersonal relationships. They are hypersensitive and exhibit excessive concern about being completely accepted without criticism. Unlike people with schizoid personality disorders, these patients want to establish relationships with others but are terrified unless they are guaranteed acceptance.

Borderline personality disorder (**choice C**) is associated with major problems with identity (e.g., gender identity, values), anger, and impulse control. Self-destructive behavior, e.g., gambling or overspending, may be present. These patients are emotionally labile and express intense feelings inappropriately.

People with dependent personality disorder (**choice D**) allow others to assume responsibility for important areas in their lives. There is a lack of self-confidence, and the priorities of others are given the most attention.

11. **The correct answer is D.** A number of issues are involved in this situation. First, the age of majority differs from state to state. As of April 1999, only two states and the District of Columbia have laws that affirm a minor's ability to obtain an abortion on her own. Twenty-five states have laws that require consent from one or both parents. All states have an option for the minor to petition the court for permission to have the abortion. These laws obviously place pregnant minors in difficulty if the laws require consent by both parents, since one may not be available and/or their whereabouts may be unknown. Girls who live in rural areas or cannot provide their own transportation have a difficult time accessing court services. Furthermore, the court system is usually much too complicated for the youth to manage on her own.

12. **The correct answer is C.** Proficiency bias occurs when the intervention under consideration is delivered with unusual skill (or incompetence) so that it cannot be reproduced in typical settings.

Ascertainment bias (**choice A**) occurs when patients with the suspected outcome are more extensively probed about their symptoms and histories than are patients without the suspected outcome.

Detection bias (**choice B**) occurs when more information is solicited from the treatment group than from the placebo group.

Recall bias (**choice D**) occurs in retrospective studies. Patients may not remember the severity of their symptoms or how much intervention occurred over the specified course of time.

Referral bias (**choice E**) occurs when the sample of patients used in a study is not typical of the general population. For example, if an academic medical center sees the most acutely ill patients admitted for bypass surgery, its overall bypass mortality rates will appear extraordinarily high.

Susceptibility bias (**choice F**) occurs when patients receive one intervention or another on the basis of the severity of their disease. For example, since sicker patients would be less likely to survive a coronary bypass operation, they might be designated to receive medical therapy instead. This, however, might result in poorer outcomes for the medical therapy group. Susceptibility bias can be avoided by randomizing subjects to different study groups.

13. **The correct answer is B.** In the Canadian system, basic health care is available to all Canadian citizens. They can select the physician they wish to see, and the federal government pays the physician on a fee-for-service basis. The fee is different for each of the provinces.

In the British system (**choice A**), physicians are on salary to the government; however, each physician is also allowed to negotiate an amount of time that they can spend in private practice for persons who want that service and can afford private fees.

Both the Indian health service (**choice C**) and the Veterans Administration (**choice E**) are socialized medicine groups. For those who are eligible, there is no charge for services rendered.

The U.S. system (**choice D**) is a collage of different reimbursement systems, including health insurance that the individual purchases, Medicare for the elderly, and Medicaid for the indigent. However, there is no universal coverage, and annually 40,000,000 persons, the majority of whom are children, are without health care coverage.

14. **The correct answer is E.** Patients with somatization disorder have many medically unexplained symptoms in multiple body systems, causing work limitation, increased visits to the physician, needless surgery, or unnecessary medical treatments. Somatization disorder is distinguished by its ego-dystonic symptoms; that is, the patient's functioning is compromised because of the unpleasantness of symptoms. It usually begins before age 30.

Body dysmorphic disorder (**choice A**) refers to the patient who is preoccupied with the belief that some part of the body is marred in looks. It usually begins in adolescence and is equally common in males and females.

Conversion disorder (**choice B**) refers to patients with neurologic complaints that are not consistent with present-day knowledge about the nervous system (e.g., anesthesia that does not run along a nerve distribution). A classic clue to this diagnosis is that the patient reveals a relative lack of concern about the symptoms, known as "la belle indifférence."

There are three types of factitious disorder (FD; **choice C**): FD with psychological symptoms, FD with medical symptoms, and chronic FD. FD with medical symptoms is different from somatization disorder. In FD, symptoms are completely fabricated, and patients often insist on hospitalization and submit to invasive procedures. They also may produce symptoms through specific acts (e.g., taking drugs). Another difference between FD and somatization disorder is that patients with FD are consciously trying to assume a sick role.

Malingering (**choice D**) refers to the situation in which a patient reports psychological or general medical symptoms to achieve some easily recognizable secondary gain. The question implied no secondary gain for the patient, therefore malingering is not the best diagnosis in this case.

15. **The correct answer is D.** Depersonalization occurs when an individual perceives that his "person" or "self" becomes detached from his body. He maintains his contact with reality and level of consciousness, as opposed to derealization (**choice E**), in which the environment seems distorted or takes on an unreal quality.

Delirium tremens (**choice A**) occurs as a withdrawal symptom in chronic alcoholics abstaining from alcohol. It is characterized by anxiety, tremor, sweating, and vivid hallucinations.

Delusions (**choice B**) are false, fixed belief systems that exist in the face of no evidence to support them and are not shared by most others.

A patient with dementia (**choice C**) has a normal level of consciousness with gradual onset of cognitive symptoms (e.g., memory disturbance) and small potential for recovery. In contrast, delirium is characterized by impaired consciousness (diminished alertness and disturbed orientation to time, place, and person), acute onset of symptoms (e.g., confusion), excessive daytime sleeping, diffuse slowing of brain waves on EEG, and full recovery in most cases.

Hallucinations (**choice F**) are perceptions that have no basis in the environmental stimuli present. Hallucinating patients are often observed to respond to internal stimuli (e.g., patients who appear to be talking to themselves are actually replying to voices heard in their heads).

An illusion (**choice G**) is when a real environmental stimulus is misperceived as something it is not.

16. **The correct answer is B.** Patients may display different expressions to different underlying emotional states based on cultural, familial, and transient circumstances. For instance, many women have been taught that they "should never be angry," so they frequently cry when they are frustrated—the natural precursor to anger.

In general, the physician should not begin by asking about specific emotional bases (**choices A, C, D, and E**). Asking the patient directly how he or she is feeling promotes patient interaction and prevents the physician from assuming a given emotion when another is present.

17. **The correct answer is C.** The rooting reflex allows puckering of the lips and sucking on objects in response to perioral stimulation. It is necessary for the child to be able to locate a nipple and ingest food. Without this reflex, the neonate cannot suckle and feed properly.

The remaining reflexes (**choices A, B, D, and E**) are crucial for later development and survival but not for immediate life.

The grasp reflex (**choice A**) occurs when pressure is exerted on the hand of the neonate. The neonate will grasp the object exerting the pressure.

The plantar reflex (**choice B**) is another name for the Babinski sign. When the lateral surface of the foot is stroked, the great toe goes up and the other toes fan.

The startle reflex (**choice D**; also called the Moro reflex) occurs when an intense sensory stimulus is received. The neonate extends and abducts the arms, then flexes and adducts them.

The tonic neck reflex (**choice E**) occurs when the head is turned; the ipsilateral leg extends and the contralateral arm and leg flex.

18. **The correct answer is C.** The reliability of a measurement refers to the ability of other researchers to reproduce the results. This can be summarized by noting that reliability = reproducibility.

The accuracy (**choice A**) of a measurement refers to the "trueness" of the measurement, i.e., how close the measured value is to the true value. It is a measure of bias. Just because another researcher could not reproduce the findings does not necessarily imply that they were inaccurate.

The power (**choice B**) of a study is best conceptualized as the probability of rejecting a null hypothesis that is in fact false. This is equal to 1 minus the probability of a type II error (1-β), since β is the probability of failing to reject a false null hypothesis.

The sensitivity (**choice D**) of a test is a measure of its ability to detect the presence of a disease in those who truly have the disease.

The validity (**choice E**) of a measurement is an index of how well the test measures what it purports to measure. The disparate results obtained by another researcher do not necessarily mean that the results are not valid.

19. **The correct answer is C.** Primary ejaculatory incompetence means that the adult male has never developed the ability to ejaculate while engaged in sexual activity with another person. It is extremely difficult to treat.

Dyspareunia (**choice A**) is painful intercourse and is easily treated by addressing the underlying medical causes that exist in the vast majority of cases.

Premature ejaculation (**choice B**) is readily addressed by the "squeeze technique."

Secondary orgasmic dysfunction (**choice D**) means there had been function but it has been lost. Any secondary sexual dysfunction is easier to treat than a primary problem.

Vaginismus (**choice E**) is often related to fear and apprehension regarding the act of penetration and is quite easily treated by behavior modification.

20. **The correct answer is C.** The courts have repeatedly ruled that adults are free to select their religious belief system and practice the tenets of that religion. If that includes refusal of certain medical procedures, that is the individual's right to choose.

Declaring an emergency and transfusing against the patient's wishes (**choice A**) is clearly not allowed. In fact, the physician undertaking such action is legally liable for assault and battery and is clearly open to a malpractice action.

Declaring the patient incompetent and performing the transfusion (**choice B**) is incorrect because the ruling of incompetence must be made by the court and not the physician. Again, the physician is open to a malpractice action if such an action were taken.

Requesting the hospital chaplain try to persuade the patient (**choice D**) is incorrect since adults in America have the right to choose their religious beliefs. Trying to dissuade them from their beliefs and impose others on them is clearly unethical.

Performing the transfusion when the patient becomes comatose (**choice E**) clearly goes against the patient's wishes. The patient's wishes were known before she became comatose, and these wishes must be followed in delivering medical care.

21. **The correct answer is B.** Brief psychotic disorder is a thought disorder of psychotic proportion (e.g., the demonstrated auditory hallucinations). There is often a precipitating event. To make this diagnosis, the patient's symptoms must have been present for at least 1 day but not more than 1 month. This duration distinguishes brief psychotic disorder from schizophrenic and schizophreniform disorders.

Bipolar disorder (**choice A**) is defined by the presence of a manic episode (characterized by an altered, intense mood, with rapid/pressured speech and hyperactivity).

Schizoaffective disorder (**choice C**) is characterized by elements of both schizophrenia (e.g., psychotic symptoms) and mood disorders (e.g., manic or depressive symptoms).

Schizophrenic disorder (**choice D**) is a chronic recurrent thought disorder often accompanied by bizarre behaviors. It usually begins in early adulthood. To make this diagnosis, the symptoms must last 6 months or more, which distinguishes it from brief psychotic and schizophreniform disorders.

Schizophreniform disorder (**choice E**) is a thought disorder of psychotic proportion with a duration between 1 and 6 months. This duration distinguishes the condition from brief psychotic disorder and schizophrenic disorder. Often, the onset of the thought disorder is as a young adult, when the person must leave the protected environment of the home and begin to assume personal responsibility for his or her life. He or she is unable to cope with the world and his/her defenses deteriorate to the point of psychosis. Typically, patients with schizophreniform disorder were unable to maintain interpersonal relationships as adolescents.

22. **The correct answer is E.** This infant is within normal limits. Infants do not begin to vocalize in the form of babbling, particularly in response to their mother's vocalizations, until about 8 weeks of age. The mother's question and concern is probably secondary to lack of experience and a bit of insecurity about her mothering skills and aptitude.

There is no evidence that this child is pulling away from human contact (autism, **choice A**), not responding to noises (**choice B**) or visual cues (**choice D**) in the environment, or lacking other developmental milestones (mental retardation indices in infants, **choice C**).

23. **The correct answer is B.** The baby is exhibiting stranger anxiety, which normally occurs between the ages of 5 and 9 months.

Let's review some other social milestones that are good to be aware of during clinical work in pediatrics:

Spontaneous smiling begins within several days after birth and disappears by 3 months. Smiling at any face occurs by 2 months, followed quickly by smiling only at familiar faces and when pleased. By 3 months, infants can imitate facial expressions. They laugh at 4 months.

Crying occurs from birth. It peaks at 6 weeks and is most frequent from 4 to 6 PM. Colic is defined as crying more than 3 hours a day for more than 3 days a week. It often spontaneously resolves by 4 months. Treatment includes holding, avoiding overstimulation, and antispasmodics.

Separation anxiety occurs between the ages of 10 and 18 months, when the infant is separated from the mother.

Between the ages of 2 months and 2 years, children might show preference for a comforting "transitional object" (e.g., a teddy bear), which is usually discarded by age 4, when the transition from dependence on the mother to independence is more complete.

24. **The correct answer is A.** The courts have repeatedly ruled that a parent's religious belief system may not be allowed to endanger the life of a child. In such an emergent situation, the physician is allowed to treat the child against the parent's wishes, although it is strongly recommended that the courts be informed of the action taken.

Discharging the mother and son from the hospital (**choice B**) is clearly punitive in nature and not in the best interest of the son. The son should be treated.

Making the patient comfortable, but not transfusing him (**choice C**), is not correct for a minor child. The courts have established the precedent that the child can be treated without fear of reprisal.

Requesting the hospital chaplain try to persuade the mother to allow the transfusion (**choice D**) is incorrect since the child can be treated against the mother's wishes.

Waiting until a court order is granted to perform the transfusion (**choice E**) is incorrect because this is an emergency, and the child needs immediate care. If one waits for the court action, the child may die before there is a ruling. Again, the courts will support the physician taking immediate action in this circumstance.

25. **The correct answer is C.** Suicide completers tend to be male, older, and white. They typically use lethal methods (e.g., guns, jumping from high places), are recently divorced or separated, live alone, have made previous suicide attempts, have a major affective disorder (major depressive disorder or bipolar disorder), and/or are alcoholic. Patients of high socioeconomic status have a higher rate of successfully committing suicide than those of lower socioeconomic status.

26. **The correct answer is B.** Projection involves attributing one's own traits, feelings, and attitudes to someone else. This swimmer's harsh criticism of her teammates' abilities is a reflection of her personal feeling of incompetence. (Doubts about her own ability are translated into doubts about her teammates' aptitude.)

Displacement (**choice A**) involves the automatic transferring of a wish or an affect from one object to a substitute. For example, a man who is angry at his wife releases his hostility by kicking the table.

Reaction formation (**choice C**) involves turning a repressed impulse or unconscious wish to its opposite. For example, a man who is attracted to his brother's wife develops an aversion to her personality.

Repression (**choice D**) occurs when the conflicting thought or feeling is automatically hidden from the person's awareness. Forgetting an emotionally charged event is an example of repression.

Sublimation (**choice E**) is a very mature mechanism that involves consciously turning socially unacceptable impulses into acceptable or more benign forms. For example, a young college girl immerses herself in athletics rather than engage in premarital sex.

27. **The correct answer is C.** The patient has schizophrenia. The key to the diagnosis of psychosis is that there has been a marked decline in the level of functioning (i.e., the man is homeless and cannot care for himself). Although hallucinations or delusions are not mentioned in the case history, the presence of disorganized speech and grossly disorganized behavior and the duration of symptoms (longer than 6 months) suggest a diagnosis of schizophrenia.

**KAPLAN** MEDICAL

In schizoaffective disorder (**choice A**), alterations in mood are present during a substantial portion of the illness.

Although schizoid personality disorder (**choice B**) produces detachment from social relationships and is characterized by restriction of emotional expression, it is not accompanied by a marked decline in occupational functioning.

Schizophreniform disorder (**choice D**) is characterized by schizophrenic-like symptoms, but the duration of symptoms is, by definition, less than 6 months.

Schizotypal personality disorder (**choice E**) is characterized by eccentricities of behavior, odd beliefs or magical thinking, and difficulties with social and interpersonal relationships. Unlike schizophrenia, schizotypal personality disorder is not characterized by a formal thought disorder.

28. **The correct answer is C.** The sensorium section of the Mental Status Examination contains information on orientation, attention-concentration, memory functioning, and other related subjects. When the examining physician discovers problems in these areas, he or she should assume there is an underlying organic/neurologic process, until proven otherwise. That is, although disruptions here can result from other conditions (**choices A, B, D, and E**), the organic possibilities should always be ruled out first.

29. **The correct answer is B.** In an obese patient, loud snoring, daytime drowsiness, and falling asleep while driving are all classic clues to the diagnosis of obstructive sleep apnea. Sleep apnea is defined as the cessation of air flow for at least 10 seconds. Obstructive apnea is the most common type and is caused by muscle atonia in the oropharynx, obstruction by the tongue or tonsils, or nasal obstruction. Contributing factors include obesity, alcohol or sedative use, and hypothyroidism.

Central sleep apnea (**choice A**) occurs when the medulla does not respond to the accumulation of $CO_2$ in the blood. It almost always occurs in children and has been considered to be one of the causes of SIDS (sudden infant death syndrome). Typically, the child is cyanotic on awakening.

Narcolepsy (**choice C**) is a chronic disorder in which there is sudden onset of REM sleep at inopportune times. Since the patient abruptly falls asleep without warning, the condition can be dangerous. You might have considered this as part of your differential diagnosis, given the complaint of suddenly falling asleep at the wheel, but the clues provided strongly imply obstructive sleep apnea as the cause.

Pavor nocturnus (**choice D**) is the technical term for night terrors. This familial disorder often co-occurs with sleepwalking. Patients suddenly sit up in bed looking terrified. They scream, are inconsolable, cannot converse, and may run from the room. Patients generally have no recollection of the event. It is usually a childhood disorder, although it occurs in some adults.

Somnambulism (**choice E**) is the technical term for sleepwalking. This familial disorder is characterized by episodes of clumsy walking that last several minutes during sleep. The syndrome usually abates by puberty.

30. **The correct answer is E.** Secobarbital is a short-acting barbiturate with considerable dependence potential. Withdrawal from short-acting barbiturates can produce anxiety, delirium, and seizures, which may be accompanied by life-threatening cardiovascular collapse.

Insomnia (**choice A**) is a complication of barbiturate withdrawal, since barbiturates are sedative/hypnotic agents; however, this complication is not serious enough to be a contraindication to abrupt cessation of the drug.

Rebound anxiety (**choice B**) would be quite likely following abrupt cessation of the barbiturate but would not constitute a sufficient danger to the patient to preclude self-detoxification.

Recidivism (**choice C**) is quite likely in drug abusers, with or without medical intervention.

Respiratory depression (**choice D**) is common with acute administration of barbiturates but would not be expected with barbiturate abstinence.

31. **The correct answer is C.** This is one of those questions for which predicting the correct answer will facilitate your selecting the appropriate answer choice. Make sure to read each choice carefully (for example, choices D and E, though both incorrect in this case, look almost identical and could cost you points if you were not reading actively).

**Choice A** refers to the crude mortality rate.

**Choice B** refers to the postnatal mortality rate.

**Choice D** is an incorrect rendering of the neonatal mortality rate, since it considers the total number of births instead of the total number of live births.

**Choice E** refers to the neonatal mortality rate.

32. **The correct answer is C.** The physician should obtain an emergency order of detention, regardless of her threats of a lawsuit. The woman clearly still has suicidal intent, demonstrated by her expressed verbalizations, and is therefore a danger to herself.

Choices **A, B,** and **D** clearly place her in a position where she can carry out her plans to terminate her life.

Sedating her (**choice E**) is the second best choice since it will prevent her from taking her life; however, sedation does not give therapists the opportunity to address the underlying motivations for her suicidal ideation.

33. **The correct answer is C.** This woman is demonstrating the symptoms of trichotillomania, which is similar to Tourette syndrome in that the behavior of hair pulling is preceded by an impulse or pressured feeling. It is unlike obsessive compulsive disorder, which is preceded by a cognition to do something. The best medication would be fluvoxamine, a serotonin specific reuptake inhibitor.

Clozapine (**choice A**) works in the dopaminergic system and has not demonstrated potential in this disorder.

Diazepam (**choice B**) works in the GABA system and likewise has demonstrated little efficacy for trichotillomania.

Lithium (**choice D**) has demonstrated only limited success in trichotillomania.

Verapamil (**choice E**) is a calcium channel blocker that has no demonstrated efficacy in this disorder.

34. **The correct answer is C.** This man is inducing signs and reporting symptoms that are all consistent with passing a kidney stone. However, he is not seeking treatment for the condition; rather, he is requesting narcotics. This is a favorite manipulation by drug-addicted persons, particularly at a time of the evening when they cannot get to their primary care physician. By providing the information that the pain is now migrating to the testicle, the patient is increasing the pressure on the physician to provide narcotics.

Antisocial personality disorder (**choice A**) is not correct since the history provides no information about past behaviors that are against society. This man may warrant such a diagnosis if the full history is obtained and support for the diagnosis is present. His requesting narcotics suggests an addiction, and many persons with substance abuse diagnoses also have antisocial personality disorders. However, there is not enough information to warrant this diagnosis at this time.

Factitious disorder (**choice B**) is the major differential diagnosis in this man since he is actively producing symptoms to obtain something. However, in factitious disorder, the individual is seeking to enter the "sick role," that is, the person obtains primary gain. However, in the malingering person, the gain is secondary (e.g., obtaining drugs or money, hiding from the police in the hospital).

Schizotypal personality disorder (**choice D**) is incorrect because disturbed interpersonal relations are not apparent in this man's background, nor are there any other signs or symptoms of the diagnosis.

Somatization disorder (**choice E**) is incorrect since this diagnosis requires multiple symptoms in multiple systems of the body; this man is presenting with only two symptoms in one system.

35. **The correct answer is A.** Classical conditioning involves the response toward one stimulus being transferred to another stimulus. For example, a patient who fears going to the doctor experiences heightened anxiety as the physician enters the room wearing a white coat. The patient's fear then becomes associated with the white coat itself, such that future exposure to this symbol evokes similar apprehension.

Extinction (**choice B**) means that when a behavior is no longer reinforced, it will disappear.

Habit hierarchies (**choice C**) are ordered statements about the probability of occurrence of behaviors. Those behaviors that have been reinforced more strongly will be more likely to occur and will therefore be ranked higher in the response hierarchy.

Negative reinforcement (**choice D**) occurs when, in response to a behavior, an aversive condition is removed rather than a positive reward being given. For example, a teenager may finally take out the garbage to stop his mother from nagging him. This is a method involved in operant conditioning (**choice E**), which is based on the relationship between a response and the consequences (reinforcement) that follow that response.

36. **The correct answer is D.** The Thematic Apperception Test is a projective test that uses pictures depicting ambiguous interpersonal situations that the examinee is asked to interpret. Psychodynamic theory suggests that since the stimuli are vague, the patient projects his or her own thoughts, feelings, and conflicts into his or her responses, providing the examiner insight into the patient's thought and memory content.

The Minnesota Multiphasic Personality Inventory (MMPI; **choice A**), which uses true and false items, is the most popular objective personality test.

The Myers-Briggs Personality Inventory (**choice B**) is based on Jungian theory and assesses basic dimensions of personality (extroversion); it is used extensively in occupational counseling. The patient selects preferred adjectives from groups of choices.

The Rorschach Test (**choice C**) is another projective test that involves asking patients to describe what they see when presented with a series of black and white inkblots.

**KAPLAN) MEDICAL**

The Type A and B Behavior Patterns Test (**choice E**) assesses the amount of "driven quality" a person has to their life. Type A's are always "running out of time." This is a verbal test that resembles an interview.

37. **The correct answer is E.** A relationship has been found between CSF levels of 5-hydroxy indoleacetic acid (5-HIAA) and impulsive aggression. 5-HIAA is a metabolite of serotonin (5-HT). Brainstem and CSF levels of 5-HIAA are decreased in individuals exhibiting impulsive aggression. Since most neurotransmitter systems work in concert with one another, the other listed systems may have secondary roles; however, serotonin is most strongly correlated with the behavior in question.

38. **The correct answer is A.** Continuous reinforcement, which means that a person is rewarded every time he or she performs a specific behavior, is the pattern of reinforcement least resistant to extinction. This is because the person soon becomes satiated with the reward and no longer performs the desired behavior to obtain it. On the other hand, behaviors established on the basis of partial reinforcement are most resistant to extinction. The rest of the answer choices are variants of partial reinforcement schedules.

    Fixed interval (**choice B**) reinforcement means that equal amounts of time must go by before the reward can be attained (e.g., if he cleans up his toys, he'll get an ice cream cone every Sunday).

    Fixed ratio (**choice C**) reinforcement means that a given number of behaviors must be done before the reward is available (e.g., he must clean up his toys at least three times before getting an ice cream cone).

    Variable interval (**choice D**) means that sometimes only 1 hour must go by, sometimes 3 hours, and so forth, before the reward is available (e.g., he might receive an ice cream cone the same night he cleaned up his toys or several days later).

    Variable ratio (**choice E**) means that sometimes a behavior is rewarded the first time, sometimes the third, etc. (e.g., sometimes he would get an ice cream cone after cleaning up his toys on only one occasion, sometimes after four occasions).

39. **The correct answer is B.** It is important that the patient know the association between his self-destructive behavior and the physical sequelae. However, it is also important for cooperation in long-term management to not make the patient defensive by labeling him an alcoholic (**choice C**).

    Equivocating with "I'm not sure" (**choice A**) or avoiding the patient's question (**choices D and E**) does not provide a basis for cooperative and mutual trust in the doctor–patient relationship.

40. **The correct answer is C.** Kubler-Ross's Death and Dying sequence is a step-wise process with five identified stages. The order in which these stages appear is the following: 1. Denial, 2. Anger, 3. Bargaining, 4. Sadness, and 5. Acceptance. "Doctor you must be wrong" is the correct answer since it reflects the patient's inability to accept the information and indicates the denial of the first stage.

    "Can you keep me alive until my daughter graduates from medical school" (**choice A**), is a statement from the third, bargaining stage.

    "Damn you doctor, you should have caught this earlier" (**choice B**) is a statement from the second or anger phase.

    "I think it is time that I make a will and say good-bye to everyone" (**choice D**) reflects the patient's acceptance of the reality and is a statement from the fifth phase (acceptance).

    "It's no use, I always lose and get the short end of the stick" (**choice E**) is a statement from the fourth phase (sadness).

41. **The correct answer is B.** In most instances in which a married person seeks sterilization, the spouse's consent is also needed. Such consent is not typically extended in cases of abortion.

    Convincing the patient to use alternative contraception (**choice A**) is inappropriate because it ignores the patient's will.

    Explaining that the chances of becoming pregnant are very low at her age (**choice C**) is factually incorrect, especially considering that she just gave birth at age 45.

    Although patient confidentiality is important, not disclosing this patient's desire for sterilization to her husband (**choice D**) violates his autonomy with regard to having children in the future. Therefore, he must be involved in the decision-making process.

42. **The correct answer is D.** This is a psychotic level disorder (the patient is hallucinating): she has a fluctuating level of consciousness and is disoriented. Also, there is a clear history of a febrile condition that developed rather rapidly, all of which suggest delirium.

    In acute stress disorder (**choice A**) a traumatic event occurs that precipitates an anxiety-type reaction, not a change in the sensorium.

    In both bipolar I disorder, manic type (**choice B**) and brief psychotic disorder (**choice C**), patients may reach a level of behavioral disruption of psychotic proportion. They do not, however, demonstrate changes in level of consciousness or major disorientation.

Persons with dementia (**choice E**) demonstrate a clear sensorium with no fluctuations in the level of consciousness. Additionally, persons with dementia predominantly show symptoms of impairment of cognitive functions (e.g., memory impairment).

43. **The correct answer is A.** People who have been injured and trapped in life-threatening conditions have the highest rates of post-disaster emotional problems.

People who are new immigrants to a given area are at heightened risk (unlike **choice B**).

People with prior emotional conditions (**choice C**) also have an increased risk, as do persons who recently lost a close relative (**choice D**), but neither of these are as traumatic as being trapped and fearing for one's life.

People at a great distance from the explosion (**choice E**) are at least risk.

44. **The correct answer is E.** This is an example of a placebo-controlled, double-blind randomized clinical trial. In this type of study, subjects with a particular disorder are randomized (the lottery) to receive either the treatment in question or a placebo. The information about whether the patient receives the treatment or the placebo is not known to either the subject or the investigator (double-blind). This type of study may be used to infer causality, i.e., if the patients taking the medication have more CD4+ T cells than the other group, it is due to the drug in question.

A case-control study (**choice A**) is a retrospective study that pairs known cases of a disease with matched controls. This type of study gives information about the importance of risk factors. The lack of a prospective design makes inferences about causality difficult.

A case report (**choice B**) is a published report of a single incidence of a disease in a subject. This is usually done for rare diseases, or for rare associations of a disease with a particular risk factor.

A cohort study (**choice C**) is an observational (non-interventional) study that tracks subjects prospectively. This type of study gives a measure of incidence of a disease.

A cross-sectional study (**choice D**) samples at a selected point in time, matching individuals with the disease with controls without the disease. The lack of a prospective design makes inferences about causality difficult.

45. **The correct answer is C.** An IQ of 53 places the individual in the upper level of moderate mental retardation. Such individuals would be expected to be able to work in a sheltered workshop situation and be assisted during times of mild social or economic stress. They can usually achieve self-maintenance in unskilled or semiskilled work under sheltered conditions. However, they do need supervision and guidance when under mild social or economic stress. As a consequence, they may do better living in a group home where there are "house-parents" on whom they can depend.

**Choices A and B** reflect expectations that are too high for a person of this IQ. However, persons with mild mental retardation can function at these levels.

**Choices D and E** are the highest expectations for severe and profound mental retardation, respectively.

46. **The correct answer is A.** Incidence is the number of new cases of a disease in a given period of time.

Lifetime expectancy (**choice B**) is the total probability of a person having a particular condition in his or her lifetime.

Lifetime prevalence (**choice C**) is the number of people who state that they have had a particular condition in their lifetime (e.g., 10% of adults state they have been alcoholic at some time in their life).

Period prevalence (**choice D**) is the number of people who have a disorder during a specified time period (longer than a calendar day or point in time).

Point prevalence (**choice E**) is the total number of cases of a condition at a given point in time.

47. **The correct answer is E.** Specificity is the proportion of persons who do not have the disease and are correctly identified by the test as being disease-free. It is given by TN/(FP + TN), where TN stands for true negatives (people who do not have the disease and test negative) and FP stands for false positives (people who do not have the disease but test positive). In this case, $95/(5 + 95) = 95/100 = 0.95$

48. **The correct answer is C.** Neuroleptic malignant syndrome (NMS) is a potentially fatal condition that can occur at any time during the course of treatment with neuroleptics. The exact etiology is unknown. Excessive muscle contraction produces muscular rigidity and is also responsible for the high temperature. The obtunded mental state and mutism are characteristic. Muscle relaxants, such as dantrolene, and dopamine agonists, such as bromocriptine, are used in the treatment of NMS.

Acute dystonia (**choice A**; prolonged contractions of muscle groups), akathisia (**choice B**; "restless legs" ), and parkinsonism (**choice D**; pill-rolling tremor and rigidity) are all extrapyramidal side effects that occur early during neuroleptic treatment.

Tardive dyskinesia (**choice E**) is a late-appearing complication of neuroleptic therapy characterized by perioral and athetoid movements.

49. **The correct answer is D.** Although electroconvulsive therapy (ECT) is highly efficacious in treating major depressions that are refractory to tricyclic antidepressants and selective serotonin reuptake inhibitors, it produces retrograde amnesia as its major side effect.

Extrapyramidal symptoms (**choice A**) are commonly produced by acute administration of antipsychotic drugs, such as phenothiazines or butyrophenones, not ECT.

Hearing loss (**choice B**) is not a common side effect of ECT.

Mania (**choice C**) is not a recognized side effect of ECT.

Rhabdomyolysis (**choice E**) does not generally occur with ECT when it is performed correctly, with the administration of skeletal muscle relaxants.

50. **The correct answer is A.** Bipolar disorder, type I, is the appropriate diagnosis because she has had repeated manic episodes. The inappropriate grandiose activity with her clients' accounts (without the benefit of consultation), decreased need for sleep, and involvement in potentially self-destructive behavior (e.g., excessive alcohol consumption) support this diagnosis.

There is no history of depressive episodes, which is mandatory for the diagnosis of bipolar disorder, type II (**choice B**).

Since her behavior is of psychotic proportion, and there is no history of depressive episodes, cyclothymic disorder (**choice C**) is incorrect.

Persons with schizophrenic disorder, paranoid type (**choice D**), have a major thought and affect disorder, and characteristically hallucinate. During an episode, they are unable to function in reality, e.g., selling and buying securities on the stock market. She demonstrates no such behavior.

The hallmark of delirium (**choice E**) is a fluctuating level of consciousness. There are no indications in the history that she is manifesting this symptom.

# STANDARD REFERENCE LABORATORY VALUES

|  | REFERENCE RANGE | SI REFERENCE INTERVALS |
|---|---|---|

**BLOOD, PLASMA, SERUM**

| | | |
|---|---|---|
| * Alanine aminotransferase (ALT, GPT at 30°C) | 8-20 U/L | 8-20 U/L |
| Amylase, serum | 25-125 U/L | 25-125 U/L |
| * Aspartate aminotransferase (AST, GOT at 30°C) | 8-20 U/L | 8-20 U/L |
| Bilirubin, serum (adult) Total // Direct | 0.1-1.0 mg/dL // 0.0-0.3 mg/dL | 2-17 μmol/L // 0-5 μmol/L |
| * Calcium, serum (Total) | 8.4-10.2 mg/dL | 2.1-2.8 mmol/L |
| * Cholesterol, serum | 140-250 mg/dL | 3.6-6.5 mmol/L |
| Cortisol, serum | 0800 h: 5-23 μg/dL // 1600 h: 3-15 μg/dL | 138-635 nmol/L // 82-413 nmol/L |
| | 2000 h: 50% of 0800 h | Fraction of 0800 h: ≤ 0.50 |
| Creatine kinase, serum (at 30°C) ambulatory | Male: 25-90 U/L | 25-90 U/L |
| | Female: 10-70 U/L | 10-70 U/L |
| * Creatinine, serum | 0.6-1.2 mg/dL | 53-106 μmol/L |
| Electrolytes, serum | | |
| Sodium | 135-147 mEq/L | 135-147 mmol/L |
| Chloride | 95-105 mEq/L | 95-105 mmol/L |
| * Potassium | 3.5-5.0 mEq/L | 3.5-5.0 mmol/L |
| Bicarbonate | 22-28 mEq/L | 22-28 mmol/L |
| Estriol ($E_3$) total, serum (in pregnancy) | | |
| 24-28 weeks // 32-36 weeks | 30-170 ng/mL // 60-280 ng/mL | 104-590 // 208-970 nmol/L |
| 28-32 weeks // 36-40 weeks | 40-220 ng/mL // 80-350 ng/mL | 140-760 // 280-1210 nmol/L |
| Ferritin, serum | Male: 15-200 ng/mL | 15-200 μg/L |
| | Female: 12-150 ng/mL | 12-150 μg/L |
| Follicle-stimulating hormone, serum/plasma | Male: 4-25 mIU/mL | 4-25 U/L |
| | Female: premenopause 4-30 mIU/mL | 4-30 U/L |
| | midcycle peak 10-90 mIU/mL | 10-90 U/L |
| | ostmenopause 40-250 mIU/mL | 40-250 U/L |
| Gases, arterial blood (room air) | | |
| $pO_2$ | 75-105 mm Hg | 10.0-14.0 kPa |
| $pCO_2$ | 33-44 mm Hg | 4.4-5.9 kPa |
| pH | 7.35-7.45 | [$H^+$] 36-44 nmol/L |
| Glucose, serum | Fasting: 70-110 mg/dL | 3.8-6.1 mmol/L |
| | 2-h postprandial: < 120 mg/dL | < 6.6 mmol/L |
| Growth hormone – arginine stimulation | Fasting: < 5 ng/mL | < 5 μg/L |
| | provocative stimuli: > 7 ng/mL | > 7 μg/L |
| Immunoglobulins, serum | | |
| IgA | 76-390 mg/dL | 0.76-3.90 g/L |
| IgE | 0-380 IU/mL | 0-380 kIU/mL |
| IgG | 650-1500 mg/dL | 6.5-15 g/L |
| IgM | 40-345 mg/dL | 0.4-3.45 g/L |
| Iron | 50-170 μg/dL | 9-30 μmol/L |
| Lactate dehydrogenase (L → P, 30°C) | 45-90 U/L | 45-90 U/L |
| Luteinizing hormone, serum/plasma | Male: 6-23 mIU/mL | 6-23 U/L |
| | Female: follicular phase 5-30 mIU/mL | 5-30 U/L |
| | midcycle 75-150 mIU/mL | 75-150 U/L |
| | postmenopause 30-200 mIU/mL | 30-200 U/L |
| Osmolality, serum | 275-295 mOsmol/kg | 275-295 mOsmol/kg |
| Parathyroid hormone, serum, N-terminal | 230-630 pg/mL | 230-630 ng/L |
| * Phosphatase (alkaline), serum (p-NPP at 30°C) | 20-70 U/L | 20-70 U/L |
| * Phosphorus (inorganic), serum | 3.0-4.5 mg/dL | 1.0-1.5 mmol/L |
| Prolactin, serum (hPRL) | < 20 ng/mL | < 20 μg/L |
| * Proteins, serum | | |
| Total (recumbent) | 6.0-7.8 g/dL | 60-78 g/L |
| Albumin | 3.5-5.5 g/dL | 35-55 g/L |
| Globulins | 2.3-3.5 g/dL | 23-35 g/L |
| Thyroid-stimulating hormone, serum or plasma | 0.5-5.0 μU/mL | 0.5-5.0 mU/L |
| Thyroidal iodine ($^{123}$I) uptake | 8-30% of administered dose/24 h | 0.08-0.30/24 h |
| Thyroxine ($T_4$), serum | 5-12 μg/dL | 64-155 nmol/L |
| Triglycerides, serum | 35-160 mg/dL | 0.4-1.81 mmol/L |
| Triiodothyronine ($T_3$), serum (RIA) | 115-190 ng/dL | 1.8-2.9 nmol/L |
| Triiodothyronine ($T_3$), resin uptake | 25-35% | 0.25-0.35 |
| * Urea nitrogen, serum (BUN) | 7-18 mg/dL | 1.2-3.0 mmol urea/L |
| * Uric acid, serum | 3.0-8.2 mg/dL | 0.18-0.48 mmol/L |

(*) Included in the Biochemical Profile (SMA-12)

| | REFERENCE RANGE | SI REFERENCE INTERVALS |
|---|---|---|
| **CEREBROSPINAL FLUID** | | |
| Cell count | 0-5 cells/mm$^3$ | 0-5 x 10$^6$/L |
| Chloride | 118-132 mmol/L | 118-132 mmol/L |
| Gamma globulin | 3-12% total proteins | 0.03-0.12 |
| Glucose | 40-70 mg/dL | 2.2-3.9 mmol/L |
| Pressure | 70-180 mm H$_2$O | 70-180 mm H$_2$O |
| Proteins, total | < 40 mg/dL | < 0.40 g/L |
| **HEMATOLOGIC** | | |
| Bleeding time (template) | 2-7 minutes | 2-7 minutes |
| Erythrocyte count | Male: 4.3-5.9 million/mm$^3$ | 4.3-5.9 x 10$^{12}$/L |
| | Female: 3.5-5.5 million/mm$^3$ | 3.5-5.5 x 10$^{12}$/L |
| Hematocrit | Male: 41-53% | 0.41-0.53 |
| | Female: 36-46% | 0.36-0.46 |
| Hemoglobin, blood | Male: 13.5-17.5 g/dL | 2.09-2.71 mmol/L |
| | Female: 12.0-16.0 g/dL | 1.86-2.48 mmol/L |
| Hemoglobin, plasma | 1-4 mg/dL | 0.16-0.62 μmol/L |
| Leukocyte count and differential | | |
| Leukocyte count | 4500-11,000/mm$^3$ | 4.5-11.0 x 10$^9$/L |
| Segmented neutrophils | 54-62% | 0.54-0.62 |
| Band forms | 3-5% | 0.03-0.05 |
| Eosinophils | 1-3% | 0.01-0.03 |
| Basophils | 0-0.75% | 0-0.0075 |
| Lymphocytes | 25-33% | 0.25-0.33 |
| Monocytes | 3-7% | 0.03-0.07 |
| Mean corpuscular hemoglobin | 25.4-34.6 pg/cell | 0.39-0.54 fmol/cell |
| Mean corpuscular hemoglobin concentration | 31-36% Hb/cell | 4.81-5.58 mmol Hb/L |
| Mean corpuscular volume | 80-100 μm$^3$ | 80-100 fl |
| Partial thromboplastin time (nonactivated) | 60-85 seconds | 60-85 seconds |
| Platelet count | 150,000-400,000/mm$^3$ | 150-400 x 10$^9$/L |
| Prothrombin time | 11-15 seconds | 11-15 seconds |
| Reticulocyte count | 0.5-1.5% of red cells | 0.005-0.015 |
| Sedimentation rate, erythrocyte (Westergren) | Male: 0-15 mm/h | 0-15 mm/h |
| | Female: 0-20 mm/h | 0-20 mm/h |
| Thrombin time | < 2 seconds deviation from control | < 2 seconds deviation from control |
| Volume | | |
| Plasma | Male: 25-43 mL/kg | 0.025-0.043 L/kg |
| | Female: 28-45 mL/kg | 0.028-0.045 L/kg |
| Red cell | Male: 20-36 mL/kg | 0.020-0.036 L/kg |
| | Female: 19-31 mL/kg | 0.019-0.031 L/kg |
| **SWEAT** | | |
| Chloride | 0-35 mmol/L | 0-35 mmol/L |
| **URINE** | | |
| Calcium | 100-300 mg/24 h | 2.5-7.5 mmol/24 h |
| Chloride | Varies with intake | Varies with intake |
| Creatinine clearance | Male: 97-137 mL/min | |
| | Female: 88-128 mL/min | |
| Estriol, total (in pregnancy) | | |
| 30 weeks | 6-18 mg/24 h | 21-62 μmol/24 h |
| 35 weeks | 9-28 mg/24 h | 31-97 μmol/24 h |
| 40 weeks | 13-42 mg/24 h | 45-146 μmol/24 h |
| 17-Hydroxycorticosteroids | Male: 3.0-10.0 mg/24 h | 8.2-27.6 μmol/24 h |
| | Female: 2.0-8.0 mg/24 h | 5.5-22.0 μmol/24 h |
| 17-Ketosteroids, total | Male: 8-20 mg/24 h | 28-70 μmol/24 h |
| | Female: 6-15 mg/24 h | 21-52 μmol/24 h |
| Osmolality | 50-1400 mOsmol/kg | |
| Oxalate | 8-40 μg/mL | 90-445 μmol/L |
| Potassium | Varies with diet | Varies with diet |
| Proteins, total | < 150 mg/24 h | < 0.15 g/24 h |
| Sodium | Varies with diet | Varies with diet |
| Uric acid | Varies with diet | Varies with diet |

# NOTES

# NOTES

# NOTES

# NOTES

# NOTES

# NOTES

# NOTES

# NOTES

# NOTES

**NOTES**

# NOTES

# NOTES

# NOTES

# NOTES

# NOTES

# NOTES

**NOTES**

# NOTES

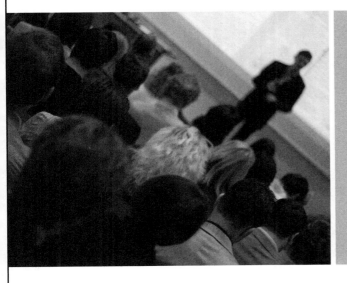
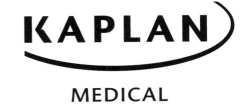

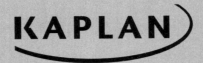

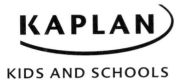
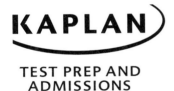
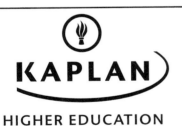
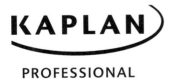